PHARMACOTHERAPY OF AFFECTIVE DISORDERS

Pharmacotherapy of Affective Disorders
Theory and Practice

Edited by

W. G. Dewhurst *and* **G. B. Baker**

Neurochemical Research Unit
Department of Psychiatry
University of Alberta
Edmonton, Canada

NEW YORK UNIVERSITY PRESS
Washington Square, New York 1985

© 1985 W.G. Dewhurst and G.B. Baker
Published in the U.S.A. by
New York University Press
Washington Square
New York, N.Y. 10003

Library of Congress Cataloging in Publication Data
Main entry under title:
Pharmacotherapy of affective disorders.
Includes bibliographies and index.
1. Affective disorders–Chemotherapy. I. Dewhurst,
W.G. (William G.) II. Baker, Glen B., 1947-
[DNLM: 1. Affective Disorders – drug therapy.
WM 171 P536]
RC537.P46 1985 616.89'18 85-3020
ISBN 0-8147-1777-2

Printed and bound in Great Britain

LIST OF CONTENTS

Preface

List of Contributors

Chapter 1   Biochemical Theories of Affective Disorders   1
G. B. Baker and W. G. Dewhurst

Chapter 2   Biological Markers in Affective Disorders   60
L. G. Huang and J. W. Maas

Chapter 3   Animal Models of Affective Disorders   108
R. D. Porsolt

Chapter 4   Observations, Reflections and Speculations on the Cerebral Determinants of Mood and on the Bilaterally Asymmetrical Distributions of the Major Neurotransmitter Systems   151
P. Flor-Henry

Chapter 5   Clinical Features of Affective Disorders I: Diagnosis, Classification, Rating Scales, Outcome and Epidemiology   185
R. C. Bland

Chapter 6   Clinical Features of Affective Disorders II: Enhancing the Productivity of Pharmacotherapeutic and Biochemical Research   231
P. Hays

Chapter 7   Monoamine Oxidase Inhibitors as Antidepressants   238
D. L. Murphy, T. Sunderland, I. Campbell, and R. M. Cohen

Chapter 8   Tricyclic Antidepressants   262
J. M. Baker and W. G. Dewhurst

Chapter 9   Recent Advances in Antidepressants   286
N. F. Damlouji, J. P. Feighner, and M. H. Rosenthal

Chapter 10	Pharmacological Approaches to Mania Y. D. Lapierre and J. Telner	312
Chapter 11	Neurobiological Basis of Antidepressant Treatments P. Blier and C. De Montigny	338
Chapter 12	Metabolism of Drugs Used in Affective Disorders M. V. Rudorfer and W. Z. Potter	382
Chapter 13	Techniques for Analysis of Drugs Used in Treatment of Affective Disorders D. F. LeGatt and G. R. Jones	449
Chapter 14	Antidepressant Plasma Concentrations and Clinical Efficacy S. A. Montgomery	512
Chapter 15	Child Depression D. R. Offord and R. T. Joffe	531
Chapter 16	The Chemotherapy of Affective Disorders in the Elderly B. Pitt	584
Index		617

PREFACE

In recent years, remarkable advances have been made not only in the pharmacotherapy of affective disorders, but in our diagnosis of such disorders and in the understanding of the mechanisms of action of the drugs used in treating them. It seems an appropriate time to gather together this information into a book which should be valuable to psychiatrists, pharmacologists and neuroscientists in general. We have compiled here chapters prepared by recognized experts in the diagnosis and treatment of affective disorders and in the action of drugs used in the pharmacotherapy of these illnesses.

Basically, the book is divided into five principal sections. In the first, which deals with basic aspects of affective disorders, there are chapters on biochemical theories, biological markers, the use of animal models, and neurotransmitter asymmetries in affective disorders. The second section deals with the diagnosis of affective disorders and consists of two chapters (5 and 6) which discuss the classification of affective disorders, the use of rating scales, and epidemiological and outcome studies. The third section contains four chapters (7-10) providing information on practical aspects of the use of various types of drugs in affective illnesses. Monoamine oxidase inhibitors, tricyclic antidepressants, second and third generation antidepressants, and antimanic agents are discussed. The fourth section concentrates on the actions and pharmacokinetics of drugs used in affective disorders and contains chapters (11-14) dealing with hypotheses on the mechanisms of action of such drugs, their metabolism, techniques employed in their analysis, and studies on the relationships between plasma concentrations and clinical efficacy. The final section, consisting of two chap-

Preface

ters, deals with the affective illnesses in special age groups, i.e. children and the elderly.

We believe that such a compilation of basic and clinical information about affective disorders fills a gap in the current literature on psychiatric illness. Where clinicians have contributed chapters, they have been encouraged to comment on observations made in everyday practice as well as review the scientific literature and to indicate how at this time they treat their patients.

Although we think that this volume provides comprehensive coverage of important areas, space limitations have not permitted discussion of some important aspects of affective illnesses. Two such areas are psychotherapy and neuropsychology. There are many texts on these topics available to the interested reader, and they have not been covered in the present book so as to permit fuller coverage of the aspects directed by the title. But that they have an important place is indicated in appropriate sections of several chapters.

We thank the contributors for their enthusiasm in preparing chapters, our colleagues for providing useful suggestions, and Mrs. C. Farley for typing the final manuscripts.

William G. Dewhurst
Professor and Chairman
Department of Psychiatry and
Co-Director
Neurochemical Research Unit

and

Glen B. Baker
Associate Professor
Department of Psychiatry and
Associate Director
Neurochemical Research Unit

University of Alberta
Edmonton, Canada

LIST OF CONTRIBUTORS

G. B. Baker
Neurochemical Research Unit, Department of Psychiatry, Clinical Sciences Building, University of Alberta, Edmonton, Alberta, Canada T6G 2G3

J. M. Baker
Alberta Pharmacy, 7004 - 98th Avenue, Edmonton, Alberta, Canada T6A 0A5

R. C. Bland
Department of Psychiatry, Clinical Sciences Building, University of Alberta, Edmonton, Alberta, Canada T6G 2G3

P. Blier
Centre de recherche en sciences neurologiques, Faculté de médecine, Université de Montréal, C. P. 6128, succursale A, Montréal, Québec, Canada H3C 3J7

I. Campbell
Clinical Neuropharmacology Branch, National Institute of Mental Health, NIH Clinical Center, Room 3D41, Bethesda, Maryland 20205, U.S.A.

R. M. Cohen
Clinical Neuropharmacology Branch, National Institute of Mental Health, NIH Clinical Center, Room 3D41, Bethesda, Maryland 20205, U.S.A.

N. F. Damlouji
Psychiatric Centers at San Diego, 5131 Garfield Street, La Mesa, California 92041, U.S.A.

W. G. Dewhurst

> Neurochemical Research Unit, Department of Psychiatry, Clinical Sciences Building, University of Alberta, Edmonton, Alberta, Canada T6G 2G3

C. De Montigny

> Centre de recherche en sciences neurologiques, Faculté de médecine, Université de Montréal, C. P. 6128, succursale A, Montréal, Québec, Canada H3C 3J7

J. P. Feighner

> Feighner Research Institute, La Mesa, California 92041, U.S.A.

P. Flor-Henry

> Alberta Hospital, P.O. Box 307, Edmonton, Alberta, Canada T5J 2J7

P. Hays

> Department of Psychiatry, Clinical Sciences Building, University of Alberta, Edmonton, Alberta, Canada T6G 2G3

L. G. Huang

> University of California at Davis, Department of Psychiatry, 2315 Stockton Boulevard, Sacramento, California 95817, U.S.A.

R. T. Joffe

> Chedoke Child and Family Centre, Chedoke-McMaster Hospitals, Chedoke Division, Box 2000, Station A, Hamilton, Ontario, Canada L8N 3Z5

G. D. Jones

> Office of the Chief Medical Examiner, P.O. Box 2257, Edmonton, Alberta, Canada T5J 2P4

Y. D. Lapierre

>Royal Ottawa Hospital, 1145 Carling Avenue, Ottawa, Ontario, Canada K1Z 7K4

D. F. LeGatt

>Department of Laboratory Medicine, University of Alberta Hospital, Edmonton, Alberta, Canada T6G 2B7

J. W. Maas

>University of Texas Health Science Center at San Antonio, 7703 Floyd Curl Drive, San Antonio, Texas 78284, U.S.A.

S. A. Montgomery

>Academic Department of Psychiatry, St. Mary's Hospital Medical School, St. Mary's Hospital, Harrow Road, London W9 3RL, U.K.

D. L. Murphy

>Clinical Neuropharmacology Branch, National Institute of Mental Health, NIH Clinical Center, Room 3D41, Bethesda, Maryland 20205, U.S.A.

D. R. Offord

>Chedoke Child and Family Centre, Chedoke-McMaster Hospitals, Chedoke Division, Box 2000, Station A, Hamilton, Ontario, Canada L8N 3Z5

B. Pitt

>German Hospital, Ritson Road, London E8 1BS, U.K.

R. D. Porsolt

>Neuropharmacology Unit, Centre de Recherche Delalande, 10 rue des Carrières, F92500 Rueil-Malmaison, France

W. Z. Potter

Unit on Clinical Psychopharmacology, Clinical Psychobiology Branch, National Institute of Mental Health, Building 10, Room 4S-239, 9000 Rockville Pike, Bethesda, Maryland 20205, U.S.A.

M. H. Rosenthal

Feighner Research Institute, La Mesa, California 92041, U.S.A.

M. V. Rudorfer

Section on Clinical Psychopharmacology, Laboratory of Clinical Science, National Institute of Mental Health, Building 10, Room 4S-239, 9000 Rockville Pike, Bethesda, Maryland 20205, U.S.A.

T. Sunderland

Clinical Neuropharmacology Branch, National Institute of Mental Health, NIH Clinical Center, Room 3D41, Bethesda, Maryland 20205, U.S.A.

J. Telner

Royal Ottawa Hospital, 1145 Carling Avenue, Ottawa, Ontario, Canada K17 7K4

1.

BIOCHEMICAL THEORIES OF AFFECTIVE DISORDERS

G. B. Baker and W. G. Dewhurst

A relatively large body of evidence now suggests that there may be a genetic vulnerability factor in many cases of primary affective disorder (review: Nurnberger and Gershon, 1984), and this has spurred on researchers to search for biochemical lesions. In this chapter, we will review the work that has been done in this area and will give information about the present status of the various hypotheses that have been put forward.

Amine Hypotheses
================

As will become evident in this review, many of the biochemical hypotheses of affective disorders have involved, directly or indirectly, biogenic amines. Some years ago, several researchers (e.g. Pare and Sandler, 1959; Everett and Tomon, 1959; Rosenblatt et al., 1960) suggested that depression could be the result of a functional deficiency of one or more brain amines at central synapses. These hypotheses were based to a large extent on observations made with reserpine and monoamine oxidase inhibitors (reviews: Weil-Malherbe, 1967; Johnstone, 1982). Not unnaturally, the two main amine hypotheses emerging concerned those amines most easily measured at the time, namely, noradrenaline (norepinephrine; NA) and 5-hydroxytryptamine (5-HT; serotonin).

The Noradrenaline (Catecholamine) Hypothesis

As stated by Schildkraut (1965), 'some, if not all, depressions are associated with an absolute or relative deficiency of catecholamines, particularly norepinephrine, at functionally important receptor sites in the brain. Elation conversely may be associated with an excess of such amines'.

It was proposed that antidepressant action of the monoamine oxidase (MAO) inhibitors and the tricyclics could be explained on the basis of this theory. The MAO inhibitors inhibit MAO, a major enzyme involved in the metabolism of NA, thus resulting in an increased availability of NA at the synaptic area. The tricyclics are certainly strong inhibitors of reuptake of NA into the nerve terminals. By blocking this reuptake mechanism, the tricyclics are making more neurotransmitter amine available in the synapse.

The intense interest in NA led a number of research groups to study the possibility that there could be abnormalities in levels of NA and/or its metabolites in brain tissue or body fluids. Most of this research has centered around MHPG (3-methoxy-4-hydroxyphenylethylene glycol), a major metabolite of NA in the CNS.

It has been reported by a number of research groups that urinary MHPG levels are lower than normal in patients with bipolar depression (Maas et al., 1973; Goodwin and Post, 1975; Garfinkel et al., 1977; Schildkraut et al., 1978; Edwards et al., 1980). There has been less agreement in studies on unipolar depressions, with low (DeLeon-Jones et al., 1975; Maas, 1978; Taube et al., 1978), normal (Goodwin and Post, 1975; Beckmann and Goodwin, 1980), or high (Garfinkel et al., 1979) urinary MHPG levels being reported. Schildkraut and co-workers have found a wide range of urinary MHPG values in patients with unipolar depression, and have also suggested that the discrepancy in findings amongst various researchers may be the result of diagnostic heterogeneity.

Levels of MHPG have also been investigated in plasma and CSF (reviews: Leckman and Maas, 1984; Post et al., 1984). A direct correspondence between MHPG concentrations in brain, cerebrospinal fluid and plasma has been demonstrated in primates (Redmond et al., 1979; Elsworth et al., 1982), and a correlation between CSF and plasma levels of this metabolite have been reported in normal human subjects (Jimerson et al., 1981). Studies on MHPG in psychiatric patients indicate high levels of plasma total MHPG in patients with a bipolar major affective disorder in the manic phase when compared to normals or depressed patients (Halaris and DeMet, 1978; Halaris, 1978; Halaris and DeMet, 1979). The same workers reported decreases in plasma total MHPG after lithium treatment and a transient increase in depressed patients following treatment with imipramine and the pyrrolidine derivative AHR-1118 (Halaris and DeMet, 1979, 1980). As Leckman and Maas (1984) have indicated, future studies on plasma MHPG should include an investigation of the following factors: free versus conjugated MHPG, and fluctuations associated with age, sex, circadian patterns and state changes in the natural history of the affective disorder.

Post et al. (1984a) have reviewed clinical and methodological variables affecting biochemical measurements of NA and its metabolites in biological samples and have also reviewed the arguments for and against these substances in lumbar CSF reflecting NA metabolism in the CNS. They conclude that concentrations of NA and MHPG in the lumbar CSF may reflect a major contribution from spinal cord NA metabolism which may be correlated with activity in rostral areas of the brain and depend in part on the activity of the locus coeruleus. Post et al. (1984) found that CSF NA is significantly elevated in manic patients relative to depressives and normal controls, but could find no significant differences in NA levels between depressed patients and controls. Studies comparing CSF MHPG levels in depressives and controls have yielded conflicting results, and these are reviewed by Post et al. (1984a). Interestingly, Jimerson et al. (1975) found that CSF concentrations of vanillylmandelic acid (VMA), another metabolite of NA, were significantly decreased in depressed patients compared to controls; in the same study, no significant difference was found in levels of VMA between manics and controls.

It has been proposed that pretreatment MHPG levels in body fluids may have predictive value in assisting the clinician to choose an appropriate antidepressant. It has been reported that depressed patients with lower than normal urinary MHPG levels respond more favorably to treatment with imipramine (Maas et al., 1972; Beckmann and Goodwin, 1975; Cobbin et al., 1979; Rosenbaum et al., 1980), desipramine (Maas et al., 1972), nortriptyline (Hollister et al., 1980) or maprotiline (Rosenbaum et al., 1980) than do depressives with high MHPG levels. Conversely, it has been reported that depressives with high pretreatment or normal MHPG levels respond better to amitriptyline than do patients with lower levels (Beckmann and Goodwin, 1975). Huang and Maas discuss such studies on MHPG in chapter 2 of this book.

Biochemical Theories of Affective Disorders

The Serotonin Hypothesis

Essentially, this hypothesis postulates a deficiency of central 5-HT as a cause of depression (Coppen, 1967; Lapin and Oxenkrug, 1969). Much of the supportive evidence is similar to that for the NA hypothesis, e.g. reserpine depletes 5-HT, MAO inhibitors prevent its destruction, and tricyclic antidepressants block its reuptake. And as with NA, searches have been made for abnormalities of 5-HT or its metabolites in the body.

Reports on urinary excretion of 5-hydroxyindole-3-acetic acid (5-HIAA), a major metabolite of 5-HT, are much less common than those for MHPG, although Ridges (1981) has proposed that urinary 5-HIAA may be useful in predicting appropriate antidepressants to use in depressed patients. Much of the work that has been done with 5-HIAA has been performed in CSF or in postmortem brain tissue. The CSF work is inconclusive, with about one-third of the groups reporting decreased CSF 5-HIAA in depressed patients (Bunney and Garland, 1981). However, van Praag (1984) has pointed out that there may be two types of depressives, one group with low and another with normal baseline concentrations. This concept seems to be borne out by the findings of other researchers as well (Asberg et al., 1976; Traskman-Bendz et al., 1981; Banki et al., 1981; Agren, 1980a,b). Van Praag (1984) suggests that decreased CSF 5-HIAA is fairly specifically related to two categories of depressed patients--a subgroup of vital (endogenous) depressions and a subgroup of schizoaffective psychoses. Higher than normal suicide rates have also been reported in depressed patients with low baseline 5-HIAA concentrations (Asberg et al., 1976; Traskman-Bendz et al., 1981).

It has been reported that there are decreases in postmortem brain region concentrations of 5-HT and 5-HIAA in suicide victims (Lloyd et al., 1974) and in depressives dying from other causes (Birkmeyer and Riederer, 1975), but Bunney and Garland (1981) have pointed out that, overall, there has not been good agreement amongst researchers on brain levels of 5-HT in postmortem tissue from depressives compared to that from normals.

As with MHPG, patterns of excretion of 5-HIAA have been used in attempts to guide treatment. Thus Ridges (1981) has found that patients with low urinary levels of 5-HIAA respond more favorably to clomipramine or maprotiline than do patients with higher 5-HIAA levels. It has also been reported that in the probenecid test, patients with lower than normal CSF 5-HIAA are more likely to respond favorably to clomipramine than to nortriptyline (van Praag, 1977; Asberg et al., 1973), and those with higher than normal 5-HIAA are likely to respond to nortriptyline or imipramine (Asberg et al., 1973). Despite these encouraging results using amine metabolites as predictors of drug response, it must be emphasized that there is much conflicting data on this subject in the literature (Sacchetti et al., 1979; Coppen et al., 1979; Spiker et al., 1980; Ananth, 1983).

Critiques of the NA and 5-HT Hypotheses

Although these hypotheses have been investigated intensively, both carry problems which have been extensively documented by Dewhurst (1968a,b, 1969) and more recently by Sulser (1982a,b), Johnstone (1982), and Sugrue (1983). These problems include the following:
(a) Discrepancy between the relatively rapid neurochemical effects of antidepressants such as the tricyclics and the time required for antidepressant efficacy, usually at least 2-3 weeks.
(b) The clinical efficacy of drugs such as iprindole and mianserin (novel or "second-generation" antidepressants) which do not inhibit MAO nor block the reuptake of NA or 5-HT.
(c) Cocaine, a potent blocker of reuptake of NA, is not an effective antidepressant.
(d) There has been a great deal of controversy over whether or not amino acid precursors of these amines are effective antidepressants.

Receptor Changes. Dewhurst had postulated a change in receptor sensitivity in depressed states as early as 1968 (a,b). And the time discrepancy mentioned in (a) above has led researchers to study the possibility that antidepressants cause changes in sensitivity and/or numbers of receptors for biogenic amines and that these changes occur over a 2-3 week period. In 1972, Ashcroft et al. suggested a modified amine hypothesis in which they stated that interactions between various neuronal systems and also alterations of post-synaptic receptor sensitivity should be considered in affective disorders. In recent years, there has been a great deal of research conducted on changes in receptors following long-term antidepressant administration. Results obtained in studies on NA-sensitive adenylate cyclase suggest that ECT and antidepressants of every class cause a down-regulation of β-adrenoreceptors (Sulser, 1982, 1983). Studies in experimental animals and experiments in humans have indicated that a variety of different treatments for depression may result in a decrease in the number of α_2 adrenoreceptors in brain (Smith et al., 1981, 1983; Cohen et al., 1982; Stanford and Nutt, 1982), leading to speculation of increased presynaptic activity in depressed patients (Crews and Smith, 1978; Siever et al., 1981). Electrophysiological studies indicate that functional responsiveness of 5-HT receptors increases following chronic antidepressant treatment (De Montigny and Aghajanian, 1978; Wang and Aghajanian, 1980; Blier and De Montigny, chapter 11 of this book), while binding experiments suggest that 5-HT$_2$ receptors are reduced in number following long-term administration of ECT and antidepressants (Snyder and Peroutka, 1984). This is an important, active area of research, and no doubt more light will be shed on the situation as research continues on subpopulations of aminergic receptors.

The discovery of specific binding sites in platelets and brain tissue for tricyclic antidepressants (Raisman et al., 1979; Langer and Briley, 1981) suggested another potential tool for studying the biochemistry of affective disorders and the mechanisms of action of antidepressant drugs. It has been proposed that the ^{3}H-imipramine binding site is closely associated with the 5-HT uptake site (Langer et al., 1980; Hrdina, 1982) and the ^{3}H-desipramine binding site with the NA uptake site (Rehavi et al, 1981; Langer et al., 1981; Hrdina, 1982). Significant decreases in the number of ^{3}H-imipramine binding sites in platelets from medication-free severely depressed patients compared to matched controls have been reported (Briley et al., 1980; Paul et al., 1981). Stanley et al. (1982) and Paul et al. (1984) observed decreased ^{3}H-imipramine binding in membranes from frontal cortex and hypothalamus, respectively, of postmortem brain tissue from patients who died as a result of suicide. Huang and Maas give further details on the use of ^{3}H-imipramine binding as a biological marker in chapter 2 of this book.

Dopamine

It has been suggested that the catecholamine dopamine (DA) may also be involved in the etiology of certain types of depression (McClure, 1973; Randrup et al., 1975). Studies in which probenecid has been used to block transport of acid metabolites out of the CSF have indicated decreased concentrations of the DA metabolite homovanillic acid (HVA) in depressed patients (Berger et al., 1980; Bowers, 1972; van Praag and Korf, 1971; van Praag et al., 1973; Sjostrom, 1973; Sjostrom and Roos, 1972). This effect is particularly pronounced in patients with retarded depression (Banki, 1977; Banki et al., 1981; Papeschi and McClure, 1971; van Praag and Korf, 1971; van Praag et al., 1973). While early studies suggested that L-DOPA, the precursor of DA, might have antidepressant properties, subsequent double-blind investigations have indicated that this effect is relatively specific for depressed patients with psychomotor retardation (Goodwin and Sack, 1974; van Praag and Korf, 1975). Nomifensine, an inhibitor of reuptake of catecholamines (particularly DA), exhibits clear antidepressant effects (Angst et al., 1974; van Schleyen et al., 1977). In a series of comprehensive papers, Willner (1983a,b,c) has discussed DA and depression, dealing with pharmacology, biochemistry, and behavioural models. Bunney and Garland (1981) have reviewed research strategies used for investigating the possible roles of NA and DA in depression and mania and of 5-HT in depression.

Trace Amines

Dewhurst (1968a,b) concluded from the results of a series of animal and human experiments that depression may be due to a functional deficiency of β-phenylethylamine (PEA) and/or tryptamine (T) in the CNS, but also emphasized changes in receptor sensitivity and psychosocial factors. Other workers subsequently proposed that there may be decreased PEA in depression (Fischer et al., 1972; Boulton and Milward, 1971; Sabelli and Mosnaim, 1974).

Tryptamine and PEA, along with a number of other amines (e.g. tyramine and octopamine), are called "trace amines" because of their low concentrations in brain compared to the catecholamines (NA and DA) and 5-HT (Usdin and Sandler, 1976). However, these amines have very rapid turnover rates, i.e. they are synthesized and metabolized very rapidly, which may be just as important physiologically as high absolute concentrations (Boulton, 1976, 1984; Dewhurst, 1984). When administered to animals in low doses, T and PEA cross the blood-brain barrier with ease and can cause marked stimulant effects (Dewhurst and Marley, 1965a,b,c).

Results of body fluid studies on levels of trace amines in affective disorders are equivocal. Lower than normal urinary PEA has been reported in depressed patients (Boulton and Milward, 1971; Sabelli et al., 1976), and Sabelli et al. (1983) have proposed that phenylacetic acid (PAA), the major metabolite of PEA, may be a reliable state marker for diagnosis of some forms of unipolar major depressive disorders. Sandler et al. (1979a) and Karoum et al. (1984) were unable to find significant differences in urinary excretion of PAA between depressives and controls, although in the same patients Sandler et al. found decreased urinary p-hydroxyphenylacetic acid and p-hydroxymandelic acid (metabolites of p-tyramine and p-octopamine, respectively) and a decreased concentration of PAA in the CSF. In a study on 15 patients undergoing treatment with MAO inhibitors, Murphy et al. (1984) found that pretreatment urinary excretion of PEA was not consistently associated with differences in severity of depression, anxiety activation or hypomania, but was negatively correlated with dysphoria and anger. However, during treatment with MAO inhibitors, increased PEA excretion was associated with decreased self-rated depression and anxiety. These workers suggested that their data might be consistent with an amended hypothesis which would relate PEA to a cluster of depression-related symptoms (e.g. dysphoria and anger), but not depressed mood alone.

Coppen et al. (1965), in a study on 13 depressives, reported that these patients displayed lower than normal urinary excretion of T, but that these levels had risen to normal on recovery. Dewhurst (1968) found that treatment of depressives with the MAO inhibitor phenelzine led to much larger increases in urine levels of T than of 5-HT or the metanephrines (amine metabolites of catecholamines).

A decrease in tyramine-conjugating ability after administration of an oral dose of p-tyramine has been observed in depression (Bonham-Carter, 1978; Harrison et al., 1983). These last-named workers found that, after the tyramine challenge, both unipolar and bipolar endogenous depressives excreted lower than normal amounts of conjugated tyramine; patients displaying atypical depressions did not differ significantly from normals in their pattern of tyramine excretion. In a study of the use of the tyramine challenge in post-partem 'four-day blues', it was shown that patients with low output of conjugated tyramine had a significantly

higher lifetime incidence of depressive illness than did those with high values (Bonham-Carter et al., 1980).
   Studies on laboratory animals have shown that administration of MAO inhibitors results in dramatic increases in brain concentrations of the trace amines, especially T and PEA, the increases being many times greater than for the catecholamines or 5-HT (Boulton et al., 1973; Saavedra and Axelrod, 1974; Boulton, 1976; Philips and Boulton, 1979; McKim et al., 1980; Philips et al., 1980; Dewhurst, 1984). Little is known about the interaction of the tricyclics and the newer antidepressant drugs with the trace amines.
   Interest in the role of trace amines has been given added impetus in recent years by reports of specific binding sites for PEA and T in brain tissue (Hauger et al., 1982; Kellar and Cascio, 1982).

Cholinergic-Adrenergic Interactions

This theory suggests that a given affective state may represent a balance between central cholinergic and adrenergic neurotransmitter activity in brain areas which regulate affect. Depression is proposed to be a disease of cholinergic dominance and mania the opposite (Janowsky et al., 1972, 1983). These researchers feel that there is a relatively large body of pharmacological evidence to support this hypothesis. Reserpine, which is known to cause depression, has central cholinomimetic effects, while many antidepressants are known to have central anticholinergic effects. It has been reported that physostigmine, a centrally active cholinesterase inhibitor, produces an inhibitory syndrome (psychomotor retardation, lethargy, anergy, sedation, slowed thoughts, decreased speech, expressionless facies, and social withdrawal; Risch and Janowsky, 1984) in human subjects (Janowsky et al., 1973a,b; Davis et al., 1976), while neostigmine, a noncentrally acting cholinesterase inhibitor, does not (Janowsky et al., 1973a,b). Administration of physostigmine has been reported to cause depression of mood in psychiatric inpatients (Janowsky et al., 1973a), in a subgroup of manics (Janowsky 1973a,b; Davis et al., 1978), in a group of euthymic bipolar patients on lithium maintenance (Oppenheimer et al., 1979), and in normal controls (Risch et al., 1981, 1983). Depression has been reported as a side effect in patients treated for a variety of disorders with precursors of acetylcholine (Tamminga et al., 1976; Davis et al., 1979).

There have been interesting developments in recent years in the use of erythrocyte choline (the precursor of acetylcholine) as a marker for affective disorders. Several researchers have observed that the antimanic drug lithium causes a dramatic accumulation of choline in the red blood cell (Jope, 1979; Hanin, 1982; Janowsky et al., 1983).

Sitarim et al. (1984) reported studies on a number of physiological responses that are believed to be mediated through cholinergic receptors, supporting the hypothesis of Janowsky and co-workers. They further postulated that muscarinic supersensitivity occurs in patients with primary affective illness when they are ill and also when they are in remission, and that muscarinic supersensitivity, as measured by the cholinergic REM Induction Test, could prove to be a measure of vulnerability to affective illness.

A recent report by Nadi et al. (1984) also seems to lend support to the idea of cholinergic overactivity in affective disorders. These workers investigated muscarinic receptors in cultured human fibroblasts and found that such cells from 18 patients with a major affective disorder had significantly higher densities of binding sites than those from 12 normal controls. Fibroblasts from 18 relatives with a history of major or minor affective disorder also displayed a higher density, while those from 5 normal relatives did not differ from controls.

Histamine

Little is known about what role this amine may have in depression; however, it has been demonstrated that several non-MAO-inhibitor antidepressants of diverse structure (tricyclics, iprindole, mianserin) act as strong blockers of histamine H_2 adenylate cyclase in brain homogenates (Green and Maayani, 1977; Kanof and Greengard, 1978), implying a blockade of H_2 receptors. Tran et al. (1978) tested a number of tricyclic antidepressants for their ability to compete with binding of ^3H-mepyramine to brain H_1 receptors. All the drugs investigated were relatively potent, with doxepin and amitriptyline being particularly effective (Snyder and Peroutka, 1984). In a recent biochemical study, Gagne et al. (1982) have reported a lower than normal urinary excretion of l-methylhistamine, a major CNS metabolite of histamine, in depressed patients.

Biochemical Theories of Affective Disorders

Amino Acids

Research on the role of amino acids in the etiology of affective illness has been going on for many years, with the emphasis being on the amino acids which are precursors of biogenic amines. Tryptophan has been the object of much of this research. There have been contradictory reports on plasma and CSF levels of tryptophan in depressed patients relative to normals (review: van Praag, 1984). Moller et al. (1980) reported a subgroup of endogenous depressives with a reduced ratio of free plasma tryptophan to other amino acids which use the same transport mechanism into the brain (phenylalanine, tyrosine, leucine, isoleucine, and valine). These patients were found to respond favourably to L-tryptophan administration. De Meyer et al. (1981) found that when depression was most severe in a group of depressives the tryptophan/competing amino acids ratio as well as total tryptophan levels were lower than in normal subjects; in addition, phenylalanine and tyrosine levels were higher than normal. These differences disappeared upon clinical improvement. A relationship between plasma free tryptophan and depressed mood in women during the first week postpartum was reported by Stein et al. (1976) and Handley et al. (1977).

Tryptophan and 5-hydroxytryptophan, both amino acid precursors of 5-HT, have been tested for antidepressant efficacy. In both cases, there have been conflicting results reported (reviews: Wirz-Justice, 1977; Young and Sourkes, 1977; Murphy et al., 1978; van Praag, 1981, 1984a,b; Baldessarini, 1984; Young, 1984). In a recent article, van Praag (1984) discusses some of the studies that have been carried out and suggests that further research should be conducted using larger doses and longer periods of administration, and that a therapeutic 'window' effect should be considered. There are several reports indicating that tryptophan potentiates the antidepressant effects of monoamine oxidase inhibitors (Coppen et al., 1963; Ayuso-Gutierrez and Lopez-Ibor, 1971; Glassman and Platman, 1969; Pare, 1973) and clomipramine (Roos, 1976; Walinder et al., 1980). van Praag (1984) has reported that the effects of clomipramine, nialamide and clorgyline are potentiated by 5-hydroxytryptophan.

The precursor amino acids for the catecholamines have also been tested for potential antidepressant activity. Although L-DOPA may produce psychomotor activation in depressives, it has been largely unsuccessful in treatment of depression (Carroll, 1972; Mendels et al., 1975; Gelenberg et al., 1982) and may produce a number of undesirable side effects (Goodwin et al., 1971; Murphy et al., 1973). High doses of L-p-tyrosine have been reported by three groups of workers to have antidepressant effects (Goldberg, 1980; Gelenberg et al., 1982; van Praag, 1983). In a recent report, Birkmayer et al. (1984) found good antidepressant efficacy with a combination of L-phenylalanine and the MAO inhibitor L-deprenyl.

Berrettini and Post (1984) have recently reviewed the evidence supporting a role for the inhibitory neurotransmitter γ-aminobutyric acid (GABA) in affective disorders. Injections of GABA into various brain regions prevented learned helplessness behaviour in rats (Sherman and Petty, 1980). Chronic, but not acute, administration of lithium to rats leads to a decreased number of GABA receptor binding sites (Maggi and Enna, 1980). Carbamazepine and sodium valproate, anticonvulsant drugs which have been used in treatment of lithium-resistant affective illness, lead to a decrease in GABA turnover in brain (Bernasconi and Martin, 1979). Chronic administration of electroconvulsive shock to rats has been reported to increase concentrations of, and decrease synthesis of, GABA in nucleus accumbens and caudate (Green et al., 1978). Clinical studies have suggested reduced CSF levels of GABA in depressed patients (Gold et al., 1980; Gerner and Hare, 1981; Kasa et al., 1982; Post et al., 1980). Antidepressant effects have been observed with the GABA agonist progabide (Morselli et al., 1980).

There have also been some studies carried out on the possible role of glycine in affective illnesses. Rosenblatt et al. (1979) studied 13 female bipolar patients and 10 female normals and found that the erythrocyte concentration of glycine was significantly elevated in the patient group. It has been proposed that such increases in glycine are related to lithium treatment rather than to the bipolar disorder per se (Deutsch et al., 1983; Shea et al., 1981; Rosenblatt et al., 1982; Pomara et al., 1983). Deutsch et al. found a significant correlation between erythrocyte glycine and levels of glycine in cerebral hemispheres of lithium-treated rats. Higher than normal CSF levels of glycine in patients taking lithium were reported by Goodnick et al. (1982).

Biochemical Theories of Affective Disorders

Enzymes

Numerous studies have been carried out on possible differences between normals and patients suffering from affective disorders with regard to activities of enzymes involved in the synthesis and metabolism of biogenic amines.

Monoamine oxidase is the enzyme which has been investigated most extensively. There is some conflicting data, particularly with regard to MAO activity in bipolar depression, and many of the results have been covered in recent review articles (Gershon, 1978; Sandler et al., 1981; Schildkraut et al., 1983; Huang and Maas, chapter 2 of this book). Mathew et al. (1981) reported that plasma levels of dopamine β-hydroxylase (DBH) were not useful for subtyping affective disorders or for predicting treatment responses with amitriptyline, nortriptyline or desipramine. The enzyme catechol-O-methyl transferase (COMT) has been investigated in erythrocytes. Dunner et al. (1971) found that erythrocyte COMT activity was less in unipolar depressive females than in bipolars and that levels in both of these groups were less than in controls. The same workers found no significant difference between male unipolar and bipolar depressives and controls. Mattson et al. (1974) observed no significant differences between unipolar and bipolar depressed patients and controls. Gershon and Jonas (1975) found no differences between unipolar and bipolar depressives with regard to erythrocyte COMT, but found that levels were significantly higher in these patients than in normals. It has been reported that there is an elevation of erythrocyte COMT in agitated depressed males (Davidson et al., 1979) and a decrease in retarded depressives (Shulman et al., 1978). Although inhibition of COMT does not influence the course of depression (Angrist et al., 1973), treatment of depressed patients with imipramine has been reported to result in a linear correlation between erythrocyte COMT activity and therapeutic response (Davidson et al., 1976). Lapierre (1982) has concluded that it seems unlikely that COMT has a direct relationship to depression *per se*, but that it may be related to associated phenomena such as motor activity.

Biochemical Theories of Affective Disorders

Adrenocorticotrophic Hormone (ACTH)/Cortisol
===

A considerable amount of research has been conducted on body fluid levels of corticosteroids. Bryson and Martin (1954) reported that urinary levels of 17-ketosteroids are increased during the depressed phase and decreased in the manic phase. Abnormal urinary levels of 17-hydroxycorticosteroids have been reported in depressed and manic phases, but there has been some disagreement as to the directions of those changes (Bunney et al., 1965; Schwartz et al., 1966; Rubin, 1967).
 Several groups have reported that levels of plasma 17-hydroxycorticosteroids, 11-hydroxycorticosteroids, and cortisol are elevated during depressed phases and are normal during phases of hypomania (Rubin, 1967; Hullin et al., 1967; Gibbons and McHugh, 1962). However increased levels of cortisol in plasma during hypomania have also been reported (Platman and Fieve, 1968). Bunney et al. (1969) found that the mean excretion of 17-hydroxycorticosteroids was significantly higher in suicidal patients than in another group of depressed patients. Fullerton et al. (1968) reported that serum and urine levels of 17-hydroxycorticosteroids were increased in cases of psychotic depression but were normal in patients with reactive depression. Sachar et al. (1970) found, in a study on depressed patients, that 9 out of 16 demonstrated an elevated production of cortisol and a return to normal upon recovery. There was little change in cortisol production in apathetic, retarded patients, mild to moderate changes in patients with marked anxiety, and pronounced changes in patients demonstrating symptoms of psychotic disorganization. Platman and Fieve (1968) reported that elevated levels of adrenocortical activity can be suppressed in many depressives by administration of dexamethasone. However, it was also observed that severely depressed patients may show resistance to this dexamethasone suppression (Carroll et al., 1968a,b; Butler and Besser, 1968). This finding of the failure of a relatively high proportion of patients with major depressive disorder to demonstrate cortisol (and ACTH) suppression after being administered dexamethasone led to the development of the dexamethasone suppression test (DST) (Carroll et al., 1981; Rubin and Marder, 1983). This test, which is described in detail by Huang and Maas in chapter 2 of this book, is thought to represent an abnormality in the hypo-

Biochemical Theories of Affective Disorders

thalamic-pituitary-adrenal (HPA) axis and is of further interest since biogenic amines such as NA and 5-HT are thought to influence release of cortisol and other hormones in that axis.

Another relationship between cortisol and tryptophan metabolism is of interest. Although there is some controversy in the literature, it has been proposed that there is an association between the use of oral contraceptives and depressive symptoms. Winston (1969) suggested that estrogen from the oral contraceptive leads to an increase in adrenal cortisol release, resulting in increased hepatic production of tryptophan oxygenase. The increased concentrations of this enzyme favour metabolism of tryptophan via a metabolic route in which the end products nicotinic acid ribonucleotide and N-methylnicotinamide are formed over the pathway which results in the formation of 5-HT. The increased metabolism of tryptophan in this manner leads to an increased requirement for pyridoxal phosphate (Vitamin B_6). This is of interest because it has been suggested that therapy with Vitamin B_6 can be useful in treating depression in women taking oral contraceptives (Winston, 1969; Baumblatt and Winston, 1970; Adams et al., 1973). Winston (1969) has also pointed out that Vitamin B_6 could, through an effect on DOPA decarboxylase, be affecting catecholamines as well as indoleamines.

Peptides Other Than ACTH

Growth Hormone (GH)

Growth hormone (GH) may prove to be a useful endocrinological marker in affective disorders since it has been demonstrated that the GH response to several challenges is blunted in certain patients with endogenous depression (Rubin and Marder, 1983). Stimuli studied have included insulin-induced hypoglycemia, amphetamine, clonidine, and desipramine (after acute administration) (Rubin and Kendler, 1977; Carroll, 1978; Rubin et al., 1979; Checkley, 1980; Brown et al., 1978; Matussek et al., 1980).

Thyrotropin-Releasing Hormone (TRH) and Thyroid-Stimulating Hormone (TSH)

The TRH test (response of TSH to administered TRH) is now used as a neuroendocrine challenge test in affective disorders and presumably reflects changes occurring in the hypothalamic-pituitary-thyroid axis. Several groups have reported that the TSH response to TRH is decreased in major unipolar depression (Prange et al., 1972; Takahashi et al., 1974; Hollister et al., 1976; Loosen et al., 1977; Kirkegaard et al., 1978; Gold et al., 1979, 1980; Extein et al., 1981, 1984). It has also been reported that TSH response to TRH is increased in bipolar depression (Gold et al., 1979, 1980), but this is more controversial (Mendlewicz et al., 1979; Amsterdam et al., 1979; Bjorum and Kirkegaard, 1979). Finally, there are preliminary reports of a decreased TSH response in mania compared to schizophrenic psychosis (Extein et al., 1980). If the TRH test does prove useful in differentiating mania from schizophrenia, this will have great benefits for psychiatric treatment since it will assist in choosing the most appropriate drug therapy (lithium or neuroleptics) and reduce the risk of producing tardive dyskinesia in misdiagnosed bipolar patients treated with long-term neuroleptics (Extein et al., 1984).

There are important relationships of this test to monoamines which have been proposed to be involved in the etiology of affective disorders. Release of TRH is stimulated by NA and DA and inhibited by 5-HT (Grimm and Reichlin, 1973; Besser et al., 1975; Chen and Meites, 1975), and thus changes in the TSH response may reflect changes in monoaminergic transmission in the CNS. Now there is also evidence indicating that TRH may be a centrally active neuromodulator outside of the hypothalamic-pituitary-thyroid axis (Renaud and Martin, 1975; Hokfelt et al., 1975; Burt and Snyder, 1975) and that it may itself exert antidepressant actions (Prange et al., 1972; Loosen and Prange, 1980). This raises the possibility that alterations in TRH release do not just reflect changes in brain monoamines but are etiologically related to affective illness (Extein et al., 1984).

Further details on the TRH-TSH test are given in chapter 2 (Huang and Maas) of this book.

Somatostatin

There is now a reasonably large body of evidence suggesting that somatostatin may have a role as a neurotransmitter and/or neuromodulator in the CNS. It has been reported to be concentrated in the synaptosomal fraction, released from brain tissue by a calcium-dependent process, and to affect the release

Biochemical Theories of Affective Disorders

and turnover of, and in turn be affected by, several neurotransmitters thought to be important in the etiology of affective illnesses (review: Rubinow et al., 1984).
  Administration of somatostatin to laboratory animals results in rather marked effects on motor activity and sleep patterns (Rezek et al., 1976, 1977). Somatostatin inhibits release of several other peptides in nervous tissue, including TSH, GH, cholecystokinin, insulin and calcitonin (Brazeau et al., 1973; Williams et al., 1979; Marco et al., 1977; Pederson et al., 1975; Rubinow et al., 1984). Gerner and Yamada (1982) found lower than normal levels of somatostatin in CSF from a group of patients with affective illness, and Rubinow et al. (1984) reported that CSF somatostatin was significantly lower in patients in the depressed state than in normals or in patients in the improved state. Rubinow et al. (1984) also found that levels of somatostatin in the CSF were positively correlated to CSF 5-HIAA and negatively correlated to CSF NA in depressed, medication-free patients.

Cholecystokinin and Bombesin

Much work remains to be done on the possible role of these two peptides in affective illnesses. They are located in areas of the brain known to be important in regulation of mood and other behavioural functions (Dockray, 1978; Saito et al., 1980; Emson et al., 1980; Moody and Pert, 1979; Brown et al., 1978) and preliminary findings indicate that they may play a role in physiological functions such as pain and regulation of appetite and digestion (Madison, 1977; Woods et al., 1981; Della-Fera and Baile, 1979; Grovum, 1981; Gibbs et al., 1976; Brown et al., 1977). Cholecystokinin fragments can inhibit DA release in mesolimbic areas (Hokfelt et al., 1980). Gerner (1984) studied cholecystokinin and bombesin in CSF from a variety of psychiatric patients and found that his data did not support a role for cholecystokinin in several major psychiatric disorders, including primary major depression and mania. A trend for decreased bombesin in depression was observed.

Vasopressin

This peptide has been reported to influence a number of functions which are abnormal in affective disorders, including memory (deWied et al., 1975), REM sleep (Weitzman et al., 1977), and the status of fluid and electrolyte balance (Robertson, 1979; Raichle and Grubb, 1978). Lithium and carbamazepine have been shown to alter vasopressin function and activity in laboratory animals and human subjects (Singer et al., 1972; Moses et al., 1976). Gold et al. (1984) reported that CSF vasopressin is lower than normal in drug-free nonpsychotic unipolar and bipolar depressives. In the group of bipolar subjects, levels were significantly lower in nonpsychotic depressed patients compared to patients studied in the manic or hypomanic phase.

Prolactin and Luteinizing Hormone

A survey of the literature reveals some contradictory findings on plasma levels of prolactin in depressives, but most studies show little or no change between depressed patients and normals (review: Checkley and Arendt, 1984). A study on prolactin suppression by L-DOPA demonstrated no differences between normals and depressives (Sachar et al., 1973). There have been conflicting reports on prolactin response to TRH in depressed patients (Ehrensing et al., 1974; Maeda et al., 1975), and abnormal prolactin responses to luteinizing hormone-releasing hormone have been observed in some depressed patients (Brambilla et al., 1978). In a preliminary study on prolactin secretion during the first 3 hours of sleep, it was found that the normal difference in prolactin secretion between pre- and postmenopausal women found in control subjects was not present amongst depressed women (F. M. Mai, B. F. Shaw, M. R. Jenner, G. Wielgosz, and D. Giles, submitted for publication).
Altman et al. (1975) have observed reduced levels of luteinizing hormone in depressed postmenopausal women compared to normal postmenopausal women.

Endorphins and Enkephalins

There has been considerable interest in the possible involvement of these endogenous opioid ligands in affective disorders. Opiate compounds are known to produce alterations in mood, motor activity, and motivation and reward behaviour. However, to date there is little agreement on whether these endogenous opioid ligands have any role in affective illnesses. Post et al. (1984) carried out comprehensive studies on patients with primary affective illness; opioid binding activity and immunoreactive

Biochemical Theories of Affective Disorders

β-endorphin in CSF were investigated. These authors concluded that CSF levels of opioid binding and immunoreactive β-endorphin are not grossly altered in manic or depressive states. They did, however, observe that opioid binding activity was correlated with the severity of anxiety in depressed patients.

Water and Minerals

Several research groups have reported that in bipolar affective illness output of water and sodium is low in the depressed phase and high in the manic phase (Klein and Nunn, 1945; Klein, 1950; Strom-Olsen and Weil-Malherbe, 1958; Crammer, 1959; Hullin et al., 1967; Rubin, 1968). Extracellular space and total body water were reported to be reduced during severe depression and to return to normal upon recovery (Dawson et al., 1956; Coppen and Shaw, 1963; Hullin et al., 1967), but they were reported as reduced, unchanged, or increased in the manic period (Dawson et al., 1956; Coppen and Shaw, 1966; Hullin, 1967). However, Russell (1960) found no significant alternations in the balance of water, sodium, or potassium during depression or upon recovery. Water and salt retention and an increase of the extracellular space following ECT have been reported (Altschule and Tillotson, 1949; Russell, 1960; Hullin et al., 1967). Anderson and Dawson (1963) found a reduced sodium/potassium ratio in verbally retarded depressives, suggesting a tendency to sodium retention.

Studies with radiolabelled sodium have suggested a decrease of 24-hour exchangeable sodium (i.e. increased retention) (Gibbons, 1960; Annual Report NIMH, 1968a,b; Baer et al., 1969). However, sodium concentrations in brains from cases of suicides have been reported to be decreased relative to brains from victims of other forms of sudden death (Shaw et al., 1969).

Gibbons (1960) and Coppen and Shaw (1966) could find no change in total or exchangeable potassium in depressed patients upon recovery. Murphy et al. (1969) reported no significant differences in whole body potassium counts between normal subjects, depressives, and manic patients. In a study on four pairs of monozygotic twins discordant for depression, it was reported that there was no difference in intracellular potassium between the sick and healthy twins, but total body water and intracellular water were significantly lower in the affected twins (Abe and Coppen, 1969).

Coppen (1960) studied the rate of transport of isotopic sodium from plasma to CSF and found that the transfer was delayed in depressed patients compared to a group of schizophrenic and other patients and that this rate returned to normal after clinical recovery. Fotherby et al. (1963) performed similar experiments but could find no differences between depressed and schizophrenic patients. Carroll et al. (1969) also studied the transfer of isotopic sodium and potassium from plasma to CSF, and concluded that there was no significant difference between controls and depressives or between pre- and post-recovery stages in the depressed patients. Glen et al. (1968), on the basis of their findings from analysis of salivary secretion, concluded that transport of sodium is reduced during both manic and depressive episodes.

Many researchers have examined electrolyte levels in patients during treatment with lithium. Lithium therapy usually leads to increased diuresis of sodium, potassium, and water on the first day, followed by several days of reduced excretion and an eventual return to normal output (Murphy et al., 1969; Baer et al., 1969; Hullin et al., 1968). Johnson et al. (1970) found no consistent changes in serum levels of electrolytes during chronic treatment with lithium. It has been reported that manic patients have a very high tolerance for lithium and retain a larger portion of the administered ion than do either normal subjects or depressives (Trautner et al., 1955; Gershon and Yuwiler, 1960; Hullin et al., 1968; Greenspan, 1968; Greenspan et al., 1968a, b). Clinical recovery during lithium therapy has been reported to be accompanied by an increase in total body and intracellular water (Mangoni et al., 1969) and an increase of 24-hour exchangeable sodium (Baer et al., 1970).

Electrolyte shifts have also been observed in adrenocortical hyperactivity or insufficiency (Fawcett and Bunney, 1967; Michael and Gibbons, 1963). Mineral metabolism is controlled or regulated by hormones of the adrenal cortex and the posterior pituitary and also by autonomic centers in the diencephalon. Biogenic amines are known to have important functions in these areas, and thus it may well be that changes in mineral metabolism are connected with the function of biogenic amines.

Ramsey et al. (1979) reported that patients with primary affective disorders have higher than normal plasma sodium, but could find no significant differences in sodium and magnesium erythrocyte levels between the two groups. These workers further observed that neither baseline concentrations of sodium and magnesium nor changes in concentrations of these cations during lithium treatment correlated with treatment response. Strzyzewski et al. (1980) studied water and electrolyte contents of plasma and erythrocytes in depressed patients and reported that initial low erythrocyte levels of sodium were characteristic of bipolar depressives. A significant increase in erythrocyte sodium was observed after imipramine treatment in a group of patients responding to this drug, while a fall in plasma calcium levels was found during the course of imipramine administration.

Changes in calcium metabolism with the disappearance of depression in patients have been indicated by the work of several research groups (Faragalla and Flach, 1970; Carman et al., 1977; Bjorum, 1972). Administration of lithium to laboratory animals has been found to affect calcium, magnesium and phosphate metabolism (Plenge and Mellerup, 1976), and it has been reported that in man lithium increases serum calcium and magnesium concentrations and decreases serum phosphate concentrations (Mellerup et al., 1976; Christiansen et al., 1976). Plenge and Rafaelsen (1982) found that treatment of patients with lithium resulted in decreased urinary calcium and phosphate excretion, while excretion of magnesium was increased. Bone mineral content decreased within the first 6 months of treatment with lithium. Carman et al. (1984) have reviewed the pharmacological evidence implicating calicum in biphasic mood disturbance and have discussed the possible involvement of the peptide calcitonin. It was proposed that a deficiency in CNS calcitonin might be involved in the etiology of mania.

Another aspect of ions that has received considerable scrutiny is membrane transport. It has been proposed that incubation of erythrocytes with lithium and an observation of subsequent cell-to-plasma lithium ratios and lithium efflux might prove useful as a biological marker (Dorus et al., 1974, 1975, 1980). However, the validity of such measurements has been questioned (Werstiuk et al., 1981; Waters et al., 1983).

Findings from erythrocytes have led to suggestions that there is a membrane abnormality in affective disorders (Mendels and Frazer, 1973). Although several groups have reported lower than normal activity of Na^+,K^+-ATPase (the sodium pump enzyme that maintains the electrical gradient across cell membranes) in erythrocytes from depressed patients (Naylor et al., 1973, 1974, 1976; Hokin-Neaverson et al., 1974; Nurnberger et al., 1981), Linnoila et al. (1983) were unable to confirm such an observation. Naylor and colleagues have also reported a positive correlation between erythrocyte Na^+,K^+-ATPase activity and mood and/or activity changes in mentally retarded patients with bipolar affective disorder and have found higher than normal plasma levels of vanadium (an endogenous inhibitor of Na^+,K^+-ATPase) in depressed and manic patients (Naylor and Smith, 1981). Linnoila et al. (1983) were unable to find a correlation between vanadium and Na^+,K^+-ATPase activity. These same workers observed a higher mean Ca^{2+}-ATPase in patients with affective disorders than in normal volunteers. Choi et al. (1981), in a study of 10 men with bipolar affective disorder treated with lithium carbonate, found that levels of erythrocyte Ca^{2+}-ATPase were depressed 2 h after lithium administration; measurements were made on days 7, 14 and 21 of the course of therapy.

Carbohydrate Metabolism
=======================

Decreased glucose tolerance was one of the earliest biochemical abnormalities reported for affective disorders (review: Weil-Malherbe, 1967). Pryce (1958a,b) reported a significant decrease in glucose tolerance in depressed patients even when the effects of age, body weight, general nutrition and lack of carbohydrate intake were taken into account, but found that in most patients glucose tolerance did not rise after recovery. Van Praag and Leijnse (1965), in a study on patients with psychotic depression, found impaired glucose tolerance, but reported that glucose tolerance increased during treatment and reached normal values upon recovery. Mueller et al. (1969) studied patients with different forms of depression, and found a lower rate of glucose utilization during endogenous depression and the depressed phase of manic-depressive psychosis than in patients with neurotic depression (whose glucose utilization was normal). In addition, these workers found that the rate of glucose utilization returned to normal in the first two groups upon recovery. Mueller et al. also found that in the patients with psychotic depression there were consistently higher plasma levels of insulin (30-60 min

after glucose injection) during the depressed phase than after recovery; these differences were not observed in the neurotic group.
Heninger and Mueller (1970) studied glucose and insulin tolerances in manic patients before and after 2 weeks of treatment with lithium, and a number of interesting observations were made. Glucose utilization tended to be higher and serum insulin levels were significantly lower before than after successful treatment. It was found that insulin sensitivity was increased in the manic phase and was reduced to the highest degree in those patients who responded most to lithium. These changes were minimal or absent in patients who did not respond to lithium.
MAO inhibitors have been reported to increase glucose utilization in depressives who responded to this chemotherapy (Van Praag and Leijnse, 1965; Cooper and Keddie, 1964; Cooper and Ashcroft, 1966). This effect seems to be specific for hydrazine compounds (Weil-Malherbe, 1972) and is probably the result of inhibition of liver gluconeogenesis (Potter et al., 1969; Triner et al., 1969; Ray et al., 1970).
Lilliker (1980) found the prevalence of diabetes mellitus to be 10% in a manic-depressive population as compared to 1.8% in the general population. Further support for an association between these two disease states was given by Fakhri et al. (1980), who found that 8 of 14 patients with diabetes mellitus showed complete remission of hyperglycemia and glycosuria after ECT. Jenike (1982) has proposed that these diabetic patients who responded to ECT were in fact endogenously depressed and the hyperglycemia and glycosuria were secondary to increased serum levels of cortisol. However, Rihmer and Arato (1982) studied serum cortisol and blood sugar in 39 patients with endogenous depression and found no significant differences between blood sugar levels of patients who were dexamethasone suppressors (i.e. low serum cortisol) and those who were nonsuppressors (high serum cortisol).

Miscellaneous Agents

Purines

Niklasson et al. (1983) analyzed the purine metabolites hypoxanthine and xanthine in the CSF of patients with major depressive disorders and found that levels of both were positively correlated to the concentrations of HVA and 5-HIAA, and that hypoxanthine was also positively linked to MHPG. The same workers reported that concentrations of hypoxanthine and xanthine were strongly related to the following variables in depressed patients: magnitude of memory disturbance, suicidal tendency, and worrying.

Prostaglandins

PGE_1 is thought to modulate intracellular calcium release, and Horrobin and Manku (1979) have suggested that production of PGE_1 in depressive patients is lower than in normals, increasing the amount of calcium released. It has been observed that tricyclic antidepressants at clinically relevant doses depress calcium release, and Horrobin and Manku suggest that this may counteract the effects of PGE_1. Linnoila et al. (1983) reported higher than normal concentrations of PGE_2 in CSF of women with unipolar depression.

S-Adenosylmethionine and Folate

It has been reported by several groups that parenteral administration of the methyl donor S-adenosylmethionine results in marked clinical improvement in depressed patients (Agnoli et al., 1976; Miccoli et al., 1978; Muscettola et al., 1982; Kufferle and Grunberger, 1982; Carney et al., 1983; Lipinski et al., 1984; Caruso et al., 1984; Reynolds et al., 1984). Further, it has been observed that the onset of action is rapid in most cases and there are no appreciable side effects other than possible induction of mania (Carney et al., 1983; Lipinski et al., 1984). It has also been reported that deficiency of folate, a compound whose metabolism and functions are closely related to S-adenosylmethionine (Reynolds et al., 1984), may be related to incidence of depressive symptoms (Reynolds, 1968; Trimble et al., 1980; Rodin and Schmaltz, 1983; Reynolds et al., 1984). These findings have led to speculation that abnormalities of methylation may have important consequences in regulation of mood.

Cholesterol

Lang and Haits (1968) proposed that serum levels of cholesterol are higher in both young and old patients with major depression than in controls. However, in a study of 192 depressed and normal subjects in which the effects of age, sex and diagnosis of major depression were investigated, Oxenkrug et al. (1983) found that age and sex influenced serum cholesterol levels, but the diagnosis of major depression did not.

Tetrahydrobiopterin

CSF levels of tetrahydrobiopterin (BH_4) have been reported to be decreased in depressed patients, and BH_4 has been found to be useful in treatment of depression (Levine and Lovenberg, 1984; Curtius et al., 1983). Blair et al. (1984) observed decreased urinary excretion of total biopterins in bipolar patients compared to normals and suggested that this indicated a reduction in BH_4 synthesis. These workers also analyzed BH_4 synthesis in post-mortem temporal cortex samples from four patients with a history of severe depression and found that the synthesis rate was significantly lower than that in control samples. This is of interest since BH_4 is a potential rate-controlling enzyme in the synthesis of 5-HT and other monoamines and is stimulated in brain preparations by 5-methyltetrahydrofolate and vitamin B_{12}.

Sleep Research

It is now well established that sleep disorders are common in patients suffering from affective illnesses. These disorders include disturbances in sleep continuity, reductions in sleep stages 3 and 4, shortened rapid-eye-movement (REM) latency, and changes in phasic REM activity (Kupfer and Perel, 1983; Kupfer and Foster, 1972; Gillin et al., 1979; Vogel et al., 1980; Coble et al., 1976). The use of manipulations of the sleep-wake cycle as a means of treating depression is now an active area of research (Gillin, 1983), and antidepressant drugs have been shown to have marked effects on REM sleep (Kupfer et al., 1979, 1982; Vogel, 1983). An exciting aspect of sleep research is the possible utilization of EEG sleep patterns for prediction of response to antidepressant drug therapy (Kupfer et al., 1980, 1981). For further information on sleep studies, see the chapter by Huang and Maas in this book.

Biochemical Theories of Affective Disorders

Genetic Markers

It has been proposed that the Xg blood group and red/green colour blindness show a close linkage with bipolar illness, but this remains a matter of controversy (Mendlewicz et al., 1979; Leckman et al., 1979; Gershon et al., 1979). A link between the human leukocyte antigen (HLA) locus and depression has also been suggested (Smeraldi et al., 1978; Weitkamp et al., 1981), but much work remains to be done in this area (Matthysse and Kidd, 1981).

Conclusion

As can be seen from the above review, research on the biochemistry of affective disorders has expanded dramatically in recent years. With the development of new neurochemical techniques, the discovery of more specific receptor ligands, and refinements in the classification of subgroups of affective disorders, exciting strides have been made in elucidating etiological factors in affective illnesses, in determining the mechanisms of action of antidepressant drugs, and in predicting responses to antidepressant drugs. It has become apparent that the original biogenic amine hypotheses were too simplistic, and that the heterogenous patient groups used in many investigations were inappropriate. As indicated in the present book, important advances have now been made in psychiatric diagnosis and neurochemical analyses. A judicious application of these techniques in comprehensive studies by multidisciplinary research groups should bode well for the understanding and treatment of affective disorders.

Acknowledgements

The authors gratefully acknowledge financial support from the Alberta Mental Health Advisory Council, the Medical Research Council of Canada, the Alberta Heritage Foundation for Medical Research, and the University of Alberta Hospital Special Services and Research Committee. The assistance of Mrs. Carolyn Farley in preparing this manuscript is much appreciated.

References

Abe, K. and Coppen, A. (1969) Personality and body composition in monozygotic twins with an affective disorder. Brit. J. Psychiatry 115, 777-780.

Adams, P. W., Wynn, Y., Rose, D. P., Seed, M., Folkard, J., and Strong, R. (1973) Effect of pyridoxine hydrochloride (Vitamin B_6) upon depression associated with oral contraception. Lancet i, 897-904.

Agnoli, A., Andreoli, V., Casacchia, M., and Cerbo, R. (1976) Effect of S-adenosyl L-methionine (SAMe) upon depressive symptoms. J. Psychiatr. Res. 13, 43-54.

Agren, H. (1980a) Symptom patterns in unipolar and bipolar depression correlating with monoamine metabolites in the cerebrospinal fluid. I. General patterns. Psychiatry Res. 3, 211-223.

Agren, H. (1980b) Symptom patterns in unipolar and bipolar depression correlating with monoamine metabolites in the cerebrospinal fluid. II. Suicide. Psychiatry Res. 3, 225-236.

Altman, N., Sachar, E. J., Gruen, P. H., Halpern, F. S., and Suminya, E. (1975) Reduced plasma LH concentration in postmenopausal depressed women. Psychosom. Med. 37, 274-276.

Altschule, M. D. and Tillotson, K. J. (1949) Effect of electro-convulsive therapy on water metabolism in psychotic patients. Am. J. Psychiatry 105, 829-832.

Amsterdam, J. D., Winokur, A., Mendels, J., and Snyder, P. (1979) Distinguishing depressive subtypes by thyrotropin response to TRH testing. Lancet ii, 904-905.

Ananth, J. (1983) Choosing the right antidepressant. Psychiatric J. Univ. Ottawa 8, 20-26.

Anderson, W. McC. and Dawson, J. (1963) Verbally retarded depression and sodium metabolism. Brit. J. Psychiatry 109, 225.

Angst, J., Koukkou, M., Bleuler-Herzog, M., and Martens, H. (1974) Ergebnisse eines offenen und einen Doppelblindversuches von Nomifensin im Vergleich zu Imipramin. Arch. Psychiat. Nervenkr. 219, 265-276.

Angrist, B., Park, S., Urcuyo, L., Roffman, M., and Greshon, S. (1973) Clinical evaluation of a possible catechol-O-methyl transferase inhibitor in endogenous depression. Curr. Ther. Res. 15, 127-132.

Annual Report (1968a) Mental Health Intramural Research Program, National Institute of Mental

Health, vol. I, p. 35.
Annual Report (1968b) Mental Health Intramural Research Program, Division of Clinical, Behavioral and Biological Research, National Institute of Mental Health, vol. II, p. 101.
Asberg, M., Bertilsson, L., Tuck, D., Cronholm, B., and Sjoqvist, F. (1973) Indoleamine metabolites in the cerebrospinal fluid of depressed patients before and during treatment with nortriptyline. Clin. Pharmacol. Ther. **14**, 277-286.
Asberg, M., Thoren, P., Traskman, L., Bertilsson, L., and Ringberger, V. (1976) 'Serotonin depression': a biochemical subgroup within the affective disorders? Science **191**, 478-480.
Ashcroft, G. W., Eccleston, D., Murray, L. G., Glen, A. I. M., Crawford, T. B. B., Pullar, I. A., Shields, P. J., Walter, D. S., Blackburn, I. M., Connechan, J., and Lonergan, M. (1972) Modified amine hypothesis for the aetiology of affective illness. Lancet **ii**, 573-577.
Axelrod, J. and Saavedra, J. M. (1974) Octopamine, phenylethanolamine, phenylethylamine and tryptamine in the brain. In: Aromatic Amino Acids in the Brain, Ciba Found. Symp., 22 (new series), Elsevier, Amsterdam, pp. 51-59.
Ayuso-Gutierrez, J. L. and Lopez-Ibor, A. J. (1971) Tryptophan and an MAOI (nialamide) in the treatment of depression. Int. Pharmacopsychiatry **6**, 92-97.
Baer, L., Durell, J., Bunney, W. E. Jr., Levy, B. S., Murphy, D. L., Greenspan, K., and Cardon, P. V. (1970) Sodium balance and distribution in lithium carbonate therapy. Arch. Gen. Psychiatry **22**, 40-44.
Baer, L., Platman, S., and Fieve, R. (1969) Aldosterone-dependent component of lithium metabolism and the effect of lithium on fluid and electrolyte balance. NIMH Workshop on Recent Advances in the Psychology of the Depressive Illnesses, Williamsburg, Va., April, 1969.
Baldessarini, R. J. (1984) Treatment of depression by altering monoamine metabolism: precursors and metabolic inhibitors. Psychopharmacol. Bull. **20**, 224-239.
Banki, C. M. (1977) Correlation between CSF metabolites and psychomotor activity in affective disorders. J. Neurochem. **28**, 255-257.
Banki, C. M., Vojnik, M., and Molnar, G. (1981a) Cerebrospinal fluid amine metabolites, tryptophan and clinical parameters in depression. Part 1.

Background variables. *J. Affec. Disorders* **3**, 81-89.

Banki, C. M., Molnar, G., and Vojnik, M. (1981b) Cerebrospinal fluid amine metabolites, tryptophan and clinical parameters in depression. Part 2. Psychopathological symptoms. *J. Affec. Disorders* **3**, 91-99.

Baumblatt, M. J. and Winston, F. (1970) Pyridoxine and the pill. *Lancet* **i**, 823-833.

Beckmann, H. and Goodwin, F. K. (1975) Antidepressant response to tricyclics and urinary MHPG in unipolar patients. *Arch. Gen. Psychiatry* **32**, 17-21.

Beckmann, H. and Goodwin, F. K. (1980) Urinary MHPG in subgroups of depressed patients and normal controls. *Neuropsychobiology* **6**, 91-100.

Berger, P. A., Faull, K. F., Kilkowski, J., Anderson, P. J., Kraemer, H., Davis, K. L., and Barchas, J. D. (1980) CSF monoamine metabolites in depression and schizophrenia. *Am. J. Psychiatry* **137**, 17 -179.

Bernasconi, R. and Martin, P. (1979) Effects of antiepileptic drugs on the GABA turnover rate. *Naunyn Schmiedeberg's Arch. Pharmacol.* **307**, 251.

Berrettini, W. H. and Post, R. M. (1984) GABA in affective illness. In: *Neurobiology of Mood Disorders* (Post, R. M. and Ballenger, J. C., eds), Williams & Wilkins, Baltimore, pp. 673-685.

Besser, G. S., Burrow, G. N., Spaulding, S. W., and Donabedian, R. (1975) Dopamine infusion acutely inhibits the TSH and prolactin response to TRH. *J. Clin. Endocrinol. Metab.* **41**, 985-988.

Birkmayer, W. and Riederer, P. (1975) Biochemical postmortem findings in depressed patients. *J. Neural. Transm.* **37**, 95-109.

Birkmayer, W., Riederer, P., Linauer, W., and Knoll, J. (1984) L-Deprenyl plus L-phenylalanine in the treatment of depression. *J. Neural Transm.* **59**, 81-87.

Bjorum, N. (1972) Electrolytes in blood in endogenous depression. *Acta psychiatr. scand.* **48**, 59-68.

Bjorum, N. and Kirkegaard, C. (1979) Thyrotropin-releasing hormone test in unipolar and bipolar depression. *Lancet* **ii**, 694.

Blair, J. A., Barford, P. A., Morar, C., Pheasant, A. E., Hamon, C. G. B., Whitburn, S. B., Leeming, R. J., Reynolds, G. P., and Coppen, A. (1984) Tetrahydrobiopterin metabolism in depression. *Lancet* **ii**, 163.

Bonham-Carter, S. M., Reveley, M. A., Sandler, M., Dewhurst, J., Little, B. C., Hayworth, J., and Priest, R. G. (1980) Decreased urinary output of conjugated tyramine is associated with lifetime vulnerability to depressive illness. Psychiatry Res. 3, 13-31.

Bonham-Carter, S. M., Sandler, M., Goodwin, B. L., Sepping, P., and Bridges, P. K. (1978) Decreased urinary output of tyramine and its metabolites in depression. Brit. J. Psychiatry 132, 125-132.

Boulton, A. A. (1976) Cerebral aryl alkyl aminergic mechanisms. In: Trace Amines and the Brain (Usdin, E. and Sandler, M., eds), Marcel Dekker, New York, pp. 22-39.

Boulton, A. A. (1984) Trace amines and the neurosciences: an overview. In: Neurobiology of the Trace Amines (Boulton, A. A., Baker, G. B., Dewhurst, W. G., and Sandler, M., eds), Humana Press, Clifton, N.J., pp. 13-24.

Boulton, A. A. and Milward, L. (1971) Separation, detection, and quantitative analysis of urinary β-phenylethylamine. J. Chromatogr. 57, 287-296.

Boulton, A. A., Philips, S. R., and Durden, D. A. (1973) The analysis of certain amines in tissues and body fluids as their dansyl derivatives. J. Chromatogr. 82, 137-142.

Bowers, M. B. (1972) Cerebrospinal fluid 5-hydroxyindoleacetic acid (5-HIAA) and homovanillic acid (HVA) following probenecid in unipolar depressives treated with amitriptyline. Psychopharmacology 23, 26-33.

Brambilla, F., Smeraldi, E., Sacchetti, E., Negri, F., Cocchi, D., and Muller, E. E. (1978) Deranged anterior pituitary responsiveness to hypothalamic hormones in depressed patients. Arch. Gen. Psychiatry 35, 1231-1238.

Brazeau, P., Vale, W., Burgus, R., Ling, N., Butcher, M., Rivier, J., and Guillemin, R. (1973) Hypothalamic polypeptide that inhibits the secretion of immunoreactive pituitary growth hormone. Science 197, 77-79.

Briley, M. S., Langer, S. Z., Raisman, R., Sechter, D., and Zarifian, E. (1980) Tritiated imipramine binding sites are decreased in platelets of untreated depressed patients. Science 209, 303-305.

Brown, M., Allen, R., Vallarreal, J., Rivier, J., and Vale, W. (1978) Bombesin-like activity: radioimmunologic assessment in biological tissues. Life Sci. 23, 2721-2728.

Brown, M., Rivier, J., and Vale, W. (1977) Bombesin: potent effects on thermoregulation in the rat. Science 196, 998-1000.

Bryson, R. W. and Martin, D. F. (1954) 17-Ketosteroid excretion in a case of manic-depressive psychosis. Lancet ii, 365-367.

Bunney, W. E. Jr., Fawcett, J. A., Davis, J. M., and Gifford, S. (1969) Further evaluation of urinary 17-hydroxycorticosteroids in suicidal patients. Arch. Gen. Psychiatry 21, 138-150.

Bunney, W. E. Jr. and Garland, B. L. (1981) Selected aspects of amine and receptor hypotheses of affective illness. J. Clin. Psychopharmacol. 1 Suppl. 6, 3S-11S.

Bunney, W. E. Jr., Hartmann, E. L., and Mason, J. W. (1965) Study of a patient with 48 hour manic-depressive cycles: II. Strong positive correlation between endocrine factors and manic defense patterns. Arch. Gen. Psychiatry 12, 619-625.

Burt, D. R. and Snyder, S. H. (1975) Thyrotropin-releasing hormone (TRH): apparent receptor binding in rat brain membranes. Brain Res. 92, 309-328.

Butler, P. W. P. and Besser, G. M. (1968) Pituitary-adrenal function in severe depressive illness. Lancet i, 1234.

Carman, J. S., Post, R. M., Goodwin, F. K., and Bunney, W. E. (1977) Calcium and the electroconvulsive therapy of severe depressive illness. Biol. Psychiatry 12, 5-17.

Carman, J. S., Wyatt, E. S., Smith, W., Post, R. M., and Ballenger, J. C. (1984) Calcium and calcitonin in bipolar affective disorder. In: Neurobiology of Mood Disorders (Post, R. M. and Ballenger, J. C., eds), Williams & Wilkins, Baltimore, pp. 340-355.

Carney, M. W. P., Martin, R., Bottiglieri, T., Reynolds, E. H., Nissenbaum, H., Toone, B. K., and Sheffield, B. F. (1983) The switch mechanism in affective illness and S-adenosylmethionine. Lancet i, 820-821.

Carroll, B. J. (1972) Monoamine precursors in the treatment of depression. Clin. Pharmacol. Ther. 12, 743-761.

Carroll, B. J. (1978) Neuroendocrine dysfunction in psychiatric disorders. In: Psychopharmacology: A Generation of Progress (Lipton, M. A., Di Mascio, A., and Killam, K. F., eds), Raven Press, New York, pp. 487-497.

Carroll, B. J., Feinberg, M., Greden, J. F., Tarika, J., Albala, A. A., Haskett, R. F., James, N. McI., Kronfol, Z., Lohr, N., Steiner, M., de Vigne, J. P., and Young, E. (1981) A specific laboratory test for the diagnosis of melancholia: standardization, validation and clinical utility. Arch. Gen. Psychiatry 38, 15-22.

Carroll, B. J., Martin, F. I. R., and Davies, B. (1968a) Resistance to suppression by dexamethasone of plasma 11-O.H.C.S. levels in severe depressive illness. Brit. Med. J. 3, 285-287.

Carroll, B. J., Martin, F. I. R., and Davies, B. (1968b) Pituitary-adrenal function in depression. Lancet i, 1373-1374.

Carroll, B. J., Stevens, L., Pope, R. A., and Davies, B. (1969) Sodium transfer from plasma to CSF in severe depressive illness. Arch. Gen. Psychiatry 21, 77-81.

Caruso, I., Fumagalli, M., Boccassini, L., Puttini, P. S., Ciniselli, G., and Cavallari, G. (1984) Antidepressant activity of S-adenosylmethionine. Lancet i, 904.

Checkley, S. A. (1980) Neuroendocrine tests of monoamine function in man: a review of basic theory and its application to the study of depressive illness. Psychol. Med. 10, 35-53.

Checkley, S. and Arendt, J. (1984) Pharmacoendocrine studies of G.H., PRL, and melatonin in patients with affective illness. In: Neuroendocrinology and Psychiatric Disorders (Brown, G. M., Koslow, S. H., and Reichlin, S., eds), Raven Press, New York, pp. 165-190.

Chen, H. J. and Meites, J. (1975) Effects of biogenic amines and TRH on release of prolactin and TSH in the rat. Endocrinology 96, 10-14.

Choi, S. J., Derman, R. M., and Lee, K. S. (1981) Bipolar affective disorder, lithium carbonate and Ca^{++} ATPase. J. Affec. Disorders 3, 77-79.

Christiansen, C., Baastrup, P. C., and Transbol, I. (1976) Lithium, hypercalcemia, hypermagnesemia, and hyperparathyroidism: Letter. Lancet ii, 969.

Cobbin, D. M., Requin-Blow, B., Williams, L. R., and Williams, W. O. (1979) Urinary MHPG levels and tricyclic antidepressant selection. Arch. Gen. Psychiatry 36, 1111-1115.

Coble, P. A., Foster, F. G., and Kupfer, D. J. (1976) Electroencephalographic sleep diagnosis of primary depression. Arch. Gen. Psychiatry 33, 1124-1127.

Cohen, R. M., Campbell, I. C., Dauphin, M., Tallman, J. F., and Murphy, D. L. (1982) Changes in - and β-adrenoreceptor densities in rat brain as a result of treatment with monoamine oxidase-inhibiting antidepressants. Neuropharmacology 21, 293-298.

Cooper, A. J. and Ashcroft, G. (1966) Potentiation of insulin hypoglycemia by M.A.O.I. antidepressant drugs. Lancet i, 407-409.

Cooper, A. J. and Keddie, K. M. G. (1964) Hypotensive collapse and hypoglycaemia after mebanazine --a monoamine oxidase inhibitor. Lancet i, 1133-1135.

Coppen, A. J. (1960) Abnormality of the blood-cerebrospinal fluid barrier of patients suffering from a depressive illness. J. Neurol. Neurosurg. Psychiat. 23, 156-161.

Coppen, A. (1967) The biochemistry of affective disorders. Brit. J. Psychiatry 113, 1237-1264.

Coppen, A., Rama Rao, V. A., Ruthven, C. R. J., Goodwin, B. L., and Sandler, M. (1979) Urinary 4-hydroxy-3-methoxyphenylglycol is not a predictor for clinical response to amitriptyline in depressive illness. Psychopharmacology 64, 95-97.

Coppen, A. and Shaw, D. M. (1963) Mineral metabolism in melancholia. Brit. Med. J. 2, 1439-1444.

Coppen, A., Shaw, D. M., and Farrell, J. P. (1963) Potentiation of the antidepressive effect of a monoamine oxidase inhibitor by tryptophan. Lancet i, 79-81.

Coppen, A., Shaw, D. M., Malleson, A., and Costain, R. (1966) Mineral metabolism in mania. Brit. Med. J. I, 71-75.

Coppen, A., Shaw, D. M., Malleson, A., Eccleston, E., and Gundy, G. (1965) Tryptamine metabolism in depression. Brit. J. Psychiatry 111, 993-998.

Crammer, J. L. (1959) Water and sodium in two psychotics. Lancet i, 1122-1126.

Crews, F. T. and Smith, C. B. (1978) Presynaptic alpha-receptor subsensitivity after long-term antidepressant treatment. Science 202, 322-324.

Curtius, H. C., Niederwieser, A., Levine, R. A., Lovenberg, W., Woggon, B., and Angst, J. (1983) Successful treatment of depression with tetrahydrobiopterin. Lancet i, 657-658.

Davidson, J. R. T., McLeod, M. N., White, H. L., and Raft, D. (1976) Red blood cell catechol-O-methyltransferase and response to imipramine in unipolar depressive women. Am. J. Psychiatry 133, 952-954.

Davidson, J. R. T., McLeod, M. N., Turnbull, C. D., White, H. L., and Feuer, E. J. (1979) Catechol-O-methyl-transferase activity and classification of depression. Biol. Psychiatry 14, 937-942.

Davis, K. L., Berger, P. A., Hollister, L. E., and Defraites, E. (1978) Physostigmine in mania. Arch. Gen. Psychiatry 35, 119-122.

Davis, K., Hollister, L. E., and Berger, P. A. (1979) Choline chloride in schizophrenia. Am. J. Psychiatry 136, 1581-1584.

Davis, K. L., Hollister, L. E., Overall, J., Johnson, A., and Train, K. (1976) Physostigmine effects on cognition and affect in normal subjects. Psychopharmacology (Berl.) 51, 23-27.

Dawson, J., Hullin, R. P., and Crocket, B. M. (1956) Metabolic variations in manic-depressive psychosis. J. Mental Sci. 102, 168-177.

DeLeon-Jones, F., Maas, J. W., Dekirmenjian, H., and Sanchez, J. (1975) Diagnostic subgroups of affective disorders and their urinary excretion of catecholamine metabolites. Am. J. Psychiatry 132, 1141-1148.

Della-Fera, M. A. and Baile, C. A. (1979) Cholecystokinin octapeptide: continuous picomole injections into the cerebral ventricles of sheep suppress feeding. Science 206, 471-473.

De Meyer, M. K., Shea, P. A., Hendrie, H. C., and Yoshimura, N. N. (1981) Plasma tryptophan and five other amino acids in depressed and normal subjects. Arch. Gen. Psychiatry 38, 642-646.

De Montigny, C. and Aghajanian, G. K. (1978) Tricyclic antidepressants: long-term treatment increases responsivity of rat forebrain neurones to serotonin. Science 202, 1303-1306.

Deutsch, S. I., Stanley, M., Peselow, E. D., and Banay-Schwartz, M. (1983) Glycine: a possible role in lithium's action and affective illness. Neuropsychobiology 9, 215-218.

Dewhurst, W. G. (1968a) New theory of cerebral amine function and its clinical application. Nature (Lond.) 218, 1130-1133.

Dewhurst, W. G. (1968b) Cerebral amine functions in health and disease. In: Studies in Psychiatry (Shepherd, M. and Davies, D. L., eds), Oxford University Press, Oxford, pp. 289-317.

Dewhurst, W. G. (1969) Amines and abnormal mood. Proc. Roy. Soc. Med. **62**, 1102-1107.

Dewhurst, W. G. (1984) Trace amines: the early years. In: Neurobiology of the Trace Amines (Boulton, A. A., Baker, G. B., Dewhurst, W. G., and Sandler, M., eds), Humana Press, New York, pp. 1-12.

Dewhurst, W. G. and Marley, E. (1965a) Methods for quantifying behaviour and cerebral activity and the effect of drugs under controlled conditions. Brit. J. Pharmacol. **25**, 671-681.

Dewhurst, W. G. and Marley, E. (1965b) The effect of α-methyl derivatives of noradrenaline, phenylethylamine and tryptamine on the central nervous system of the chicken. Brit. J. Pharmacol. **25**, 682-704.

Dewhurst, W. G. and Marley, E. (1965c) Action of sympathomimetic and allied amines on the central nervous system of the chicken. Brit. J. Pharmacol. **25**, 705-727.

deWied, D., Bohus, B., and van Wimersma Greidanus, T. J. B. (1975) Memory deficit in rats with hereditary diabetes insipidus. Brain Res. **85**, 152-156.

Dockray, G. J. (1978) Cholecystokinin-like peptides in brain. In: Gut Hormones (Bloom, S. R. and Grossman, M. I., eds), Churchill-Livingstone, New York and Edinburgh, pp.

Dorus, E., Pandey, G. N., Frazer, A., and Mendels, J. (1974) Genetic determinant of lithium ion distribution. Arch. Gen. Psychiatry **31**, 463-465.

Dorus, E., Pandey, G. N., and Davis, J. M. (1975) Genetic determinant of lithium ion distribution. Arch. Gen. Psychiatry **32**, 1097-1102.

Dorus, E., Pandey, G. N., Shaughnessey, R., and Davis, J. (1980) Lithium transport across the RBC membrane: a study of genetic factors. Arch. Gen. Psychiatry **37**, 80-81.

Dunner, D. L., Cohn, C. K., Gershon, E. S., and Goodwin, F. K. (1971) Differential catechol-O-methyl transferase activity in unipolar and bipolar affective illness. Arch. Gen. Psychiatry **32**, 348-353.

Edwards, D. J., Spiker, D. G., Neil, J. F., Kupfer, D. J., and Rizk, M. (1980) MHPG excretion in depression. Psychiatry Res. **2**, 295-305.

Ehrensing, R. H., Kastin, A. J., Schach, D. S., Friesen, H. G., Vargas, J. R., and Schally, A. V. (1974) Affective state and thyrotropin and prolactin responses after repeated injections of thyrotropin releasing hormone in depressed pa-

tients. *Am. J. Psychiatry* **131**, 714-718.
Elsworth, J. D., Redmond, D. E., and Roth, R. H. (1982) Plasma and cerebrospinal fluid 3-methoxy-4-hydroxyphenylethylene glycol (MHPG) as indices of brain norepinephrine metabolism in primates. *Brain Res.* **235**, 115-124.
Emson, P. C., Hunt, S. P., Rehfeld, J. F., Golterman, N., and Fahrenkrug, J. (1980) Cholecystokinin and vasoactive intestinal polypeptide in the mammalian CNS: distribution and possible physiological roles. In: *Neural Peptides and Neuronal Communication* (Costa, E. and Trabucchi, M., eds), Raven Press, New York, pp. 63-74.
Everett, G. M. and Tomon, J. E. P. (1959) Mode of action of Rauwolfia alkaloids and motor activity. In: *Biological Psychiatry* (Masserman, J. H., ed.), Grune & Stratton, New York, pp. 75-81.
Extein, I., Pottash, A. L. C., and Gold, M. S. (1981) The thyrotropin-releasing hormone test in the diagnosis of unipolar depression. *Psychiatry Res.* **5**, 311-316.
Extein, I., Pottash, A. L. C., Gold, M. S., and Cowdry, R. W. (1984) Changes in TSH response to TRH in affective illness. In: *Neurobiology of Mood Disorders* (Post, R. M. and Ballenger, J. C., eds), Williams & Wilkins, Baltimore, pp. 297-310.
Extein, I., Pottash, A. L. C., Gold, M. S., and Martin, D. M. (1980) Differentiating mania from schizophrenia by the TRH test. *Am. J. Psychiatry* **137**, 981-982.
Fakhri, O., Fadhli, A. A., and el Rawi, R. M. (1980) Effect of electroconvulsive therapy on diabetes mellitus. *Lancet* **ii**, 775-777.
Faragala, F. F. and Flach, F. F. (1970) Studies of mineral metabolism in mental depression. I. The effects of imipramine and electric convulsive therapy on calcium balance and kinetics. *J. Nerv. Ment. Dis.* **151**, 120-129.
Fawcett, J. A. and Bunney, W. E. Jr. (1967) Pituitary adrenal function and depression. An outline for research. *Arch. Gen. Psychiatry* **16**, 517-535.
Fischer, E., Spatz, H., Heller, B., and Reggiani, H. (1972) Phenylethylamine content of human urine and rat brain, its alteration in pathological conditions and after drug administration. *Experientia* **15**, 307-308.
Fotherby, K., Ashcroft, G. W., Affleck, J. W., and Forrest, A. D. (1963) Studies on sodium transfer and 5-hydroxyindoles in depressive illness. *J. Neurol. Neurosurg. Psychiat.* **26**, 71-73.

Fullerton, D. T., Wenzel, F. J., Lohrenz, F. M., and Fahs, H. (1968) Circadian rhythm of adrenal cortical activity in depression. II. A comparison of types in depression. Arch. Gen. Psychiatry 19, 682-688.

Gagne, M. A., Wollin, A., Navert, H., and Pinard, G. (1982) Anomaly of histamine methylation in endogenous depression. Progr. Neuro-Psychopharmacol. & Biol. Psychiat. 6, 483-486.

Garfinkel, P. E., Warsh, J. J., and Stancer, H. C. (1977) CNS monoamine metabolism in bipolar affective disorders. Arch. Gen. Psychiatry 34, 735-739.

Garfinkel, P. E., Warsh, J. J., and Stancer, H. C. (1979) Depression: new evidence in support of biological differentiation. Am. J. Psychiatry 136, 535-539.

Gelenberg, A. J., Gibson, C. J., and Wojcik, J. D. (1982) Neurotransmitter precursors for the treatment of depression. Psychopharmacol. Bull. 18, 7-18.

Gerner, R. H. (1984) Cerebrospinal fluid cholecystokinin and bombesin in psychiatric disorders and normals. In: Neurobiology of Mood Disorders (Post, R. M. and Ballenger, J. C., eds), Williams & Wilkins, Baltimore, pp. 388-392.

Gerner, R. H. and Hare, T. A. (1981) CSF GABA in normals, depression, schizophrenia, mania, and anorexia nervosa. Am. J. Psychiatry 138, 1098-1101.

Gerner, R. H. and Yamada, T. (1982) Altered neuropeptide concentrations in cerebrospinal fluid of psychiatric patients. Brain Res. 238, 298-302.

Gershon, E. S. (1978) The search for genetic markers in affective disorders. In: Psychopharmacology: A Generation of Progress (Lipton, M. A., Di Mascio, A., and Killam, K. F., eds), Raven Press, New York, pp. 1197-1212.

Gershon, E. S. and Jonas, W. Z. (1975) Erythrocyte soluble catechol-O-methyl transferase activity in primary affective disorder: a clinical and genetic study. Arch. Gen. Psychiatry 32, 1351-1356.

Gershon, E. S., Targum, S. D., Matthysse, S., and Bunney, W. E. (1979) Color blindness not closely linked to bipolar illness. Report of a new pedigree series. Arch. Gen. Psychiatry 36, 1423-1430.

Gershon, S. and Yuwiler, A. (1960) Lithium ion: a specific psychopharmacological approach to the treatment of mania. J. Neuropsychiatry 1, 229-241.

Gibbons, J. L. (1960) Total body sodium and potassium in depressive illness. Clin. Sci. 19, 133-138.

Gibbons, J. L. and McHugh, P. R. (1962) Plasma cortisol in depressive illness. J. Psychiat. Res. 1, 162-171.

Gibbs, J., Falasco, J. D., and McHugh, P. R. (1976) Cholecystokinin-decreased food intake in rhesus monkeys. Am. J. Physiol. 230, 15-18.

Gillin, J. C. (1983) The sleep therapies of depression. Progr. Neuro-Psychopharmacol. & Biol. Psychiat. 7, 351-364.

Gillin, J. C., Duncan, W., Pettigrew, K. D., Frankel, B. L., and Snyder, F. (1979) Successful separation of depressed, normal and insomnic subjects by EEG sleep data. Arch. Gen. Psychiatry 36, 85-90.

Glassman, A. H. and Platman, S. R. (1969) Potentiation of a monoamine oxidase inhibitor by tryptophan. J. Psychiatr. Res. 7, 83-88.

Glen, A. I. M., Ongley, G. C., and Robinson, K. (1968) Diminished membrane transport in manic-depressive psychosis and recurrent depression. Lancet ii, 241-243.

Gold, B. I., Bowers, M. B. Jr., Roth, R. H., and Sweeney, D. W. (1980) GABA levels in CSF of patients with psychiatric disorders. Am. J. Psychiatry 137, 362-364.

Gold, M. S., Pottash, A. L. C., Davies, R. D., Ryan, N., Sweeney, D., and Martin, D. (1979) Distinguishing unipolar and bipolar depression by thyrotropin release test. Lancet ii, 411-413.

Gold, M. S., Pottash, A. L. C., Ryan, N., Sweeney, D., Davies, R., and Martin, D. (1980) TRH-induced TSH response in unipolar, bipolar, and secondary depressions: possible utility in clinical assessment and differential diagnosis. Psychoneuroendocrinology 5, 147-155.

Gold, P. W., Ballenger, J. C., Robertson, G. L., Weingartner, H., Rubinow, D. R., Hoban, M. C., Goodwin, F. K., and Post, R. M. (1984) Vasopressin in affective illness: direct measurement, clinical trials, and response to hypertonic saline. In: Neurobiology of Mood Disorders (Post, R. M. and Ballenger, J. C., eds), Williams & Wilkins, Baltimore, pp. 323-339.

Goldberg, I. K. (1980) L-Tyrosine in depression. Lancet ii, 364.

Goodnick, P. J., Evans, H. E., Dunner, D. L., and Fieve, R. R. (1982) Lithium and amino acids. Am. J. Psychiatry 139, 538-539.

Goodwin, F. K., Murphy, D. L., Brodie, H. K. H., and Bunney, W. E. Jr. (1971) Levo-DOPA: Alterations in behavior. Clin. Pharmacol. Ther. 13, 383-396.

Goodwin, F. K. and Post, R. M. (1975) Studies of amine metabolites in affective illness and in schizophrenia: a comparative analysis. In: Biology of Major Psychoses (Freedman, D. X., ed.), Raven Press, New York, pp. 299-332.

Goodwin, F. K. and Sack, R. L. (1974) Central dopamine function in affective illness: evidence from precursors, enzyme inhibitors, and studies of central dopamine turnover. In: Neuropsychopharmacology of Monoamines and Their Regulatory Enzymes (Usdin, E., ed.), Raven Press, New York, pp. 261-279.

Green, A. R., Peralta, E., Hong, J. S., Mao, C. C., Atterwill, C. K., and Costa, E. (1978) Alterations in GABA metabolism and met-enkephalin content in rat brain following repeated electroconvulsive shocks. J. Neurochem. 31, 607-618.

Green, J. P. and Maayani, S. (1977) Tricyclic antidepressant drugs block histamine H_2 receptors in brain. Nature (Lond.) 269, 164-165.

Greenspan, K. (1968) Clinical pharmacology and pending biochemical questions of lithium therapy. Dis. Nerv. Sys. 29, 178-181.

Greenspan, K., Green, R., and Durell, J. (1968a) Retention and distribution patterns of lithium, a pharmacological tool in studying the pathophysiology of manic-depressive psychosis. Am. J. Psychiatry 125, 512-519.

Greenspan, K., Goodwin, F. K., Bunney, W. E. Jr., and Durell, J. (1968b) Lithium ion retention and distribution. Patterns during acute mania and normothymia. Arch. Gen. Psychiatry 19, 664-673.

Grimm, Y. and Reichlin, J. S. (1973) Thyrotropin-releasing hormone (TRH): neurotransmitter regulation of secretion by mouse hypothalamic tissue in vitro. Endocrinology 93, 626-631.

Grovum, W. L. (1981) Factors affecting the voluntary intake of food by sheep, 3. The effect of intravenous infusions of gastrin, cholecystokinin and secretin on motility of the reticulo-remun and intake. Brit. J. Nutr. 45, 183-201.

Halaris, A. E. (1978) Plasma 3-methoxy-4-hydroxyphenylglycol in manic psychosis. Am. J. Psychiatry 135, 493-494.

Halaris, A. E. and DeMet, E. M. (1978) Noradrenaline metabolism in a manic-depressive patient. Lancet i, 670.

Halaris, A. E. and DeMet, E. M. (1979) Studies of norepinephrine metabolism in manic and depressive states. In: Catecholamines: Basic and Clinical Frontiers (Usdin, E., Kopin, I. J., and Barchas, J., eds), Pergamon Press, New York, pp. 1866-1868.

Halaris, A. E. and DeMet, E. M. (1980) Open trial evaluation of a pyrrolidine derivative (AHR-1118) on norepinephrine metabolism. Progr. Neuro-Psychopharmacol. 4, 43-49.

Handley, S. L., Dunn, T. L., Baker, J. M., Cockshott, C., and Gould, S. (1977) Mood changes in puerperium and plasma tryptophan and cortisol concentrations. Brit. Med. J. 11, 18-22.

Hanin, I. (1982) RBC choline as a potential marker in psychiatric and neurologic disease. In: Proceedings of the Conference on Biologic Markers in Psychiatry and Neurology (Usdin, E. and Hanin, I., eds.), Pergamon Press, Oxford, pp. 187-192.

Harrison, W. M., Cooper, T. B., Quitkin, F. M., Liebowitz, M. R., McGrath, P. J., Stewart, J. W., and Klein, D. F. (1983) Tyramine sulfate excretion test in depressive illness. Psychopharmacol. Bull. 19, 503-504.

Hauger, R. L., Skolnick, P., and Paul, S. M. (1982) Specific [^{3}H]-β-phenylethylamine binding sites in rat brain. Eur. J. Pharmacol. 83, 147-148.

Heninger, G. R. and Mueller, P. S. (1970) Carbohydrate metabolism in mania. Arch. Gen. Psychiatry 23, 310-319.

Herzberg, B. N., Johnson, A. L., and Brown, S. (1970) Depressive symptoms and oral contraceptives. Brit. Med. J. 4, 142-145.

Hokfelt, T., Fuxe, K., Johansson, O., Jeffcoate, S., and White, N. (1975) Thyrotropin-releasing hormone containing nerve terminals in certain brain stem nuclei and the spinal cord. Neurosci. Lett. 1, 133-139.

Hokfelt, T., Johansson, O., Ljungdahl, A., Lundberg, J. M., and Schultzberg, M. (1980) Peptidergic neurones. Nature (Lond.) 284, 515-521.

Hokin-Neaverson, M., Spiegel, D. A., and Lewis, W. C. (1974) Deficiency of erythrocyte sodium pump activity in bipolar manic-depressive psychosis. Life Sci. 15, 1739-1748.

Hollister, L. E., Davis, K. L., and Berger, B. A. (1980) Subtypes of depression based on excretion of MHPG and response to nortriptyline. Arch. Gen. Psychiatry 37, 1107-1110.

Hollister, L. E., Kenneth, L. D., and Berger, P. A. (1976) Pituitary response to thyrotropin-releasing hormone in depression. Arch. Gen. Psychiatry 33, 1393-1396.

Horrobin, D. F. and Manku, M. S. (1980) Possible role of prostaglandin E_1 in the affective disorders and in alcoholism. Brit. Med. J. 280, 1363-1366.

Hrdina, P. D. (1982) Tricyclic antidepressants: differences in high affinity binding of (^{3}H)-desipramine and (^{3}H)-imipramine in the brain. In: New Vistas in Depression (Langer, S. Z., Takahashi, R., and Briley, M., eds), Pergamon Press, Oxford, p. 125-132.

Hullin, R. P., Bailey, A. D., McDonald, R., Dransfield, G. A., and Milne, H. B. (1967a) Variations in body water during recovery from depression. Brit. J. Psychiatry 113, 573-583.

Hullin, R. P., Bailey, A. D., McDonald, R., Dransfield, G. A., and Milne, H. B. (1967b) Body water variations in manic-depressive psychosis. Brit. J. Psychiatry 113, 584-592.

Hullin, R. P., Bailey, A. D., McDonald, R., Dransfield, G. A., and Milne, H. B. (1967c) Variations in 11-hydroxycorticosteroids in depression and manic-depressive psychosis. Brit. J. Psychiatry 113, 593-600.

Hullin, R. P., Swinscoe, J. C., McDonald, R., and Dransfield, G. A. (1968) Metabolic balance studies on the effect of lithium salts in manic-depressive psychosis. Brit. J. Psychiatry 114, 1561-1574.

Janowsky, D. S., Davis, J. M., El-Yousef, M. K., and Sekerke, H. J. (1973a) Acetylcholine and depression. Psychosom. Med. 35, 458.

Janowsky, D. S., El-Yousef, M., Davis, J. M., and Sekerke, H. J. (1972) A cholinergic-adrenergic hypothesis of mania and depression. Lancet ii, 632-635.

Janowsky, D. S., El-Yousef, M. K., Davis, J. M., and Sekerke, H. J. (1973b) Parasympathetic suppression of manic symptoms by physostigmine. Arch. Gen. Psychiatry 28, 542-547.

Janowsky, D. S., Risch, S. C., and Gillin, J. T. (1983) Adrenergic-cholinergic balance and the treatment of affective disorders. Progr. Neuro-Psychopharmacol. & Biol. Psychiat. 7, 297-307.

Jenike, M. A. (1982) ECT and diabetes mellitus. Am. J. Psychiatry 139, 136.

Jimerson, D. C., Ballenger, J. C., Lake, C. R., Post, R. M., Goodwin, F. R., and Kopin, I. J. (1981) Plasma and CSF MHPG in normals. Psychopharmacol. Bull. **17**, 86-87.

Jimerson, D. C., Gordon, E. K., Post, R. M., and Goodwin, F. K. (1975) Central noradrenergic function in man: vanillylmandelic acid in CSF. Brain Res. **99**, 434-439.

Johnson, G., Maccario, M., Gershon, S., and Korein, J. (1970) The effects of lithium on electroencephalogram, behavior and serum electrolytes. J. Nerv. Men. Dis. **151**, 273-289.

Johnstone, E. C. (1982) Affective disorders. In: Disorders of Neurohumoural Transmission (Crow, T. J., ed.), Academic Press, New York, pp. 255-286.

Jope, R. S. (1979) Effects of lithium treatment in vitro and in vivo on acetylcholine metabolism in rat brain. J. Neurochem. **33**, 487-495.

Kanof, P. D. and Greengard, P. (1978) Brain histamine receptors as targets for antidepressant drugs. Nature (Lond.) **272**, 329-333.

Karoum, F., Torrey, E. F., Murphy, D. L., and Wyatt, R. J. (1984) The origin, drug interaction, urine, plasma and CSF concentrations of phenylacetic acid in normal and psychiatric patients. In: Neurobiology of the Trace Amines (Boulton, A. A., Baker, G. B., Dewhurst, W. G., and Sandler, M., eds), Humana Press, Clifton, N.J., pp. 457-473.

Kasa, K., Otsuki, S., Yamamoto, M., Sato, M., Kuroda, H., and Ogawa, N. (1982) CSF GABA and HVA in depressive disorders. Biol. Psychiatry **17**, 877-883.

Kellar, K. J. and Cascio, C. S. (1982) [^{3}H]-Tryptamine: high affinity binding sites in rat brain. Eur. J. Pharmacol. **78**, 475-478.

Kirkegaard, C., Bjorum, N., Cohn, D., and Lauridsen, U. B. (1978) Thyrotopin-releasing hormone stimulation test in manic depressive illness. Arch. Gen. Psychiatry **35**, 1017-1021.

Klein, R. (1950) Clinical and biochemical investigations in a manic-depressive with short cycles. J. Mental Sci. **96**, 293-297.

Klein, R. and Nunn, R. F. (1945) Clinical and biochemical analysis of a case of manic-depressive psychosis showing regular weekly cycles. J. Mental Sci. **91**, 79-88.

Kufferle, B. and Grunberger, J. (1982) Early clinical double-blind study with S-adenosyl-L-methionine: a new potential antidepressant. In: Typical and Atypical Antidepressants: Clinical Practice (Costa, E. and Racagni, G., eds), Raven Press, New York, pp. 175-180.

Kupfer, D. J. and Foster, F. G. (1972) Interval between onset of sleep and rapid eye movement sleep as an indicator of depression. Lancet ii, 684-685.

Kupfer, D. J. and Perel, J. (1983) Application of sleep investigations in understanding antidepressant drug-clinical drug interactions. In: Frontiers in Neuropsychiatric Research (Usdin, E., Goldstein, M., Friedhoff, A. J., and Georgotas, A., eds), Macmillan Press, London, pp. 275-286.

Kupfer, D. J., Spiker, D. G., Coble, P. A., and McPartland, R. J. (1979) Amitriptyline and EEG sleep in depressed patients. I: Drug effect. Sleep 1, 148-159.

Kupfer, D. J., Spiker, D. G., Coble, P. A., Neil, J. F., Ulrich, R. F., and Shaw, D. H. (1980) Depression, EEG sleep and clinical response. Comp. Psychiatry 21, 212-220.

Kupfer, D. J., Spiker, D. G., Coble, P. A., Neil, J. F., Ulrich, R. F., and Shaw, D. H. (1981) Sleep and treatment prediction in endogenous depression. Am. J. Psychiatry 138, 429-434.

Kupfer, D. J., Spiker, D. G., Rossi, A., Coble, P. A., Shaw, D. H., and Ulrich, R. F. (1982) Nortriptyline and EEG sleep in depressed patients. Biol. Psychiatry 17, 535-546.

Lang, S. and Haits, G. (1968) Blutserumcholesterinwerte bei depression. Das Deutsche Gesundheitswesen 23, 82-84.

Langer, S. Z. and Briley, M. (1981) High affinity [^{3}H]imipramine binding: a new biological tool for studies in depression. Trends Neurosci. 4, 28-31.

Langer, S. Z., Moret, C., Raisman, R., Dubocovich, M. L., and Briley, M. (1980) High affinity (^{3}H)-imipramine binding in rat hypothalamus: association with uptake of serotonin but not norepinephrine. Science 210, 1133-1135.

Langer, S. Z., Raisman, R., and Briley, M. (1981) High affinity (^{3}H)-DMI binding is associated with neuronal noradrenaline uptake in the periphery and the central nervous system. Eur. J. Pharmacol. 72, 423-424.

Lapierre, Y. D. (1982) Neurotransmitter functions in depression. Prog. Neuro-Psychopharmacol. & Biol.

Psychiat. **6**, 639-644.
Lapin, I. P. and Oxenkrug, G. F. (1969) Intensification of the central serotoninergic processes as a possible determinant of the thymoleptic effect. Lancet **i**, 132-136.
Leckman, J. F., Gershon, E. S., McGinniss, M. H., Targum, S. D., and Dibble, E. D. (1979) New data do not suggest linkage between Xg blood group and bipolar illness. Arch. Gen. Psychiatry **36**, 1435-1441.
Leckman, J. F. and Maas, J. W. (1984) Plasma MHPG: relationship to brain noradrenergic systems and emerging clinical applications. In: Neurobiology of Mood Disorders (Post, R. M. and Ballenger, J. C., eds), Williams & Wilkins, Baltimore, pp. 529-538.
Levine, R. A. and Lovenberg, W. (1984) CSF tetrahydrobiopterin levels in patients with affective disorders. Lancet **i**, 283.
Lilliker, S. L. (1980) Prevalence of diabetes in a manic-depressive population. Comp. Psychiatry **21**, 270-275.
Linnoila, M., Karoum, F., and Potter, W. Z. (1983a) Effects of antidepressant treatments on dopamine turnover in depressed patients. Arch. Gen. Psychiatry **40**, 1015-1017.
Linnoila, M., MacDonald, E., Reinila, M., Leroy, A., Rubinow, D. R., and Goodwin, F. K. (1983b) RBC membrane adenosine triphosphatase activities in patients with major affective disorders. Arch. Gen. Psychiatry **40**, 1021-1026.
Linnoila, M., Whorton, A. R., Rubinow, D. R., Cowdry, R. W., Ninan, P. T., and Waters, R. N. (1983c) CSF prostaglandin levels in depressed and schizophrenic patients. Arch. Gen. Psychiatry **40**, 405-406.
Lipinski, J. F., Cohen, B. M., Frankenburg, F., Tohen, M., Waternaux, C., Altesman, R., Jones, B., and Harris, P. (1984) Open trial of S-adenosylmethionine for treatment of depression. Am. J. Psychiatry **141**, 448-450.
Lloyd, K. J., Farley, I. J., Deck, J. H. N., and Hornykiewicz, O. (1974) Serotonin and 5-hydroxyindoleacetic acid in discrete areas of the brainstem of suicide victims and control patients. Adv. Biochem. Psychopharmacol. **11**, 387-397.
Loosen, P. T. and Prange, A. J. Jr. (1980) Thyrotropin releasing hormone (TRH): a useful tool for psychoendocrine investigation. Psychoneuroendocrinology **5**, 63-80.

Loosen, P. T., Prange, A. J. Jr., Wilson, I. C., Lara, P., and Pettus, C. (1977) Thyroid stimulating hormone response after thyrotropin-releasing hormone in depressed, schizophrenic and normal women. Psychoneuroendocrinology 2, 137-148.

Maas, J. W. (1978) Clinical and biochemical heterogeneity of depressive disorders. Ann. Intern. Med. 88, 556-663.

Maas, J. W., Dekirmenjian, H., and De Leon-Jones, F. (1973) The identification of depressed patients who have a disorder of norepinephrine metabolism and/or disposition. In: Frontiers in Catecholamine Research--Third International Catecholamine Symposium (Usdin, E. and Snyder, S., eds), Pergamon Press, New York.

Maas, J. W., Fawcett, J. A., and Dekirmenjian, H. (1972) Catecholamine metabolism, depressive illness and drug response. Arch. Gen. Psychiatry 26, 252-262.

Maddison, S. (1977) Intraperitoneal and intracranial cholecystokinin depresses operant responding for food. Physiol. Behav. 19, 819-824.

Maeda, K., Kato, Y., and Ohgo, S. et al. (1975) GH and prolactin release after injection of TRH in patients with depression. J. Clin. Endocrinol. Metab. 40, 501-505.

Maggi, A. and Enna, S. J. (1980) Regional alterations in rat brain neurotransmitter systems following chronic lithium treatment. J. Neurochem. 34, 888-892.

Mangoni, A., Andreoli, V., Cabibbe, F., and Mandelli, V. (1969) Body fluids distribution in manic and depressed patients treated with lithium carbonate. Abst. 2nd Int. Meet. Int. Soc. Neurochem., Milan, p. 279.

Marco, J., Hedo, J. A., and Villanueva, M. L. (1977) Inhibitory effect of somatostatin on human pancreatic polypeptide secretion. Life Sci. 21, 739-742.

Mathew, R. J., Ho, B. T., Davis, C., Taylor, D., and Rock, J. (1981) Depression, antidepressants and plasma DBH. Psychiatry Res. 5, 331-334.

Matthysse, S. and Kidd, K. K. (1981) Evidence of HLA linkage in depressive disorders. New Engl. J. Med. 305, 1301-1306.

Mattson, B., Mjorndal, T., Oreland, L., and Perris, C. (1974) Catechol-O-methyltransferase and plasma monoamine oxidase in patients with affective disorders. Acta psychiatr. scand., Suppl. 255, 187-193.

Matussek, N. (1980) Neurobiology of depression in relation to pharmacological-biochemical properties of antidepressants. Curr. Med. Res. and Opin. **6**, 5-12.

McClure, D. J. (1973) The role of dopamine in depression. Can. Psychiatr. Assoc. J. **18**, 309-312.

McKim, H. R., Calverley, D. G., Philips, S. R., Baker, G. B., and Dewhurst, W. G. (1980) The effects of tranylcypromine on the levels of some cerebral amines in rat diencephalon. In: Recent Advances in Canadian Neuropsychopharmacology (Grof, P. and Saxena, B., eds), S. Karger, Basel, pp. 7-13.

Mellerup, E. T., Lauritsen, B., Dam, H., and Rafaelsen, O. J. (1976) Lithium effects on diurnal rhythm of calcium, magnesium, and phosphate metabolism in manic-melancholic disorder. Acta psychiatr. scand. **53**, 360-370.

Mendels, J. and Frazer, A. (1973) Intracellular lithium concentration and clinical response: towards a membrane theory of depression. J. Psychiatr. Res. **10**, 9-18.

Mendels, J., Stinnert, J. L., Burns, D., and Frazer, A. (1975) Amine precursors and depression. Arch. Gen. Psychiatry **32**, 22-30.

Mendlewicz, J., Linkowski, P., and Brauman, H. (1979) TSH responses to TRH in women with unipolar and bipolar depression. Lancet **ii**, 1079-1080.

Mendlewicz, J., Linkowski, P., Guroff, J. J., and van. Praag, H. M. (1979) Color blindness linkage to bipolar manic-dpressive illness. Arch. Gen. Psychiatry **36**, 1442-1449.

Miccoli, L., Porro, V., and Bertolino, A. (1978) Comparison between the antidepressant activity of S-adenosylmethionine (SAMe) and that of some tricyclic drugs. Acta Neurol. **33**, 243-255.

Michael, R. P. and Gibbons, J. L. (1963) Interrelationships between the endocrine system and neuropsychiatry. Int. Rev. Neurobiol. **5**, 243-302.

Moller, S. E., Kirk, L., and Honore, P. (1980) Relationship between plasma ratio of tryptophan to competing amino acids and the response to L-tryptophan treatment in endogenously depressed patients. J. Affec. Disorders **2**, 47-59.

Moody, T. W. and Pert, C. B. (1979) Bombesin-like peptides in rat brain: quantitation and biochemical characterization. Biochem. Biophys. Res. Commun. **90**, 7-14.

Morselli, P. L., Bossi, L., Henry, J. F., Zarifian, E., and Bartholini, G. (1980) On the therapeutic action of SL 76 002, a new GABA-mimetic agent.

Brain Res. Bull. **5** Suppl. 2, 411-415.
Moses, A. M., Miller, M., and Streeten, D. H. P. (1976) Pathophysiologic and pharmacologic alterations in the release and action of ADH. *Metabolism* **25**, 697-721.
Mueller, P. S., Heninger, G. R., and McDonald, R. K. (1969) Insulin tolerance test in depression. *Arch. Gen. Psychiatry* **21**, 587-594.
Mueller, P. S., Heninger, G. R., and McDonald, R. K. (1969) Intravenous glucose tolerance test in depression. *Arch. Gen. Psychiatry* **21**, 470-477.
Murphy, D. L., Campbell, I. C., and Costa, J. L. (1978) The brain serotonergic system in the affective disorders. *Progr. Neuro-Psychopharmacol.* **2**, 1-31.
Murphy, D. L., Goodwin, F. K., Brodie, H. K. H., and Bunney, W. E. Jr. (1973) L-Dopa dopamine, and hypomania. *Am. J. Psychiatry* **130**, 79-82.
Murphy, D. L., Goodwin, F. K., and Bunney, W. E. Jr. (1969) Potassium, sodium and aldosterone in manic-depressive patients: changes in relation to clinical state and lithium administration. *NIMH Workshop on Recent Advances in the Psychobiology of the Depressive Illnesses*, Williamsburg, Va., April, 1969.
Murphy, D. L., Karoum, F., Alterman, I., Lipper, S., and Wyatt, R. J. (1984) Phenylethylamine, tyramine and other trace amines in patients with affective disorders: associations with clinical state and antidepressant drug treatment. In: *Neurobiology of the Trace Amines* (Boulton, A. A., Baker, G. B., Dewhurst, W. G., and Sandler, M., eds), Humana Press, Clifton, N.J., pp. 499-514.
Muscettola, G., Galzenati, M., and Balbi, A. (1982) SAMe versus placebo: a double blind comparison in major depressive disorders. In: *Typical and Atypical Antidepressants: Clinical Practice* (Costa, E. and Racagni, G., eds), Raven Press, New York, pp. 151-156.
Nadi, N. S., Nurnberger, J. I., and Gershon, E. S. (1984) Muscarinic cholinergic receptors on skin fibroblasts in familial affective disorder. *N. Engl. J. Med.* **311**, 225-230.
Naylor, G. J., Dick, D. A. T., and Dick, E. G. (1976) Erythrocyte membrane cation carrier, relapse rate of manic-depressive illness and response to lithium. *Psychol. Med.* **6**, 257-263.
Naylor, G. J., Dick, D. A. T., Dick, E. G., LePoidevin, D., and Whyte, S. F. (1973) Erythrocyte membrane cation carrier in depressive illness. *Psychol. Med.* **3**, 502-508.

Naylor, G. J., Dick, D. A. T., Dick, E. G., and Moody, J. P. (1974) Lithium therapy and erythrocyte membrane cation carrier. Psychopharmacologia (Berl.) 37, 81-86.

Naylor, G. J. and Smith, A. H. W. (1981) Vanadium: a possible aetiological factor in manic-depressive illness. Psychol. Med. 11, 249-256.

Niklasson, F., Agren, H., and Hallgren, R. (1983) Purine and monoamine metabolites in cerebrospinal fluid: parallel purinergic and monoaminergic activation in depressive illness? J. Neurol. Neurosurg. Psychiat. 46, 255-260.

Nurnberger, J. I. and Gershon, E. S. (1984) Genetics of affective disorders. In: Neurobiology of Mood Disorders (Post, R. M. and Ballenger, J. C., eds), Williams & Wilkins, Baltimore, pp. 76-101.

Nurnberger, J., Jimerson, D., Simmons, S., et al. (1981) Red cell Na^+-K^+-ATPase: correlation with plasma cortisol and use of the two measurements as markers of affective disorder. In: Biological Research at the Interface with Psychiatric Practice, Society of Biological Psychiatry, New Orleans, p. 91.

Oppenheimer, G., Ebstein, R., and Belmaker, R. (1979) Effects of lithium on the physostigmine-induced behavioral syndrome and plasma cyclic GMP. J. Psychiatr. Res. 14, 133-138.

Oxenkrug, G. F., Branconnier, R. J., Harto-Truax, N., and Cole, J. O. (1983) Is serum cholesterol a biological marker for major depressive disorder? Am. J. Psychiatry 140, 920-921.

Papeschi, R. and McClure, D. J. (1971) Homovanillic acid and 5-hydroxyindoleactic acid in cerebrospinal fluid in depressed patients. Arch. Gen. Psychiatry 25, 354-358.

Pare, C. M. B. (1973) Potentiation of monoamine-oxidase inhibitors by tryptophan. Lancet ii, 527-528.

Pare, C. M. B. and Sandler, M. J. (1959) A clinical and biochemical study of a trial of iproniazid in the treatment of depression. J. Neurol. Neurosurg. Psychiat. 22, 247-251.

Paul, S. M., Rehavi, M., Skolnick, P., Ballenger, J. C., and Goodwin, F. K. (1981) Depressed patients have decreased binding of tritiated imipramine to platelet serotonin "transporter". Arch. Gen. Psychiatry 38, 1315-1317.

Paul, S. M., Rehavi, M., Skolnick, P., and Goodwin, F. K. (1984) High affinity binding of antidepressants to biogenic amine transport sites in human brain and platelet: studies in depression. In: Neurobiology of Mood Disorders (Post, R. M. and Ballenger, J. C., eds), Williams & Wilkins, Baltimore, pp. 846-853.

Pederson, R. A., Dryburgh, J. R., and Brown, J. C. (1975) The effect of somatostatin on release and insulinotropic action of gastric inhibitory polypeptide. Can. J. Physiol. Pharmacol. 53, 1200-1205.

Philips, S. R., Baker, G. B., and McKim, H. R. (1980) Effects of tranylcypromine on the concentration of some trace amines in the diencephalon and hippocampus of the rat. Experientia 36, 241-242.

Philips, S. R. and Boulton, A. A. (1979) The effects of monoamine oxidase inhibitors on some arylalkylamines in rat striatum. J. Neurochem. 33, 159-167.

Platman, S. R. and Fieve, R. R. (1968a) Biochemical aspects of lithium in affective disorders. Arch. Gen. Psychiatry 19, 659-663.

Platman, S. R. and Fieve, R. R. (1968b) Lithium carbonate and plasma cortisol response in the affective disorders. Arch. Gen. Psychiatry 18, 591-594.

Plenge, P. and Mellerup, E. T. (1976) Lithium effects of serum calcium, magnesium and phosphorus in rats. Psychopharmacologia (Berl.) 49, 187-190.

Plenge, P. and Rafaelsen, O. J. (1982) Lithium effects on calcium, magnesium and phosphate in man: effects on balance, bone mineral content, faecal and urinary excretion. Acta psychiat. scand. 66, 361-373.

Pomara, N., Banay-Schwartz, M., Block, R., Stanley, M., and Gershon, S. (1983) Elevation of RBC glycine and choline levels in geriatric patients treated with lithium. Am. J. Psychiatry 140, 911-913.

Post, R. M., Ballenger, J. C., Hare, T. A., Goodwin, F. K., Lake, C. R., Jimerson, D. C., and Bunney, W. E. Jr. (1980) CSF GABA in normals and patients with affective disorder. Brain Res. Bull. 5 Suppl. 2, 755-759.

Post, R. M., Jimerson, D. C., Ballenger, J. C., Lake, C. R., Uhde, T. W., and Goodwin, F. K. (1984a) Cerebrospinal fluid norepinephrine and its metabolites in manic-depressive illness. In: Neurobiology of Mood Disorders (Post, R. M. and Ballenger, J. C., eds), Williams & Wilkins, Baltimore, pp. 539-553.

Post, R. M., Pickar, D., Ballenger, J. C., Naber, D., and Rubinow, D. R. (1984b) Endogenous opiates in cerebrospinal fluid: relationship to mood and anxiety. In: Neurobiology of Mood Disorders (Post, R. M. and Ballenger, J. C., eds), Williams & Wilkins, Baltimore, pp. 356-368.

Potter, W. Z., Zaharko, D. S., and Beck, L. V. (1969) Possible role of hydrazine group in hypoglycemia associated with the use of certain monoamine oxidase inhibitors (MAOIs). Diabetes 18, 538-541.

Prange, A. J. Jr., Wilson, I. C., Lara, P. P., Alltop, L., and Breese, G. (1972) Effects of thyrotropin-releasing hormone in depression. Lancet ii, 999-1022.

Pryce, I. G. (1958a) Melancholia, glucose tolerance and body weight. J. Mental Sci. 104, 421-427.

Pryce, I. G. (1958b) The relationship between glucose tolerance, body weight and clinical state in melancholia. J. Mental Sci. 104, 1079-1092.

Raichle, M. D. and Grubb, R. L. Jr. (1978) Regulation of brain water permeability by centrally released vasopressin. Brain Res. 143, 191-194.

Raisman, R., Briley, M., and Langer, S. Z. (1979) Specific tricyclic antidepressant binding sites in rat brain. Nature (Lond.) 281, 148-150.

Ramsey, T. A., Frazer, A., and Mendels, J. (1979) Plasma and erythrocyte cations in affective illness. Neuropsychobiology 5, 1-10.

Randrup, A., Munkvad, I., Fog, R., Gerlach, J., Molander, L., Kjellberg, B., and Scheel-Kruger, J. (1975) Mania, depression and brain dopamine. In: Current Developments in Psychopharmacology, vol. 2 (Essman, W. B. and Valzelli, L., eds), Spectrum Publications, New York, pp. 206-248.

Ray, P. D., Hanson, R. L., and Lardy, H. A. (1970) Inhibition by hydrazine of gluconeogensis in the rat. J. Biol. Chem. 245, 690-696.

Redmond, D. E. Jr., Roth, R. H., Hattox, S. E., Stogin, J. M., and Baulu, J. (1979) 3-Methoxy-4-hydroxyphenylethyleneglycol (MHPG) in monkey brain, CSF, and plasma during naloxone precipitated morphine abstinence. Neurosci. Abstr. 5, 348.

Rehavi, M., Skolnick, P., Hulihan, B., and Paul, S. M. (1981) High affinity binding of (^{3}H)-desipramine to rat cerebral cortex: relationship to tricyclic antidepressant-induced inhibition of norepinephrine uptake. Eur. J. Pharmacol. 70, 597-599.

Renaud, L. P. and Martin, J. P. (1975) Thyrotropin releasing hormone (TRH): depressant action on central neuronal activity. Brain Res. 86, 150-154.

Reynolds, E. H. (1968) Mental effects of anticonvulsants, and folic acid metabolism. Brain 91, 197-214.

Reynolds, E. H., Carney, M. W. P., and Toone, B. K. (1984) Methylation and mood. Lancet ii, 196-198.

Rezek, M., Havlicek, V., Hughes, K. R., and Friesen, H. (1977) Behavioural and motor excitation and inhibition induced by the administration of small and large doses of somatostatin into the amygdala. Neuropharmacology 16, 157-162.

Rezek, M., Havlicek, V., Hughes, K. R., and Friesen, H. (1976) Cortical administration of somatostatin (SRIF): effect on sleep and motor behavior. Pharmacol. Biochem. Behav. 5, 73-77.

Ridges, A. P. (1981) Amine metabolism and the prediction of response to dothiepin and other antidepressant medications. Proc. 8th Meet. Int. Soc. Neurochem., p. 227.

Rihmer, Z. and Arato, M. (1982) Depression and diabetes mellitus: a study of the relationship between serum cortisol and blood sugar levels in patients with endogenous depression. Neuropsychobiology 8, 315-318.

Risch, S. C. and Janowsky, D. S. (1984) Cholinergic-adrenergic balance in affective illness. In: Neurobiology of Mood Disorders (Post, R. M. and Ballenger, J. C., eds), Williams & Wilkins, Baltimore, pp. 652-663.

Risch, S. C., Kalin, N. H., and Janowsky, D. S. (1981a) Cholinergic challenges in affective illness: behavioral and neuroendocrine correlates. J. Clin. Psychopharmacol. 1, 186-192.

Risch, S. C., Kalin, N. H., and Murphy, D. L. (1981b) Neurochemical mechanisms in the affective disorders and neurochemical correlates. J. Clin. Psychopharmacol. 1, 180-185.

Robertson, G. L. (1979) The physiopathology of ADH secretion. In: Clinical Neuroendocrinology: A Pathophysiological Approach (Tolis, G., LaBrie, F., Martin, J. B., and Naftolin, F., eds), Raven Press, New York, pp. 247-260.

Rodin, E. and Schmaltz, S. (1983) Folate levels in epileptic patients. In: Advances in Epileptology (Parsonage, M., Grant, R. H. E., Craig, A. G., and Ward, A. A., eds), Raven Press, New York, pp. 143-150.

Roos, B. E. (1976) Tryptophan, 5-hydroxytryptophan, and tricyclic antidepressants in the treatment of depression. Monogr. Neural Sci. 3, 23-25.

Rosenbaum, A. H., Schatzberg, A., Maruta, T., Orsulak, P. J., Cole, J. O., Grab, E. L., and Schildkraut, J. J. (1980) MHPG as a predictor of antidepressant response to imipramine and maprotiline. Am. J. Psychiatry 137, 1090-1092.

Rosenblatt, S., Chanley, J. D., Sobotka, H., and Kaufman, M. R. (1960) Interrelationship between electroshock, the blood-brain barrier, and catecholamines. J. Neurochem. 5, 172-176.

Rosenblatt, S., Gaull, G. E., Chanley, J. D., Rosenthal, J. S., Smith, H., and Sarkozi, L. (1979) Amino acids in bipolar affective disorders: increased glycine levels in erythrocytes. Am. J. Psychiatry 136, 672-674.

Rosenblatt, S., Leighton, W. P., and Chanley, J. D. (1982) Elevation of erythrocyte glycine levels during lithium treatment of affective disorders. Psychiatry Res. 6, 203-214.

Rubin, R. T. (1967) Adrenal cortical activity changes in manic-depressive illness. Influence on intermediary metabolism of tryptophan. Arch. Gen. Psychiatry 17, 671-679.

Rubin, R. T. (1968) Multiple biochemical correlates of manic-depressive illness. J. Psychosomatic Res. 12, 171-180.

Rubin, R. T. and Kendler, K. S. (1977) Psychoneuroendocrinology: fundamental concepts and correlates in depression. In: Depression: Clinical Biological and Psychosocial Perspectives (Usdin, E., ed.), Brunner/Mazel, New York, pp. 122-138.

Rubin, R. T. and Marder, S. R. (1983) Biological markers in affective and schizophrenic disorders: a review of contemporary research. In: Affective and Schizophrenic Disorders: New Approaches to Diagnosis and Treatment (Zales, M. R., ed.), Brunner/Mazel, New York, pp. 53-100.

Rubin, R. T., Poland, R. E., and Hays, S. E. (1979) Psychoneuroendocrine research in endogenous depression: a review. In: Biological Psychiatry Today (Obiols, J., Ballus, C., Gonzales Monclus, E., and Pujol, J., eds), Elsevier-North Holland, Amsterdam, pp. 684-688.

Rubinow, D. R., Gold, P. W., Post, R. M., Ballenger, J. C., and Cowdry, R. W. (1984) Somatostatin in patients with affective illness and in normal volunteers. In: Neurobiology of Mood Disorders (Post, R. M. and Ballenger, J. C., eds), Williams & Wilkins, Baltimore, pp. 369-387.

Rubinow, D. R., Post, R. M., Gold, P. W., Ballenger, J. C., and Wolff, E. A. (1984) The relationship between cortisol and clinical phenomenology of affective illness. In: Neurobiology of Mood Disorders (Post, R. M. and Ballenger, J. C., eds), Williams & Wilkins, Baltimore, pp. 271-289.

Russell, G. F. M. (1960) Body weight and balance of water, sodium and potassium in depressed patients given electro-convulsive therapy. Clin. Sci. 19, 327-336.

Sabelli, H. C., Fawcett, J., Gusovsky, F., Javaid, J., Edwards, J., and Jeffries, J. (1983) Urinary phenyl acetate: a diagnostic test for depression. Science 220, 1187-1188.

Sabelli, H. C., Fawcett, J., Javaid, J., and Bagri, S. (1983) The methylphenidate test for differentiating desipramine-responsive from nortriptyline-responsive depression. Am. J. Psychiatry 140, 212-214.

Sabelli, H. C. and Mosnaim, A. D. (1974) Phenylethylamine hypothesis of affective behavior. Am. J. Psychiatry 131, 695-699.

Sabelli, H. C., Mosnaim, A. D., Vazquez, A. J., Giardina, W. J., Borison, R. L., and Pedemonte, W. A. (1976) Biochemical plasticity of synaptic transmission: a critical review of Dale's principle. Biol. Psychiatry 11, 481-522.

Sacchetti, E., Allaria, E., Negri, F., Biondi, P. A., Smeraldi, E., and Cazzullo, C. L. (1979) 3-Methoxy-4-hydroxyphenylglycol and primary depression: clinical and pharmacological considerations. Biol. Psychiatry 14, 473-484.

Sachar, E. J., Frantz, A. G., Altman, N., and Sassin, J. (1973) Growth hormone and prolactin in unipolar and bipolar depressed patients: responses to hypoglycaemia and L-dopa. Am. J. Psychiatry 130, 1362-1367.

Sachar, E. J., Hellman, L., Fukushima, D. K., and Gallagher, T. F. (1970) Cortisol production in depressive illness. Arch. Gen. Psychiatry 23, 289-298.

Saito, A., Sankaran, H., Goldfine, I., and Williams, J. A. (1980) Cholecystokinin receptors in the brain: characterization and distribution. Science 208, 1155-1156.

Sandler, M., Bonham-Carter, S. M., and Walker, P. L. (1984) Tyramine and depressive illness. In: Neurobiology of the Trace Amines (Boulton, A. A., Baker, G. B., Dewhurst, W. G., and Sandler, M., eds), Humana Press, New York, pp. 487-498.

Sandler, M., Reveley, M. A., and Glover, V. (1981) Human platelet monoamine oxidase activity in health and disease: a review. J. Clin. Pathol. 34, 292-302.

Sandler, M., Ruthven, C. J. R., Goodwin, B. L., and Coppen, A. (1979a) Decreased cerebrospinal fluid concentration of free phenylacetic acid in depressive illness. Clin. Chim. Acta 93, 169-171.

Sandler, M., Ruthven, C. R. J., Goodwin, B. L., Reynolds, G. P., Rao, V. A. R., and Coppen, A. (1979b) Deficient production of tyramine and octopamine in cases of depression. Nature (Lond.) 278, 357-358.

Schildkraut, J. J. (1965) The catecholamine hypothesis of affective disorders: a review of supporting evidence. Am. J. Psychiatry 122, 509-522.

Schildkraut, J. J., Orsulak, P. J., LaBrie, R. A., Schatzberg, A. F., Gudeman, J. E., Cole, J. O., and Rohde, W. A. (1978) Toward a biochemical classification of depressive disorders II: application of multivariate discriminant function analysis to data on urinary catecholamines and metabolites. Arch. Gen. Psychiatry 35, 1436-1439.

Schildkraut, J. J., Schatzberg, A. F., Mooney, J. J., and Orsulak, P. J. (1983) Depressive disorders and the emerging field of psychiatric chemistry. In: Psychiatry Update, vol. II, American Psychiatric Press, Inc., Washington, D.C., pp. 457-471.

Schwartz, M., Mandell, A. J., Green, R., and Ferman, R. (1966) Mood, motility and 17-hydroxycorticoid excretion: a polyvariable case study. Brit. J. Psychiatry 112, 149-156.

Shaw, D. M., Frizel, D., Camps, F. E., and White, S. (1969) Brain electrolytes in depressive and alcoholic suicides. Brit. J. Psychiatry 115, 69-79.

Shea, P. A., Small, J. C., and Hendrie, H. C. (1981) Elevation of choline and glycine in red cells of psychiatric patients due to lithium treatment. Biol. Psychiatry 16, 825-830.

Sherman, A. D. and Petty, F. (1980) Neurochemical basis of the action of antidepressants on learned helplessness. Behav. Neural. Biol. 30, 119-134.

Shulman, R., Griffiths, J., and Diewold, P. (1978) Catechol-O-methyl transferase activity in patients with depression illness and anxiety states. Brit. J. Psychiatry 132, 133-138.

Siever, L. J., Insel, T., and Uhde, T. (1981) Noradrenergic challenges in the affective disorders. J. Clin. Psychopharmacol. 1, 193-206.

Singer, I., Rotenberg, D., and Puschett, J. (1972) Lithium-induced nephrogenic diabetes insipidus: in vivo and in vitro studies. J. Clin. Invest. 51, 1081-1091.

Sitaram, N., Gillin, J. C., and Bunney, W. E. Jr. (1984) Cholinergic and catecholaminergic receptor sensitivity in affective illness: strategy and theory. In: Neurobiology of Mood Disorders (Post, R. M. and Ballenger, J. C., eds), Williams & Wilkins, Baltimore, pp. 629-651.

Sjostrom, R. (1973) 5-Hydroxyindoleacetic acid and homovanillic acid in cerebrospinal fluid in manic-depressive psychosis and the effect of probenecid treatment. Eur. J. Clin. Pharmacol. 6, 75-80.

Sjostrom, R. and Roos, B. E. (1972) 5-Hydroxyindoleacetic acid and homovanillic acid in cerebrospinal fluid in manic-depressive psychosis. Eur. J. Clin. Pharmacol. 4, 170-176.

Smeraldi, E., Negri, F., Melica, A. M., and Scorza-Smeraldi, R. (1978) HLA system and affective disorders: a sibship genetic study. Tissue Antigens 12, 270-274.

Smith, C. B., Garcia-Sevilla, J. A., and Hollingsworth, P. J. (1981) Alpha$_2$ adrenoreceptors in rat brain are decreased after long-term tricyclic antidepressant drug treatment. Brain Res. 210, 413-418.

Smith, C. B., Hollingsworth, P. J., Garcia-Sevilla, J. A., and Zis, A. P. (1983) Platelet alpha$_2$ adrenoreceptors are decreased in number after antidepressant therapy. Prog. Neuro-Psychopharmacol. & Biol. Psychiat. 7, 241-247.

Snyder, S. H. and Peroutka, S. J. (1984) Antidepressants and neurotransmitter receptors. In: Neurobiology of Mood Disorders (Post, R. M. and Ballenger, J. C., eds), Williams & Wilkins, Baltimore, pp. 686-697.

Spiker, D. G., Edwards, D., Hanin, I., Neil, J. F., and Kupfer, D. J. (1980) Urinary MHPG and clinical response to amitriptyline in depressed patients. Am. J. Psychiatry 137, 1183-1187.

Stanford, S. C. and Nutt, D. J. (1982) Comparison of the effects of repeated electroconvulsive shock on α_2- and β-adrenoreceptors in different regions of rat brain. Neuroscience 7, 1753-1757.

Stanley, M., Virgilio, J., and Gershon, S. (1982) Tritiated imipramine binding sites are decreased in the frontal cortex of suicides. Science 216, 1337-1339.

Stein, G., Milton, F., Bebbington, P., Wood, K., and Coppen, A. (1976) Relationship between mood disturbances and free and total plasma tryptophan in postpartum women. Brit. Med. J. 2, 457.

Strom-Olsen, R. and Weil-Malherbe, H. (1958) Humoral changes in manic-depressive psychosis with particular reference to the excretion of catechol amines in urine. J. Mental Sci. 104, 696-704.

Strzyzewski, W., Rybakowski, J., and Kapelski, Z. (1980) Investigations on electrolyte and water contents in plasma and red blood cells in the course of thymoleptic treatment of depressive syndromes. Neuropsychobiology 6, 121-127.

Sugrue, M. F. (1983) Do antidepressants possess a common mechanism of action? Biochem. Pharmacol. 32, 1811-1817.

Sulser, F. (1982a) Giovanni Lorenzini Foundation Lecture--Antidepressant drug research: its impact on neurobiology and psychobiology. In: Typical and Atypical Antidepressants: Molecular Mechanisms (Costa, E. and Racagni, G., eds), Raven Press, New York, pp. 1-20.

Sulser, F. (1982b) Regulation and adaptation of central norepinephrine receptor systems: modification by antidepressant treatments. Psychiatr. J. Univ. Ottawa 7, 196-203.

Sulser, F. (1983) Deamplification of noradrenergic signal transfer by antidepressants: a unified catecholamine-serotonin hypothesis of affective disorders. Psychopharmacol. Bull. 19, 300-304.

Takahashi, R., Nakahara, T., and Sakurai, Y. (1974) Emotional stress and biochemical responses of manic-depressive patients. Psychoneuroendocrinology, pp. 58-66.

Takahashi, S., Kindo, H., Yoshimura, M., and Ochi, Y. (1974) Thyrotropin responses to TRH in depressive illness: relation to clinical subtypes and prolonged duration of depressive episode. Folia Psychiatr. Neurol. Jpn. 28, 335-365.

Tamminga, C., Smith, R. C., Chang, S., Naraszti, J. S., and Davis, J. M. (1976) Depression associated with oral choline. Lancet ii, 905.

Taube, S. L., Kirstein, L. S., Sweeney, D. R., Heninger, G. R., and Maas, J. W. (1978) Urinary 3-methoxy-4-hydroxyphenylglycol and psychiatric diagnosis. Am. J. Psychiatry 135, 78-82.

Tran, V. T., Chang, R. S. L., and Snyder, S. H. (1978) Histamine H_1 receptors identified in mammalian brain membranes with ^{3}H-mepyramine. Proc. Natl. Acad. Sci. U.S.A. 75, 6290-6294.

Traskman-Bendz, L., Asberg, M., Bertilsson, L., and Sjostrand, L. (1981) Monoamine metabolites in CSF and suicidal behavior. Arch. Gen. Psychiatry 38, 631-636.

Trautner, E. M., Morris, R., Noack, C. H., and Gershon, S. (1955) The excretion and retention of ingested lithium and its effect on the ionic balance of man. Med. J. Austral. 2, 280-291.

Trimble, M. R., Corbett, J., and Donalldson, D. (1980) Folic acid and mental symptoms in children with epilepsy. J. Neurol. Neurosurg. Psychiat. 43, 1030-1034.

Triner, L., Verosky, M., Papayoanou, J., and Nahas, G. G. (1969) The effect of some monoamine oxidase inhibitors on gluconeogenesis. Life Sci. 81, 1281-1290.

Usdin, E. and Sandler, M. (eds) (1976) Trace Amines and the Brain. Marcel Dekker, New York.

van Praag, H. M. (1977) Significance of biochemical parameters in the diagnosis, treatment and prevention of depressive disorders. Biol. Psychiatry 12, 101-131.

van Praag, H. M. (1981) Central monoamines and the pathogenesis of depression. In: Handbook of Biological Psychiatry, vol. I, part IV (van Praag, H. M., Lader, M. H., Raphaelson, L. J., and Sachar, E. J., eds), Marcel Dekker, New York, pp. 159-205.

van Praag, H. M. (1982) Serotonin precursors in the treatment of depression. In: Serotonin in Biological Psychiatry (Ho, B. T., et al., eds), Raven Press, New York, pp. 259-286.

van Praag, H. M. (1983) In search of the mode of action of antidepressants. 5-HTP/tyrosine mixtures in depressions. Neuropharmacology 22, 433-440.

van Praag, H. M. (1984a) Depression, suicide, and serotonin metabolism in the brain. In: Neurobiology of Mood Disorders (Post, R. M. and Ballenger, J. C., eds), Williams & Wilkins, Baltimore, pp. 601-618.

van Praag, H. M. (1984b) Studies on the mechanism of action of serotonin precursors in depression.

Psychopharmacol. Bull. **20,** 599-602.
van Praag, H. M. and Korf, J. (1971) Retarded depression and dopamine metabolism. Psychopharmacology **19,** 199-203.
van Praag, H. M. and Korf, J. (1975) Central monoamine deficiency in depression: causative or secondary phenomenon? Pharmacopsychiatry **8,** 321-326.
van Praag, H. M., Korf, J., and Schut, T. (1973) Cerebral monoamines and depression. An investigation with the probenecid technique. Arch. Gen. Psychiatry **28,** 827-831.
van Praag, H. M. and Leijnse, B. (1965) Depression, glucose tolerance, peripheral glucose uptake and their alterations under the influence of antidepressive drugs of the hydrazine type. Psychopharmacologia (Berl.) **8,** 67-78.
van Praag, H. M. and Leijnse, B. (1966) Some aspects of the metabolism of glucose and of the nonesterified fatty acids in depressive patients. Psychopharmacologia (Berl.) **9,** 220-233.
van Scheylen, J. D., van Praag, H. M., and Korf, J. (1977) Controlled study comparing nomifensine and clomipramine in unipolar depression, using the probenecid technique. Brit. J. Clin. Pharmacol. **4,** 1795-1845.
Vogel, G. W. (1983) Evidence for REM sleep deprivation as the mechanism of action of antidepressant drugs. Progr. Neuro-Psychopharmacol. & Biol. Psychiatr. **1,** 343-349.
Vogel, G. W., Vogel, F., McAbee, R. S., and Thurmond, A. J. (1980) Improvement of depression by REM sleep deprivation. Arch. Gen. Psychiatry **37,** 247-253.
Walinder, J., Carlsson, A., Persson, R., and Wallin, L. (1980) Potentiation of the effect of antidepressant drugs by tryptophan. Acta psychiatr. scand. **61(S-390),** 243-249.
Wang, R. Y. and Aghajanian, G. K. (1980) Enhanced sensitivity of amygdaloid neurons to serotonin and norepinephrine after chronic antidepressant treatment. Commun. Psychopharmacol. **4,** 83-90.
Waters, B., Thakar, J., and Lapierre, Y. (1983) Erythrocyte lithium transport variables as a marker for manic-depressive disorder. Neuropsychobiology **9,** 94-98.
Weil-Malherbe, H. (1967) The biochemistry of the functional psychoses. In: Advances in Enzymology, vol. 29 (Nord, F. F., ed.), Interscience Publishers, New York, pp. 479-553.

Weil-Malherbe, H. (1972) In: Handbook of Neurochemistry, vol. 7 (Lajtha, A., ed.), Plenum Press, New York, pp. 371-416.
Weitkamp, L. R., Stancer, H. C., Persad, E., Flood, C., and Guttormsen, S. (1981) Depressive disorders and HLA: a gene or chromosome 6 that can affect behavior. New Engl. J. Med. 305, 1301-1306.
Weitzman, R. E., Fisher, D. W., Minisek, S., Ling, N., and Guilleman, F. (1977) Beta-endorphin stimulates secretion of arginine vasopressin in vivo. Endocrinology 101, 1643-1645.
Werstiuk, E., Rathbone, M. P., and Grof, P. (1981) Phloretin-sensitive lithium transport in erythrocytes of affectively ill patients: intraindividual reproducibility. Prog. Neuropsychopharmacol. 5, 503-506.
Williams, G. A., Hargis, G. K., Ensinck, J. W., Kukreja, S. C., Bower, E. N., Chertow, B. S., and Handerson, W. J. (1979) Role of endogenous somatostatin in the secretion of parathyroid hormone and calcitonin. Metabolism 28, 950-954.
Willner, P. (1983a) Dopamine and depression: a review of recent evidence. I. Empirical studies. Brain Res. Rev. 6, 211-224.
Willner, P. (1983b) Dopamine and depression: a review of recent evidence. II. Theoretical approaches. Brain Res. Rev. 6, 225-236.
Willner, P. (1983c) Dopamine and depression: a review of recent evidence. III. The effects of antidepressant treatments. Brain Res. Rev. 6, 237-246.
Winston, F. (1969) Oral contraceptives and depression. Lancet i, 1209.
Wirz-Justice, A. (1977) Theoretical and therapeutic potential of indoleamine precursors. Neuropsychobiology 3, 199-233.
Woods, S. C., West, D. B., Stein, L. J., McKay, L. D., Lotter, E. C., Porte, S. G., Kenney, N. J., and Porte, E. Jr. (1981) Peptides and the control of meal size. Diabetologia 20, 305-313.
Young, S. N. (1984) Monoamine precursors in the affective disorders. In: Advances in Human Psychopharmacology, vol. 3 (Burrows, G. D. and Werry, J. S., eds), JAI Press Inc., Greenwich, CT, pp. 251-285.
Young, S. N. and Sourkes, T. L. (1977) Tryptophan in the central nervous system: regulation and significance. Adv. Neurochem. 2, 133-191.

2.

BIOLOGIC MARKERS IN AFFECTIVE DISORDERS

L. G. Huang and J. W. Maas

Introduction
============

A major aim of current clinical research conducted in the affective and schizophrenic disorders has been the identification of reliable biologic or pharmacologic probes that may correlate with state or trait characteristics of these disorders, provide diagnostic tools in complex clinical presentations, aid in treatment selection, and serve as predictors of clinical response.
    In general, biologic markers for the affective disorders have been better defined than those for the schizophrenic disorders, with the former having more reliable and clear-cut biologic correlates of the disease state both for diagnosis and response prediction. Biologic markers of the affective disorders comprise the neuroendocrine axis consisting of sleep studies, the protirelin challenge test (blunted TSH response), the dexamethasone suppression test, the growth hormone and prolactin response, and cortisol hypersecretion. The biogenic amine markers comprise monoamine oxidase (MAO) activity, 5-hydroxyindole-3-acetic acid (5-HIAA) correlation with depression and suicide, ^{3}H-imipramine binding, 3-methoxy-4-hydroxyphenylglycol (MHPG) correlation with depressive state and treatment selection, and the red blood cell lithium (RBC-Li) ratio in bipolar disorders.
    Where the data permit, each biologic marker will be reviewed from the aspect of its specificity, sensitivity and reliability in diagnosis of primary endogenous depression, bipolar mania and bipolar depression; possible correlation with trait characteristics; and as a tool useful for treatment selection and treatment response. The pathophysiologic

implications and correlations between each psychobiologic marker will be explored.

^{3}H-Imipramine Binding

The biogenic amine theory of affective disorders postulates that depression is related to a deficiency in catecholamine and/or 5-hydroxytryptamine (5-HT; serotonin) transmission at the synapse (Schildkraut and Kety, 1967). Mania, in contrast, has been thought to be associated with excess noradrenergic function. Lithium inhibition of norepinephrine (noradrenaline; NA) efflux from pre-synaptic neurons provides partial support for the hypothesis that mania is related to excess catecholaminergic function (Katz et al., 1968). The theory of catecholaminergic or serotonergic deficient transmission in depression is also in part supported by the finding that traditional antidepressants either block the reuptake of NA and/or 5-HT into pre-synaptic neurons (Glowinski and Axelrod, 1964) or, in the case of the MAO inhibitors, block the intraneuronal degradation of these amines (Barchas et al., 1977). The above does not, however, satisfactorily explain the mechanism of action of all antidepressants in that some of the newer atypical antidepressants, viz. iprindole, mianserin, and viloxazine, do not block NA or 5-HT reuptake (Rosloff and Davis, 1974; Bevan et al., 1975; Lippmann and Pugsley, 1976; Baumann and Maitre, 1977). In addition, chronic tricyclic treatment has been shown also to downregulate brain post-synaptic β-adrenoceptors, as demonstrated by decreased binding of β-^{3}H-dihydroaprenolol (Charney et al., 1981a; Raisman et al., 1980). The mode of action of tricyclic antidepressants may, therefore, be more complex than simple monoamine reuptake blockade. If the actual mode of antidepressant action is post-synaptic and involves down-regulation of receptors, the lag time of 2-4 weeks before such receptor alteration may be a factor in the comparable lag in clinical improvement.

Commonly known receptors involved in neurotransmission are the $α_1$ and $α_2$ adrenoceptors, the β-adrenoceptor, the H_1 and H_2-histaminic receptors, the serotonergic receptor and muscarinic cholinoceptors, and the benzodiazepine receptors (Langer and Briley, 1981; Langer and Raisman, 1983). A search for a receptor site of action of tricyclic antidepressants led to the discovery of a high affinity, rapidly reversible, specific imipramine binding site in the rat brain (Charney et al., 1981b; Raisman et al., 1979). This was hypothesized as a possible receptor site of action of the tricyclic antidepressants. The binding was not directly related to known neurotransmitter receptor systems, with the possible exception of the 5-HT reuptake system (Langer and Briley, 1981; Palkovits et al., 1981; Langer et al., 1980b; Paul et al., 1980). The binding sites possessed many of the properties usually associated with the specific site of action of a drug (Raisman et al., 1980). The binding was saturable and competitive, and Scatchard analysis gave a straight line, indicating a single population of non-interacting binding sites (Raisman et al., 1980). The specific binding was unevenly distributed in the rat brain, being highest in the hypothalamus and amygdala and lowest in the cerebellum (Raisman et al., 1980; Palkovits et al., 1981). No specific binding was detected in peripheral organs low in serotonergic function but high in noradrenergic function, such as the heart and vas deferens (Raisman et al., 1980). Similar binding sites were subsequently found in platelets from several animal species, including man (Paul et al., 1980; Briley et al., 1979; Langer et al., 1980a).

The inhibition of ^{3}H-imipramine binding to rat cerebral cortex and to human platelet membranes was virtually identical as measured by the high correlation between IC$_{50}$ values for inhibition of ^{3}H-imipramine binding for the two tissues for a series of 25 drugs (r = 0.81, p < 0.001) (Langer et al., 1980a). The IC$_{50}$ value is that concentration of a drug that inhibits receptor binding by 50%. The ^{3}H-imipramine binding site is associated with, but not identical with, the presynaptic 5-HT reuptake systems (Langer and Briley, 1981; Palkovits et al, 1981; Langer et al, 1980b; Paul et al., 1980). The density of ^{3}H-imipramine binding sites parallels the endogenous levels of 5-HT, being low to undetectable in organs with noradrenergic innervation (Langer and Briley, 1981; Palkovits et al., 1981). There is no relationship with levels of dopamine. A close parallelism exists between the potency of a series of drugs for inhibition of 5-HT uptake in the rat hypothalamus and the potency of inhibition of ^{3}H-imipramine binding (Langer and Briley, 1981; Langer et al., 1980b; Arbilla et al., 1981). Further evidence that the 5-HT uptake system and ^{3}H-imipramine binding are related but not identical comes from a study of patients with alcoholic cirrhosis but no depressive disorder, who had a decrease in 5-HT uptake into platelets but normal values for ^{3}H-imipramine binding (Langer and Briley, 1981).

^{3}H-Imipramine binding in postmortem human brains had properties essentially identical to those described in rat brain (Rehavi et al., 1980; Langer and Briley, 1981). Binding sites in human platelets were next found to have identical properties to rat brain ^{3}H-imipramine binding (Paul et al., 1980; Briley et al., 1979; Langer et al., 1980b).

Chronic treatment with imipramine or desipramine was found to decrease ^{3}H-imipramine binding in rat cerebral cortex and cat hypothalamus and platelets (Raisman et al., 1980; Langer and Raisman, 1983), as reflected in a significant reduction in B_{max} (maximum number of binding sites) with no change in Kd (affinity constant). Tricyclic antidepressants inhibit ^{3}H-imipramine binding, with the degree of inhibition paralleling their clinical potency in terms of average therapeutic doses (Arbilla et al., 1981). The degree of affinity of the tricyclic antidepressant is proportional to the degree of methylation (Mellerup et al., 1982), secondary amine tricyclics having lower affinities. Non-tricyclic antidepressants have a mechanism of action that is not correlated significantly with inhibition of ^{3}H-imipramine binding (Langer and Raisman, 1983; Arbilla et al., 1981).

Given that the platelet ^{3}H-imipramine binding sites have properties virtually identical to cortical binding sites, the accessibility of the platelet system to study makes it an appealing system for investigations in patients with affective disorders. Decreased binding in brain and platelets of depressed patients has been reported by several groups (Langer et al., 1981; Paul et al., 1981; Perry et al., 1983; Raisman et al., 1981; Briley et al., 1980a; Briley et al., 1980b; Asarch et al., 1980). This consisted of a 20-50% reduction in the maximum number of binding sites (B_{max}) with no significant difference in Kd between the depressed patients and age- and sex-matched controls (Raisman et al., 1981; Briley et al., 1980a; Asarch et al., 1980).

B_{max} and the reduction in B_{max} in depressed patients were found to be independent of sex but not necessarily of age, as reduction in B_{max} but not Kd has been found to occur with increasing age (Langer and Briley, 1981; Arbilla et al., 1981). The decrease, however, was significant only in patients over seventy (Langer et al., 1980a). The reduction in B_{max} in depressed patients appears to be independent of the severity of depression and to remain low in the face of clinical improvement (Perry et al., 1983; Briley et al., 1980b). ^{3}H-Imipramine binding remained stable over at least a 4-week time span (Langer and Briley, 1981).

Similar reductions in ^{3}H-imipramine binding were seen in bipolar depressed, unipolar depressed, and reactively depressed patients examined separately. The length of the drug-free washout period (less than 30 days versus longer than 30 days) also was found not to affect B_{max} (Perry et al., 1983). However, the mean Kd for the patients with shorter washout periods was significantly higher (Perry et al., 1983).

Perry et al. (1983) studied ^{3}H-imipramine binding in the hippocampus and occipital cortex of postmortem brains of depressed patients as compared tc age-matched patients with no psychiatric disorders and patients with Alzheimer's disease. A significant reduction was again found in B_{max} and not Kd in brains from depressed patients. No change in binding was found in the Alzheimer's patients. No difference in binding was observed between patients treated with tricyclic antidepressants at the time of their death and untreated cases (Perry et al., 1983). Mellerup et al. (1982), in contrast, found B_{max} to be higher in a series of manic-melancholic patients as compard to euthymic manic-melancholic patients, normal controls, and psychiatric controls (Mellerup et al., 1982). Differences in patient population, current and previous medications, diagnostic procedure, or enzymatic procedure may be partial explanations for these discrepant findings.

Drugs like fluoxetine and femoxitine, which inhibit 5-HT uptake, potently inhibit ^{3}H-imipramine binding (Raisman et al., 1980; Raisman et al., 1979; Rehavi et al., 1980). Lesions of the dorsal raphe, a site rich in 5-HT function, diminish by 40% ^{3}H-imipramine binding, and similarly reduce 5-HT content (Palkovits et al., 1981). ^{3}H-Imipramine binding is not altered by inhibition of NA uptake (Langer et al., 1980b). In contrast to the clinical results to date, tricyclic treatment in rats and cats decreases platelet and brain ^{3}H-imipramine binding. Other antidepressant interventions have also been shown to decrease ^{3}H-imipramine binding. In rats, electroshock treatments and 72-hour paradoxical sleep deprivation, tools with antidepressant effects in man, significantly decrease B_{max} in the cortex (Langer and Briley, 1981) and hypothalamus (Langer et al., 1981; Mogilnicka et al., 1980) without affecting Kd.

The lack of change in ^{3}H-imipramine binding seen in humans with tricyclic antidepressant treatment and with clinical improvement may represent the net result of two counteracting effects, the tricyclic-induced inhibition of binding cancelling the possible increase in B_{max} with clinical improvement (Langer and Briley, 1981). Decreased ^{3}H-imipramine binding might be an indicator of increased diathesis toward the development of an affective disorder, regardless of subtype (Langer and Briley, 1981). It may represent a compensatory mechanism in those persons predisposed, by means of a genetically determined deficiency in 5-HT transmission, against the development of an affective disorder. Low ^{3}H-imipramine binding might therefore indicate a vulnerability toward the development of an affective disorder. Whether it may be a tool useful in implementing or monitoring antidepressant treatment remains to be established.

Similar studies have found that ^{3}H-desipramine labels the neuronal NA uptake mechanism. It is present only in noradrenergically innervated tissues, being absent in platelets. Chemical sympathectomy with 6-hydroxydopamine decreases ^{3}H-desipramine binding sites (Grob et al., 1981; Hrdina et al., 1981) but does not affect the ^{3}H-imipramine binding site. Drugs which inhibit NA uptake potently inhibit ^{3}H-desipramine binding (Raisman et al., 1982). The ^{3}H-desipramine binding site is at present a little studied research tool which has not yet been associated with any disease state.

In summary, there is a general consensus that platelet and brain ^{3}H-imipramine binding is decreased from 20-50% in primary endogenous, bipolar, and reactive depressions. There are no studies to date in secondary depressions. The decrease appears to be a fixed trait factor in that correlations do not exist with severity of depressions and changes in binding do not occur with clinical improvement. All clinical studies to date have used patients previously treated with antidepressant drugs, and thus it is possible that decreased binding may wholly, or in part, be due to prior tricyclic treatment rather than be a trait marker for a depressive disorder. Thus a study of depressed patients with no prior tricyclic antidepressant treatment history would possibly help to deal with the issue of decreased ^{3}H-imipramine binding being an artifact of previous treatment rather than an indication of a diathesis toward the development of an affective syndrome.

Should these studies indicate that the ^{3}H-imipramine binding site is not an artifact of previous drug treatment, the important question remaining is whether the ^{3}H-imipramine binding site and the 5-HT reuptake site are contiguous and functionally related. Such a functional interrelationship has not as yet been shown to exist.

5-HT uptake is deficient in depressive disorders, and ^{3}H-imipramine binding by consensus is also decreased. Functional separation of the two sites would show whether decreased ^{3}H-imipramine binding is simply another expression of decreased serotonergic function in depression or is a trait marker in and of itself. Finally, studies as to whether decreased ^{3}H-imipramine binding exists in first degree relatives of depressed patients would also be of interest in dealing with questions of the genetics of depressive disorders.

5-HT, 5-HIAA, and 5-HT Uptake in Depression

The evidence that 5-HT modulates mood is largely indirect. Reserpine, which produces depression, depletes neurons of dopamine (DA), 5-HT, and NA (Carlsson et al., 1957). Coppen (1967) specifically linked depression and mania to alterations in the 5-HT system. Now a more recent hypothesis is that the serotonergic system may play a more 'permissive' role in affective disorders and, by making the monoamine systems more vulnerable, may predispose to depressive states. Maas (1975) postulated that biochemically discrete depressions exist--one determined by an underfunctional noradrenergic system, the other due to a serotonergic deficit.

Alterations in the 5-HT system relate not only to major affective disorders but also to other disorders with disturbed mood, including suicide and aggressive behavior. Work to date on the serotonergic system in depression has focused around five major biochemical abnormalities:
1. autopsy data on 5-HT and its metabolites in brains from suicidal and/or depressed patients, revealing decreased serotonergic activity in certain regions of the brain;
2. study of 5-HT metabolites (5-HIAA) in CSF of depressed patients showing that low CSF 5-HIAA is correlated with suicidal behavior;
3. 5-HT uptake in human blood platelets used as a parallel to neuronal function;
4. ^{3}H-imipramine binding and 5-HT uptake in human

platelets and neurons;
5. neuroendocrine measures of 5-HT activity.

Postmortem studies of the brains of suicidal depressed patients have revealed in the majority decreased 5-HT and/or 5-HIAA content (Shaw et al., 1967; Bourne et al., 1968). More recent reports studied 5-HT and 5-HIAA concentrations in brain regions rich in serotonergic activity. 5-HIAA in the raphe has been found to be decreased in postmortem brains (Lloyd et al., 1974). Postmortem analysis of 5-HIAA and 5-HT in human brains conducted by Beskow et al. (1976) indicated lowered 5-HIAA levels in suicide victims in 6 of 8 parts of the brain studied. However, a decrease in 5-HIAA was found to occur with time lapse since death. When the time of death to postmortem analysis was controlled for, no significant difference in 5-HIAA levels was found between suicide victims and controls (Beskow et al., 1976).

Studies of CSF 5-HIAA levels in depressed patients as compared to controls have assessed baseline differences across groups and also after probenecid treatment. Probenecid blocks the transport of 5-HIAA out of CSF across the blood-brain barrier and thus provides a measure of the turnover of the serotonergic system. About half of the studies have linked low CSF 5-HIAA with depression (Ashcroft et al., 1966; Dencker et al., 1966; van Praag and Korf, 1971; Coppen et al., 1972), whereas others found no significant differences (Brodie et al., 1973; Goodwin et al., 1973; Ashcroft et al., 1973). Similarly, after probenecid treatment some investigators have reported low 5-HIAA accumulations (van Praag et al., 1970; van Praag and Korf, 1971; Goodwin et al., 1977) while others found no significant differences (Korf et al., 1983; Berger et al., 1980).

Asberg et al. (1976) reported that a bimodal distribution existed in CSF 5-HIAA and that those in the low mode attempted suicide more often than those in the high mode; furthermore, the suicide attempts were of a more violent nature (hanging, shooting, gassing). 5-HIAA was thus thought to be a predictor of suicide, and of a more violent means. Goodwin et al. (1977) and van Praag (1982) also found a bimodal CSF 5-HIAA distribution using probenecid, though a larger recent study did not find a bimodal distribution (Koslow et al., 1983).

Low CSF 5-HIAA has also been correlated with aggression and impulsivity (Brown et al., 1982) as well as suicide. Subjects with low 5-HIAA had higher scores on aggression on the psychopathic deviate scale of the MMPI. Levels of aggression were associated with a history of suicidal behavior and correlated with decreased CSF 5-HIAA. In a recent, particularly thorough study, Koslow et al. (1983) reported significant sex and age differences in levels of CSF 5-HIAA, thereby possibly contributing to the bimodal distributions found earlier by Asberg et al. Koslow et al. found that depressed women had significantly higher levels of CSF 5-HIAA than did depressed males whereas this sex difference was not found with the healthy controls. Further, when the depressed group was separated into unipolar and bipolar groups, the sex effects for CSF 5-HIAA were found only with the unipolar patients (Koslow et al., 1983).

5-HIAA may be a trait factor in depressive illnesses in that several investigators (Coppen et al., 1972; van Praag, 1980; Post et al., 1980) showed no change in CSF 5-HIAA with improvement in depression. Other studies, however, have shown a decrease in 5-HIAA with antidepressant treatment. A high correlation exists between identical and fraternal twins in CSF 5-HIAA, indicating that this might be a genetically controlled factor. Thus, 5-HIAA may be partially genetically controlled and be a state- or phase-independent indication of a diathesis toward developing an affective disorder. Normals with low CSF 5-HIAA have an increased family incidence of depression (Sedvall et al., 1980).

Blood platelets take up 5-HT by a process similar to that in CNS neurons and, due to their accessibility, have been extensively studied in affective disorders. 5-HT uptake is significantly reduced (decreased V_{max} but no change in Km) among patients with affective disorder, particularly bipolar patients (Meltzer et al., 1981; Coppen et al., 1978). A significant (30-40%) decrease in ^{3}H-imipramine binding sites occurs in brains of suicide victims, and this is similar to the reduction in 5-HT reuptake in platelets (Stanley et al., 1982; Paul et al., 1981; Goodwin and Post, 1983).

In summary, postmortem studies of brains of suicide deaths as compared to controls have suggested a decrease in 5-HIAA concentrations when the hindbrain and the raphe sections are examined. A limitation exists, however, in these studies in terms of the accuracy of the retrospective diagnosis, the variations in the nutritional and medicinal treatment of and the terminal status of the patients, and the time elapsed from death to assay. The study of Beskow et al. (1976) bears this out in that, when time elapsed from death to tissue sampling is statistically controlled for, a decrease in brain 5-HIAA is no longer present in suicide brains as compared to controls.

In the studies utilizing CSF 5-HIAA, it is not clear how much of the 5-HIAA produced from different brain regions enters the CSF nor how accurately the 5-HIAA concentrations in the lumbar sac reflect brain contribution since spinal neurons also produce 5-HIAA. A concentration gradient does exist in CSF 5-HIAA, with the lowest levels occurring in the lumbar area. For these reasons CSF 5-HIAA may or may not serve as a marker of events in 5-HT brain neurons. In addition, the results of studies of CSF 5-HIAA and depression have been contradictory and the effects of a variety of confounding variables such as sex, age, and type of depression have not always been taken into account. As a result, at this juncture it is not possible to make a clear statement re CSF 5-HIAA being increased or decreased in depression.

Studies of 5-HT receptor response to effective antidepressant treatment have not consistently shown changes in the densities of 5-HT receptors (Charney et al., 1981a). By contrast, several lines of evidence indicate that antidepressant drugs which act pharmacologically on the serotonergic system do, with time, reduce the density of the β-adrenergic receptors (Barbaccia et al., 1983).

Preclinical studies have also found evidence for a facilitative effect of serotonergic neurons on sympathetic activity (McCall and Humphrey, 1982; Janowsky et al., 1972). These data have led to theoretical concepts that propose a disturbed serotonergic system in some depressed patients, but with that system acting through the noradrenergic system to produce depression (Sulser et al., 1983). Thus, 5-HT system disturbances in depression may not independently alter mood, but may do so through interaction with noradrenergic systems.

3-Methoxy-4-Hydroxyphenylglycol (MHPG)

In 1968 it was initially reported that levels of 3-methoxy-4-hydroxyphenylglycol (MHPG) were lower in depressed patients than in normal healthy subjects, whereas other NA metabolites such as normetanephrine and metanephrine did not significantly differ between these two groups (Maas et al., 1968). This finding was of particular interest because it had been demonstrated that MHPG is the principal metabolite of NA in brain and hence this finding provided some support for the earlier erected hypothesis which suggested that depressive states were characterized by a deficiency of brain NA. Since that initial report, a continuing series of investigations of MHPG has been pursued by a diverse group of investigators. In general the directions of study have been four-fold. In the first of these, investigations of the routes of metabolism of NA in brain have been intensified and particular attention has been paid to the formation of other metabolites such as vanillylmandelic acid (VMA) and 3,4-dihydroxyphenylglycol (DHPG). A second group of studies have dealt with issues having to do with the degree to which measures of MHPG in plasma or urine may reflect events in noradrenergic neurons within the central nervous system. The third area of study has concerned itself with whether or not levels of MHPG in urine or plasma differ between depressed patients and healthy subjects or between different subtypes of depressed patients. Finally, the fourth area of focus has been that of the use of MHPG as a predictor of the type of response which depressed patients will have to tricyclic antidepressant drug treatment. Each of these areas has been reviewed in the past (for example, see Maas, 1983) and a review of all of them would represent a major review paper in and of itself. For this reason, the material in this section will deal only with MHPG as a biological marker which may predict a response to treatment with the tricyclic antidepressant drugs.

Following the initial report that MHPG in urine of depressed patients was lower as compared with that of normal, healthy controls, patients who were being treated with tricyclic antidepressants were studied and it was serendipitously found that those patients who had low urinary MHPG's prior to drug treatment with imipramine or desmethylimipramine subsequently showed marked improvement, whereas those patients who had high values of this metabolite failed to respond to drug treatment (Maas, J. W., Fawcett, J., and Dekermenjian, H., presented at American Psychiatry Association Meeting, Boston, 1968). A replication study was performed by this same group of investigators and the results were combined and published in 1972 (Maas et al., 1972). Subsequent to this finding, Schildkraut (1973) reported that patients who had high values of urinary MHPG responded favorably to treatment with amitriptyline. Beckman and Goodwin (1975) next looked at a group of patients who had received amitriptyline and another group who had received imipramine in relationship to their pretreatment values of urinary MHPG and their subsequent type of therapeutic response. Their results confirmed the earlier reports of Maas et al., as well as those of Schildkraut (1973), i.e., they found that high levels of urinary MHPG were associated with a favorable response to amitriptyline whereas low levels of the same metabolite were associated with a favorable response to imipramine. These findings were felt to have potentially practical utility in developing a more rational treatment of depressed patients as well as in assisting in the further refinement of amine-aiming theories of depression. For example, given these findings as well as some of the known modes of action of amitriptyline and imipramine or NA, it was hypothesized that there may be both noradrenergic and serotonergic type depressions.

Subsequent work in this area has supported the original findings of a relationship between low pretreatment urinary MHPG and response to imipramine, but the findings regarding amitriptyline and treatment response remain controversial. This area is briefly reviewed next. Cobbin et al. (1979) noted the findings by Maas et al. (1972), Schildkraut (1973), and Beckman and Goodman (1975) and examined the utility of using MHPG in a regular clinical setting. This study was of importance because the earlier studies had been done on research units and had paid particular attention to problems of collecting complete 24-hour urine specimens, etc. In contrast the Cobbin et al. (1979) study posed the question as to whether or not, if the urinary MHPG test was applied in a more routine clinical setting, one could improve the efficacy of tricyclic antidepressant treatment. The findings with both drugs did, in fact, indicate that with the use of urinary MHPG in choosing a particular antidepressant drug treatment, efficacy was enhanced.

Rosenbaum et al. (1980) looked at MHPG as a predictor of antidepressant response to imipramine and maprotiline. They also found that lower values of urinary MHPG were predictive of a favorable response to imipramine. The results with maprotiline were similar, i.e. low values of MHPG were associated with a favorable response, and this is of particular interest because maprotiline is a relatively potent drug in blocking the reuptake of NA into noradrenergic neurons. Hollister et al. (1980) also found that low pretreatment levels of urinary

MHPG were associated with an increased incidence of response of depressed patients to nortriptyline.

A recent report from the National Institute of Mental Health - Clinical Research Branch, Collaborative Program on the Psychobiology of Depression - Biological Studies has also supported the earlier findings that low urinary MHPG is associated with a subsequent favorable response to imipramine, but this study has extended the earlier findings in that other amines and neurotransmitter metabolites as well as sub-types of depressions were examined in terms of their association with the therapeutic response type (Maas et al., in press). Briefly, the findings from this study indicate that low urinary MHPG predicts a favorable response to imipramine and perhaps amitriptyline in bipolar but not unipolar depressed patients. Further, when the pretreatment values of other amines and metabolites in relationship to the subsequent categorization of patients as responders or nonresponders was examined using an analysis of covariance method, it was found that CSF MHPG, urinary NA, normetanephrine, VMA, and MHPG pretreatment values were significantly lower in the subsequently recovered than in the nonrecovered group. Again, this was found only with the bipolar group. It thus appears that in this bipolar group there is some abnormality in noradrenergic system function which is detected by the measurement of NA or its metabolites and that this abnormality is correctable by treatment with tricyclic antidepressant drugs. However, these findings were clearer for imipramine than for amitriptyline because, as was noted by chance, the number of bipolar subjects assigned to treatment with the amitriptyline group was quite small and hence did not lend itself easily to the examination of the question of relationships between bipolar depressive illness, pretreatment metabolite values, and subsequent response to amitriptyline, and this area remains one which will require further investigation.

Two other studies have been done in which relationships between pretreatment urinary MHPG and subsequent response to amitriptyline have been reported. Sacchetti et al. (1976) found no relationship between urinary MHPG and response to amitriptyline but the number of subjects examined in this study was small. In addition, Coppen et al. (1979) also reported no relationship between urinary MHPG and subsequent response to amitriptyline.

In summary, the available data suggest that low values of urinary MHPG are associated with a favorable response to imipramine. All investigations performed to date are in agreement on this point. Subsequent work has suggested, however, that this finding is chiefly associated with bipolar depression. In the case of amitriptyline the results are less clear and the relationship between urinary MHPG and the response of patients to this drug will require further examination, with particular reference to the testing of an adequate number of bipolar depressed patients. Values of urinary MHPG may also be associated with treatment response to other antidepressant drugs, *viz.* maprotiline and nortriptyline.

Platelet MAO Activity

Platelet MAO is an insoluble mitochondrial enzyme which catabolizes the biogenic amines (Kopin, 1964). Central nervous system MAO consists of the A and B forms, based on the differential inhibitory effects of clorgyline (Johnston, 1968). MAO type A is inhibited by clorgyline and oxidatively deaminates NA and 5-HT; type B is inhibited preferentially by deprenyl and catabolizes phenylethylamine (Knoll and Magyar, 1972; Yang and Neff, 1973). The human platelet is a pure source of MAO B (Donnelly and Murphy, 1977) and, being an easily accessible source of MAO, has been studied in numerous diseases ranging from alcoholism to schizophrenia to affective disorders (Sandler et al., 1981). Platelet MAO is increased in megaloblastic anemia and reduced in iron deficiency anemia. The consensus of the data indicates that platelet MAO activity is reduced in alcoholism and schizophrenia as compared to controls (Sandler et al., 1981). Tricyclic antidepressants in high doses (Edwards and Burns, 1974; Sullivan et al., 1977b) and neuroleptics (Chojnacki et al., 1981; DeLisi et al., 1981) have been reported to inhibit platelet MAO activity. Therefore, a possible neuroleptic-induced reduction in platelet MAO activity in schizophrenia in some studies needs to be considered. The significance and consistency of this finding remains to be established. Low platelet MAO activity in college student volunteers has been associated with increased vulnerability to psychiatric disorder as evidenced by an increased incidence of psychiatric counselling, criminal convictions, and an increased family incidence of suicide attempts (Buchsbaum et al., 1976). Subsequent studies found a correlation of low platelet MAO activity

...tion-seeking behavior (Donnelly et al., ...er et al., 1978).

...s of platelet MAO activity in affective disorders require a division of depressions studied into bipolar and unipolar groups. Murphy and Weiss in 1972 first reported a reduction in platelet MAO activity in bipolar depressed patients. There is variability in the literature in that Belmaker et al. (1976) reported an increase in platelet MAO activity in remitted bipolar patients with the substrates benzylamine and tryptamine, but the patients studied were all receiving lithium, which appears to increase MAO (Meltzer et al., 1982; Bockar et al., 1974). Reveley et al. (1981) also reported higher platelet MAO activity in bipolar and unipolar depressed women while on $LiCO_3$ treatment as compared to controls. Elevated platelet MAO activity has also been reported (Orsulak et al., 1978) in schizophrenia-related depressions characterized by chronic asocial behavior. Edwards et al. (1978) reported no difference with tryptamine as the substrate in platelet MAO activity between bipolar, unipolar, and control patients, but did find greater variance in the bipolar patients. Sullivan et al. (1977a) reported that lithium-refractory manic patients had lower platelet MAO activity than lithium responders. Mann (1979) reported high and low platelet MAO activity in unipolar vs bipolar depressed patients, respectively, and only with tryptamine as the substrate. The differences persisted with remission.

There appears to be more unanimity among unipolar depressed patients in that consistent elevations have been reported as compared to controls (Nies et al., 1974; Edwards et al., 1978; Landowski, 1975; Mann, 1979). White et al. (1980) reported elevated MAO activity in nonendogenous depression, whereas Gudeman et al. (1982) found platelet MAO activity to be directly correlated with the symptoms of depression and anxiety on the Hamilton rating scale. White et al. (1980) found high platelet MAO activity in nonendogenously depressed females as compared to control females. There is a consensus in the literature that females have higher MAO activity than males (Murphy et al., 1976; Robinson et al., 1971).

In summary, platelet MAO activity is decreased in schizophrenia and alcoholism. How much of this reduction in schizophrenics is due to neuroleptic treatment artifact is unknown. There is little consensus as to whether platelet MAO activity is raised or lowered in bipolar depressions; disparate findings have occurred with different substrates. The contradictory findings may be due to assay conditions, heterogeniety of patients, drug effects, or heterogeniety of platelet MAO in bipolar disorders. More consensus is available in the literature on unipolar disorders of increased platelet MAO activity. There are few studies of platelet MAO and diagnostic distinctions into primary, secondary, and reactive depressions, or the familial spectrum depressions of Winokur (1974). The finding by Gudeman et al. (1982) of high MAO activity in patients rated higher on anxiety and depression is compatible with the clinical observation that MAO inhibitors are efficacious in phobic depressions. Further studies are clearly needed in bipolar depressions, with patients rigidly classified, and with substrate and assay standardization to eliminate the disparities known to exist currently.

Erythrocyte Lithium Ratio
========================

Lithium is an effective agent in the treatment and prophylaxis of bipolar affective disorder and in the prophylaxis of recurrent unipolar depressions. Its mode of action remains unclear, since it affects several discrete neurotransmitter systems independently (Katz et al., 1968). That there may be a disorder of cell membrane function in affective disorders is less speculative as several authors have reported an abnormality in the erythrocyte (red blood cell, RBC) membrane transport of lithium (Frazer et al., 1978; Ramsey et al., 1979; White et al., 1979; Rybakowski et al., 1981; Dorus et al., 1979; Ostrow et al., 1978). The RBC lithium ratio is defined as the ratio of the concentration of lithium in the RBC to that in the plasma (Ostrow et al., 1978; Ramsey et al., 1979). The lithium ratio is relatively stable over time in a particular individual, has large individual variations, and is partly under genetic control (Dorus et al., 1975; Mendlewicz et al., 1978, Frazer et al., 1978). It is reportedly independent of plasma lithium concentration (Flemenbaum et al., 1978). However, the lithium ratio along with the lithium-sodium countertransport system has been reported to be reversibly diminished by the administration of lithium (Ostrow et al., 1978; Rybakowski et al., 1978). There are indications that the lithium ratio and the corresponding abnormalities in the lithium-sodium countertransport mechanism, which will be discussed later, may be transmitted as a Mendelian dominant trait under autosomal control (Ostrow et al., 1978). Initial studies into the lithium ratio and affective disorders have indicated that bipolar patients have significantly higher mean RBC lithium ratios in vivo than do normal individuals (Dorus et al., 1979); it was thus suggested early on that a cell membrane defect may be involved in the pathogenesis of bipolar illness (Dorus et al., 1979). The RBC lithium ratio has subsequently been linked to prognosis and to side effects and has been described as a trait factor which persists regardless of the clinical state and may indicate a diathesis towards the development of an affective disorder (Dorus et al., 1979). RBC lithium concentration more accurately reflects brain lithium levels than do plasma lithium levels (Mendels and Frazer, 1973).

The first report of the lithium ratio in 13 depressed men found good intrasubject stability in the lithium ratio over time and higher lithium ratios among responders to lithium than nonresponders (0.56 ± 0.03 vs 0.39 ± 0.02, $p < .005$) (Mendels and Frazer, 1973). Subsequent analysis, when this earlier finding could not be replicated in a later study conducted by the same investigators, indicated that the responders and those with the higher lithium ratio were mainly bipolar patients while nonresponders and those with a lower lithium ratio were mainly unipolar depressed patients (Ramsey et al., 1979; Frazer et al., 1978). They subsequently reported that bipolar patients, regardless of whether they were currently manic, hypomanic or depressed, had higher mean lithium ratios than did unipolar patients or control subjects. However, a significant overlap existed between the bipolar and unipolar patients. Therefore, the lithium ratio cannot be solely relied upon to make the diagnosis of unipolar or bipolar illness (White et al., 1979).

Some authors have reported that responders to lithium have high lithium ratios (Flemenbaum et al., 1978), but others have failed to replicate these findings (Frazer et al., 1978). Part of the difficulty in these disparate findings is due to the variability in patient sampling and to variability in the assays. Some authors have used in vitro lithium assays to determine the RBC lithium ratio on patients who were drug-free. In contrast, other authors have determined the lithium ratios on patients currently treated with lithium. Others have reached an intermediate point in which they sample the lithium ratio 10 to 12 hours after discontinuation of lithium. Other sources for these discrepant findings come from the use of direct versus the indirect determination of the lithium ratio. The direct method measures the concentration of lithium in a hemolysate of packed erythrocytes whereas the indirect method measures the difference between a whole blood lithium concentration and plasma lithium concentration (Frazer et al., 1978). The combination of these difficulties results in some discrepant findings in the literature. However, in the majority of studies bipolar patients do have elevated mean lithium ratios (Frazer et al., 1978; Ramsey et al., 1979).

Studies of the *in vitro* lithium ratio in first-degree relatives of bipolar patients have also indicated that those relatives with a history of major and minor affective disorders have significantly higher mean lithium ratios than do relatives with no history of affective disorders (Dorus et al., 1979). The differences in these studies were found not to be attributable to variations in age, sex, alcoholism, or previous psychotropic medications. When the lithium ratios in relatives of patients with affective illness were compared to those of 291 normal controls sampled, the ratios were significantly higher than those in control subjects (Dorus et al., 1979).

There is also a trend in the unipolar and bipolar patients for females to have a higher lithium ratio than males (Ramsey et al., 1979; Lyttkens et al., 1973). Higher lithium ratios have been reported in both primary and secondary affective illness. White et al. (1979) reported lithium ratios to be significantly higher in manics than in schizophrenics. They found that although there was a tendency for the lithium ratio to increase with plasma lithium, the ratio remained the highest in the manics.

Three processes govern the lithium distribution across the RBC: (1) the phloretin-sensitive sodium-lithium countertransport system governing lithium efflux against its electrochemical gradient, (2) passive diffusion down the lithium electrochemical gradient, and (3) the ouabain-sensitive sodium-potassium transport with lithium substituting at the potassium site (Ostrow et al., 1978; Greil et al., 1977). Of these three, the sodium-lithium counter-transport system is the main determinant of the lithium ratio, transporting lithium out of the RBC into plasma against its electrochemical gradient, resulting in a final ratio of between .3 and .5 in the lithium ratio intracellularly to that of plasma concentration (Greil et al., 1977; Ostrow et al., 1978).

The countertransport mechanism itself has been measured and found to be inversely proportional to the lithium ratio: the lower the activity of the countertransport system, the higher the intracellular lithium concentration and thus the higher the lithium ratio (Greil et al., 1977). The countertransport mechanism has been reported to be significantly lower in affective disorders, with low levels more frequently reported in manics (Rybakowski et al., 1981). The mean countertransport values were reported by one author to be lower in affectively disordered patients who are in remission than in controls (Rybakowski et al., 1978). The countertransport mechanism is under genetic control. The resultant hypothesis is that a subgroup of bipolar patients have a hereditary deficiency in their countertransport system, leading to high RBC lithium ratios (Dorus et al., 1979). Lithium has been reported to inhibit this countertransport system along with its reversible inhibition of the lithium ratio by 35-40% (Ostrow et al., 1978).

Rybakowski et al. (1981) reported significantly lower levels of the countertransport mechanism during an episode of affective illness, with the lowest levels reported frequently in bipolar manics. The level of the countertransport mechanism before lithium therapy is an excellent predictor of the subsequent *in vivo* lithium ratio. Countertransport was found by Ostrow et al. (1978) to be deficient in approximiately one-fourth of bipolar patients but not in controls, schizophrenic patients or unipolar depressives.

If a membrane abnormality is inherited in bipolar illness, the abnormality is likely to be in the lithium-sodium countertransport mechanism in which, in the absence of lithium, sodium is exchanged for sodium across the RBC. This might be a trait characteristic and may indicate that one of the actions of lithium is the stabilization of the RBC membrane.

There is consensus in the literature in that the lithium ratio has consistently been reported to be higher in bipolar manics. Methodological problems as described above remain in that values have been variably reported in patients with varying drug states, and varying assay procedures have been used. That lithium does repress the countertransport mechanism and thereby increases the lithium ratio needs to be considered in evaluating past studies. If the lithium ratio is indeed a marker of a membrane abnormality in bipolar illness, it is unclear why the ratio would not fluctuate according to state changes. That such state changes have not been found might be due to assay methods or drug interference.

Electroencephalographic Sleep Studies

The diagnosis of affective illness, particularly primary endogenous depression, has traditionally been based on characteristic clinical mood and neurovegetative symptoms of dysphoria, anorexia, weight loss, psychomotor retardation or agitation, loss of libido, together with loss of interest and social withdrawal. One of the cardinal symptoms of affective disorder is sleep disturbance, and the diagnosis of a major depressive disorder or bipolar disorder is rarely made without some clinical evidence of the following characteristics: reduced total sleep time, increased sleep latency (time between lying down and actual sleep onset), reduced sleep efficiency (the percent time spent asleep while in bed), increased intermittent awakenings, and early morning awakening (Spiker et al., 1978; Gillin, 1983). Of all the psychobiologic markers investigated to date, electroencephalographic sleep studies, in particular REM latency and REM density (Feinberg et al., 1981), may provide the most specific, sensitive, and reliable markers of the primary endogenous depressed state and may be reliable predictors of relapse and treatment responsiveness.

The basic aspects of sleep architecture on which current findings are based include a division into REM (rapid eye movement) periods and non-REM periods (NREM). NREM sleep consists of stages 1, 2, 3, 4 (Karacan and Bertelson, 1980). Sleep is comprised of four to six NREM-REM cycles, with REM onset occurring every 90 minutes. Fifty percent of total normal sleep time is in stage 2, 25% in REM, 20% in stages 3 and 4 (slow-wave sleep), and less than 5% in stage 1. REM sleep is associated with dreaming and autonomic arousal, along with rapid, jerking eye movements. Most psychotropic drugs suppress REM sleep, leading to a REM rebound on withdrawal consisting of decreased REM latency, shortened NREM intervals, and an increase in the number and length of REM periods (Karacan and Bertelson, 1980).

Biologic Markers in Affective Disorders

Recent research has advanced the field and has eliminated earlier conflicts in data based on differing patient selection, differing medication status, and inclusion of first night sleep data which are often in the phase of adaptation. Patients have been free of all medications for at least 2 weeks, diagnostically standardized with separation of unipolar from bipolar depression and primary from secondary depression, and the sleep parameters actually measured have been better standardized.

The following is a definition of terms from current research which will be used here. Sleep latency is the time between lying down and actual onset of sleep; REM latency is the time between sleep onset and the first REM period; slow wave sleep comprises stages 3 and 4; sleep efficiency is the ratio of total sleep time (TST) to total time in bed (TIB) x 100. REM density is the percentage of REM sleep to TST (Gillin, 1983).

Findings in depressions are of long sleep latency, intermittent awakenings, shortened REM latency, early morning awakening, decreased sleep efficiency, and decreased slow wave sleep (Gillin, 1983; Karacan and Bertelson, 1980; Kupfer et al., 1982a). Gillin et al. (1979a) successfully separated insomniac, primary depressed patients from normal controls using REM latency, REM density, and REM index. They correctly classified 100% of normals, 72% of depressed patients, and 77% of the insomniacs by using total sleep time, total recording period, sleep efficiency, sleep latency, early morning awake time, and REM %. In contrast to normal patients, depressed patients showed greater early morning awake time, shorter REM latency, less total sleep time, prolonged sleep latency, more intermittent awake time, less slow wave (delta) sleep, less sleep efficiency, and greater REM density.

The limitations to the use of short REM latency as a psychobiologic marker for the primary depressed state is that it has been reported in some schizophrenic patients, some manic patients, and some natural short sleepers (Gillin, 1983; Gillin et al., 1979a). Drug withdrawal states (heroin abstinence) may also result in REM rebound and shortened REM latency (Howe et al., 1980).

Gillin et al. (1979a) found that TST, total recording period, sleep efficiency, sleep latency, awake time, and EMA distinguished depressed from normal patients. REM time and REM %, along with total sleep time and sleep efficiency, separated insomniac and depressed patients. Despite the diagnostic association of short REM latency with primary depression, approximately one-third of depressed patients had an REM latency within one standard deviation of the normal mean (Karacan and Bertelson, 1980).

The above sleep alterations have been strongly associated with primary depressions, particularly endogenous depressions, and are proposed as psychobiologic markers (Kupfer, 1976). In the absence of psychopharmacologic interventions, the changes correlated with the depressive state are stable across time. Short REM latency and decreased delta sleep in particular persist in the absence of drug intervention or spontaneous remission (Coble et al., 1979). TST, delta sleep, sleep efficiency, and REM latency decrease as a function of age (Gillin et al., 1981). When age is covaried out, depressed patients have a shorter REM latency. Cairns et al. (1980) reported a case study in which sleep efficiency declined from 72% to 43% prior to clinical relapse. Tricyclic nonresponders demonstrate differences in the second half of the REM period as compared to partial and complete responders (Kupfer et al., 1982a).

Shortened REM latency has been linked to the muscarinic supersensitivity model in that cholinergic agents (physostigmine and arecholine) shorten the REM-to-REM interval, and patients in remission, when infused with arecholine, enter the next REM cycle more rapidly than do controls (Sitaram et al., 1977; Gillin et al., 1979b). It is thus hypothesized that depression is associated with cholinergic supersensitivity: an increased ratio of cholinergic to noradrenergic activity (Janowsky et al., 1972).

In summary, recent sleep research has utilized drug-free patients, has better standardized sleep variables, and has eliminated the first night adaptation phase. Consistent findings are of a strong association of decreased REM latency with primary endogenous depression, with high sensitivity and specificity. Discriminant analysis of sleep variables can accurately separate depressed from insomniac patients, from schizophrenic and manic patients, and primary endogenous depressions from secondary depressions. The correlation of short REM latency with depression is stable across time in the absence of pharmacologic intervention. Decreased sleep efficiency in a patient otherwise clinically euthymic may herald the onset of relapse. Whether REM latency may also be a predictor of relapse is unclear. Consistent sleep findings have not been found in schizophrenic disorders. REM latency has been associated with severity of depression in psychotic depressions. Data in schizoaffective disorders are less well elucidated, and whether REM latency remains a valid marker of depression in schizoaffective depressions needs to be established.

Dexamethasone Suppression Test

The dexamethasone suppression test (DST) is a laboratory procedure that has been used in psychiatry to investigate hypothalamic-pituitary-adrenal abnormalities in affective disorders. The DST has been used as an aid in differential diagnosis, in estimating prognosis, and investigated as to its usefulness in medication choice. The use of the DST in the clinical management of depression remains controversial. The DST involves the administration of 1 or 2 mg of synthetic dexamethasone at 11 p.m., followed by blood sampling of plasma cortisol at either 8 a.m. or 4 p.m. the next day. Nonsuppression is defined by plasma cortisol levels of 5 µg/dl or higher within a 24-hour period after dexamethasone administration (Carroll et al., 1976a). Cortisol secretion has a diurnal rhythm, with the nadir occurring between 4 p.m. and midnight and the peak in the morning hours, around 9 a.m. (Gwirtsman et al., 1982). It is thought that plasma cortisol acts as a negative feedback inhibitor of hypothalamic release of CRF, leading to a decrease in adrenal cortisol production.

Neuroendocrine research into the hypothalamic-pituitary-adrenocortical (HPA) axis has been extensive in the last 15 years, since cortisol hypersecretion in depression was first demonstrated in urine (Carpenter and Bunney, 1971; Shopsin and Gershon, 1971) and blood (Sachar, 1975; Carroll, 1976c). Conflicting results on CSF cortisol exist (Traskman et al., 1980; Carroll, 1976d; Jimerson et al., 1980). Dexamethasone nonsuppressors may be a subset of the cortisol hypersecreters (Carroll et al., 1976a,b; Sachar et al., 1980; Amsterdam et al., 1982), although not all studies agree (Stokes et al., 1984). Escape from suppression in response to the DST has been proposed as a biologic marker for depression (Carroll et al., 1976a,b). Carroll et al. (1976a,b) found that a subgroup of 'endogenomorphic' depressions or melancholics demonstrate escape from suppression in the late morning. Other groups have confirmed the phenomenon of 'escape' from suppression, and generally nonsuppression has been shown by the majority of studies to occur in about one-half or less of depressed patients. Initial studies reported nonsuppression in only 0-4% of control populations consisting of normal volunteers, schizophrenics, manics, drug abusers, and character disorders (Carroll, 1976c; Shopsin and Gershon, 1971; Carroll et al., 1976b; Stokes et al., 1975; Carroll et al., 1981a; Gold et al., 1981). Early studies indicated a 50-65% sensitivity and a 96% specificity for the DST in endogenous depression (Carroll et al., 1981a; Gold et al., 1981). These studies (Carroll, 1982) indicated a higher rate of nonsuppression in primary in contrast to secondary depression (65/146 vs 0/42) (Schlesser et al., 1980). Later studies have indicated that nonsuppression may be seen in schizoaffective schizophrenia, depressed type, and in some patients with borderline personality disorder (Carroll et al., 1981b). The results of the NIMH collaborative study also indicate that the incidence of non-suppression in normal and schizophrenic subjects is significant, i.e. approximately 15%. Also 37.5% of patients with obsessive-compulsive disorder (Insel et al., 1982) show cortisol nonsuppression. Patients with panic disorder and agoraphobia have also been found to have a 30% incidence of non-suppression (3/10 patients) even though no symptoms of depression were present. The DST non-suppression is attributable to causes other than the panic attacks (Curtis et al., 1982). Non-suppression on the DST has been reported in up to 30% of chronic schizophrenic patients (Dewan et al., 1982).

Carroll et al. (1976a,b) reported that a small number of patients had complete nonsuppression on the DST, whereas others demonstrated early escape from suppression, e.g. post-dexamethasone levels less than 5 µg/dl at 8 a.m. but greater than 5 or 6 µg/dl at the 4 p.m. blood sampling.

DST nonsuppression as indicated by Carroll and associates may be also of prognostic value (Carroll, 1982) in that reversion to normal suppression accompanies clinical improvement and appears to precede clinical symptoms of improvement. Greden and associates (1980) reported that continued nonsuppression occurred in those patients who relapsed quickly after treatment was discontinued, compared to those who remained well (Greden et al., 1980). They studied 14 depressed patients for up to 36 months: 10 initially demonstrated DST nonsuppression, which normalized with clinical improvement. Four patients had persistent abnormal DST's. Eight of the 10 who had normalized on followup remained symptom-free, while all of the patients who demonstrated DST nonsuppression relapsed within 6-8 weeks.

Amsterdam et al. (1981) partially confirmed the above findings in that 1 of 2 endogenously depressed patients who had a persistent abnormal DST rapidly relapsed on reduction of tricyclic medications, whereas the second case report revealed normalization of a previous abnormal DST test during a recurrence of depression.

Several factors may produce a false positive on the DST: drugs such as phenytoin, barbiturates, meprobamate, glutethemide, methyprylon, methaqualone, and carbamazepine which accelerate metabolism of dexamethasone, cardiac failure, renal failure, disseminated cancer, serious infections, recent major trauma or surgery, fever, nausea, dehydration, and temporal lobe disease, pregnancy, high-dose steroid therapy, Cushing's disease, and diabetes mellitus. Extreme weight loss, malnutrition, anorexia nervosa, alcohol abuse and alcohol withdrawal also produce false positives (Carroll, 1982). False negatives are produced by Addison's disease, hypopituitarism, long-term synthetic steroid therapy, indomethacin, and possibly benzodiazepine (high dose) therapy. Lithium, tricyclic antidepressants, neuroleptics, MAO inhibitors, and chloral hydrate do not interfere with the DST.

Carroll's initial results indicated that only endogenous depressions were associated with abnormal DST's, whereas nonendogenously depressed patients showed normal DST results (Carroll et al., 1981a; Carroll et al., 1980). As was noted previously, this degree of specificity has not been found by all investigators.

Controversy exists over the relationship between an abnormal DST and the selection of antidepressant drugs or treatment responsiveness to antidepressants (Greden et al., 1981). To date there is no convincing evidence that nonsuppression on the DST is an aid in the prediction of treatment response (Greden et al., 1981) in that most studies find no association between the DST and response to tricyclic antidepressants.

Coryell and Schlesser (1981) and Carroll et al. (1981b) reported that patients who committed suicide had a history of an abnormal DST, whereas there was a lower rate of an abnormal DST in matched, nonsuicidal depressed patients. The linkage between the DST and suicide risk in other diagnostic groups with a high suicide risk, such as schizophrenics and alcoholics, has not been found (Coryell and Schlesser, 1981). It was postulated by Bunney et al. (1969) that the hypothalamic-pituitary-adrenal dysfunction associated with primary affective illness is more likely to involve suicides than other types.

Targum et al. (1982b) found a strong association of DST nonsuppression when endogenously depressed patients were categorized according to the familial pure depressive disease (FPDD) vs depressive spectrum disease (DSD), with 69% of FPDD having abnormal DST's in contrast to 13% of patients with DSD. The DSD group had the lowest incidence of abnormal DST's of all other unipolar depressed groups. Schlesser et al. (1979, 1980) found nonsuppression in 76% of patients classified as FPDD in contrast to 7% of those with DSD. The DST is not helpful in distinguishing depression from dementia, in that an abnormal DST occurred in almost 50% of patients with senile dementia, Alzheimer's type (Carroll, 1982; Spar and Gerner, 1982; Raskind et al., 1982).

The DST is not useful in distinguishing unipolar from bipolar depression (Sachar et al., 1980a). Abnormal DST's have been reported in patients (series of 3) with bipolar mixed states, with reversion to normal suppression with clinical improvement (Krishnan et al., 1983).

Regulation of the HPA axis involves an interaction of catecholamines and indoleamines in the limbic-hypothalamic-adrenal system. NA is known to exert a tonic inhibition of the HPA axis, likely by inhibition of release of corticotrophic-releasing factor (CRF) (Sachar et al., 1980a,b; Schlesser et al., 1979). The hypothesis is that nonsuppression on the DST in depressed patients reflects deficiency of the NA system in the limbic-hypothalamic-adrenal system (Carroll, 1978; Sachar et al., 1980b). 5-HT activates the HPA system, and the diurnal rhythm for 5-HT and cortisol coincides (Collu, 1977). It has been postulated that the observed deficiency in brain 5-HT in depressed patients is secondary to a primary abnormality of cortisol secretion (Prange et al., 1976).

In summary, nonsuppression in the DST is not specific to endogenous depression but has been found in nonendogenous depression, panic disorders, schizoaffective disorder, organic brain syndrome, obsessive-compulsive disorder, and at a moderate rate in normals. This limits the clinical utility of the DST for the diagnosis of endogenous depression. On the other hand, the test clearly has value as a research tool in biological psychiatry.

Serum TSH Response to TRH (Protirelin Test)

Thyrotropin-releasing hormone (TRH) is a tripeptide produced by the hypothalamus and some peripheral organs (Loosen and Prange, 1982) which stimulates release of thyrotropin (TSH), prolactin, and growth hormone from the anterior pituitary (Loosen and Prange, 1982). The TSH response to TRH is one of a series of neuroendocrine tests which has been evaluated in the last 10 years to probe neurochemical abnormalities in affective disorders.

TRH is carried via the hypophyseal portal venous system to the anterior pituitary where it primarily stimulates release of thyroid-stimulating hormone (TSH), which then stimulates secretion of thyroxine (T_4) and triiodothyronine (T_3) by the thyroid gland (Sternbach et al., 1982). Peripheral levels of T_3 and T_4 are regulated by feedback inhibition of TSH at the anterior pituitary (Sternbach et al., 1982).

Intravenous administration of TRH produces a rise in TSH which peaks at 15-45 minutes and returns to baseline in 2-4 hours (Hershman, 1980). The TRH stimulation test consists of giving an IV bolus of 500 µg of TRH over 30 seconds following an overnight fast, with blood sampling for the TSH rise being performed at 15-minute intervals for up to 60 minutes. The rise of TSH in normal controls averages 15 µU/ml (Hershman, 1980). A blunted TSH response to TRH has been defined as having values of less than 5 µU/ml by most sources (Hershman, 1980). Side effects of TRH administration include a metallic taste, nausea, warmth, headache, chest tightness, dry mouth, desire to urinate, or an unpleasant genital sensation (Sternbach et al., 1982). In man, TRH administration produces relaxation and mood elevation in and of itself (Loosen and Prange, 1982) and has been used as attempted treatment of depression and mania.

In 1972 Prange first reported a blunted TSH response to TRH infusion in some unipolar depressed patients (Prange et al., 1972). This has been corroborated by several laboratories, and, in general, 25-35% of endogenously depressed patients display a blunted TSH response, in contrast to a significantly lower incidence in nondepressed patients, schizophrenics, and normal controls (Loosen and Prange,

1982; Sternbach et al., 1982; Kirstein, 1982; Gold et al., 1980). The criteria for an abnormal TSH response differs between centers. Some use a threshold criterion of change in TSH of less than 7 µU/ml in differentiating endogenously depressed patients from other psychiatric groups (Extein et al., 1981; Gold et al., 1980).

Several factors may blunt TSH response to TRH: hypercortisolemia (Otsuki et al., 1973), increasing age (Extein et al., 1981), and sex (men have less change in TSH). Lithium, secondary to drug-induced hypothyroidism, augments the TSH response to TRH (Lauridsen et al., 1974). Others have noted, however, that plasma cortisol levels are not correlated with a blunted TSH response (Gold et al., 1980; Kirkegaard and Carroll, 1980). Dopamine and L-Dopa lower serum TSH and blunt the TSH response to TRH (Besses et al., 1975). Aspirin, barbiturates and opiates also blunt the TSH response (Kirkegaard et al., 1977).

The TSH response to TRH has been found to be abnormal in unipolar and bipolar depression, as well as in mania (Sternbach et al., 1982). Normal TSH responses are seen in schizophrenics and personality disorders (Sternbach et al., 1982). Blunted TSH responses are also seen in 25% of abstinent and withdrawing alcoholics (Prange and Loosen, 1980). Blunted TSH responses in depression are not related to severity of disease and are not due to hypothyroidism (Sternbach et al., 1982). TSH response to TRH has been found to be reduced in manic patients (Takahashi et al., 1974). McLarty found exaggerated TSH responses in 21 manic patients taking lithium, but this was probably due to lithium-induced hypothyroidism (McLarty et al., 1975). Tanimoto found that lithium treatment augmented previously normal TSH responses to TRH in manics when the patients were placed on lithium (Tanimoto et al., 1981). TSH response to TRH has been found to be somewhat diminished in manic patients (Kirkegaard et al., 1978). Others found a significant difference in that most unipolar (77%) but few bipolar depressed patients (17%) demonstrated a blunted TSH response (Kirstein et al., 1982). Kirstein also found that a switch in bipolar depressives was preceded by a change in the TSH response from a normal to a blunted one.

The protirelin test may be useful in distinguishing mania from schizophrenia, with the maximal TSH response lower in manic than in schizophrenic patients or controls (Extein et al., 1982a). A considerable overlap has been noted, however, between the manic and schizophrenic groups. The stated sensitivity of the protirelin test is 60%, with a specificity of 85%.

The TSH response to TRH is blunted in unipolar and bipolar depressed patients as compared to normal controls (Linkowski et al., 1981). There is no difference between the maximum change in TSH between the unipolar and bipolar patients. The protirelin test does not distinguish between subtypes of unipolar depressions using the criteria of Winokur (Targum et al., 1982a). Extein found no relationship between tricyclic response and either the DST or the protirelin response (Extein et al., 1982b).

The TSH blunting to TRH and nonsuppression on the DST test may be independent phenomena. Simultaneous diminished TSH response and DST nonsuppression in a series of 54 patients with major depressive disorder occurred in only 11% of patients (Targum et al., 1982b). Fewer than half of blunted TSH responses normalize when patients are in remission (Targum, 1983). The protirelin test may be useful in predicting clinical course in that those patients whose blunting normalized sustained their clinical remission at 6 month followup whereas 65% of those who displayed persistent blunted response relapsed within 6 months (Targum, 1983).

NA and DA stimulate, and 5-HT inhibits, TRH release (Ettigi and Brown, 1977). The above findings are partially consistent with the catecholaminergic hypothesis of mania in that in mania catecholaminergic excess may lead to increased TRH release and subsequent 'desensitization' of pituitary-thyroid axis. Why blunted TSH response occurs in depression is still unclear.

That a blunted TSH response occurs in 25-35% of endogenously depressed patients has been corroborated by several laboratories. Whether this blunted TSH response has diagnostic specificity for primary endogenous depression is less clear, as protirelin challenge blunting is seen in schizophrenics, bipolar and unipolar depressives, manics, and also approximately 25% of withdrawing alcoholics. As such, the protirelin test currently cannot distinguish bipolar depression from unipolar depressions or separate bipolar depression from mania or mixed states. The TSH response is slightly lower in manics than in schizophrenics and might be of diagnostic aid in complicated presentations. The diagnostic specificity here, however, is still limited due to the existent large overlap between the two groups.

The protirelin challenge test has not been used in discriminating primary from secondary depressions. The TSH response is not useful in predicting drug treatment outcome, and is only slightly better in predicting relapse in that the majority of patients will have a normal TSH response. Only the minority of patients who have a blunted TSH response which normalizes might be reliably predicted to be less prone for relapse. The DST and TSH tests are simultaneously abnormal in only a small minority of patients and do not covary. As such, abnormalities in the TSH and HPA axes appear to be independent.

References

Amsterdam, J. D., Winokur, A., and Caroff, S. (1981) Dexamethasone suppression test as a prognostic tool: two case reports. Am. J. Psychiatry 138, 979-980.

Amsterdam, J. D., Winokur, A., Caroff, S. N., and Conn, J. (1982) The dexamethasone suppression test in outpatients with primary affective disorder and healthy control subjects. Am. J. Psychiatry 139, 287-291.

Arbilla, S., Briley, M., Cathala, F., Langer, S. Z., Pornin, C., and Raisman, R. (1981) Parallel changes in [^{3}H]-imipramine binding sites in cat brain and platelets following chronic treatment with imipramine. Brit. J. Pharmacol. 72, 154-155.

Asarch, K. B., Shih, J. C., and Kulscar, A. (1980) Decreased ^{3}H-imipramine binding in depressed males and females. Commun. Psychopharmacol. 4, 425-432.

Asberg, M., Traskman, L., and Thoren, P. (1976) 5-HIAA in the cerebrospinal fluid. A biochemical suicide predictor? Arch. Gen. Psychiatry 33, 1193-1197.

Ashcroft, G. W., Blackburn, I. M., and Eccleston, D. (1973) Changes on recovery in the concentration of tryptophan and the biogenic amine metabolites in the cerebrospinal fluid of patients with affective disorders. Psychol. Med. 3, 319-325.

Ashcroft, G. W., Crawford, T. B., Eccleston, D., Sharman, D. F., Macdougall, E. J., Stanton, J. B., and Binns, J. K. (1966) 5-Hydroxyindole compounds in the cerebrospinal fluid of patients with psychiatric or neurological diseases. Lancet ii, 1049-1052.

Barbaccia, M. L., Brunello, N., Chuang, D. M., and Costa, E. (1983) On the mode of action of imipramine: relationships between serotonergic axon terminal function and down regulation of β-adrenergic receptors. Neuropharmacology 22, 373-383.

Barchas, J. D., Berger, P., Ciaranello, R., and Elliot, G. (1977) Psychopharmacology - From Theory to Practice, Oxford University Press, New York.

Baumann, P. A. and Maitre, L. (1977) Blockade of presynaptic receptors and of amine uptake in the rat brain by the antidepressant mianserin. Naunyn-Schmiedeberg's Arch. Pharmacol. 300, 31-37.

Beckman, H. and Goodwin, F. (1975) Antidepressant response to tricyclics and urinary MHPG in unipolar patients: clinical response to imipramine or amitriptyline. Arch. Gen. Psychiatry 32, 17-21.
Belmaker, R. H., Ebbesen, K., Ebstein, R., and Rimon, R. (1976) Platelet monoamine oxidase in schizophrenia and manic-depressive illness. Brit. J. Psychiatry 129, 227-232.
Berger, P. A., Faull, K. F., Kilkowski, J., Anderson, P. J., Kraemer, H., Davis, K. L., and Barchas, J. D. (1980) CSF monoamine metabolites in depression and schizophrenia. Am. J. Psychiatry 137, 174-180.
Beskow, J., Gottfries, C. G., Roos, B. E., and Winblad, B. (1976) Determination of monoamines and monoamine metabolites in the human brain: post mortem studies in a group of suicides and in a control group. Acta psychiatr. scand. 53, 7-20.
Besses, G. S., Burrow, G. N., Spaulding, S. W., and Donabedian, R. K. (1975) Dopamine infusion acutely inhibits the TSH and prolactin response to TRH. J. Clin. Endocrinol. Metab. 41, 985-988.
Bevan, P., Bradshaw, C. M., and Szabadi, E. (1975) Effects of iprindole on responses of single corticol and caudate neurones to monoamines and acetylcholine. Brit. J. Pharmacol. 55, 17-25.
Bockar, J., Rath, R., and Heninger, G. (1974) Increased human platelet monoamine oxidase activity during lithium carbonate therapy. Life Sci. 15, 2109-2118.
Bourne, H. R., Bunney, W. E. Jr., Colburn, R. W., Davis, J. M., Davis, J. N., Shaw, D. M., and Coppen, A. J. (1968) Noradrenaline, 5-hydroxytryptamine and 5-hydroxyindoleacetic acid in hindbrains of suicidal patients. Lancet ii, 805-808.
Briley, M. S., Raisman, R., and Langer, S. Z. (1979) Human platelets possess high-affinity binding sites for ^{3}H-imipramine. Eur. J. Pharmacol. 58, 347-348.
Briley, M. S., Langer, S. Z., Raisman, R., Sechter, D., and Zarifian, E. (1980a) Tritiated imipramine binding sites are decreased in platelets of untreated depressed patients. Science 209, 303-305.
Briley, M. S., Raisman, R., Sechter, D., Zarifian, E., and Langer, S. Z. (1980b) ^{3}H-Imipramine binding in human platelets: a new biochemical parameter in depression. Neuropharmacology 19, 1209-1210.

Brodie, H. K. H., Sack, R., and Siever, L. (1973) Clinical studies of L-5-hydroxytryptophan in depression. In: *Serotonin and Behavior* (Barchas, J. and Usdin, E., eds), Academic Press, New York, pp. 549-627.

Brown, G., Ebert, M., Goyer, P., Jimerson, D., Klein, W., Bunney, W., and Goodwin, F. (1982) Aggression, suicide, and serotonin: relationships to CSF amine metabolites. *Am. J. Psychiatry* **139**, 741-746.

Buchsbaum, M. S., Coursey, R. D., and Murphy, D. L. (1976) The biochemical high risk paradigm: behavioral and familial correlates of low platelet monoamine oxidase activity. *Science* **194**, 339-341.

Bunney, W. E., Fawcett, J. A., Davis, J., and Gifford, S. (1969) Further evaluation of urinary 17-hydroxycorticosteroids in suicidal patients. *Arch. Gen. Psychiatry* **21**, 138-150.

Cairns, J., Waldron, J., Maclean, A. W., and Knowles, J. B. (1980) Sleep and depression, a case study of EEG sleep prior to relapse. *Can. J. Psychiatry* **25**, 259-263.

Carlsson, A., Rosengren, E., Bertler, D., and Nissen, J. (1957) Effect of reserpine on the metabolism of catecholamines. In: *Psychotropic Drugs* (Garattini, S. and Getti, V., eds), Elsevier, Amsterdam, p. 125.

Carpenter, W. T. Jr. and Bunney, W. E. Jr. (1971) Adrenal corticol activity in depressive illness. *Am. J. Psychiatry* **128**, 31-40.

Carroll, B. J. (1978) Neuroendocrine function in psychiatric disorders. In: *Psychopharmacology: A Generation of Progress* (Lipton, M. A., DiMascio, A., and Killam, K. F., eds), Raven Press, New York, pp. 489-491.

Carroll, B. J. (1982) Use of the dexamethasone suppression test in depression. *J. Clin. Psychiatry* **43**, 44-50.

Carroll, B. J., Curtis, G. C., and Mendels, J. (1976a) Neuroendocrine regulation in depression. II. Discrimination of depressed from nondepressed patients. *Arch. Gen. Psychiatry* **33**, 1051-1058.

Carroll, B. J., Curtis, G. C., and Mendels, J. (1976b) Neuroendocrine regulation in depression limbic system-adrenocortical dysfunction. *Arch. Gen. Psychiatry* **33**, 1039-1044.

Carroll, B. J. (1976c) Limbic system-adrenal cortex regulation in depression and schizophrenia. *Psychosom. Med.* **38**, 106-121.

Carroll, B. J., Curtis, G. C., and Mendels, J. (1976d) Cerebrospinal fluid and plasma free cortisol concentrations in depression. Psychol. Med. 76, 235-244.

Carroll, B. J., Feinberg, M., Greden, J. F., Tarika, J., Albala, A. A., Haskett, R. F., James, N. M., Kronfol, Z., Lohr, N., Skiner, M., deVigne, J. P., and Young, E. (1981a) A specific laboratory test for the diagnosis of melancholia; standardization, validation, and clinical utility. Arch. Gen. Psychiatry 38, 15-22.

Carroll, B. J., Feinberg, M., Greden, J. F., Haskett, R. F., James, N. M., Steiner, M., and Tarika, J. (1980) Diagnosis of endogenous depression: comparison of clinical research and neuroendocrine criteria. J. Affec. Disorders 2, 177-194.

Carroll, B. J., Greden, J. F., and Feinberg, M. (1981b) Suicide, neuroendocrine dysfunction, and CSF 5-HIAA concentrations in depression. In: Recent Advances in Neuropsychopharmacology: Proc. 12th Congress of the Collegium Internationale Neuropsychopharmacologicum (Anguist, B., ed.), Permagon Press, Oxford, pp. 302-315.

Charney, D. S., Menkes, D. B., and Heninger, G. R. (1981a) Receptor sensitivity and the mechanism of actions of antidepressant treatment, implications for the etiology and therapy of depression. Arch. Gen. Psychiatry 38, 1160-1180.

Charney, D. S., Heninger, G. R., Sternberg, D. E., Redmond, D. E., Leckman, J. F., Maas, J. W., and Roth, R. H. (1981b) Presynaptic adrenergic receptor sensitivity in depression: the effect of long-term desipramine treatment. Arch. Gen. Psychiatry 38, 1334-1340.

Chojnacki, M., Kralik, P., Allen, R. H., Ho, B. T., Schoolar, J. C., and Smith, R. C. (1981) Neuroleptic-induced decrease in platelet MAO activity of schizophrenic patients. Am. J. Psychiatry 138, 838-840.

Cobbin, D. M., Requin-Blow, B., and Williams, L. R. (1979) Urinary MHPG levels and tricyclic antidepressant drug selection. Arch. Gen. Psychiatry 36, 1111-1118.

Coble, P. A., Kupfer, D. J., Spiker, D. G., Neil, J. F., and McPartland, R. J. (1979) EEG sleep in primary depression, a longitudinal placebo study. J. Affec. Disorders 1, 131-138.

Collu, R. (1977) Role of central cholinergic and aminergic neurotransmitters in the control of anterior pituitary hormone secretion. In: Clinical Neuroendocrinology (Martini, L. and Besser, G. M., eds), Academic Press, New York, pp. 55-56.

Coppen, A. (1967) The biochemistry of affective disorder. Brit. J. Psychiatry 113, 1237-1264.

Coppen, A., Prange, A. J. Jr., Whybrow, P. C., and Noguera, R. (1972) Abnormalities of indoleamines in affective disorders. Arch. Gen. Psychiatry 26, 474-478.

Coppen, A., Rama Rao, V. A., Ruthven, C. R. J., Goodwin, B. L., and Sandler, M. (1979) Urinary 4-hydroxy-3-methoxyphenylglycol is not a predictor for clinical response to amitriptyline in depressive illness. Psychopharmacology 64, 95-97.

Coppen, A., Swade, C., and Wood, K. (1978) Platelet 5-hydroxytryptamine accumulation in depressive illness. Clin. Chim. Acta 87, 165-168.

Coryell, W. and Schlesser, M. A. (1981) Suicide and dexamethasone suppression test in unipolar depression. Am. J. Psychiatry 138, 1120-1121.

Curtis, G. C., Cameron, O. G., and Nesse, R. M. (1982) The dexamethasone suppression test in panic disorder and agoraphobia. Am. J. Psychiatry 139, 1043-1046.

DeLisi, L. E., Wise, C. D., Bridge, T. P., Rosenblatt, J. E., Wagner, R. L., Morihisa, J., Karson, C., Potkin, S. G., and Wyatt, R. J. (1981) A probable neuroleptic effect on platelet monoamine oxidase in chronic schizophrenic patients. Psychiatry Res. 4, 95-107.

Deneker, S. J., Malm, U., Roos, B. E., and Werdinius, B. (1966) Acid monoamine metabolites of cerebrospinal fluid in mental depression and mania. J. Neurochem. 13, 1545-1548.

Dewan, M. J., Pandurangi, A. K., Boucher, M. L., Levy, B. F., and Major, L. F. (1982) Abnormal dexamethasone suppression test results in chronic schizophrenic patients. Am. J. Psychiatry 139, 1501-1503.

Donnelly, C. H. and Murphy, D. L. (1977) Substrate and inhibitor-related characteristics of human platelet monoamine oxidase. Biochem. Pharmacol. 26, 853-858.

Donnelly, E. F., Murphy, D. L., Waldman, I. N., Buchsbaum, M. S., and Coursey, R. D. (1979) Psychological characteristics corresponding to low versus high platelet monoamine oxidase activity. Biol. Psychiatry 14, 375-383.

Dorus, E., Pandey, G. N., and Davis, J. M. (1975) Genetic determinant of lithium ion distribution. An in vitro and in vivo monozygotic-dizygotic twin study. Arch. Gen. Psychiatry 32, 1097-1102.

Dorus, E., Pandey, G. N., Shaughnessy, R., Gaviria, M., Val, E., Ericksen, S., and Davis, J. M. (1979) Lithium transport across red cell membrane: a cell membrane abnormality in manic-depressive illness. Science 205, 932-934.

Edwards, D. J. and Burns, M. O. (1974) Effects of tricyclic antidepressants upon human platelet monoamine oxidase. Life Sci. 15, 2045-2058.

Edwards, D. J., Spiker, D. G., Kupfer, D. J., Foster, G., Neil, J. F., and Abrams, L. (1978) Platelet monoamine oxidase in affective disorders. Arch. Gen. Psychiatry 35, 1433-1446.

Ettigi, P. G. and Brown, G. M. (1977) Psychoneuroendocrinology of affective disorder: an overview. Am. J. Psychiatry 134, 493-501.

Extein, I., Pottash, A. L., Gold, M. S., and Cowdry, R. W. (1982a) Using the protirelin test to distinguish mania from schizophrenia. Arch. Gen. Psychiatry 39, 77-81.

Extein, I., Kirstein, L. S., Pottash, A. L., and Gold, M. S. (1982b) The dexamethasone suppression and thyrotropin-releasing hormone tests and response to treatment in unipolar depression. Int. J. Psychiatry in Medicine 12, 267-274.

Extein, I., Pottash, A. L., Gold, M. S., and Martin, D. M. (1980) Differentiating mania from schizophrenia by the TRH test. Am. J. Psychiatry 137, 981-982.

Extein, I., Pottash, A. L., and Gold, M. S. (1981) Neuroendocrine diagnostic test in psychiatry. J. Med. Serv., N.J. 78, 731-734.

Feinberg, M., Gillin, J. C., Carroll, B. J., Greden, J. F., and Zis, A. P. (1981) EEG studies of sleep in the diagnosis of depression. Biol. Psychiatry 17, 305-316.

Flemenbaum, A., Weddige, R., and Miller, J. Jr. (1978) Lithium erythrocyte/plasma ratio as a predictor of response. Am. J. Psychiatry 135, 336-338.

Frazer, A., Mendels, J., Brunswick, D., London, J., Pring, M., Ramsey, T. A., and Rybakowski, J. (1978) Erythrocyte concentrations of the lithium ion: clinical correlates and mechanisms of action. Am. J. Psychiatry 135, 1065-1069.

Gillin, J. C. (1983) Sleep studies in affective illness: diagnostic, therapeutic and pathophysiological implications. Psychiatric Annals 13, 367-

382.
Gillin, J. C., Duncan, W. C., Murphy, D. L., Post, R. M., Wehr, T. A., Goodwin, F. K., Wyatt, R. J., and Bunney, W. E. Jr. (1981) Age-related changes in sleep in depressed and normal subjects. Psychiatry Res. 4, 73-78.
Gillin, J. C., Duncan, W., Pettigrew, K. D., Frankel, B. L., and Snyder, F. (1979a) Successful separation of depressed, normal, and insomniac subjects by EEG sleep data. Arch. Gen. Psychiatry 36, 85-90.
Gillin, J. C., Sitarim, N., and Duncan, W. (1979b) Muscarinic supersensitivity: a possible model for the sleep disturbance of primary depression? Psychiatry Res. 1, 17-22.
Glowinski, J. and Axelrod, J. (1964) Inhibition of uptake of tritiated noradrenaline in the intact rat brain by imipramine and structurally related compounds. Nature (Lond.) 204, 1318-1319.
Gold, M. S., Pottash, A. L., Extein, I., and Sweeney, D. R. (1981) Diagnosis of depression in the 1980's. J. Am. Med. Assoc. 245, 1562-1564.
Gold, M. S., Pottash, A. L., Ryan, N., Sweeney, D. R., Davies, R. K., and Martin, D. M. (1980) TRH induced TSH response in unipolar, bipolar, and secondary depressions: possible utility in clinical assessment and differential diagnosis. Psychoneuroendocrinology 5, 147-155.
Goodwin, F. K. and Post, R. M. (1983) 5-Hydroxytryptamine and depression: a model for the interaction of normal variance with pathology. Brit. J. Clin. Pharmacol. 15, 393S-405S.
Goodwin, F. K., Post, R. M., Dunner, D. L., and Gordon, E. K. (1973) Cerebrospinal fluid amine metabolites in affective illness: the probenecid technique. Am. J. Psychiatry 130, 73-79.
Goodwin, F. K., Rubovets, R., Jimerson, D. C., and Post, R. M. (1977) Serotonin and norepinephrine 'subgroups' in depression: metabolite findings and clinical pharmacological correlations. Sci. Proc. Am. Psychiat. Ass. 130, 108.
Greil, W., Eisenried, F., Becker, B. F., and Duhm, J. (1977) Interindividual differences in the Na^+ dependent Li^+-countertransport system and in the Li^+-distribution ratio across the red cell membrane among Li^+-treated patients. Psychopharmacology 53, 19-26.
Greden, J. F., Albala, A. A., Haskett, R. F., James, N. M., Goodman, L., Steiner, M., and Carroll, B. J. (1980) Normalization of dexamethasone suppression test: a laboratory index of recovery from

endogenous depression. Biol. Psychiatry 15, 449-458.
Greden, J. F., Kronfol, Z., Gardner, R., Feinberg, M., Mukhopadhyay, S., Albala, A. A., and Carroll, B. J. (1981) Dexamethasone suppression test and selection of antidepressant medications. J. Affec. Disorders 3, 389-396.
Grob, H., Gothert, M., Ender, H. P., Schumann, H. J. (1981) ^{3}H-Imipramine binding sites in the rat brain: selective localization on serotonergic neurones. Naunyn Schmiedeberg's Arch. Pharmacol. 317, 310-314.
Gudeman, J. E., Schatzberg, A. F., Samson, J. A., Orsulak, P. J., Cole, J. O., and Schildkraut, J. J. (1982) Toward a biochemical classification of depressive disorders, VI: Platelet MAO activity and clinical symptoms in depressed patients. Am. J. Psychiatry 139, 630-633.
Gwirtsman, H., Gerner, R. H., and Sternbach, H. (1982) The overnight dexamethasone suppression test: clinical and theoretical review. J. Clin. Psychiatry 43, 321-327.
Hershman, J. M. (1980) Control of thyrotropin secretion. In: Radio-Immunoassay of Hormones, Proteins, and Enzymes: Proceedings of the International Symposium (Albertini, A., ed.), Gardone Riviera, May 8-10, 1980, Excerpta Medica, Amsterdam, pp. 13-22.
Hollister, L. E., Davis, K. L., and Berger, P. A. (1980) Subtypes of depression based on excretion of MHPG and response to nortriptyline. Arch. Gen. Psychiatry 37, 1107-1110.
Howe, R. C., Hegge, F. W., and Phillips, J. L. (1980) Acute heroin abstinence in man: II. Alterations in rapid eye movement (REM) sleep. Drug and Alcohol Dependence 6, 149-161.
Hrdina, P. D., Elson-Hartman, K., Roberts, D. C. S., and Pappas, B. A. (1981) High affinity [^{3}H]-desipramine binding in rat cerebral cortex decreases after selective lesions of noradrenaline neurons with 6-hydroxydopamine. Eur. J. Pharmacol. 73, 373-376.
Insel, T. R., Kalin, N. H., Guttmacher, L. B., Cohen, R. M., and Murphy, D. L. (1982) The dexamethasone suppression test in patients with primary obsessive-compulsive disorder. Psychiatry Res. 6, 153-160.
Janowsky, D. S., el-Yousef, M. K., Davis, J. M., and Sekerke, H. J. (1972) A cholinergic-adrenergic hypothesis of mania and depression. Lancet ii, 632-635.

Jimerson, D. C., Post, R. M., Van Kammen, D. P., Skyler, J. S., Brown, G. L., and Bunney, W. E. Jr. (1980) Cerebrospinal fluid cortisol levels in depression and schizophrenia. Am. J. Psychiatry 137, 979-980.

Johnston, J. P. (1968) Some observations upon a new inhibitor of monoamine oxidase in brain tissue. Biochem. Pharmacol. 17, 1285-1297.

Karacan, I. and Bertelson, A. D. (1980) Sleep EEG in depression. J. Clin. Psychiatry 41, 40-44.

Katz, R. I., Chase, T. N., and Kopin, I. J. (1968) Evoked release of norepinephrine and serotonin from brain slices: inhibition by lithium. Science 162, 466-467.

Kirkegaard, C., Bjorum, N., Cohn, D., Faber, J., Lauridsen, U. B., and Nerup, J. (1977) Studies of the influence of biogenic amines and psychoactive drugs on the prognostic value of the TRH stimulation test in endogenous depression. Psychoendocrinology 2, 131-136.

Kirkegaard, C., Bjorum, N., Cohn, D., and Lauridsen, U. B. (1978) TRH stimulation test in manic depressive illness. Arch. Gen. Psychiatry 35, 1017-1021.

Kirkegaard, C. and Carroll, B. J. (1980) Dissociation of TSH and adrenocortical disturbances in endogenous depression. Psychiatry Res. 3, 253-264.

Kirstein, L., Gold, M. S., Extein, I., Martin, D., and Pottash, A. L. (1982) Clinical correlates of the TRH infusion test in primary depression. J. Clin. Psychiatry 43, 191-194.

Knoll, J. and Magyar, K. (1972) Some puzzling pharmacological effects of monoamine oxidase inhibitors. In: Monoamine Oxidase - New Vistas (Costa, E. and Sandler, M., eds), Raven Press, New York, pp. 393-408.

Kopin, I. J. (1964) Storage and metabolism of catecholamines: the role of monoamine oxidase. Pharmacol. Rev. 16, 179-191.

Korf, J., van den Burg, W., and van den Hoofdakker, R. H. (1983) Acid metabolites and precursor amino acids of 5-hydroxytryptamine and dopamine in affective and other psychiatric disorders. Psychiatria Clinica 16, 1-16.

Koslow, S., Maas, J. W., Bowden, C., Davis, J., Hanin, I., and Javaid, J. (1983) CSF and urinary biogenic amines and metabolites in depression and mania: a controlled univariate analysis. Arch. Gen. Psychiatry 40, 999-1010.

Krishnan, R. R., Maltbie, A. A., and Davidson, J. R. (1983) Abnormal cortisol suppression in bipolar patients with simultaneous manic and depressive symptoms. Am. J. Psychiatry 140, 203-205.

Kupfer, D. J. (1976) REM latency: a psychobiologic marker for primary depressive disease. Biol. Psychiatry 11, 159-174.

Kupfer, D. (1982) Interaction of EEG sleep, antidepressants, and affective disease. J. Clin. Psychiatry 43, 30-35.

Kupfer, D. J., Shaw, D. H., Ulrich, R., Coble, P. A., and Spiker, D. G. (1982) Application of automated REM analysis in depression. Arch. Gen. Psychiatry 39, 569-573.

Landowski, J., Lysiak, W., and Angielski, S. (1975) Monoamine oxidase activity in blood platelets from patients with cyclophrenic depressive syndromes. Biochem. Med. 14, 347-354.

Langer, S. Z., Briley, M. S., Raisman, R., Henry, J. F., and Morselli, P. L. (1980a) Specific ^{3}H-imipramine binding in human platelets: influence of age and sex. Naunyn Schmiedeberg's Arch. Pharmacol. 313, 189-194.

Langer, S. Z., Moret, C., Raisman, R., Dubocovich, M. L., and Briley, M. (1980b) High affinity [^{3}H]-imipramine binding in rat hypothalamus: association with uptake of serotonin but not norepinephrine. Science 210, 1133-1135.

Langer, S. Z. and Briley, M. (1981) High affinity ^{3}H-imipramine binding: a new biological tool for studies in depression. Trends Neurosci. 4, 28-31.

Langer, S. Z. and Raisman, R. (1983) Binding of [^{3}H]-imipramine and [^{3}H]-desipramine as biochemical tools for studies in depression. Neuropharmacology 22, 407-413.

Langer, S. Z., Sette, M., and Raisman, R. Association of ^{2}H-imipramine binding with serotonin uptake and of ^{2}H-desipramine binding with noradrenaline uptake: potential research tools in depression. Proceedings of the 3rd International Meeting on Clinical Pharmacology in Psychiatry (in press).

Langer, S. Z., Zarifian, E., Raisman, M., and Sechter, D. (1981) High affinity binding of ^{3}H-imipramine in brain and platelets and its relevance to the biochemistry of affective disorders. Life Sci. 29, 211-220.

Lauridsen, U. B., Kirkegaard, C., and Nerup, J. (1974) Lithium and the pituitary-thyroid axis in normal subjects. J. Clin. Endocrinol. Metab. 39, 383-385.

Linkowski, P., Brauman, H., and Mendlewicz, J. (1981) Thyrotropin response to thyrotropin-releasing hormone in unipolar and bipolar affective illness. J. Affec. Disorders **3**, 9-16.

Lippmann, W. and Pugsley, T. A. (1976) Effects of viloxazine, an antidepressant agent, on biogenic amine uptake mechanisms and related activities. Can. J. Physiol. Pharmacol. **54**, 494-509.

Lloyd, K. G., Farley, I. J., Deck, J. H., and Hornykiewicz, O. (1974) Serotonin and 5-hydroxyindoleacetic acid in discrete areas of the brainstem of suicide victims and control patients. Adv. Biochem. Psychopharmacol. **11**, 387-397.

Loosen, P. T. and Prange, A. J. Jr. (1982) Serum thyrotropin response to thyrotropin-releasing hormone in psychiatric patients: a review. Am. J. Psychiatry **139**, 405-416.

Lyttkens, L., Soderberg, U., and Wetterberg, L. (1973) Increased lithium erythrocyte/plasma ratio in manic-depressive psychosis. Lancet **i**, 40.

Maas, J. W., Fawcett, J. A., and Dekirmenjian, H. (1968) 3-Methoxy-4-hydroxyphenylglycol (MHPG) excretion in depressive states. Arch. Gen. Psychiatry **19**, 147-162.

Maas, J. W., Fawcett, J. A., and Dekirmenjian, H. (1972) Catecholamine metabolism, depressive illness, and drug response. Arch. Gen. Psychiatry **26**, 252-262.

Maas, J. W. (1975) Biogenic amines and depression. Arch. Gen. Psychiatry **32**, 1357-1361.

Maas, J. W. (ed.) (1983) MHPG: Basic Mechanisms and Psychopathology. Academic Press.

Maas, J. W., Koslow, S. H., Katz, M. M., Gibbons, R. L., Bowden, C. L., Robins, E., and Davis, J. Pretreatment neurotransmitter metabolites and tricyclic antidepressant drug response. Am. J. Psychiatry (in press).

Mann, J. (1979) Altered platelet monoamine oxidase activity in affective disorders. Psychol. Med. **9**, 729-736.

McCall, R. B. and Humphrey, S. J. (1982) Involvement of serotonin in the central regulation of blood pressure: evidence for a facilitative effect on sympathetic nerve action. J. Pharmacol. Exp. Therap. **222**, 94-102.

McLarty, D. G., O'Boyle, J. H., Spencer, C. A., and Radcliffe, J. G. (1975) Effects of lithium on hypothalamic-pituitary-thyroid function in patients with affective disorders. Brit. Med. J. **3**, 623-626.

Mellerup, E. T., Plenge, P., and Rosenberg, R. (1982) ^{3}H-Imipramine binding sites in platelets from psychiatric patients. Psychiatry Res. 7, 221-227.

Meltzer, H. Y., Arora, R. C., Baber, R., and Tricou, B. J. (1981) Serotonin uptake in blood platelets of psychiatric patients. Arch. Gen. Psychiatry 38, 1322-1326.

Meltzer, H. Y., Tueting, P., and Jackman, H. (1982) The effect of lithium on platelet monoamine oxidase activity in bipolar and schizoaffective disorders. Brit. J. Psychiatry 140, 192-198.

Mendels, J. and Frazer, A. (1973) Intracellular lithium concentration and clinical response: towards a membrane theory of depression. J. Psychiatric Res. 10, 9-18.

Mendlewicz, J., Verbanck, P., Linkowski, P., and Wilmotte, J. (1978) Lithium accumulation in erythrocytes of manic-depressive patients--an in vivo twin study. Brit. J. Psychiatry 133, 436-444.

Mogilnicka, E., Arbilla, S., Depoortere, H., and Langer, S. Z. (1980) Rapid-eye-movement sleep deprivation decreases the density of ^{3}H-dihydroalprenolol and ^{3}H-imipramine binding sites in the rat cerebral cortex. Eur. J. Pharmacology 65, 289-292.

Murphy, D. L. and Weiss, R. (1972) Reduced monoamine oxidase activity in blood platelets from bipolar depressed patients. Am. J. Psychiatry 128, 1351-1357.

Murphy, D. L., Wright, C., Buchsbaum, M., Nichols, A., Costa, J. L., and Wyatt, R. J. (1976) Platelet and plasma amine oxidase activity in 680 normals: sex and age differences and stability over time. Biochem. Med. 16, 254-265.

Nies, A., Robinson, D. S., Harris, L. S., and Lamborn, K. R. (1974) Comparison of monoamine oxidase substrate activities in twins, schizophrenics, depressives, controls. In: Neuropsychopharmacology of Monoamines and Their Regulatory Enzymes (Usdin, E., ed.), Raven Press, New York, pp. 59-70.

Orsulak, P. J., Schildkraut, J. J., Schatzberg, A. F., and Herzog, J. M. (1978) Differences in platelet monoamine oxidase activity in subgroups of schizophrenic and depressive disorders. Biol. Psychiatry 13, 637-647.

Ostrow, D. G., Pandey, G. M., Davis, J. M., Hurt, S. W., and Tosteson, D. C. (1978) A heritable disorder of lithium transport in erythrocytes of a subpopulation of manic-depressive patients. Am. J. Psychiatry **135**, 1070-1078.

Otsuki, M., Dakoda, M., and Baba, S. (1973) Influence of glucocorticoids on TRF-induced TSH response in man. J. Clin. Endocrinology and Metabolism **36**, 95-102.

Palkovits, M., Raisman, R., Briley, M., and Langer, S. Z. (1981) Regional distribution of ^{2}H-imipramine binding in rat brain. Brain Res. **210**, 493-498.

Paul, S. M., Rehavi, M. S., Skolnick, P., Ballenger, J. C., and Goodwin, F. K. (1981) Depressed patients have decreased binding of tritiated imipramine to platelet serotonin transporter. Arch. Gen. Psychiatry **38**, 1315-1317.

Paul, S. M., Rehavi, M. L., Nurnberger, J. I., Gershon, E., Skolnick, P., and Goodwin, F. K. Concordance of ^{3}H-imipramine binding but not of serotonin uptake in platelets from monozygotic twins. Psychiatry Res. (in press).

Paul, S. M., Rehavi, M., Skolnick, P., and Goodwin, F. K. (1980) Demonstration of specific 'high affinity' binding sites for [^{3}H]-imipramine on human platelets. Life Sci. **26**, 953-959.

Perry, E. K., Marshall, E. F., Blessed, G., Tomlinson, B. E., and Perry, R. H. (1983) Decreased imipramine binding in the brains of patients with depressive illness. Brit. J. Psychiatry **142**, 188-192.

Post, R. M., Ballenger, J. C., and Goodwin, F. K. (1980) Cerebrospinal fluid studies of neurotransmitter function in manic and depressive illness. In: The Neurobiology of Cerebrospinal Fluid, vol. 1 (Wood, J. H., ed.), Plenum Press, New York, pp. 685-717.

Prange, A. J. Jr. and Loosen, P. T. (1980) Some endocrine aspects of affective disorders. J. Clin. Psychiatry **41**, 29-34.

Prange, A. J., Wilson, I. C., Breese, G. R., et al. (1976) Hormonal alterations of imipramine response: a review. In: Hormones, Behavior and Psychopathology (Sachar, E. J., ed.), Raven Press, New York, pp. 41-67.

Prange, A. J. Jr., Wilson, I. C., Alltop, L. B., Breese, G. R., and Lara, P. P. (1972) Effects of thyrotropin-releasing hormone in depression. Lancet **ii**, 999-1002.

Raisman, R., Briley, M., and Langer, S. Z. (1979) Specific tricyclic antidepressant binding sites in rat brain. Nature (Lond.) 281, 148-150.

Raisman, R., Briley, M. S., and Langer, S. Z. (1980) Specific tricyclic antidepressant binding sites in rat brain characterized by high affinity ^{3}H-imipramine binding. Eur. J. Pharmacol. 61, 373-380.

Raisman, R., Sechter, D., Briley, M. S., Zarifian, E., and Langer, S. Z. (1981) High affinity ^{3}H-imipramine binding in platelets from untreated and treated depressed patients compared to healthy volunteers. Psychopharmacology 75, 368-371.

Raisman, R., Sette, M., Pimoule, C., Briley, M., and Langer, S. Z. (1982) High-affinity [^{3}H]-desipramine binding in the peripheral and central nervous system: a specific site associated with the neuronal uptake of noradrenaline. Eur. J. Pharmacol. 78, 345-351.

Ramsey, T. A., Frazer, A., Mendels, J., and Dyson, W. L. (1979) The erythrocyte lithium-plasma lithium ratio in patients with primary affective disorder. Arch. Gen. Psychiatry 36, 457-461.

Raskind, M., Peskind, E., Rivard, M. F., Veith, R., and Barnes, R. (1982) Dexamethasone suppression test and cortisol coriodian rhythm in primary degenerative dementia. Am. J. Psychiatry 139, 1468-1471.

Rehavi, M., Paul, S. M., Skolnick, P., and Goodwin, F. K. (1980) Demonstration of specific high affinity binding sites for [^{3}H]-imipramine in human brain. Life Sci. 26, 2273-2279.

Reveley, M. A., Glover, V., Sandler, M., and Coppen, A. (1981) Increased platelet monoamine oxidase activity in affective disorders. Psychopharmacology 73, 257-260.

Robinson, D. S., Davis, J. M., Nies, A., Ravaris, C. L., and Sylvester, D. (1971) Relations of sex and aging to monoamine oxidase activity of human brain, plasma, and platelets. Arch. Gen. Psychiatry 24, 536-539.

Rosenbaum, A. H., Schatzberg, A. F., Marota, T., et al. (1980) MHPG as a predictor of antidepressant response to imipramine and maprotiline. Am. J. Psychiatry 137, 1090-1092.

Rosloff, B. N. and Davis, J. M. (1974) Effect of iprindole on norepinephrine turnover and transport. Psychopharmacologia (Berl.) 40, 53-64.

Rybakowski, J., Frazer, A., and Mendels, J. (1978) Lithium efflux from erythrocytes incubated in vitro during lithium carbonate administration.

Commun. Psychopharmacol. **2**, 105-112.
Rybakowski, J., Potak, E., and Strzyzewski, W. (1981) The activity of the lithium-sodium countertransport system in erythrocytes in depression and mania. J. Affec. Disorders **3**, 59-64.
Sacchetti, E., Smeraldi, E., Cagnasso, M., et al. (1976) MHPG, amitriptyline and affective disorders: a longitudinal study. Int. Pharmacopsychiatry **11**, 157-162.
Sachar, E. J. (1975) Twenty-four-hour cortisol secretory patterns in depressed and manic patients. Prog. Brain Res. **42**, 81-91.
Sachar, E. J., Asnis, G., Halbreich, U., Nathan, R. S., and Halpern, F. (1980a) Recent studies in the neuroendocrinology of major depressive disorders. Psychiatric Clinics of North America **3**, 313-326.
Sachar, E. J., Asnis, G., Nathan, R. S., Halbreich, U., Tabrizi, M. A., and Halpern, F. S. (1980b) Dextroamphetamine and cortisol in depression. Morning plasma cortisol suppressed. Arch. Gen. Psychiatry **37**, 755-757.
Sandler, M., Reveley, M. A., and Glover, V. (1981) Human platelet monoamine oxidase activity in health and disease: a review. J. Clin. Pathol. **34**, 292-302.
Schildkraut, J. J. (1973) Norepinephrine metabolites as biochemical criteria for classifying depressive disorders and predicting response to treatment: preliminary findings. Am. J. Psychiatry **130**, 695-698.
Schildkraut, J. J. and Kety, S. S. (1967) Biogenic amines and emotion. Science **156**, 21-37.
Schlesser, M. A., Winokur, G., and Sherman, B. M. (1979) Genetic subtypes of unipolar primary depressive illness distinguished by hypothalamic-pituitary-adrenal axis activity. Lancet **i**, 731-741.
Schlesser, M. A., Winokur, G., and Sherman, B. M. (1980) Hypothalamic-pituitary-adrenal axis activity in depressive illness: its relationship to classification. Arch. Gen. Psychiatry **37**, 737-743.
Schoder, C., Zahn, T. P., Murphy, D. L., and Buchsbaum, M. S. (1978) Psychological correlates of monoamine oxidase activity in normals. J. Nerv. Ment. Dis. **166**, 177-186.
Sedvall, G., Fyro, G., Gullberg, B., Nyback, H., Wiesel, F. A., and Wode-Helgodt, B. (1980) Relationships in healthy volunteers between concentrations of monoamine metabolites in cerebrospin-

al fluid and family history of psychiatric morbidity. Brit. J. Psychiatry 136, 366-374.

Sette, M., Raisman, R., Briley, M., and Langer, S. Z. (1981) Localization of tricyclic antidepressant binding sites on serotonin nerve terminals. J. Neurochem. 37, 40-42.

Shaw, D. M., Camps, F. E., and Eccleston, E. G. (1967) 5-Hydroxytryptamine in the hindbrain of depressive suicides. Brit. J. Psychiatry 113, 1407-1411.

Shopsin, B. and Gershon, S. (1971) Plasma cortisol response to dexamethasone suppression in depressed and control patients. Arch. Gen. Psychiatry 24, 320-326.

Sitaram, N., Mendelson, W. B., Wyatt, R. J., and Gillin, J. C. (1977) The time-dependent induction of REM sleep and arousal by physostigmine infusion during normal human sleep. Brain Res. 122, 562-567.

Spar, J. E. and Gerner, R. (1982) Does the dexamethasone suppression test distinguish dementia from depression? Am. J. Psychiatry 139, 238-240.

Spiker, D. G., Coble, P., Cofsky, J., Foster, F. G., and Kupfer, D. J. (1978) EEG sleep and severity of depression. Biol. Psychiatry 13, 485-488.

Stanley, M., Virgilio, J., and Gershon, S. (1982) Tritiated imipramine binding sites are decreased in the frontal cortex of suicides. Science 216, 1337-1339.

Sternbach, H., Gerner, R. H., and Gwirtsman, H. E. (1982) The thyrotropin releasing hormone stimulation test: a review. J. Clin. Psychiatry 43, 4-6.

Stokes, P. E., Pick, G. R., Stoll, M. P., and Nunn, W. D. (1975) Pituitary adrenal function in depressed patients: resistance to dexamethasone suppression. J. Psychiatric Res. 12, 271-281.

Stokes, P. E., Stoll, P. M., Koslow, S. H., Maas, J. W., Davis, J. M., Swann, A. C., and Robins, E. (1984) Pretreatment hypothalamic-pituitary-adrenocortical function in depressed patients and comparison groups: a multi-center study. Arch. Gen. Psychiatry 41, 257-267.

Sullivan, J. L., Cavenar, J. O. Jr., Maltbie, A., and Stanfield, C. (1977a) Platelet-monoamine-oxidase activity predicts response to lithium in manic-depressive illness. Lancet ii, 1325-1327.

Sullivan, J. L., Dackis, C., and Stanfield, C. (1977b) In vivo inhibition of platelet MAO activity by tricyclic antidepressants. Am. J. Psychiatry 134, 188-190.

Sulser, F., Janowsky, J., Okada, F., Manier, B. H., and Mobley, P. L. (1983) Regulation of recognition and action function of norepinephrine (NE) receptor-coupled adenylate cyclase system in brain: implications for the therapy of depression. Neuropharmacology 22, 425-431.

Takahashi, S., Kondo, H., Yoshimura, M., and Ochi, Y. (1974) Thyrotropin responses to TRH in depressive illness: relation to clinical subtypes and prolonged duration of depressive episode. Folia Psychiatr. Neurol. Japon. 28, 355-365.

Tanimoto, K., Maeda, K., Yamaguchi, N., Chihara, K., and Fujita, T. (1981) Effect of lithium on prolactin response to TRH in patients with manic state. Psychopharmacology 72, 129-133.

Targum, S. (1983) Neuroendocrine challenge studies. Psychiatric Annals 13, 385-395.

Targum, S. D., Byrnes, S. M., and Sullivan, A. C. (1982a) The TRH stimulation test in subtypes of unipolar depression. J. Affec. Disorders 4, 29-34.

Targum, S. D., Byrnes, S. M., and Sullivan, A. C. (1982b) Subtypes of unipolar depression distinguished by the dexamethasone suppression test. J. Affec. Disorders 4, 21-27.

Targum, S. D., Sullivan, A. C., and Byrnes, S. M. (1982c) Neuroendocrine interrelationships in major depressive disorder. Am. J. Psychiatry 139, 282-286.

Traskman, L., Tybring, G., Asberg, M., Bertilsson, L., Lantto, O., and Schalling, D. (1980) Cortisol in the CSF of depressed and suicidal patients. Arch. Gen. Psychiatry 37, 761-767.

van Praag, H. M. (1980) Central monoamine metabolism in depression. Comp. Psychiatry 21, 30-43.

van Praag, H. M. (1982) Depression, suicide and the metabolism of serotonin in the brain. J. Affec. Disorders 4, 275-290.

van Praag, H. M. and Korf, J. (1971) A pilot study of some kinetic aspects of the metabolism of 5-hydroxytryptamine in depressed patients. Biol. Psychiatry 3, 105-112.

van Praag, H. M., Korf, J., and Puite, J. (1970) 5-hydroxyindoleacetic acid levels in the cerebrospinal fluid of depressive patients treated with probenecid. Nature (Lond.) 225, 1259-1260.

White, K., Bohart, R., and Eaton, E. (1979) RBC lithium uptake ratios in manics, schizophrenics, and normals. Biol. Psychiatry 14, 663-669.

White, K., Shih, J., Fong, T., Young, H., Gelfand, R., Boyd, J., Simpson, G., and Sloane, R. B. (1980) Elevated platelet monoamine oxidase activity in patients with nonendogenous depression. Am. J. Psychiatry **137,** 1258-1259.

Winokur, G. (1974) The division of depressive illness into depression spectrum disease and pure depressive disease. Int. Pharmacopsychiatry **9,** 5-13.

Yang, H. Y. and Neff, N. H. (1973) β-Phenylethylamine: a specific substrate for type B monoamine oxidase of brain. J. Pharmacol. Exp. Therap. **187,** 365-371.

3.

ANIMAL MODELS OF AFFECTIVE DISORDERS

R. D. Porsolt

Introduction

Perhaps the first question which could be asked in a chapter about animal models of affective disorders is why have animal models at all? This fundamental question will not be addressed in detail here as it has already been largely dealt with by others (McKinney and Bunney, 1969; Kornetsky, 1977; McKinney, 1977; Robbins and Sahakian, 1980; Reite et al., 1983). None the less, several points deserve to be mentioned. On the one hand it seems evident that many aspects of human affective disorders would be almost impossible to model in animals. For example, it is difficult to imagine convincing animal analogues for pessimism, guilt, self-depreciation or suicidal ideation which characterise human depressive illness. The same would be true for the expansiveness, flight of ideas and pressure of speech often experienced in mania. On the other hand, much of the basic and applied research into the origins and treatment of affective illness could not be performed in the absence of animal models which attempt to imitate the clinical syndrome.

In general animal models enable the rigorous investigation of basic mechanisms and variables which could not be evaluated in man for obvious ethical and/or practical reasons. Among the kinds of experiment excluded in man on ethical grounds are those using profoundly aversive stimulation, invasive techniques (implantation, ablation, chemical or electrical brain stimulation), or those requiring sacrifice of the subjects. It should none the less be emphasized that animal experiments are not entirely free of ethical constraints either, which creates a special problem for depression research where, by definition, the animals are not rendered happy. This aspect should be borne in mind by the animal modeller who should always attempt to use methods which provide a maximum of information for a minimum of discomfort to the animal. Apart from ethical considerations, the use of animal models has practical advantages as, for example, in the study of genetic or developmental variables which can be followed in lower animals on a time scale which would not be feasible in man for prospective studies. Furthermore, animal models, although frequently a gross oversimplification of the clinical realities, also frequently serve a heuristic purpose in stimulating research around particular topics (e.g. 'learned helplessness', 'separation') or suggest novel hypotheses which are open to experimental testing. A final and more pragmatic point is that animal models, even primitive ones, often represent the only means we possess to discover new and better treatments; this is particularly true for the search for new antidepressant drugs.

Even the most promising animal models of affective disorder, however, will never completely encompass all that is included under that term in man. This is perfectly understandable but unfortunately frequently forgotten. A model is by its nature an oversimplification of a more complex reality--it is never the real thing. Recognition of this fact does not, however, preclude the necessity of subjecting any proposed model to a detailed evaluation to determine at least its relative validity and thereby the limits to its usefulness as a research tool. McKinney (1977) has proposed four criteria for validating animal models:
1. Similarity of inducing conditions.
2. Similarity of behavioural state produced.
3. Similarity of underlying neurobiological mechanisms.
4. Similarity of clinically effective treatment techniques.

It can be seen immediately that even these limited criteria demand information, in particular that concerning inducing conditions and underlying mechanisms, which is at present scarcely available. Somewhat more is known concerning symptomatology and we do have fairly reliable information about the efficacy of certain treatments. Additional factors which should be borne in mind when evaluating the utility of a particular model are reproducibility, objectivity of behavioural assessment, procedural simplicity, rapidity and cost.

Animal Models of Affective Disorders

The present chapter attempts to provide a critical review of available animal models of affective disorder in the light of the above factors. In what follows there is an admittedly heavy emphasis on the analysis of drug effects. This is so partly because of my own particular interests as a behavioural pharmacologist. A more important reason is that the analysis of drug and other treatment effects, the fourth criterion of McKinney (1977), constitutes the area in which most information is currently available.

Separation Models of Depression

Separation-Induced Despair in Primates

Perhaps the most convincing animal analogue of depression is the despair syndrome described in monkeys. Similar to the depressive syndromes sometimes observed in young children separated from their mothers (Bowlby, 1977), marked signs of depression can be induced in young monkeys separated from their mothers (Hinde and Spencer-Booth, 1971; Kaufmann and Rosenblum, 1967; Seay and Harlow, 1965) or their cage mates (Suomi et al., 1970) or after confinement in 'vertical chambers' (Suomi and Harlow, 1972). The syndrome consists typically of two phases, first a high level of agitation and vocalisation ('protest phase'), followed within a few days by a marked reduction in play and social activities with increases in huddling and self-directed behaviour ('despair' phase). Recovery usually occurs spontaneously, if not immediately, when the precipitating conditions are terminated. Whereas maternal separation induces depression only in monkeys up to 9 months old and becomes less effective as the monkeys grow up and naturally become more independent of their mothers (Harlow and Harlow, 1965), peer separation, especially in animals reared together from birth, has been used repeatedly to induce depressions over longer periods of time (Suomi et al., 1970). The most effective method for inducing depression, however, appears to be confinement in 'vertical chambers'. Severe depressive symptoms lasting up to one year have been induced in infant monkeys, 45 days old, after 6 weeks of confinement (Suomi and Harlow, 1972), whereas somewhat milder depressive behaviours (passivity, contact clinging) have been induced in 3-year-old monkeys which, at this age, are usually resistant to peer separation

procedures (McKinney et al., 1972).
Monkey depression not only bears a striking behavioural resemblance to some aspects of human depression but can also be alleviated by antidepressant treatments such as imipramine (Suomi et al., 1978) and desipramine (Hrdina et al., 1979), whereas treatment with the neuroleptic chlorpromazine is without effect (Moran and McKinney, 1975). Repeated electroconvulsive shock (ECS) has also been found effective in increasing general activity and decreasing submissive behaviour in young monkeys which had been exposed during early life to prolonged vertical chamber confinement (Lewis and McKinney, 1976). Furthermore, a more recent finding showing positive effects with low doses of alcohol (Kraemer et al., 1981) provides suggestive evidence for the euphoria which can be induced after consumption of moderate amounts of alcohol.

Depression-like symptoms are not an invariable response to separation in primates where species, age and prior experimental history all appear to play a role (Mineka and Suomi, 1978). Even in the young rhesus monkey, which appears to be the most susceptible, several authors have failed to observe convincing signs of depression in all animals after separation from the mother (Gunnar et al., 1981; Lewis et al., 1976) or peers (Porsolt, 1983b) or even after confinement in vertical chambers for up to 8 days (Porsolt, 1983b). That such individual differences exist, as they do in man, is probably an indication of the validity of the model but limit its practical utility. Encouraging new findings suggest, however, that monkeys with relatively low levels of CSF noradrenaline (NA) are more likely to show a severe despair response to social separation (Kraemer et al., 1983), and that the behaviour occurring during social separation is accompanied by a wide variety of marked physiological changes (Gunnar et al., 1981; Reite and Snyder, 1982). Investigation of the biochemical and physiological correlates of despair behaviour in primates appears, therefore, to be a promising line of research in this area.

Separation-Induced Vocalisations in Primates and Other Animals

Although 'despair' behaviour has mainly been studied in primates, 'protest' vocalisations have been observed in a wide range of young animals including chicks (Panksepp et al., 1980a,b), guinea pigs

(Panksepp et al., 1980a), rats (Hofer, 1975), cats (Rheingold and Eckerman, 1971) and dogs (Panksepp et al., 1980a; Scott, 1975). Some authors (Panksepp et al., 1980b; Scott, 1975) have suggested that even 'protest' vocalisations might serve as a model of at least some aspects of depression. In support of this suggestion, Scott (1975) found that vocalisations in beagle puppies were suppressed by acute injections of imipramine at doses which had no other effects on behaviour; other dog breeds, however, showed considerably less marked effects with imipramine. Suomi et al. (1981) also mention unpublished experiments in which infant rhesus monkeys treated with imipramine showed a less marked protest response than controls when subjected to a peer separation. In contrast to the findings of Scott (1975) and Suomi et al. (1981), we found that imipramine, after acute or sub-chronic treatment, did not decrease but, if anything, increased separation-induced vocalisations in young rhesus monkeys (Porsolt et al., 1984). Although our study differed from that described by Suomi et al. (1981) in that they administered imipramine chronically over a 60-day period covering two separations and reunions, Suomi et al. (1981) reported that vocalisations decreased even at the beginning of treatment. In general, the pharmacology of separation-induced vocalisations has not been widely studied. Some authors (Panksepp et al., 1980a) have shown that separation-induced vocalisations in chicks, guinea pigs and puppies are reduced by opiates and endogenous opioids and that these effects can be antagonised by naloxone. In one study the same authors (Panksepp et al., 1980b) showed that imipramine reduced vocalisations in chicks but only at clearly neurotoxic doses.

Conclusions

From the above it can be seen that separation-induced 'despair' behaviour in monkeys, although cumbersome to manipulate and not always reproducible, satisfies many of the criteria required of an animal model of depression. It is induced in conditions which at least heuristically are thought capable of precipitating depressive episodes in man. The symptoms observed bear a striking resemblance to behaviours which would be described as depressive in humans. The syndrome seems furthermore to respond to certain treatments known to alleviate human depression, and preliminary experiments suggest a further parallel between man and monkeys in the CSF levels of NA, which can sometimes serve to discriminate normal from depression-prone individuals. On the other hand the status of 'protest' vocalisations, although highly reproducible, remains uncertain for the present.

Learned Helplessness

Behavioural Aspects

Another animal model that has gained wide interest in recent years is Seligman's 'learned helplessness' (Seligman, 1975; Maier and Seligman, 1976; Hellhammer, 1983). According to this model, animals and even humans, when exposed to aversive situations over which they have no control, suffer decreased motivation to respond, cognitive deficits which interfere with new learning, and emotional disruption--first anxiety and then, with increased exposure to the precipitating conditions, depression. As a consequence, the subjects' ability to respond adaptively to subsequent traumatic events is diminished. For example, dogs, when given a series of inescapable shocks, were unable on a later occasion to learn the responses necessary to escape from shocks of the same intensity. Instead of trying to escape they simply lay down and whined. Similar learning deficits have been observed in experiments in man and have been accompanied by mood changes similar to those occurring in clinical depression. The deficits observed are examples of 'learned helplessness' which, according to Seligman, results from the organism's having learned that the situation is uncontrollable. Contrary to this position, Glazer and Weiss (1976) have argued that 'learned helplessness' is due to the subjects' having learned competing responses during exposure to inescapable shocks which interfere with subsequent active escape learning. Whatever the theoretical explanation, the 'learned helplessness' model has stimulated considerable research both in man and in animals and has recently been widened to provide a cognitive account of depression in man (Abramson et al., 1978).

In animals the induction of 'learned helplessness' is usually studied by means of the so-called triadic design. In this procedure three animals are tested simultaneously. The first animal is subjected to aversive stimulation from which it can learn to escape by performing an appropriate response. The second animal is yoked to the first, that is, it receives the same aversive stimulation without the possibility of terminating it; termination occurs when the first animal successfully performs the escape response. The third animal receives no aversive treatment. Later all animals are tested on a new task. 'Learned helplessness' is demonstrated if the yoked animals show deficits in learning compared with the non-yoked animals. The triadic design is thus an elegant way of demonstrating that the deficits result from the animal's inability to control the aversive stimulation rather than from simply having received it.

In addition to dogs, 'learned helplessness' has been demonstrated in a wide variety of animals including mice, rats, fish and pigeons (Seligman, 1975). In rodents 'learned helplessness' has been rather more difficult to demonstrate than in dogs. In standard learning tasks where escape from shock requires a simple response such as a single lever press or fleeing to the other side of a shuttle box, only minor performance deficits (e.g. increases in latency), but no failure to learn ('helplessness'), have been observed in animals pre-exposed to inescapable shock. Substantial 'helplessness' has, however, been observed in rodents where the learning tasks were made more difficult, for example, by requiring a rat to perform multiple lever presses or to run back and forth more than once in a shuttle box to escape shock (Maier and Seligman, 1976).

Pharmacological and Biochemical Aspects

Recently several authors have described the effects of psychotropic drugs on the escape deficits induced by pre-exposure to inescapable electric shock. Leshner et al. (1979) showed that repeated injection of desipramine reduced the high latencies observed in a shuttle box in rats previously exposed to inescapable shocks without affecting latencies in non-shocked animals. Similarly, Sherman et al. (1979) showed that chronic, but not acute, administration of imipramine prevented failures in the acquisition of a 'jump up' escape task in rats previously exposed to inescapable shock. This effect was correlated with concentrations of imipramine and its principal metabolite desipramine, not only in the whole brain (Sherman et al., 1979) but particularly in the frontal neocortex (Petty et al., 1982). In further studies, using a bar-pressing task, the same authors (Sherman et al., 1982) showed that a wide variety of antidepressants--including tricyclics, monoamine oxidase inhibitors (MAOIs), and atypical antidepressants such as iprindole and mianserin--also reversed 'learned helplessness', as did ECS. Minor tranquillisers (chlordiazepoxide, diazepam, lorazepam, ethanol), neuroleptics (chlorpromazine, haloperidol) or psychostimulants (amphetamine, caffeine) were ineffective. Reversal of 'helplessness' was observed after local injections of desipramine into the frontal neocortex, of γ-aminobutyric acid (GABA) into the hippocampus or lateral geniculate body or of serotonin (5-hydroxytryptamine; 5-HT) into the frontal neocortex or septum, suggesting highly localised and neurochemically specific sites of action; in contrast, direct injection of NA in any of the regions studied had no effect on established 'learned helplessness' (Sherman and Petty, 1980). Further evidence for a role for GABA was the finding that hippocampal release of GABA was diminished in 'helpless' animals, an effect which was attenuated by chronic treatment with imipramine whereas chronic treatment with imipramine increased hippocampal GABA release in naive animals (Sherman and Petty, 1982).

In contrast to the neurochemical findings of Petty's group, which suggest that injection of 5-HT, at least into some brain areas, decreases 'learned helplessness', some recent pharmacological findings suggest that 'learned helplessness' can be aggravated by increasing brain levels of 5-HT by systemic administration of its precursors L-tryptophan and 5-hydroxytryptophan (5-HTP) (Brown et al., 1982). Other findings, again in contrast to Petty's group, implicate mainly catecholamine function, with little or no role for brain 5-HT. For example, Anisman and his co-workers (Anisman et al., 1979a,b) reported that treatment with the catecholamine precursor L-DOPA decreased escape deficits in mice after inescapable shock whereas treatment with the 5-HT precursor 5-HTP was without effect. Conversely, escape deficits were enhanced by reserpine, a depletor of catecholamines and 5-HT, and by alpha-methyl-para-tyrosine (AMPT), which specifically depletes catecholamines, but not by the specific 5-HT depletor p-chlorophenylalanine (PCPA). Escape deficits were also enhanced by the dopamine (DA) receptor blockers haloperidol and pimozide. Consistent with these pharmacological findings were the results of biochemical determinations which showed that exposure to inescapable shock decreased the concentrations of hypothalamic NA but did not affect hypothalamic 5-HT

(Anisman and Sklar, 1979). Similarly, Weiss et al. (1981) showed that exposure to severe inescapable shocks caused marked decreases in brain levels of NA in rats, particularly in the brain stem and hypothalamus, without greatly affecting DA or 5-HT levels.

It is not at present possible to determine the reasons for these apparently discrepant findings. Marked procedural differences are probably largely responsible (Brown et al., 1982). None the less, the kinds of experiments undertaken provide a good example of how such models could be useful in attempts to unravel complex functions and mechanisms. They also suggest the advantages of studying the neurochemical actions of drugs in models of pathological, as opposed to normal, states.

Conclusions

Concerning 'learned helplessness' as a model of depression, it is clear that the model has stimulated an important quantity of research concerning both the aetiology, treatment and even prevention of depression. Furthermore, animal 'helplessness' in its most marked forms, as observed for example in the intractably pathological behaviour of some dogs exposed to inescapable electric shocks, undoubtedly resembles certain aspects of clinical depression. On the other hand the term 'helplessness' seems overly dramatic for describing the rather milder performance deficits observed in rodents. More generally, it can be questioned whether the considerable cognitive ramifications of 'learned helplessness' theory provide a sufficiently parsimonious account of the behaviours observed in most animal experiments with 'learned helplessness'.

Stress Models of Depression
===========================

Acute Swim Stress: 'Behavioural Despair'

One of the classic ways of inducing stress in small animals is to force them to swim in water from which they cannot escape. Rats or mice forced to swim in this way will, after an initial period of vigorous activity, adopt a characteristic immobile posture and make no further movements apart from those necessary to keep their heads above the water. This immobile behaviour was first observed in rats during learning experiments in a water maze (see Porsolt,

1981). Rats were plunged into the water at one end of the maze and required to find the exit at the other end within 10 minutes. Most rats found the exit quite easily but some, after swimming around for some time without finding the exit, ceased struggling altogether and remained floating passively in the water. It seemed that for these rats the situation intuitively appeared inescapable (cf. Seligman, 1975) and that they had 'given up hope'. In subsequent experiments rats (Porsolt et al., 1977b), and also mice (Porsolt et al., 1977a), were forced to swim in narrow cylinders where there was no possibility of escape and immobility could be induced rapidly and reliably.

Immobility is decreased by most clinically active antidepressants, including tricyclics, MAOIs and various atypical agents such as bupropion, danitracene, doxepin, iprindole, mianserin, pizotifen, trazodone and viloxazine, which possess little or no effects in classical pharmacological tests for antidepressant activity (Porsolt et al., 1978a; Gorka and Wojtasik, 1980; Porsolt, 1981). Furthermore, the amount of immobility observed and the effects thereon of imipramine depend on the strain of animal employed (Porsolt et al., 1978b), suggesting, as in man, the importance of a genetic component. The effects observed with antidepressants do not appear simply to be due to increased motor activity because the doses which reduce immobility generally decrease motor activity (Porsolt et al., 1978a); antidepressants appear in particular to prolong the escape-directed behaviour observed at the beginning of a test session (Kitada et al., 1981; Nomura et al., 1982). Thus antidepressants can be distinguished from two classes of false positives, psychostimulants (amphetamine, caffeine) and anticholinergics (atropine, scopolamine), which increase locomotor activity (Porsolt et al., 1978a; Sansone and Hano, 1979) and cause generalised motor stimulation throughout the duration of the forced swimming test (Kitada et al., 1981; Nomura et al., 1982). Immersion in water, even at 25 or 35°C, causes marked hypothermia, but the effects of antidepressants do not seem to be due to antagonism of hypothermia because, unlike in the reserpine test, doses of imipramine which reduce immobility actually potentiate forced swimming-induced hypothermia (Porsolt et al., 1979b). Furthermore, in a related behavioural model where immobility is induced by suspending mice by the tail, thereby avoiding immersion-induced hypothermia, closely analogous pharmacological results have been obtained (Steru et al., 1984). In contrast to antidepressants, minor tranquillisers (chlordiazepoxide, diazepam) do not affect immobility whereas classical neuroleptics (chlorpromazine, haloperidol, pimozide) enhance it (Porsolt et al., 1978a, 1979a). Immobility is, however, reduced by some non-classical neuroleptics such as clozapine (Browne, 1979), t-chlorprothixene (Browne, 1979), sulpiride and carpipramine (Mercier et al., 1979), an effect which could be due to antidepressant or 'disinhibitory' effects of these atypical compounds (Deniker et al., 1980). Potential false positives in the procedure include, however, antihistamines (Wallach and Hedley, 1979; Rogoz et al., 1981), subconvulsive doses of convulsants (Betin et al., 1982) and several neuropeptides (Kastin et al., 1978). False negatives include specific 5-HT uptake blockers (Porsolt et al., 1979a) and beta-adrenergic stimulants (Porsolt et al., 1979a; Przegalinski et al., 1980; Frances et al., 1983) in rats, although 5-HT uptake blockers appear to be active in mice (Porsolt et al., 1977a; Browne, 1979).

Immobility in rats appears to be mediated primarily through dopaminergic and noradrenergic mechanisms. It is reduced by agents which increase noradrenergic or dopaminergic activity and is generally enhanced by agents which reduce activity in these two systems (Porsolt et al., 1979a). The action of tricyclic antidepressants is potentiated by agents which accelerate the release of NA by blockade of presynaptic alpha-adrenergic receptors (Zebrowska-Lupina, 1980) and is attenuated by agents which decrease noradrenergic activity either by stimulating presynaptic alpha-receptors (Zebrowska-Lupina, 1980) or blocking postsynaptic alpha-receptors (Borsini et al., 1981). In contrast, increasing central 5-HT activity either has no effect or even increases immobility (Borsini et al., 1981; Gorka et al., 1979; Porsolt et al., 1979a).

These conclusions based on pharmacological data are consistent with available biochemical data. An early experiment by Ruther et al. (1966) showed a marked decrease in NA levels but an increase in 5-HT levels in the brains of rats swum to exhaustion in cold water (15°C); these neurochemical effects as well as the marked behavioural depression observed after swimming were reversed by pretreatment with desipramine but enhanced by pretreatment with 5-HTP. Similarly, intracerebral injection of NA, and to a lesser extent DA, reversed the depression of exploratory activity observed after rats had been forced to swim in cold water (15°C) for 20 minutes, whereas intracerebral injection of 5-HT decreased activity even further (Stone and Mendlinger, 1974). A more recent experiment showed that forced swimming for shorter periods (two 6-minute sessions separated by a 5-minute interval) in cold water (sic) caused a slight decrease in medullary NA levels with a marked increase in 3-methoxy-4-hydroxyphenylethylene glycol sulfate (MOPEG-SO$_4$; MHPG-SO$_4$) levels, effects which were prevented by pretreatment with desipramine or (+)-amphetamine (Bareggi et al., 1978). Similarly, Miyauchi et al. (1981), following our own procedure in rats, observed marked increases in MOPEG-SO$_4$ in various brain regions, particularly the septum after 50 minutes' forced swimming at 25°C. These effects were counteracted by acute and chronic administration of amitriptyline or desipramine.

In conclusion, 'behavioural despair' represents an explicit attempt to mimic in rodents some aspects of human depression and is sensitive to a wide variety of clinically effective antidepressant treatments. Repeated treatment is more effective than acute treatment, but there are both false positives and false negatives. It is evident that marked parallels exist between this model and Seligman's 'learned helplessness'; both require that animals be exposed to aversive stimulation from which there is no escape. Moreover, in so far as comparable data are available, both models respond in a similar way to pharmacological treatment and appear to depend on similar neurochemical substrates. Unlike 'learned helplessness', however, the 'behavioural despair' model does not make assumptions concerning cognitive and motivational factors and the dependent variable, immobility, is simpler to define and manipulate than the various learning deficits studied in 'learned helplessness' procedures. It remains to be seen whether 'behavioural despair' will be useful for identifying novel antidepressants or for elucidating some of the neurochemical mechanisms of depressive illness.

Chronic Stress Models

In contrast to the 'behavioural despair' model, which employs an acute exposure to swim stress, other authors have investigated the behavioural and neuroendocrine consequences of prolonged exposure to aversive stimulation.

The Hatotani Model.
Hatotani and co-workers (Hato-

tani et al., 1977, 1979) forced female rats to run inside revolving drums until exhaustion on three separate occasions separated by 24-hour rest periods. In a majority of the animals this procedure caused a marked decrease in subsequent spontaneous running behaviour together with disruption of circadian activity rhythms and abolition of oestrus cycles for periods up to 6 weeks. In addition, it was noted that 'depressed' rats, although eating and drinking normally, were hyper-reactive and aggressive and showed ptosis and instability of sleep. These effects were accompanied by a decreased turnover rate of catecholamines in the nerve terminals of the ascending NA system. In animals that recovered spontaneously, NA turnover rates were similar to those observed in control animals. Preliminary drug experiments indicate that repeated administration of imipramine, but not chlorpromazine, causes a recovery in spontaneous activity and a return of oestrus cycles (Hatotani et al., 1981). These studies, although only at an early stage, appear particularly interesting, firstly because a relatively lasting state is induced with individual differences in recovery rates, and secondly because the altered behaviour is accompanied by neuroendocrinological changes (e.g. abolition of oestrus cycles) which are also observed in clinical depression (Deniker et al., 1980).

The Katz Model. Another chronic stress model is that proposed by Katz and co-workers (Katz, 1981, 1982, 1983). Rats, when exposed to acute stress (1 hour exposure to 95 dB white noise), show an increase in open field activity and an elevation in plasma corticosterone levels. When exposed to chronic intermittent stress, including food and water deprivations, electric shocks, cold swims, tail pinches and shaker stress over a three-week period, there is a decrease in basal open field activity and in the activation response to acute noise stress together with an increase in defecation, suggesting increased emotionality. Chronic stress also results in an elevation in basal corticosterone levels, with a further increase when the animals are challenged with acute noise stress. Another effect of chronic stress is a decrease in consumption of sucrose or saccharin which may be related to the hedonic deficits frequently observed in depression. Preliminary studies indicate that chronic stress causes decreases in brain levels of adrenaline and NA (Katz, 1983). Repeated administration during the chronic stress of antidepressants including tricyclics, MAOIs and atypical agents (bupropion, iprindole, mianserin), as well as ECS, restores both basal activity in the open field and the activation response to acute noise stress. Corticosterone levels are also normalised as is the consumption of saccharin. In contrast, repeated treatment with amphetamine, scopolamine, haloperidol or oxazepam, or acute administration of imipramine, is ineffective. Partial 'antidepressive' effects are, however, observed with the antihistamine tripelennamine.

Taken together, the results presently available with this model indicate that the behavioural changes observed resemble certain aspects of depression (reduced general activity, blunted response to environmental stimuli, increased emotionality, decreased consummatory behaviour). Furthermore, the behavioural phenomena are accompanied by neuroendocrine changes which have also been described in human depression (Rubin and Poland, 1983). As in humans, the behavioural and neuroendocrine changes are corrected by chronic, but not acute, treatment with various antidepressant agents, but are not affected by psychostimulants, anticholinergics, neuroleptics or minor tranquillisers. Further information concerning the duration of the behavioural changes and their neurochemical correlates would be of great theoretical interest. On the other hand, the model is rather cumbersome, and it is difficult to imagine convincing human parallels to the severe stresses required to induce the condition.

Chronic Social Isolation. Another model which would fit within the category of chronic stress is that described by Garzon and co-workers (Garzon et al., 1979; Garzon and del Rio, 1981). Rats, placed in isolation at weaning and maintained alone for 10-12 months, develop a complex behavioural syndrome characterised by marked hyperactivity, flight from the experimenter, compulsive digging, crouched posture and vocalisations. Hyperactivity is reduced by acute administration of tricyclics, MAOIs and atypical antidepressants (iprindole, mianserin, nomifensine, salbutamol, trazodone and viloxazine) but not by neuroleptics, minor tranquillisers or amphetamine in non-neurotoxic doses. The model thus appears to respond in a fairly selective manner to antidepressants. Its relation to depression is less clear, however, because hyperactivity would not appear to be a symptom typical of depression except perhaps for agitated depressions. The model would appear more akin to the isolation syndromes observed in mice (Valzelli, 1973) and monkeys (Harlow and McKinney, 1971)[1], which are not generally thought to model depressive illness. Further major disadvantages of the model are that the rats must be isolated for at least 10 months for the hyperactivity to appear and that the hyperactivity disappears if the animals are handled, thereby limiting the model's usefulness for repeated testing of different drugs or for studying the effects of chronic treatment.

Drug Models of Depression
================

The following section discusses models where different pharmacological agents are used to induce behavioural changes intended to imitate aspects of depression. Most of these models were developed as pharmacological test procedures for the identification of novel antidepressant agents. As such they suffer from inherent circularity in that they were adopted largely because they had been found sensitive to the effects of known antidepressants. As a consequence they are unlikely to discover antidepressant drugs with mechanisms of action greatly different from those of the reference compounds used to establish them as tests. This problem is illustrated by the existence of several compounds, for example iprindole, mianserin and trazodone, which show little or no activity in these drug-based tests but which are clinically active as antidepressants. A further disadvantage of drug-based models is that the mechanisms of action of the inducing drugs is rarely completely understood and may have little to do with the pathological processes involved in depressive illness. None the less, many of these models have been highly productive in the development of new antidepressants, mainly other tricyclic compounds and MAOIs but also atypical compounds such as bupropion (Soroko et al., 1977), nomifensine (Hoffman, 1973) and viloxazine (Greenwood, 1975).

— — —

1. The 'isolation' syndrome in monkeys is not to be confused with the 'separation' syndrome discussed in a previous section (see Kraemer et al., 1983).

Furthermore, the knowledge, even if imperfect, of their mechanisms of action has been able to throw light not only on the mechanism of action of some antidepressants but has also served as a source of hypotheses concerning depressive illness itself.

Reserpine Syndrome

The syndrome induced by reserpine and related compounds is the model most widely used in experimental pharmacology for the detection of antidepressant drugs. Interest in the psychotropic effects of reserpine arose from the clinical observation that some patients treated with reserpine for hypertension developed clear signs of clinical depression. Although the validity of reserpine-induced depression in man has been seriously questioned (Bein, 1978), indirect support for the notion is provided by the observation that rhesus monkeys chronically treated with reserpine show behavioural signs similar to those induced by separation procedures (McKinney et al., 1971). The fact that most clinically active antidepressant drugs antagonise some or all of the symptoms induced by reserpine provides empirical evidence for the validity of the reserpine model. Reserpine and related compounds, among their other actions, deplete intraneuronal vesicular stores of biogenic amines such as DA, NA and 5-HT, resulting in lower brain levels of these neurotransmitter substances. Indeed, it was this action of reserpine which was at the origin of the amine hypothesis of depression (Schildkraut and Kety, 1967) which has dominated thinking in this field over the last two decades.

The extensive literature on the effects of reserpine and their antagonism by antidepressants has been reviewed in detail elsewhere (Garattini and Jori, 1967; Colpaert et al., 1975; Gouret et al., 1977) and only the major outline and pitfalls will be dealt with here. The most striking feature of reserpine-based tests is their diversity both in terms of the symptoms studied and experimental protocols followed. As a result many inconsistencies exist and it is difficult to generalise between different experimental findings.

A first potential variable is the compound used to induce the so-called reserpine syndrome. Apart from reserpine itself, the two most widely used compounds are the two benzoquinolizine derivatives tetrabenazine and its water-soluble analogue Ro 4-1284. Although tetrabenazine and Ro 4-1284 produce symptoms similar to those induced by reserpine, their effects are more rapid in onset, shorter in duration and relatively more pronounced in the CNS than in the periphery. Furthermore, tetrabenazine appears to have a stronger depleting action on central DA and NA whereas reserpine appears to have a preferential effect on central 5-HT (Quinn et al., 1959; Kuczenski, 1977). A systematic comparison of tetrabenazine and reserpine antagonism using a wide range of antidepressants has not been undertaken.

Reserpine-like compounds induce a variety of symptoms including sedation, hypothermia, ptosis, miosis, diarrhea, hypersalivation, lacrimation, gastric hypersecretion, and bradycardia (Garattini and Jori, 1967). The symptoms most frequently studied in antagonism tests are sedation, hypothermia and ptosis. Whereas sedation and hypothermia are largely central in origin, ptosis is probably due to sympatholytic actions in the periphery (Fielden and Green, 1965) and would thus appear less valid as a model of depression. A further effect of reserpine-like compounds which is almost certainly of central origin is the induction of ponto-geniculo-occipital (PGO) spikes in curarised animals (Jalfre et al., 1970).

Procedures used have varied very widely and quite subtle differences can markedly change the results obtained. Gouret et al. (1977) have shown that factors such as the dose of reserpine used, its route of administration, and the observation time can critically determine whether a test compound is found active or not. Different effects are observed depending on whether reserpine is administered before or after the test compound. For example, when imipramine is administered before reserpine, prolonged hyperthermia is observed, whereas when it is administered to already reserpinised animals their lowered body temperature is restored to normal (Garattini and Jori, 1967). In most tests currently used, the test compound is administered before reserpine (Colpaert et al., 1975; Howard et al., 1981). Species differences can also be important. Whereas tricyclic antidepressants prevent reserpine-induced sedation in the rat and even cause behavioural excitation (Garattini and Jori, 1967; Howard et al., 1981), conflicting findings have been reported in the mouse; some studies have reported an antagonism (Howard et al., 1981), whereas the comprehensive study by Colpaert et al. (1975) showed that all the 24 tricyclic antidepressants tested were inactive in preventing Ro 4-1284-induced sedation. A further problem concerning the validity of the reserpine model is that it is based on the acute effects of antidepressants whereas clinically these drugs are effective only after chronic treatment. Indeed it has been shown that chronic treatment with imipramine or desipramine was no more effective than acute treatment in reversing reserpine-induced hypothermia (Garattini and Jori, 1967).

In view of the above, it is difficult to draw general conclusions concerning the reserpine syndrome as an animal model of depression. Ptosis, although probably a peripheral effect, appears to detect the greatest number of clinically effective antidepressants, including substances such as mianserin and trazodone (Gouret et al., 1977) which are generally regarded as false negatives in most reserpine procedures. There are, on the other hand, many false positives including psychostimulants, anticholinergics, antihistamines, analgesics, and peripherally acting sympathomimetics (Colpaert et al., 1975). With parameters more closely dependent on central effects (hypothermia, sedation, PGO spikes), the number of false positives tends to decrease, but there is a corresponding increase in false negatives (Gouret et al., 1977). In general, MAOIs appear to show clearer antagonism and reversal of most reserpine parameters than do tricyclic or atypical antidepressants (Colpaert et al., 1975).

Syndrome Induced by Alpha-Methyl-p-Tyrosine (AMPT)

One amine depletion model which has apparently not aroused much interest as a potential model of depression is the behavioural syndrome induced by AMPT. AMPT is an inhibitor of tyrosine hydroxylase and causes specific depletion of brain levels of DA and NA by inhibition of their synthesis. These effects are accompanied by marked decreases in spontaneous and conditioned behaviour. When given in high doses, AMPT produces 'despair-like' behaviour in monkeys (Redmond et al., 1971). More interestingly, lower doses of AMPT which by themselves are without behavioural effect potentiate the 'despair' response to separation in infant monkeys, particularly in animals subjected to repeated separations (Kraemer and McKinney, 1979). Similarly, AMPT has been reported to potentiate 'learned helplessness' in mice (Anisman et al., 1979a) and 'behavioural despair' in rats (Porsolt et al., 1979a). Despite these positive indications for AMPT, clinical reports of depression associated with its use are rare, although the compound has been used for the treatment of mania (Kraemer and McKinney, 1979). Systematic interaction studies with antidepressants have not been undertaken.

5-HT-Induced Behavioural Depression

Aprison and his colleagues (Aprison et al., 1978; Nagayama et al., 1981) have proposed, in contrast to the classical monoamine hypothesis, that at least some kinds of depression might be due to an excess of 5-HT in the synaptic cleft, with resulting subsensitivity of the post-synaptic 5-HT receptor. The same authors suggest that one of the mechanisms of action of antidepressant drugs might be to increase 5-HT receptor sensitivity, perhaps by receptor blockade. In support of their hypothesis they have reported that acute injections of several antidepressants including amitriptyline, imipramine, iprindole and mianserin, like the 5-HT receptor antagonist methysergide, block the depression of operant responding induced by the 5-HT precursor 5-HTP whereas the depression of responding is enhanced by fluoxetine, a relatively specific inhibitor of 5-HT uptake.

The findings are interesting in that they would confirm an antidepressant action for iprindole and mianserin and suggest an alternative, postsynaptic, mechanism of action for imipramine and amitriptyline.' The findings are, moreover, consistent with biochemical studies showing a selective displacement by tricyclics of the binding of [^{3}H]-LSD and [^{3}H]-5-HT to central receptors (Ogren et al., 1979) and microiontophoretic studies indicating an increase in 5-HT receptor sensitivity after chronic treatment with tricyclic and atypical antidepressants (de Montigny and Aghajanian, 1978). Furthermore, the proposed mechanism might explain the antidepressant activity of other atypical compounds such as pizotifen and trazodone whose primary acute action appears to be blockade of postsynaptic 5-HT receptors (Maj, 1979).

Other findings, however, suggest limits to the generality of Aprison's hypothesis. In contrast to tricyclics, acute treatment with MAOIs does not block 5-HT mediated stereotyped behaviour and tremor, whereas after chronic treatment 5-HT-induced behaviour is blocked by MAOIs but not tricyclics (Lucki and Frazer, 1982). Further, in contrast to the increased sensitivity of 5-HT receptors demonstrated after chronic antidepressant treatment (de

Montigny and Aghajanian, 1978) the binding of [^{3}H]-5-HT to 5-HT receptors is decreased after chronic administration of MAOIs but unchanged after repeated administration of tricyclics (Lucki and Frazer, 1982). The findings of Aprison's group would also suggest that fluoxetine would either possess no antidepressant activity or might even aggravate depression, whereas available clinical findings suggest that fluoxetine is active as an antidepressant (Cohn, 1983).

Clonidine-Induced Behavioural Depression

Clonidine is an alpha-adrenergic receptor stimulant which is thought to act preferentially at presynaptic receptor sites, thereby reducing the release of NA. In addition to its marked cardiovascular effects, clonidine causes hypothermia, analgesia and marked sedation. This latter effect, which is probably related to a decrease in central NA activity, has incited several authors to use clonidine-induced hypoactivity as a test model for antidepressant drugs. The model would appear to be of particular interest for detecting mianserin-like drugs because mianserin is thought to act through a specific inhibition of presynaptic alpha-adrenergic receptors (Robson et al., 1978) and is almost without effect in most classical tests for antidepressant activity. Robson et al. (1978) reported that mianserin antagonised clonidine-induced decreases in conditioned avoidance behaviour, and other authors have described antagonism of clonidine-induced hypoactivity by mianserin and also by tricyclic antidepressants and MAOIs (Gower and Marriott, 1980; Green et al., 1982; Kostowski and Malatynska, 1983; Passarelli and Scotti de Carolis, 1983). Repeated treatment with tricyclics is more effective than a single treatment in reversing the sedative and EEG effects of clonidine, as is also true with ECS (Heal et al., 1981; Passarelli and Scotti de Carolis, 1983). Unfortunately, conflicting results have also been reported in which clonidine-induced decreases in locomotor activity of self-stimulation behaviour could not be antagonised by mianserin (Delini Stula et al., 1979; Hunt et al., 1981) or other antidepressants (Passarelli and Scotti de Carolis, 1983; von Voigtlander et al., 1978) after acute or chronic administration, although von Voigtlander et al. (1978) reported antagonism of clonidine-induced hypothermia after chronic but not acute antidepressant treatment. In view of these contradictory findings it is too early to judge whether clonidine-induced hypoactivity could serve as a valid model or a useful test for antidepressant activity.

Neuroleptic-Induced Sedation and Catalepsy

The most prominent behavioural effects of neuroleptics are a decrease in spontaneous activity and, at higher doses, production of catalepsy. Antagonism of these effects has been used by some authors as a test for antidepressant activity. Indeed, the catalepsy induced by chlorpromazine, prochlorperazine or chlorprothixene is more potently antagonised by tricyclics and MAOIs than that induced by reserpine (Zetler, 1963). Amphetamine is also active in this model whereas neuroleptics and minor tranquillisers are not (Zetler, 1963). Although this model may possess sensitivity and selectivity at least equal to that of some reserpine models, it has not been widely used in preclinical pharmacology. This is perhaps surprising because neuroleptics, like reserpine-like compounds, have occasionally been associated with depressive symptoms in man (Helmchen and Hippius, 1967).

Behavioural Depression after Amphetamine Withdrawal

Acute treatment with amphetamine causes release of catecholamines and stimulation of motor activity whereas long-term treatment leads to eventual catecholamine depletion; marked decreases in motor activity are observed when amphetamine is withdrawn (Kokkinidis et al., 1980; Leith and Barrett, 1976; Lynch and Leonard, 1978; Seltzer and Tongre, 1975). Amphetamine withdrawal after chronic abuse has also been associated with signs of depression in man (Jaffe, 1980). In animals previously submitted to repeated amphetamine treatment, post-amphetamine decreases in motor activity (Lynch and Leonard, 1978; Seltzer and Tongre, 1975) and self-stimulation behaviour (Kokkinidis et al., 1980) have been counteracted by amitriptyline, imipramine, mianserin and pargyline after acute, but particularly after repeated, administration. Although these findings must be extended, the amphetamine withdrawal model would appear to be promising, especially as it does not depend directly on a drug-drug interaction.

Other Pharmacological Models

This final section briefly mentions several empirically based pharmacological tests which are currently used for the detection of antidepressant activity in novel compounds. These test models differ from those described in the previous sections in that they make no attempt, implicit or explicit, to imitate depressive illness. For this reason it is doubtful whether they can be considered as models at all, but they have none the less been found useful for characterising the pharmacological activity of potential antidepressants. Included among these test models are the mouse-killing behaviour (Vogel, 1975), passive avoidance deficits in bulbectomised rats (Cairncross et al., 1978), kindled amygdaloid convulsions (Babington, 1977) and apomorphine-induced hypothermia (Puech et al., 1981), together with the potentiation by antidepressants of the effects of yohimbine, amphetamine and various biogenic amines--DA, NA and 5-HT (Sanghvi and Gershon, 1977). For a more detailed discussion of these models see Porsolt (1983a).

Major risks of these models are that they are either too closely predicated on existing hypotheses about the origins of depression (e.g. the amine potentiation tests) or, at the other extreme, are based on what may be merely fortuitous pharmacological relationships (e.g. mouse-killing, bulbectomy-induced passive avoidance deficits). On the other hand, it is interesting to note that three of these models (kindled amygdaloid convulsions, mouse-killing, bulbectomy) directly implicate a role for the amygdala which is consistent with certain notions concerning the neuro-anatomical locus of dysfunction in depressive illness (see Jalfre and Porsolt, 1984).

Animal Models of Mania

Introduction

In contrast to the multitude of models which have been proposed for depression, there have been relatively few specific attempts to model mania in animals. This is probably because mania has a much lower incidence than the various forms of depression and causes less direct suffering to the individuals concerned (Weissman and Boyd, 1983). Animal models of mania have been extensively reviewed by Murphy (1977) and Robbins and Sahakian (1980), and only the most prominent ones will be dealt with here. As mentioned in the Introduction to this chapter, certain aspects of mania, for example expansiveness, flight of ideas and pressure of speech, would be difficult to translate into animal terms. Other aspects such as hyperactivity and irritability would appear to present less of a problem. Robbins and Sahakian (1980) have ingeniously proposed that euphoria or elation could be regarded operationally as a reduction in the threshold for reinforcement or reward, but the validity of this proposition requires rigorous testing in man. A more indirect approach would be to study the behavioural effects in animals of treatments known to induce euphoria in man.

As with depression models, a major criterion for evaluating the validity of models of mania is the specificity with which they respond to treatments known to reduce mania in man. This problem is perhaps more simple for mania than for depression because at present there appears to be only one specific antimanic treatment, lithium (Deniker et al., 1980). Other treatments, including neuroleptics, AMPT, PCPA, physostigmine, and, more recently, carbamazepine have been used but their efficacy and, in particular, their specificity have not been clearly established. Another approach would be to study the effects of agents known to precipitate or aggravate mania in man (e.g. tricyclic and MAOI antidepressants or sleep deprivation) to see whether they potentiate the behavioural phenomena in animals.

Drug-Induced Hyperactivity

Hyperactivity can be induced by many drug treatments including psychostimulants (either alone or in combination with minor tranquillisers or anticholinergics), morphine, MAOIs, monoamine precursors (either alone or in combination with MAOIs), combinations of antidepressants with reserpine-like compounds, and lysergic acid (LSD). Only some of these have specifically been proposed as models of mania and are dealt with in more detail below.

Antidepressant/Reserpine Combinations. In one of the earliest animal models of mania, Matussek and Linsmayer (1968) reported that the hyperactivity induced in rats by desipramine followed by Ro 4-1284 could be antagonised by prior treatment with lithium, with a more marked effect after chronic lithium treatment. That hyperactivity can be induced by combining an antidepressant with a depressogenic agent is interesting because it seems to provide an animal analogue of antidepressant-induced switches to mania. Amphetamine, however, also antagonised desipramine + Ro 4-1284 hyperactivity, a paradoxical finding, and subsequent experiments have not confirmed the antagonism by lithium of hyperactivity induced by combinations of reserpine-like agents with tricyclic (d'Encarnacao and Anderson, 1970) or MAOI antidepressants (Furukawa et al., 1975).

Amphetamine-Induced Hyperactivity. Amphetamine and related compounds increase locomotor activity and at higher doses induce stereotyped behaviour. In man in addition to their psychomotor activating effect they can also cause marked euphoria. From their review of the available literature Robbins and Sahakian (1980) concluded that the hyperactivity induced by amphetamine can be antagonised by lithium but that this is not the case with the stereotyped behaviour which, if anything, is enhanced. Neuroleptics antagonise both effects of amphetamine (Kreiskott, 1980). These findings are interesting because on the one hand they suggest a dissociation between hyperactivity and stereotyped behaviour, which is traditionally thought to model schizophrenia, and on the other hand a dissociation between the effects of lithium, a relatively specific antimanic agent, and neuroleptics, which are used to treat both schizophrenia and mania (Deniker et al., 1980). A further link between amphetamine-induced hyperactivity and mania is provided by the observation described in a previous section that withdrawal of amphetamine after chronic treatment induces a depression-like state in man and in animals, suggesting, as in human bipolar illness, an intimate relation between the two states. In addition to the above effects, amphetamine has been shown to enhance the reinforcing properties of electrical brain stimulation (Liebman and Segal, 1976), which is consistent with the notion of Robbins and Sahakian (1980) that thresholds for reward are lowered in mania; it should be pointed out, however, that lithium did not antagonise this effect of amphetamine. The effects of amphetamine can be potentiated by most classical antidepressants (Moller Nielsen, 1980), suggesting a parallel with the clinical capacity of these drugs to aggravate mania. Finally, experiments in depressed patients have shown that amphetamine-induced euphoria can be attenuated by treatment with lithium (Van Kammen and Murphy, 1975). Taken together, these findings suggest that amphetamine-induced hyperactivity represents a potential model of mania which deserves further detailed attention.

Morphine-Induced Hyperactivity. Another pharmacological agent which possesses clear euphoric action in man is morphine. Acute administration of morphine to animals induces marked hyperactivity which differs from amphetamine-induced hyperactivity by the presence of a greater reactivity to environmental stimulation ('irritability'?) and rapid transitions between bursts of locomotion and periods of sedation. Like amphetamine, morphine reduces the threshold for rewarding electrical brain stimulation (Esposito and Kornetsky, 1977). Hyperactivity and the change in the self-stimulation threshold have both been reported to be antagonised by lithium (Carroll and Sharp, 1971; Liebman and Segal, 1976), although negative findings have also been described (Sanghvi and Gershon, 1973). Hyperactivity is also antagonised, however, by the narcotic antagonist nalorphine (Carroll and Sharp, 1972) which is not reputed to possess antimanic effects in man. Furthermore, repeated administration of morphine leads to the development of tolerance, with marked withdrawal symptoms when the drug is stopped. It is not clear how these changes might find direct clinical parallels. Finally, one study in man (Jasinski et al., 1977) showed that lithium was ineffective in blocking morphine-induced euphoria, throwing doubt on the relevance of this phenomenon as an example of mania.

Brain Stimulation Models

Electrical stimulation of the brain in man can produce elation, flight of ideas, pressure of speech and hypersexual behaviour (Delgado, 1976), all of which bear a clear resemblance to mania. Thus, behaviour induced by electrical brain stimulation could be considered a potential model of mania. Non-contingent brain stimulation should not, however, be confused with intracerebral self-stimulation behaviour where the stimulation is a consequence of a particular behaviour and serves as a reinforcement, although changes in the threshold for ICSS may sometimes provide evidence that a manic-like state has been induced (see above). Low level electrical brain stimulation produces in animals a variety of effects including increased activity and consummatory behaviour (Valenstein, 1976) and neurological symptoms such as convulsions (Babington, 1977), particularly after repeated testing ('kindling'). The behaviours elicited appear to be frequently of a repetitive, stereotyped nature, recalling more the effects of high doses of amphetamine. Electrically induced behavioural changes do not appear to have been much investigated with drugs, in particular lithium.

Brain Lesion Models

Although mania as occurring in manic-depressive illness has not been associated with brain damage, the manic-like behaviour sometimes observed in patients subjected to leucotomy suggests that the behavioural syndromes resulting from certain brain lesions may serve as potential models of mania. Lesions to various brain areas (frontal cortex, hippocampus, caudate nucleus, globus pallidus, nucleus accumbens, ventral tegmental area, and the raphe nucleus) can all result in heightened activity (see Robbins and Sahakian, 1980), but a detailed pharmacological investigation, particularly with lithium, does not appear to be available. Another syndrome is induced by lesions to the septum, where animals, although not hyperactive, show marked irritability and hyperreactivity to environmental stimulation. Although the septal syndrome appears to be antagonised by lithium (Mukherjee and Pradhan, 1976), it is also antagonised by many other psychotropic compounds, including neuroleptics, minor tranquillisers, antidepressants, analgesics and anticholinergics (Decsi and Nagy, 1975), suggesting that the syndrome is by no means specific.

Receptor Hypersensitivity Models

Neuronal receptors can be rendered hypersensitive by continued pharmacological blockade or by destruction of afferent nerve terminals. Behaviourally, receptor hypersensitivity is indicated by an increased sensitivity to receptor agonists or to environmental stimuli ('irritability'). Recently two models of receptor hypersensitivity have been proposed and have been found sensitive to the effects of lithium.
    Pert et al. (1978) rendered rat DA receptors hypersensitive by administering haloperidol over a three-week period, followed by challenge with apomorphine and then sacrifice for estimation of DA receptor binding. Concurrent treatment with lithium not only decreased subsequent hypersensitivity to apomorphine but prevented the increase in $[^3H]$-spiroperidol binding observed after pretreatment

with haloperidol alone. Petty and Sherman (1981) induced catecholamine receptor hypersensitivity by intraventricular injection of 6-hydroxydopamine, a neurotoxin which specifically destroys catecholamine nerve terminals. The resulting hyperreactivity to electric footshock was prevented by chronic lithium, ECS and chlorpromazine, but was enhanced by imipramine.

These findings are only at a preliminary stage but appear worthy of further investigation, particularly concerning the apparently prophylactic effects observed with lithium.

Positive Contrast Effects

One class of behavioural phenomena which initially appeared promising as potential models for 'elation' and 'depression' are the so-called positive and negative contrast effects observed when animals are suddenly subjected to a change in the density or quality of reinforcement. In a typical example (Baltzer et al., 1979) rats were trained on a bar-pressing task and on some days received large rewards (4 pellets) and on other days small rewards (1 pellet). During each test session the animals were subjected to brief periods where the other reinforcement condition was instated. Sudden increases in the density of reinforcement caused marked increases in the rate of responding (positive contrast), whereas sudden decreases caused depression of responding (negative contrast). Preliminary pharmacological results indicated that the tricyclic derivative maprotiline enhanced positive contrast ('elation') whereas positive contrast was reduced by chlorpromazine, amylobarbitone and two benzodiazepines (chlordiazepoxide, diazepam). Imipramine and the type B MAOI pargyline were without effect on positive contrast, but imipramine, as well as amylobarbitone and the two benzodiazepines, reduced negative contrast ('depression'). Although lithium was not tested, these pharmacological findings suggest that, contrary to initial hopes, positive and negative contrast phenomena do not respond in a predictable way to agents which could be expected to enhance or decrease manic or depressive behaviour.

Conclusion

From the above brief review it is apparent that of the several models proposed only a few can be retained as viable models of mania and that considerable further testing is required before establishing their relative validity or usefulness. Although amphetamine-induced hyperactivity, but not stereotypy, satisfies many of the required criteria, it is evident that not all forms of drug-induced hyperactivity are equivalent. One promising line of research would be the investigation of behavioural phenomena occurring when treatment with potentially depressogenic agents is stopped, which could provide a kind of mirror image to the depression-like behaviour occurring after cessation or treatment with euphorigenic agents.

General Conclusions

The present chapter has critically reviewed existing animal models of affective disorder. From this review it is apparent that a wide variety of behavioural phenomena have been proposed as models and that many of them have been subjected to and have even satisfied several of the criteria for validity and utility. Where should we go from here?

One aspect which this review has not really addressed, but which is no doubt crucial for further advance in this field, is the heterogeneity of affective illness. Clinical heterogeneity has two consequences for the development of animal models. First, it is unlikely that any one model will ever represent all facets of the illness. Indeed, a major problem with existing models is that they all tend to model a limited range of symptoms. This is probably a necessary consequence of all modelling approaches but constitutes an important limitation. Recent discussions of this problem (Robbins and Sahakian, 1980; Carroll, 1983; Reite et al., 1983) have pleaded for a broadening of modelling approaches to cover a wider variety of core symptoms. In the case of depression, these should include loss of interest, anhedonia, disturbed psychomotor regulation, sadness, disturbances in sleep, appetite, cognition and biological rhythms in addition to biochemical and neurophysiological parameters. In the case of mania, in addition to hyperactivity, irritability and euphoria, symptoms should include sleeplessness, distractibility, impaired discrimination and decreased response to risk. Although most of the models discussed above touch some of these aspects, a multi-parameter approach has not yet been systematically adopted. A second consequence of clinical heterogeneity is that it is unlikely that any particular treatment will be universally effective. Indeed, there are suggestions in the clinical literature (e.g. Deniker et al., 1980) that certain kinds of depression respond differently to different kinds of antidepressant. Furthermore, there is always a variable proportion of patients who are therapy-resistant. Thus, to assume, as the present review implicitly does, that compounds can be classified as either effective or ineffective represents a rather gross oversimplification. Unfortunately, after 25 years of clinical use of antidepressant and antimanic agents, firm clinical evidence which could guide a more selective approach in pharmacology is not as yet available.

A particular weakness of presently available models of depression is that they appear mainly to model reactive rather than endogenous depression. As yet no examples of apparently spontaneous depression in animals have been described with cyclic or even bipolar characteristics. On the other hand, there have been experiments which report strain differences in susceptibility to inducers, and marked individual differences have also been observed in primates. It is possible that the distinction reactive/endogenous is somewhat artificial and that there really exists a continuum on which some individuals are particularly susceptible to life events which for others are insignificant (Paykel, 1983). If this is true, one potentially fruitful line of research would be selective breeding of animals found sensitive to the inducing conditions of a particular model. Another possible research direction would be the selection of animal species which clearly exhibit affective behaviours such as sadness and joy.

I should like to conclude this chapter with a plea which is unusual in an article of this kind, a plea for the use of intuition, anecdotal evidence and even anthropomorphism in the search for newer and better animal models of affective illness. Although it is only infrequently acknowledged, most of the existing animal models, apart from non-imitative empirically based models, started from rather casual observations of animal behaviour with a concerted attempt by the observer to 'understand' the behaviour in terms of the circumstances which provoked it. What has characterised the scientific development of these models is their subsequent subjection to rigorous testing procedures to establish their relative validity. In other words, it is not the source of the idea which is important but the manner in which, afterwards, the idea is put to experimental test. Without the judicious use of intuition and anthropomorphism it is doubtful whether many of the models presently under investigation would ever have come into existence.

Acknowledgements

I thank Dr. Maurice Jalfre for critically reading the manuscript and Miss Francoise Latour for typing the text.

References

Abramson, L. Y., Seligman, M. E. P., and Teasdale, J. D. (1978) Learned helplessness in humans: critique and reformulation. J. Abnorm. Psychol. **87**, 49-74.

Anisman, H., Irwin, J., and Sklar, L. S. (1979a) Deficits of escape performance following catecholamine depletion: implications for behavioral deficits induced by uncontrollable stress. Psychopharmacology **64**, 163-170.

Anisman, H., Remington, G., and Sklar, L. S. (1979b) Effect of inescapable shock on subsequent escape performance: catecholaminergic mediation of response initiation and maintenance. Psychopharmacology **61**, 107-124.

Anisman, H. and Sklar, L. S. (1979) Catecholamine depletion in mice upon re-exposure to stress: mediation of the escape deficits produced by inescapable shock. J. Comp. Physiol. Psychol. **93**, 610-625.

Aprison, M. H., Takahashi, R., and Tachiki, K. (1978) Hypersensitive serotonergic receptors involved in clinical depression--a theory. In: Neuropharmacology and Behavior (Haber, B. and Aprison, M. H., eds), Plenum, New York, pp. 23-53.

Babington, R. G. (1977) The pharmacology of kindling. In: Animal Models in Psychiatry and Neurology (Hanin, I. and Usdin, E., eds), Pergamon Press, Oxford, pp. 141-149.

Baltzer, V., Huber, H., and Weiskrantz, L. (1979) Effects of various drugs on behavioral contrast using a double-crossover procedure. Behav. Neur. Biol. **27**, 330-341.

Bareggi, S. R., Markey, K., and Paoletti, R. (1978) Effects of amphetamine, electrical stimulation and stress on endogenous MOPEG-SO$_4$ levels in rat brain. Pharmacol. Res. Commun. **10**, 65-73.

Bein, H. J. (1978) Prejudices in pharmacology and pharmacotherapy: reserpine as a model for experimental research in depression. Pharmakopsychiat. Neuro-psychopharmakol. **11**, 289-293.

Betin, C., de Feudis, F. V., Blavet, N., and Clostre, F. (1982) Further characterization of the behavioral despair test in mice: positive effects of convulsants. Physiol. Behav. **28**, 307-311.

Borsini, F., Bendotti, C., Velkov, V., Rech, R., and Samanin, R. (1981) Immobility test: effects of 5-hydroxytryptaminergic drugs and role of catecholamines in the activity of some antidepressants. J. Pharm. Pharmacol. 33, 33-37.

Bowlby, J. (1977) The making and breaking of affectional bonds. I. Aetiology and psychopathology in the light of attachment theory. Brit. J. Psychiatry 130, 201-210.

Brown, L., Rosellini, R. A., Samuels, O. B., and Riley, E. P. (1982) Evidence for a serotonergic mechanism of the learned helplessness phenomenon. Pharmacol. Biochem. Behav. 17, 877-883.

Browne, R. G. (1979) Effects of antidepressants and anticholinergics in a mouse 'behavioural despair' test. Eur. J. Pharmacol. 58, 331-334.

Cairncross, K. O., Cox, B., Forster, C., and Wren, A. F. (1978) A new model for the detection of antidepressant drugs: olfactory bulbectomy in the rat compared with existing models. J. Pharmacol. Meth. 1, 131-143.

Carroll, B. J. (1983) Neurobiologic dimensions of depression and mania. In: The Origins of Depression: Current Concepts and Approaches (Angst, J., ed.), Springer Verlag, Berlin, pp. 163-186.

Carroll, B. J. and Sharp, P. T. (1971) Rubidium and lithium: opposite effects on amine-mediated excitement. Science 172, 1355-1357.

Carroll, B. J. and Sharp, P. T. (1972) Monoamine mediation of the morphine-induced activation of mice. Brit. J. Pharmacol. 46, 124-139.

Cohn, J. B. (1983) Fluoxetine hydrochloride in the treatment of major depressive disorder. Proc. 7th World Congr. Psychiat., Vienna, Abstr. F662.

Colpaert, F. C., Lennaerts, F. M., Niemegeers, C. J. E., and Janssen, P. A. J. (1975) A critical study on Ro-4-1284 antagonism in mice. Arch. Int. Pharmacodyn. Ther. 215, 40-90.

Decsi, L. and Nagy, J. (1975) Septum-lesioned rats in pharmacological investigations: a re-evaluation. Acta Physiol. Acad. Sci. Hung. 46, 71-78.

Delgado, J. M. R. (1976) New orientations in brain stimulation in man. In: Brain-Stimulation Reward (Wauquier, A. and Rolls, E. T., eds), North Holland/Elsevier, New York, pp. 481-503.

Delini Stula, A., Baumann, P., and Buch, O. (1979) Depression of exploratory activity by clonidine in rats as a model for the detection of relative pre- and post-synaptic central noradrenergic receptor selectivity of alpha-adrenolytic drugs. Naunyn Schmiedeberg's Arch. Pharmacol. 307, 115-

122.
de Montigny, C. and Aghajanian, G. K. (1978) Tricyclic antidepressants: long-term treatment increases responsivity of rat forebrain neurons to serotonin. Science 202, 1303-1306.

d'Encarnacao, P. S. and Anderson, K. (1970) Effects of lithium pretreatment on amphetamine and DMI tetrabenazine produced psychomotor behavior. Dis. Nerv. Sys. 31, 494-496.

Deniker, P., Ginestet, D., and Loo, H. (1980) Maniement des Medicaments Psychotropes, Doin Editeurs, Paris.

Esposito, R. and Kornetsky, C. (1977) Morphine lowering of self-stimulation thresholds: lack of tolerance with long-term administration. Science 195, 189-191.

Fielden, R. and Green, A. L. (1965) Validity of ptosis as a measure of the central depressant action of reserpine. J. Pharm. Pharmacol. 17, 185-186.

Frances, H., Poncelet, M., Danti, S., Goldschmidt, P., and Simon, P. (1983) Psychopharmacological profile of clenbuterol. Drug Dev. Res. 3, 349-356.

Furukawa, T., Ushizima, I., and Ono, N. (1975) Modification by lithium of behavioral responses to methamphetamine and tetrabenazine. Psychopharmacology (Berl.) 42, 243-248.

Garattini, S. and Jori, A. (1967) Interactions between imipramine-like drugs and reserpine on body temperature. In: Antidepressant Drugs (Garattini, S. and Dukes, M. N. G., eds), Excerpta Medica Foundation, Amsterdam, pp. 179-193.

Garzon, J. and del Rio, J. (1981) Hyperactivity induced in rats by long-term isolation: further studies on a new animal model for the detection of antidepressants. Eur. J. Pharmacol. 74, 287-294.

Garzon, J., Fuentes, J. A., and del Rio, J. (1979) Antidepressants selectively antagonize the hyperactivity induced in rats by long-term isolation. Eur. J. Pharmacol. 59, 293-296.

Glazer, H. I. and Weiss, J. M. (1976) Long-term and transitory interference effects. J. Exp. Psychol. Anim. Behav. Proc. 2, 191-201.

Gorka, Z. and Wojtasik, E. (1980) The effect of antidepressants on behavioral despair in rats. Pol. J. Pharmacol. Pharm. 32, 463-468.

Gorka, Z., Wojtasik, E., Kwiatek, H., and Maj, J. (1979) Action of serotonomimetics in the behavioral despair test in rats. Commun. Psychopharmacol. **3**, 133-136.

Gouret, C., Mocquet, G., Coston, A., and Raynaud, G. (1977) Interaction de divers psychotropes avec cinq effets de la reserpine chez la souris et chez le chat. J. Pharmacol. (Paris) **8**, 330-350.

Gower, A. J. and Marriott, A. S. (1980) The inhibition of clonidine-induced sedation in the mouse by antidepressant drugs. Brit. J. Pharmacol. **69**, 287P-288P.

Green, A. R., Heal, D. J., Lister, S., and Molyneux, S. (1982) The effect of acute and repeated desmethylimipramine administration on clonidine-induced hypoactivity in rats. Brit. J. Pharmacol. **75**, 33P.

Greenwood, D. T. (1975) Animal pharmacology of viloxazine (Vivalan). J. Intern. Med. Res. **3**, Suppl. 3, 18-30.

Gunnar, M. R., Gonzalez, C. A., Goodlin, B. L., and Levine, S. (1981) Behavioral and pituitary-adrenal responses during a prolonged separation period in infant rhesus macaques. Psychoneuroendocrinology **6**, 66-75.

Harlow, H. F. and Harlow, M. K. (1965) The affectional systems. In: Behavior of Non-Human Primates, vol. 2 (Schrier, A. M., Harlow, H. F., and Stollnitz, F., eds), Academic Press, New York, pp. 287-334.

Harlow, H. F. and McKinney, W. T. (1971) Non-human primates and psychoses. J. Aut. Child. Schiz. **1**, 368-375.

Hatotani, N., Nomura, J., Inoue, K., and Kitayama, I. (1979) Psychoendocrine model of depression. Psychoneuroendocrinology **4**, 155-172.

Hatotani, N., Nomura, J., and Kitayama, I. (1981) Changes of monoamines in the animal model for depression. Proc. 3rd World Congr. Biol. Psychiatry, Stockholm, Abstract n°: S154.

Hatotani, N., Nomura, J., Yamaguchi, T., and Kitayama, I. (1977) Clinical and experimental studies on the pathogenesis of depression. Psychoneuroendocrinology **2**, 115-130.

Heal, D. J., Akagi, H., Bowdler, J. M., and Green, A. R. (1981) Repeated electroconvulsive shock attenuates clonidine-induced hypoactivity in rodents. Eur. J. Pharmacol. **75**, 231-237.

Hellhammer, D. (1983) Learned helplessness: an animal model revisited. In: The Origins of Depression: Current Concepts and Approaches (Angst, J., ed.), Springer Verlag, Berlin, pp. 147-162.

Helmchen, H., and Hippius, H. (1967) Depressive syndrome im verlauf neuroleptischer therapie. Ner-

venarzt **38**, 455-458.
Hinde, R. A. and Spencer-Booth, Y. (1971) Effects of brief separations from mothers on rhesus monkeys. Science **173**, 111-118.
Hofer, M. A. (1975) Studies on how early maternal separation produces behavioral change in young rats. Psychosom. Med. **37**, 245-264.
Hoffmann, I. (1973) 8-Amino-2-methyl-4-phenyl-1,2,3,4,-tetrahydroisoquinoline, a new antidepressant. Arzneim. Forsch. **23**, 45-50.
Howard, J. L., Soroko, F. E., and Cooper, B. R. (1981) Empirical behavioral models of depression with an emphasis on tetrabenazine antagonism. In: Antidepressants: Neurochemical, Behavioral and Clinical Perspectives (Enna, S. J., Malick, J. B., and Richelson, E., eds), Raven Press, New York, pp. 107-120.
Hrdina, P. D., von Kulmiz, P., and Stretch, R. (1979) Pharmacological modification of experimental depression in infant macaques. Psychopharmacology **64**, 89-93.
Hunt, G. E., Atrens, D. M., and Johnson, G. F. S. (1981) The tetracyclic antidepressant mianserin: evaluation of its blockade of pre-synaptic alpha-adrenoceptors in a self-stimulation model using clonidine. Eur. J. Pharmacol. **70**, 59-63.
Jaffe, J. H. (1980) Drug addiction and drug abuse. In: The Pharmacological Basis of Therapeutics (Gilman, A. G., Goodman, L. S., and Gilman, A., eds), MacMillan, New York, pp. 535-584.
Jalfre, M. and Porsolt, R. D. (1984) Antidepressants and the limbic system. In: Psychopharmacology of the Limbic System (Zarifian, E. and Trimble, M., eds), Wiley, New York (in press).
Jalfre, M., Monachon, M. A., and Haefely, W. (1970) Pharmacological modification of benzoquinolizine-induced geniculate spikes. Experientia **26**, 691.
Jasinsky, D. R., Nutt, J. G., Haertzen, C. A., Griffith, J. D., and Bunney, W. E. (1977) Lithium: effects on subjective functioning and morphine-induced euphoria. Science **195**, 582-584.
Kastin, A., Scollan, E. L., Ehrensing, R. H., Schally, A. V., and Coy, D. H. (1978) Enkephalin and other peptides reduce passiveness. Pharmacol. Biochem. Behav. **9**, 515-519.
Katz, R. J. (1981) Animal models and human depressive disorders. Neurosci. Biobehav. Rev. **5**, 231-277.
Katz, R. J. (1982) Animal model of depression: pharmacological sensitivity of a hedonic deficit. Pharmacol. Biochem. Behav. **16**, 965-982.

Katz, R. J. (1983) Stress, conflict and depression. In: The Origins of Depression: Current Concepts and Approaches (Angst, J., ed.), Springer Verlag, Berlin, pp. 121-132.
Kaufmann, I. C. and Rosenblum, L. A. (1967) Depression in infant monkeys separated from their mothers. Science 155, 1030-1031.
Kitada, Y., Miyauchi, T., Satoh, A., and Satoh, S. (1981) Effects of antidepressants in the rat forced swimming test. Eur. J. Pharmacol. 72, 145-152.
Kokkinidis, L., Zacharko, R. M., and Predy, P. A. (1980) Post-amphetamine depression of self-stimulation responding from the substantia nigra: reversal by tricyclic antidepressants. Pharmacol. Biochem. Behav. 13, 379-383.
Kornetsky, C. (1977) Animal models: promises and problems. In: Animal Models in Psychiatry and Neurology (Hanin, I. and Usdin, E., eds), Pergamon Press, Oxford, pp. 1-7.
Kostowski, W. and Malatynska, E. (1983) Antagonism of behavioural depression produced by clonidine in the mongolian gerbil: a potential screening test for antidepressant drugs. Psychopharmacology 79, 203-208.
Kraemer, G. W., Ebert, M., Lake, C. R., and McKinney, W. T. (1983a) Interactive effects of drugs and social separation on CNS catecholamine metabolism in rhesus monkeys. Proc. 5th Catecholamine Symposium, Goteborg, Abstract n° 276.
Kraemer, G. W., Ebert, M. H., and McKinney, W. T. (1983b) Separation models and depression. In: The Origins of Depression: Current Concepts and Approaches (Angst, J., ed.), Springer Verlag, Berlin, pp. 133-146.
Kraemer, G. W., Lin, D. H., Moran, E. C., and McKinney, W. T. (1981) Effects of alcohol on the despair response to peer separation in rhesus monkeys. Psychopharmacology 73, 307-310.
Kraemer, G. W. and McKinney, W. T. (1979) Interactions of pharmacological agents which alter biogenic amine metabolism and depression. J. Affec. Disorders 1, 33-54.
Kreiskott, H. (1980) Behavioral pharmacology of antipsychotics. In: Psychotropic Agents, Part I: Antipsychotics and Antidepressants (Hoffmeister, F. and Stille, G., eds), Springer Verlag, Berlin, pp. 59-88.
Kuczenski, R. (1977) Differential effects of reserpine and tetrabenazine on rat striatal synaptosomal dopamine biosynthesis and synaptosomal dopa-

mine pools. J. Pharmacol. Exp. Ther. **201**, 357-367.

Leith, N. J. and Barrett, R. J. (1976) Amphetamine and the reward system: evidence for tolerance and post-drug depression. Psychopharmacology **46**, 19-25.

Leshner, A. I., Remler, H., Biegon, A., and Samuel, D. (1979) Desmethylimipramine (DMI) counteracts learned helplessness in rats. Psychopharmacology **66**, 207-208.

Lewis, J. K. and McKinney, W. T. (1976) The effect of electrically induced convulsions on the behavior of normal and abnormal rhesus monkeys. Dis. Nerv. Sys. **37**, 687-693.

Lewis, J. K., McKinney, W. T., Young, L. D., and Kraemer, G. W. (1976) Mother-infant separation in rhesus monkeys as a model of human depression. A reconsideration. Arch. Gen. Psychiatry **33**, 699-705.

Liebman, J. M. and Segal, D. S. (1976) Lithium differentially antagonises self-stimulation facilitated by morphine and (+)-amphetamine. Nature (Lond.) **260**, 161-163.

Lucki, I. and Frazer, A. (1982) Prevention of the serotonin syndrome in rats by repeated administration of monoamine oxidase inhibitors but not by tricyclic antidepressants. Psychopharmacology **77**, 205-211.

Lynch, M. A. and Leonard, B. E. (1978) Effect of chronic amphetamine administration on the behaviour of rats in the open field apparatus: reversal of post-withdrawal depression by two antidepressants. J. Pharm. Pharmacol. **30**, 798-799.

Maier, S. F. and Seligman, M. E. P. (1976) Learned helplessness: theory and evidence. J. Exp. Psychol. **105**, 3-46.

Maj, J. (1979) Pharmacological spectrum of some new antidepressants. In: Neuropsychopharmacology (Dumont, G., ed.), Pergamon Press, Oxford, pp. 161-170.

Matussek, N. and Linsmayer, M. (1968) The effect of lithium and amphetamine on desmethylimipramine--Ro 4-1284 induced motor hyperactivity. Life Sci. **7**, 371-375.

McKinney, W. T. (1977) Biobehavioral models of depression in monkeys. In: Animal Models in Psychiatry and Neurology (Usdin, E. and Hanin, I., eds), Pergamon Press, Oxford, pp. 117-126.

McKinney, W. T. and Bunney, W. E. (1969) Animal model of depression. Review of evidence: implications for research. Arch. Gen. Psychiatry **21**,

240-248.
McKinney, W. T., Eising, R. G., Moran, E. C., Suomi, S. J., and Harlow, H. F. (1971) Effects of reserpine on the social behavior of rhesus monkeys. Dis. Nerv. Syst. 32, 735-741.
McKinney, W. T., Suomi, S. J., and Harlow, H. F. (1972) Repetitive peer separation of juvenile-age rhesus monkeys. Arch. Gen. Psychiatry 27, 200-203.
Mercier, J., Scotto, A. M., and Dessaigne, S. (1979) L'action desinhibitrice de certains neuroleptiques est-elle previsible experimentalement? C. R. Soc. Biol. 173, 788-796.
Mineka, S. and Suomi, S. J. (1978) Social separation in monkeys. Psychol. Bull. 85, 1376-1400.
Miyauchi, T., Kitada, Y., and Satoh, S. (1981) Effects of acutely and chronically administered antidepressants on the brain regional 3-methoxy-4-hydroxyphenylethyleneglycol sulphate in the forced swimming rat. Life Sci. 29, 1921-1928.
Moller Nielsen, I. V. (1980) Tricyclic antidepressants: general pharmacology. In: Psychotropic Agents, Part I: Antipsychotics and Antidepressants (Hoffmeister, F. and Stille, G., eds), Springer Verlag, Berlin, pp. 399-414.
Moran, E. C. and McKinney, W. T. (1975) Effects of chlorpromazine on the vertical chamber syndrome in rhesus monkeys. Arch. Gen. Psychiatry 32, 1409-1413.
Mukherjee, B. P. and Pradhan, S. N. (1976) Effects of lithium on septal hyperexcitability and muricidal behavior in rats. Res. Commun. Psychol. Psychiat. Behav. 1, 241-247.
Murphy, D. L. (1977) Animal models for mania. In: Animal Models in Psychiatry and Neurology (Hanin, I. and Usdin, E., eds), Pergamon Press, Oxford, pp. 211-226.
Nagayama, H., Hintgen, J. N., and Aprison, M. H. (1981) Post-synaptic action by four antidepressive drugs in an animal model of depression. Pharmacol. Biochem. Behav. 15, 125-130.
Nomura, S., Shimizu, J., Kinjo, M., Kametani, H., and Nakazawa, T. (1982) A new behavioural test for antidepressant drugs. Eur. J. Pharmacol. 83, 171-175.
Ogren, S. O., Fuxe, K., Agnati, L. F., Gustafsson, J. A., Jansson, G., and Holm, A. C. (1979) Re-evaluation of the indoleamine hypothesis of depression. Evidence for a reduction of functional activity of central 5-HT systems by antidepressant drugs. J. Neural Transm. 46, 85-103.

Panksepp, J., Herman, B. H., Vilberg, T., Bishop, P., and de Eskinazi, F. G. (1980a) Endogenous opioids and social behavior. Neurosci. Biobehav. Rev. **4**, 473-487.

Panksepp, J., Meeker, R., and Bean, N. J. (1980b) The neurochemical control of crying. Pharmacol. Biochem. Behav. **12**, 437-443.

Passarelli, F. and Scotti de Carolis, A. (1983) Effects of chronic treatment with imipramine, trazodone and electroshock on the behavioural and electroencephalographic modifications induced by clonidine in the rat. Neuropharmacology **22**, 785-789.

Paykel, E. S. (1983) Recent life events and depression. In: The Origins of Depression: Current Concepts and Approaches (Angst, J., ed.), Springer Verlag, Berlin, pp. 91-106.

Pert, A., Rosenblatt, J. E., Sivit, C., Pert, C. B., and Bunney, W. E. (1978) Long-term treatment with lithium prevents the development of dopamine receptor supersensitivity. Science **201**, 171-173.

Petty, F., Saquitne, J. L., and Sherman, A. D. (1982) Tricyclic antidepressant drug action correlates with its tissue levels in anterior neocortex. Neuropharmacology **21**, 475-477.

Petty, F. and Sherman, A. D. (1981) A pharmacologically pertinent animal model of mania. J. Affec. Disorders **3**, 381-387.

Porsolt, R. D. (1981) Behavioral despair. In: Antidepressants: Neurochemical, Behavioral and Clinical Perspectives (Enna, S. J., Malick, J. B., and Richelson, E., eds), Raven Press, New York, pp. 121-139.

Porsolt, R. D. (1983a) Pharmacological models of depression. In: The Origins of Depression: Current Concepts and Approaches (Angst, J., ed.), Springer Verlag, Berlin, pp. 313-330.

Porsolt, R. D. (1983b) Failure of repeated peer separations to induce depression in infant rhesus monkeys. Drug Dev. Res. **3**, 567-572.

Porsolt, R. D., Anton, G., Blavet, N., and Jalfre, M. (1978a) Behavioural despair in rats: a new model sensitive to antidepressant treatments. Eur. J. Pharmacol. **47**, 379-391.

Porsolt, R. D., Bertin, A., Blavet, N., Deniel, M., and Jalfre, M. (1979a) Immobility induced by forced swimming in rats: effects of agents which modify central catecholamine and serotonin activity. Eur. J. Pharmacol. **57**, 201-210.

Porsolt, R. D., Bertin, A., and Jalfre, M. (1977a) Behavioural despair in mice: a primary screening test for antidepressants. Arch. Int. Pharmacodyn. Ther. **229,** 327-336.

Porsolt, R. D., Bertin, A., and Jalfre, M. (1978b) Behavioural despair in rats and mice: strain differences and the effects of imipramine. Eur. J. Pharmacol. **51,** 291-294.

Porsolt, R. D., Deniel, M., and Jalfre, M. (1979b) Forced swimming in rats: hypothermia, immobility and the effects of imipramine. Eur. J. Pharmacol. **57,** 431-436.

Porsolt, R. D., Le Pichon, M., and Jalfre, M. (1977b) Depression: a new animal model sensitive to antidepressant treatments. Nature (Lond.) **266,** 730-732.

Porsolt, R. D., Roux, S., and Jalfre, M. (1984) The effects of imipramine on separation-induced vocalizations in young rhesus monkeys. Pharmacol. Biochem. Behav. (in press).

Przegalinski, E., Baran, L., and Kedrek, G. (1980) The central action of salbutamol, a beta-agonist with a potential antidepressant activity. Pol. J. Pharmacol. Pharm. **32,** 485-493.

Puech, A. J., Chermat, R., Poncelet, M., Doare, L., and Simon, P. (1981) Antagonism of hypothermia and behavioural response to apomorphine: a simple, rapid and discriminating test for screening antidepressants and neuroleptics. Psychopharmacology **75,** 84-91.

Quinn, G. P., Shore, P. A., and Brodie, B. B. (1959) Biochemical and pharmacological studies of Ro 1-9569 (tetrabenazine), a non-indole tranquillizing agent with reserpine-like effects. J. Pharmacol. Exp. Ther. **127,** 103-109.

Redmond, D. E., Maas, J. W., Kling, A., and Dekirmenjian, H. (1971) Changes in primate social behavior after treatment with alpha-methyl-para-tyrosine. Psychosom. Med. **33,** 97-113.

Reite, M. L., Anders, T. F., Greil, W., Hellhammer, D., Henn, F. A., Katz, R. J., Kaufmann, I. C., Kraemer, G. W., Linden, M., McGuire, M. T., McKinney, W. T., Nissen, G., and Porsolt, R. D. (1983) Animal models. In: The Origins of Depression: Current Concepts and Approaches (Angst, J., ed.), Springer Verlag, Berlin, pp. 405-423.

Reite, M. L. and Snyder, D. S. (1982) Physiology of maternal separation in a bonnet macaque. Am. J. Primatol. **2,** 115-120.

Rheingold, H. L. and Eckerman, C. O. (1971) Familiar, social and non-social stimuli and the kitten's response to a strange environment. Devel. Psychobiology **4**, 78-89.

Robbins, T. W. and Sahakian, B. J. (1980) Animal models of mania. In: Mania--an Enduring Concept (Belmaker, R. and van Praag, H. M., eds), Spectrum, New York, pp. 143-216.

Robson, R. D., Antonaccio, M. J., Saelens, J. K., and Liebman, J. (1978) Antagonism by mianserin and classical alpha-adrenoceptor blocking drugs of some cardiovascular and behavioral effects of clonidine. Eur. J. Pharmacol. **47**, 431-442.

Rogoz, Z., Skuza, G., and Sowinska, H. (1981) Effects of antihistaminic drugs in tests for antidepressant action. Pol. J. Pharmacol. Pharm. **33**, 321-335.

Rubin, R. T. and Poland, R. E. (1983) Neuroendocrine function in depression. In: The Origins of Depression: Current Concepts and Approaches (Angst, J., ed.), Springer Verlag, Berlin, pp. 205-220.

Ruther, E., Ackenheil, M., and Matussek, N. (1966) Beitrag zum noradrenalin und serotonin stoffwechsel im rattenhirn nach stresszustanden. Arzneim. Forsch. **16**, 261-263.

Sanghvi, I. S. and Gershon, S. (1973) Rubidium and lithium: evaluation as antidepressant and antimanic agents. Res. Commun. Chem. Pathol. Pharmacol. **6**, 293-300.

Sanghvi, I. S. and Gershon, S. (1977) Animal test models for prediction of clinical antidepressant activity. In: Animal Models in Psychiatry and Neurology (Hanin, I. and Usdin, E., eds), Pergamon Press, Oxford, pp. 157-171.

Sansone, M. and Hano, J. (1979) Enhancement by chlordiazepoxide of the anticholinergic-induced locomotor stimulation in mice. Psychopharmacology **64**, 181-184.

Schildkraut, J. J. and Kety, S. S. (1967) Biogenic amines and emotion. Science **156**, 21-30.

Scott, J. P. (1975) Effects of psychotropic drugs on separation distress in dogs. In: Neuropsychopharmacology (Boissier, J. R., Hippius, H., and Pichot, P., eds), Excerpta Medica, Amsterdam, pp. 735-745.

Seay, B. and Harlow, H. F. (1965) Maternal separation in the rhesus monkey. J. Nerv. Ment. Dis. **140**, 434-441.

Seligman, M. E. P. (1975) Helplessness: On Depression, Development and Death, Freeman, San Francisco.

Seltzer, V. and Tongre, S. R. (1975) Methylamphetamine withdrawal as a model for the depressive state: antagonism of post-amphetamine depression by imipramine. J. Pharm. Pharmacol. 27, 16P.

Sherman, A. D., Allers, G. L., Petty, F., and Henn, F. A. (1979) A neuropharmacologically relevant animal model of depression. Neuropharmacology 18, 891-893.

Sherman, A. D. and Petty, F. (1980) Neurochemical basis of the action of antidepressants on learned helplessness. Behav. Neur. Biol. 30, 119-134.

Sherman, A. D. and Petty, F. (1982) Additivity of neurochemical changes in learned helplessness and imipramine. Behav. Neur. Biol. 35, 344-353.

Sherman, A. D., Saquitne, J. L., and Petty, F. (1982) Specificity of the learned helplessness model of depression. Pharmacol. Biochem. Behav. 16, 449-454.

Soroko, F. E., Mehta, N. B., Maxwell, R. A., Ferris, R. M., and Schroeder, D. H. (1977) Bupropion hydrochloride [(±)-alpha-t-butylamino-3-chloropropiophenone HCl]: a novel antidepressant agent. J. Pharm. Pharmacol. 29, 767-770.

Steru, L., Chermat, R., Thierry, B., and Simon, P. (1984) Tail suspension induced immobility: a new test for screening antidepressants in mice. Psychopharmacology (in press).

Stone, E. A. and Mendlinger, S. (1974) Effects of intraventricular amines on motor activity in hypothermic rats. Res. Commun. Chem. Pathol. Pharmacol. 7, 549-556.

Suomi, S. J. and Harlow, H. F. (1972) Depressive behavior in young monkeys subjected to vertical chamber confinement. J. Comp. Physiol. Psychol. 180, 11-18.

Suomi, S. J., Harolow, H. F., and Domek, C. J. (1970) Effect of repetitive infant-infant separation of young monkeys. J. Abnorm. Psychol. 76, 161-172.

Suomi, S. J., Kraemer, G. W., Baysinger, C. M., and Delizio, R. D. (1981) Inherited and experiential factors associated with individual differences in anxious behavior displayed by rhesus monkeys. In: Anxiety: New Research and Changing Concepts (Klein, D. F. and Rabkin, J., eds), Raven Press, New York, pp. 179-199.

Suomi, S. J., Seaman, S. F., Lewis, J. K., Delizio, R. D., and McKinney, W. T. (1978) Effects of imipramine treatment on separation-induced social disorders in rhesus monkeys. Arch. Gen. Psychi-

atry **35**, 321-325.
Valenstein, E. (1976) The interpretation of behavior evoked by brain stimulation. In: Brain-Stimulation Reward (Wauquier, A. and Rolls, E. T., eds), North Holland/Elsevier, New York, pp. 557-575.
Valzelli, L. (1973) The 'isolation syndrome' in mice. Psychopharmacology **31**, 305-320.
Van Kammen, D. P. and Murphy, D. L. (1975) Attenuation of the euphoriant and activating effects of d- and l-amphetamine by lithium carbonate treatment. Psychopharmacology **44**, 215-224.
Vogel, J. R. (1975) Antidepressants and mouse-killing. In: Industrial Pharmacology, Vol. 2: Antidepressants (Fielding, S. and Lal, H., eds), Futura, New York, pp. 99-112.
von Voigtlander, P. F., von Triezenberg, H. G., and Losey, E. G. (1978) Interactions between clonidine and antidepressant drugs: a method for identifying antidepressant-like agents. Neuropharmacology **17**, 375-381.
Wallach, M. B. and Hedley, L. R. (1979) The effects of antihistamines in a modified behavioral despair test. Commun. Psychopharmacol. **3**, 35-39.
Weiss, J. M., Goodman, P. A., Losito, B. G., Corrigan, S., Charry, J. M., and Bailey, W. H. (1981) Behavioural depression produced by an uncontrollable stressor: relationship to norepinephrine, dopamine and serotonin levels in various regions of rat brain. Brain Res. Rev. **3**, 167-205.
Weissman, M. M. and Boyd, J. H. (1983) The epidemiology of bipolar and nonbipolar depression: rates and risks. In: The Origins of Depression: Current Concepts and Approaches (Angst, J., ed.), Springer Verlag, Berlin, pp. 27-38.
Zebrowska-Lupina, I. (1980) Presynaptic alpha-receptors and the action of tricyclic antidepressant drugs in behavioural despair in rats. Psychopharmacology **71**, 169-172.
Zetler, G. (1963) Die antikataleptische wirksamkeit einiger antidepressiva (thymoleptika). Arzneim. Forsch. **13**, 103-109.

4.

OBSERVATIONS, REFLECTIONS AND SPECULATIONS ON THE CEREBRAL DETERMINANTS OF MOOD AND ON THE BILATERALLY ASYMMETRICAL DISTRIBUTIONS OF THE MAJOR NEUROTRANSMITTER SYSTEMS

P. Flor-Henry, M.D.

I will, in this chapter, review the general organisation of the neural systems determining mood states and attempt to integrate topographic aspects with the emerging knowledge on the asymmetrical distribution of the major neurotransmitter systems.
    It has been shown that in the mammalian and in the avian brain the left hemisphere is specialised for communicative functions and the right hemisphere for spatial and emotional (including sexual and aggressive) functions. From a general systems theory perspective, three functional principles are necessary and sufficient to account for the general characteristics of a linked double-brain system:
    1. Intra-hemispheric activation
    2. Contralateral inhibition
    3. Inter-hemispheric coupling
       (Denenberg, 1980, 1981)
    A general finding, invariant across several species (i.e. in rodents, chicks and in homo sapiens: see Flor-Henry, 1983a), demonstrates that emotionality, aggression and sexual arousal, all dependent on right hemispheric systems, are modulated by inhibitory influences originating in the left hemisphere. Neuro-hormonal interactions are of critical importance in the development of (some) lateralised neural assemblies as, for example, song control in the male canary is testosterone-dependent: the left syrinx is heavier and has a higher acetylcholine esterase content than the right syrinx, differences which disappear in the castrated male or which can be induced by testosterone in females thus made to vocalise. Here we have a left-brain-testosterone-cholinergic interaction.
    A dramatic example of right brain-catecholamine interaction is provided by Robinson (1979): lateralised cerebral infarcts were produced in the rat by

ligation of the right and left middle cerebral arteries. Rats with left brain infarcts showed no behavioral changes and no alterations in hemispheric and striatal catecholamine concentrations. Following right hemispheric infarcts a syndrome of emotional hyperactivity of 3 weeks duration supervened which was associated with a 30% reduction in hemispheric noradrenaline (NA) concentration (in both injured and non-injured cortices) and a 20% reduction in striatal dopamine (DA).

In male mice high fetal estrogen concentrations correlate with increased adult sexual activity and decreased aggression (vom Saal et al., 1983). However, in newborn female rats exposure of the left hypothalamus to estrogens (intrahypothalamic implants) results in defeminised development while exposure of the right hypothalamus to estrogens leads to masculinised behavior. Testosterone masculinises both male and female rodents (Nordeen and Yahr, 1982). The balance between androgens and estrogen has even structural neuroanatomical implications in the mammalian brain: posterior regions of the right hemisphere cortex of the male rat are thicker than in the female and, conversely, the homologous area in the left hemisphere of the female rat is larger. Ovariectomy after birth in female rats alters their cortical anatomy in the direction of the male rat (i.e. because of the absence of estrogens; hence adrenal cortex-derived androgens act unopposed; Diamond, 1980).

In humans a left hemisphere-testosterone interaction is suggested by the two independent studies of dextrals and sinistrals carried out by Geschwind and Behan (1982), who found that learning disabilities were 12 times more frequent in sinistrals than in dextrals and 3 times more common in their relatives. Further there was a significantly increased incidence of auto-immune disease in sinistrals (11%) compared to dextrals (4%). The link between the (male) susceptibility to learning disability, developmental dyslexia type and the correlated sinistrality and susceptibility to auto-immune disease (Hashimoto thyroiditis, ulcerative colitis and Coeliac disease) is thought to be testosterone supersensitivity which simultaneously slows the developmental pace of the left hemisphere (hence sinistrality) and suppresses fetal thymus activity and T lymphocytes. Geschwind remarks that the paradox that females rather than males are prone to auto-immune disorders can be explained by the fact that testosterone has been shown to suppress auto-immune diseases.

There are other curious associations between sinistrality and central neurotransmitter functions. For example, Buchsbaum (1977) in 375 normals reported that platelet monoamine oxidase (MAO) activity was reduced in normal, male sinistrals. This has quite recently been confirmed by von Knorring (1984, personal communication) in a large sample. Von Knorring and Oreland (1983) studied the personality correlates associated with high and low platelet MAO activity in an unselected sample consisting of 1,129, 18-year-old males, conscripted for military service. They confirmed the observations of Buchsbaum et al. (1976, 1980) relating low MAO activity to social extraversion, impulsivity, 'sensation-seeking behavior' and suicidal attempts. Similarly, in a study of a German rural population, Demisch et al. (1982) found in males a significant linear correlation between MAO activity and introversion. No such correlation could be established in women. In the large Swedish series, von Knorring 'very clearly demonstrates that left-handers have low platelet MAO activity'. It is thought that platelet MAO activity reflects cerebral serotonin turnover since positive correlations have been established between MAO activity and CSF 5-hydroxyindoleacetic acid (5-HIAA) (Oreland et al., 1981) and since associations have been found intracerebrally between serotonin (5-hydroxytryptamine, 5-HT) and MAO activity (Adolfsson et al., 1978).

Sai-Halasz et al. (1958) administered intravenous dimethyltryptamine to 30 experimental subjects, all physicians. They found a significant excess of transient left-sided neurological abnormalities: hyper-reflexia and Babinski. Subjectively, spatial illusions, disturbances of body schemata and subjective time, and euphoria were present. The mental symptoms induced by the short-lived hallucinogen occurred synchronously with the neurological signs. In view of the fact that serotonin is chemically so closely related to dimethyltryptamine, the right hemispheric lateralisation of serotoninergic systems, in a functional sense, is clearly demonstrated. If we recall that Gottfries et al. (1974) reported a correlation between the amplitude of evoked responses in the right hemisphere and CSF concentration of 5-HIAA, and that Laurian et al. (1983) found a preponderance of right hemispheric spectral EEG indicators in depression after 25 mg of amitriptyline, a tricyclic interacting principally with serotoninergic systems, a definite relationship emerges between MAO activity, serotonin and right hemispheric functions. There is an interesting observation by Brown et al. (1979) which relates aggression in soldiers with various types of personality disorders to low CSF concentrations of 5-HIAA --a significant negative correlation. Von Knorring and Oreland (1983) note that MAO activity in healthy controls and in patients with bipolar affective psychoses is exactly identical; it is only slightly lower in major depressive syndromes, but falls markedly in personality disorders with depressed mood. The general associations of low platelet MAO activity thus are the following: impulsivity, extraversion, psychopathic type personality deviation, characterological forms of dysphoric mood, acting-out type suicidal attempt behavior and sinistrality <u>in the male</u>.

If we accept with van Praag (1984) that reduced MAO activity leads to decreased serotonin turnover (rather than the reverse) and if we accept that serotonin is essentially an <u>inhibitory</u> neurotransmitter (i.e. the myoclonus in post anoxic encephalopathy is abolished by the serotonin precursor L-5-hydroxytryptophan, which increases the concentration of intracerebral serotonin, cf. Chadwick et al., 1978: in animals, increasing serotoninergic functions leads to diminished food intake and reduced sexual activity, cf. Shaw, 1978) then the problem of the associations of low MAO activity can be reformulated in the following way: why does a relative defect of central neural inhibition correlate with sinistrality, extraversion, dysphoric mood, and aggression only in the male? Consideration of the differential hemispheric organisation of the male and female brain can perhaps provide the answer.[1]

In its simplest expression, <u>relative</u> to each other, the male brain is hypofunctional for dominant, and hyperfunctional for non-dominant functions, while the reverse is true for the female brain, hyperfunctional for dominant and hypofunctional for non-dominant functions. Further, the female brain is more bilateral and has a higher degree of interhemispheric 'coupling' than the male brain:

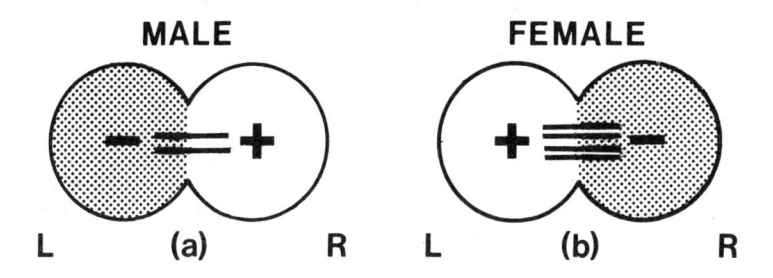

Brain Mood Systems - Neurotransmitters - Asymmetry

MALE   **FEMALE**

L   (a)   R   L   (b)   R

We see that, since the initial state is different in (a) and (b), then in principle a generalised loss of central inhibition will have quite different consequences in (a) and (b): if we take the case of left brain inhibition of right brain systems in the male the initial functional asymmetry will be accentuated:

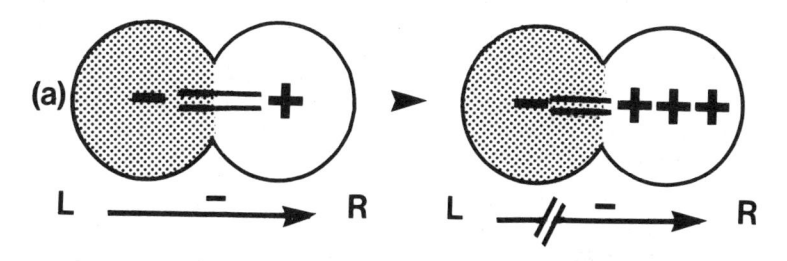

(a)

In females, whose level of MAO activity is higher than males in any case, either there will be no effect on account of the 'stronger' left hemispheric state and because of the greater degree of interhemispheric coupling, or if an effect does occur it will be of opposite directionality:

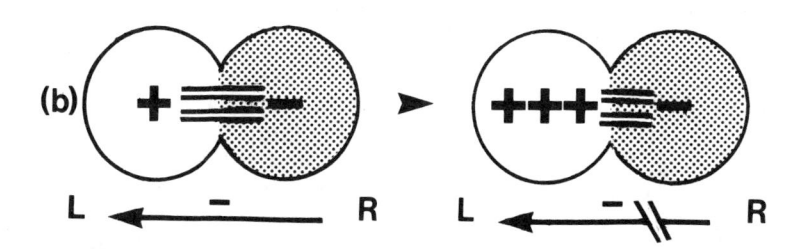

(b)

The model assumes that, even though serotonin-ergic systems are biased towards the non-dominant hemisphere, the first consequences of disturbed serotonin-mediated neural inhibition will occur in the neurophysiologically less stable hemisphere. This representation is obviously tentative and exploratory. It does explain why the association of low MAO activity with sinistrality and dysphoric psychopathic instability is seen only in males: there is now abundant evidence that the pattern of cerebral organisation of psychopathy (a male syndrome itself associated with sinistrality) is characterised by discrete left hemisphere dysfunction and normal or superior right hemispheric state (Flor-Henry, 1973, 1974; Yeudall et al., 1981; Fedora and Fedora, 1983; Nachshon, 1983). Further, certain predictions, open to experimental verification, can be made: chronic schizophrenia, characterised by dysfunctional hypofunction of the left and right hemispheric preponderance in low MAO individuals, should be associated with males rather than females, while 'acute schizophrenia' or manic-hypomanic states characterised by dysfunctional hypoactivation of the right hemisphere and left hemispheric preponderance (cf. Flor-Henry, 1978b; Gruzelier, 1981) should have a higher frequency in females with low MAO activity.

Many observations have accumulated which show that emotional stability and mood regulation are more precarious in the sinistral than in the dextral brain organisation. Orme (1970) measured emotional instability in 300 school girls from an approved school and compared the 23 (7.6%) who were left-handed with the 277 right-handed, both groups being of comparable, normal intelligence. Although the right-handed school girls were significantly more unstable than the 143 controls, the left-handed group was significantly more unstable than the right-handed one. Hicks and Pellegrini (1978) studied 266 college students with a modification of Annett's handedness inventory and with the Taylor Manifest Anxiety scale. Comparing the 35 most sinistral students with the 35 who were totally dextral, it was found that the sinistral group scored significantly higher for anxiety than the dextrals. Davidson and Schaffer (1983) measured anxiety in 538 college students and evaluated the personality test scores as a function of sex and of handedness. Dextral females were more anxious than dextral males. Comparing the most anxious with the least anxious groups, 4 of 7 of the high anxiety subjects were

left-handed against only 2 of the 33 low anxiety individuals, a very significant difference (p = 0.0006).
There is evidence that in the manic-depressive syndrome, more generally in the bipolar psychoses including the schizo-affective forms, there is also increased sinistrality. Lishman and McMeekan (1976) found the frequency of inconsistent sinistrality in the bipolar syndromes to be 12%, or twice the general population incidence. In a series of 115 consecutive psychotics studied some years ago (Flor-Henry, 1976) we found exactly the same incidence of sinistrality in bipolar states, particularly in their excited phases, as did the London group. In their studies of bipolar psychoses Sackeim and Decina (1983) have shown that sinistrality has very fundamental implications to the manic-depressive syndrome. Their sample consisted of 113 bipolar psychotics (62 bipolar I and 51 bipolar II). In the total sample 24.7% were sinistral, in the bipolar I group 32.25%, and in the bipolar II group 15.69%. The difference between bipolar I and II was significant.
Confirming Lishman and McMeekan's observation, the sinistrality was not associated with increased familial sinistrality. It was, however, strongly associated with family history for affective disorders: 55% for dextrals and 84% for sinistrals for the total group. The effect was particularly pronounced for bipolar I, 49% in dextrals and 89% in sinistrals. Remarkably, Sackeim and Decina found when they investigated 31 children between the ages of 7 and 14 years, born to bipolar parents (compared to 18 children born to healthy parents, matched for age, sex and full scale I.Q.) a significant excess of sinistrality in the children of the manic-depressives: 29% versus 5% in the controls (p < 0.05). Further, the children of the sick parents exhibited a significant decrement of performance I.Q. relative to verbal I.Q. There was a trend whereby the left-handed children of bipolar I parents showed the largest verbal/performance discrepancy. 32% of the bipolar children received a clinical diagnosis, depression in about half, and expansiveness, exhibitionism and egocentrism in the other half. The 'expansive' children had greater verbal/performance discrepancy than the depressed children. In the absence of familial sinistrality, left-handedness is often compensatory to subtle damage to the dominant hemisphere, leading to varying degrees of shifts of language processing to the non-dominant hemisphere.

This in turn interferes with the visuo-spatial processing functions in that hemisphere, hence the decrement in performance abilities. Simultaneously, because of the left brain dysfunction, the left brain inhibition of right brain systems is disrupted, releasing abnormal activation, the expressions of which are dysphoric mood, depression and impaired visuo-spatial efficiency. More perplexing is the situation where bipolar subjects, who have no familial excess of sinistrality but familial loading for affective illness, produce offspring who are both sinistral and have attenuated forms of bipolar disturbance in childhood. Perhaps the clue to this paradox lies in the fact of bipolarity.

Here a digression into the nature of the different brain states which determine depression, mania and the overall cerebral regulation of mood becomes necessary. The evidence available a few years ago (Flor-Henry, 1978b, 1979, 1983b) led to the conclusion that the neural systems which determine emotion are

> Orbital and mesial frontal bilaterally and non-dominant frontotemporal: an asymmetrical anterior limbic system which is shifted towards non-dominant limbic axis in homo sapiens on account of the linguistic-verbal specialisation of its dominant counterpart. The neural substrate for emotion, normal and abnormal, is predominantly non-dominant, but its regulation is a function of both the dominant and non-dominant regions for different emotions. The right and left controlling systems are themselves under active reciprocal interaction through transcallosal neural inhibition. In this manner, anger, euphoria, paranoid mood are evoked when the non-dominant hemisphere no longer controls the dominant systems, together with verbal motor disinhibition. When on the other hand the non-dominant regions are no longer under dominant control, the emotional-catastrophic reaction, dysphoric emotions of anxiety and sadness are released. When the cerebral disorganisation is principally restricted to the non-dominant hemisphere, the depressive phase of the manic-depressive syndrome supervenes. At a certain threshold the dominant hemisphere becomes activated, triggering the manic phase. If the contralateral perturbation becomes more extensive, reaching the dominant temporal regions, then the thought-disordered manias or the

schizo-affective states are induced.

A number of different techniques--neurophysiological, carotid barbiturisation, dichotic, lateral saccadic eye movements, motoric laterality--in psychosis are all convergent and demonstrate that psychotic phenomena are associated not only with a disruption of verbal and spatial functions but also with complex alterations in the organisation of cerebral cognitive laterality (Flor-Henry and Koles, 1980). In a recent confirmation by Silberman et al. (1983) it is shown in a tachistoscopic study that whereas normal dextral men and women have the expected left hemisphere advantage for verbal processing, dextral depressed women demonstrated right hemisphere superiority. According to the method of analysis, cognitive laterality can be shown to be reduced, more bilaterally or contralaterally shifted, depending partly on the psychosis of the cognitive conditions studied. Thus we were led to the view that

> if it is accepted that normal cerebral functions require the simultaneous stabilising of each hemisphere through transcallosal neural inhibition originating in the opposite hemisphere--and that in particular the maintenance of specific cognitive hemispheric specialisation presupposes the contralateral inhibition of potentially rival specialised systems in the opposite side of the brain--then it is clear that the laterality hypothesis of the endogenous psychoses immediately accounts for these phenomena. The extent to which the bilaterally asymmetrical hemispheric dysfunction (determining the psychosis) interferes with ipsilateral cognitive mechanisms--and the extent to which this process abolishes transcallosal neural inhibition--will at the same time be the basis for, and limit the degree of, laterality shifts possible in psychosis (Flor-Henry and Koles, 1980).

This basic representation has since been confirmed. The essential observations are that non-irritative lesions of the <u>left</u> hemisphere evoke dysphoric mood and depression, and those of the <u>right</u> hemisphere evoke euphoria, while the situation is reversed in the case of irritative (i.e. ictal) lesions when <u>depression</u> relates to <u>right</u> and <u>euphoria</u> to <u>left</u> hemispheric activation (Sackeim et al., 1982; Flor-

Henry, 1983f for review).

Induced sadness and euphoria have been shown in normal subjects to be also related to right and left frontal activation, respectively, with techniques measuring regional alpha power desynchronisation (i.e. Tucker et al., 1981; Schaffer et al., 1983). A recent study (Reuter-Lorenz et al., 1983), using a tachistoscopic hemifield presentation-reaction time paradigm, even demonstrated a left hemisphere effect for the recognition of happy faces and a right hemisphere effect for the recognition of sad faces in both dextrals and non-inverted left-handers, the opposite occurring in inverted sinistrals!

Some specialists, Tucker et al. (1981) and Gainotti (1983) for example, consider that both positive and negative emotions are derivative of right hemispheric systems. Jerre Levy (1983) has clearly exposed this position. Euphoric or positive emotions are related to high levels of arousal, negative or depressed mood to low levels of arousal in the right hemisphere: regional right frontal desynchronisation in sadness indicates not increased activation of that hemisphere but increased inhibitory suppression of arousal, the regulation of cerebral arousal hinging on right parietal cortical systems linked in a positive feedback with mid-brain reticular networks. Certainly there is wide agreement that the fundamental specialisation of the dominant hemisphere relates to sequential analysis and selective attention, that of the non-dominant hemisphere to arousal and to simultaneous processing. However, to view the right frontal system as the key centre of cerebral inhibition is hardly justified since psychophysiological data dependent on habituation characteristics and on the directionality of electrodermal amplitude asymmetry to an orienting stimulus in hemiparkinsonism and in unilateral brain lesions right and left indicate that the left hemisphere is inhibitory and the right hemisphere excitatory (Gruzelier, 1981; Mintz and Myslobodsky, 1983). Further, the idea that positive emotions reflect increased right hemisphere arousal is not compatible with the observations that right hemispherectomies alone are associated with euphoria, or with the euphoric consequences of transient inactivation of the right hemisphere with either unilateral ECT or right carotid barbiturisation. Nor is the idea that negative emotions are due to reduced right hemisphere arousal consistent with the fact that in temporal lobe epilepsy both autonomic auras (epigastric) and auras of dysphoric mood are significantly associated with right temporal lobe epilepsy (Gupta et al., 1983). Positron Emission Topographic studies of depression reveal increased metabolism of deoxyglucose in the right hemisphere (Hawkins et al., 1983). By contrast at least one observation relates amphetamine-induced euphoria to increased left hemispheric cerebral blood flow (Risberg et al., 1980). Sackeim (1984, personal communication), following repeated episodes of mania in a single patient, also found a left hemispheric increase in blood flow, compared to the normothymic phases.

The evolutionary evidence reviewed earlier and the constant association of the emotional-catastrophic reaction with left frontal lesions suggest that the overall regulation of mood is left hemisphere dependent. This was confirmed in an elegant experiment by Buck and Duffy (1980) who showed in the comparison of left hemisphere-damaged (aphasic), right hemisphere-damaged patients, and controls that facial-gestural affective responses in the left brain-damaged patients were <u>greater</u> than in the controls, these being reduced in the right brain-damaged group—a clear demonstration of left hemisphere inhibition of right hemisphere affective modulation disrupted by left frontal lesions.

Neurological studies in recent years focussing on aprosodias have established that the understanding and expression of the affective modulations of language depend on the integrity of neural sets in the right hemisphere exactly homologous with Wernicke and Broca areas in the left, respectively. Thus the flat, blunted monotonous voice of a right brain-damaged subject may hide the intensity of a pre-existing, independent endogenous depression. Ross and Rush (1981) in an important paper give a detailed examination of the neuroanatomy of depression in brain-damaged patients after right and left strokes and with <u>pre-existing</u> depressions consequently modified and 'masked' by the subsequent brain lesion(s). They conclude that the 'verbal expression of a depressive verbal-cognitive set requires an intact Broca and Wernicke area' whereas the internal representation of depression depends on the integrity of Wernicke's area alone. Thus patients with localised left hemisphere deficit may be totally unaware of a nevertheless treatable depression with secondary irritability, insomnia, anorexia, etc. Neurotic forms of depression are quite different from the psychotic forms. The overall severity of dysfunction is much less, the overlap with normals much greater, and there is evidence in a subgroup, particularly in the male, of dominant rather than non-dominant dysfunction (Fromm-Auch, 1983; Flor-Henry et al., 1983g). The concept of 'verbal-cognitive' depressions, with a primary locus in the dominant hemisphere and secondary transcallosal right hemisphere disturbance, becomes important here.

The study of the location of lesions in stroke patients, which the widespread application of CAT scan radiological techniques has made very precise, has revealed the importance of the antero-posterior gradient of dysfunction in the genesis of abnormal mood states after right and left cerebrovascular accidents. Robinson and his collaborators (Robinson and Price, 1982; Lipsey et al., 1983; Robinson et al., 1983) have found that both the incidence and severity of depression after strokes is determined by a left frontal localisation. The intensity of the depression is correlated with lesion size. For the left hemisphere lesion group as a whole, the presence or absence of aphasia was unrelated to the probability or intensity of depression. A significant negative correlation was found between the Hamilton Depression score and the distance of the lesion away from the anterior pole of the frontal lobe in the left hemisphere. Although globally, depression was only significantly related to left frontal injury and unrelated to right hemisphere or brain-stem lesions, when the right hemisphere alone was considered then depression was significantly correlated with posterior and euphoric reactions with anterior location. Finset (1982), who had examined mood changes following right hemisphere strokes, also noted that depressive mood only occurred after posterior lesions with intact right frontal lobes. Consequently the following antero-posterior and right-left interactions in the neuroanatomy of mood states are suggested:

DEPRESSION

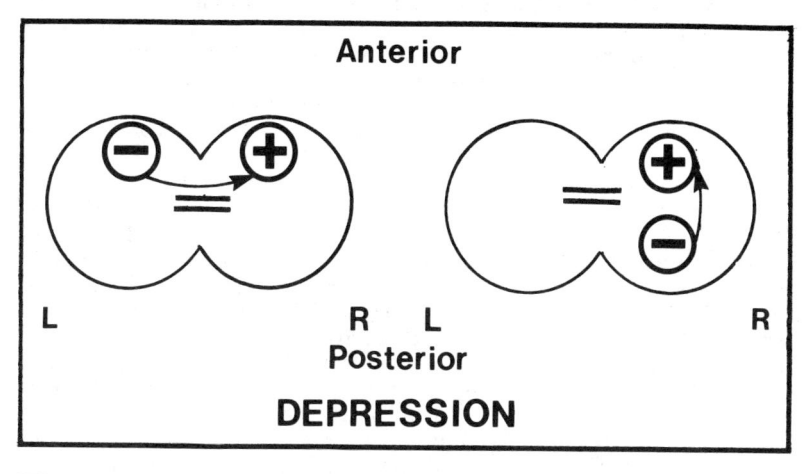

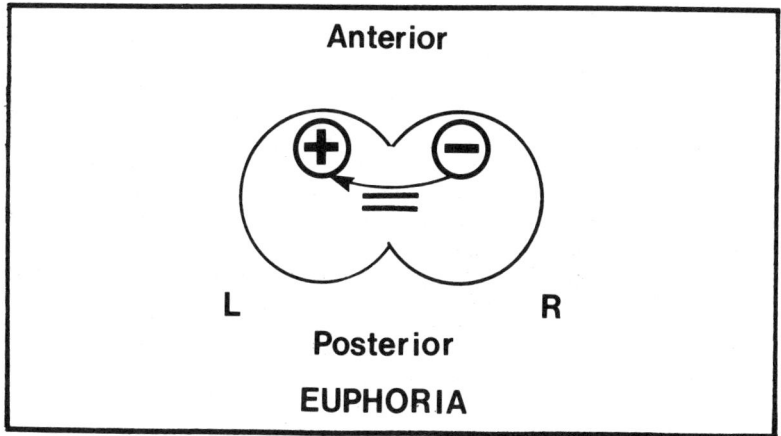

EUPHORIA

We note that the schematic representation above, which summarises the empirical findings of the four investigations of the effects on mood of CVA lesion localisation, emphasises the bilateral frontal non-dominant hemispheric asymmetrical organisation of the cerebral systems determining mood which was developed quite independently. Further, in the conditions associated with depression it is worthy of emphasis that the right frontal zone is always intact. Similarly, for euphoric reactions to be induced the left frontal zone is intact. These observations are consistent with the model of abnormal frontal activation, left-sided for positive and right-sided for negative emotions, as destroyed tissue in a CVA cannot be abnormally activated. The contralateral inhibitory projections, however, will be disrupted. Again these studies eloquently document the fundamental importance of the dominant frontal system in the overall regulation of affect.

It is clear that the recognition of the importance of the antero-posterior gradient requires a supplementary hypothesis, that of posterior-anterior intrahemispheric systems of inhibition. In the organisation of the cerebral mood systems these are apparently less important than the right/left systems of reciprocal influences. Theoretically, one might expect a parallel system of posterior-anterior intra-hemispheric inhibition in the left hemisphere which, with Wernicke-type posterior temporal-parietal lesions, would 'release' euphoria through left frontal disinhibition.

The special importance of the left frontal and right posterior cerebral regions in depression is revealed in the curious finding of Uytenhoef et al. (1983) of a state-dependent left frontal hypervascularisation and right posterior hypovascularisation in major depressive disorders which emerged in their regional cerebral blood flow study of major and minor depressives, normothymic bipolar patients and healthy controls.

Let us now turn to the cerebral dynamics of unipolar and bipolar psychoses. Several experimental approaches indicate that with the deepening of depression (and increasing right hemisphere dysfunction) there is induced at a certain threshold contralateral dominant hemispheric disorganisation. This is suggested by:

1. The fact that in dextral depressives the degree of left hemisphere language competence is inversely correlated with depth of depression during intracarotid barbiturisation (Hommes and Panhuyssen, 1970).
2. The fact that depressions not responding to tricyclics but ECT-responsive fail to show the expected right ear superiority to verbal stimuli on dichotic stimulation before treatment: it returns after treatment and with recovery (Moscovitch et al., 1981).
3. The fact that in depression there is an increase in the acoustic threshold for the left ear (right hemisphere effect) which returns to

normal after recovery (Sackeim et al., 1983). However, when psychomotor retardation supervenes in depression the acoustic threshold for the right ear is increased (left hemisphere effect) (Bruder et al., 1980).
4. In the majority of cases of symptomatic mania secondary to neurological lesions (non-irritative), cerebral tumours are usually associated with right hemisphere localisation (Cohen and Niska, 1980).
5. Psychometric studies indicate a significant decrement of performance relative to verbal I.Q. in both psychotic depression and mania. The effect is stronger for mania than depression. Hence a functional disorganisation of the right hemisphere, more pronounced in mania than depression, is implicated (Flor-Henry et al., 1983g).
6. Both neuropsychological (Flor-Henry et al., 1983g) and power spectral EEG parameters (Flor-Henry et al., 1983h) indicate that the pattern of cerebral disorganisation in mania and schizophrenia is very similar, although the severity of dysfunction is less in mania.
7. During spatial processing in mania (n = 75) the right hemisphere leads the left hemisphere while in psychotic depression (n = 63) the left hemisphere leads the right (Flor-Henry et al., 1984).

When we examined the statistical quantitative EEG configurations of unmedicated bipolar psychoses (n = 78) compared to unipolar psychoses (n = 55), grouping together the excited and inhibited forms of each category, the few statistical differences found on univariate analysis were all related to the left parietal zone. The power and variance in this area were significantly reduced in the alpha frequencies (eyes closed) and the logarithm of the right/left parietal coefficient of variation ratio was positive in unipolar and negative in bipolar psychoses. There were no significant differences between the two groups in the eyes-open or in the two verbal-cognitive conditions. During the spatial task the phase lead of the parietal zone, with respect to the right temporal region, was significantly more pronounced in the bipolar syndromes (Flor-Henry, 1983e). These findings suggest that in bipolar states there is a greater left hemisphere activation than in unipolar states (reduced left parietal alpha power) and that the balance in relative hemispheric activation, right/left, is shifted in opposite directionality (negative and positive log. of right/left c.v. ratios). The left parietal neuroelectric set, however, does not interact with verbal, but with spatial cognitive processing, underlining the fundamental importance of right hemispheric function in both unipolar and bipolar psychoses.

If we contrast the clinical symptomatology of the extreme manifestations of the bipolar syndromes, the frenetic hypermotility, speech acceleration and euphoric exaltation of mania with the psychomotor retardation, the paucity of speech or the mutism and functional paralysis of depressive stupor, an immediate conclusion is evident. Since the cerebral systems which determine speech, euphoria and (bilateral) motility all are left hemisphere-dependent, the opposition between the excited and inhibited phases of the bipolar psychoses are determined by left hemispheric activation in the former and inhibition in the latter. If, as the evidence available to date suggests, in both unipolar and bipolar illnesses of endogenous type the primary locus of dysfunction is in the right hemisphere, then the theoretical expectation is that, other conditions being equal, individuals with 'stronger' left hemispheric functions will be less susceptible to induced left hemispheric disorganisation than individuals with 'weaker' left hemispheric systems. In other words, unipolar syndromes should be more frequent in women than in men and bipolar syndromes should, statistically, be more common in men than in women. There are indications that this is so. Winokur et al. (1983) examined the sex ratios of unipolar and bipolar affective disorders in 14 studies of bipolar probands and their relatives. These authors conclude that

> The data are highly consistent in demonstrating that
> 1. Females are more frequently affected than males.
> 2. Among affected females the ratio of unipolar depression to bipolar illness is about 2:1.
> 3. Among affected males, the ratio of bipolar to unipolar illness is approximately 1:1.

Given the left hemisphere vulnerability of the male relative to the female and the right hemisphere vulnerability of the female compared to the male, further theoretical expectations immediately follow: depression, being right hemisphere dependent, should be more frequent in women than in men; and mania, being left hemisphere dependent, should be more frequent in men than in women. Winokur et al. (1983) conclude unambiguously: 'Thirteen of the fourteen studies showed evidence of more depression than mania in females, and 13 of 13 showed more unipolar depression in females than in males, ($p < 0.002$) . . . females were more likely to be depressed than manic, and females were more likely to be depressed than males'. The Iowa workers cite the studies of lifetime risk for bipolar and unipolar illness of Boyd and Weissman (1981) which indicate that female depressives in the general population far outnumber female manics and that female depressives far outnumber male depressives. Exactly in accordance with the gender-related lateralised hemispheric vulnerability of the dominant hemisphere in the male and of the non-dominant hemisphere in the female is the finding that, on neuropsychological indices, only males exhibit asymmetrical dysfunction (L > R) in schizophrenia and mania, and only females (R > L) in psychotic depression. Schizophrenia and mania in women and depression in men are associated with more symmetrical bilateral dysfunction (Flor-Henry et al., 1983g).

So let us consider again the paradox of Sackeim: bipolar probands show an excess of sinistrality, their parents have an excess of affective illness but not of sinistrality, yet the children of the bipolar probands have an excess both of bipolar illness and sinistrality. Here the genetic predisposition is for affective illness but the sinistrality is non-genetic, hence acquired. Developmental or birth-perinatal events have been responsible for subtle left hemisphere disorganisation, one manifestation of which is sinistrality, another the consequent verbal/performance discrepancy and a third the bipolarity itself. It is relevant to note in this context that the age of onset of bipolar forms is significantly younger than unipolar forms and that the evolution towards chronicity and deterioration is much greater with bipolar than unipolar syndromes.

There is now increasing evidence that the severe, chronic depressions of endogenous type, and the schizo-affective, bipolar and some manic psychoses of early onset are characterised by structural brain changes: ventricular dilatation and/or cortical atrophy. The effect below the ages of 50-60 is not age-related. The first unequivocal report was that of von Nagy (1963) who examined the pneumoencephalographic findings of 260 chronic schizophrenics and 133 manic-depressives, all females under the age of 50. Whereas cerebral atrophy was present in 58% of the schizophrenic group taken as a whole and in 80% of the chronic types with defect, abnormal pneumoencephalographic patterns occurred in 23% of all manic-depressives and in 78% of those with chronic affective syndromes. Pearlson and Veroff (1981) showed by CAT scan examination the presence of a significant increase in ventricular size in 16 manic-depressives compared to age-matched controls, 25% of the group showing evidence of cortical atrophy as well. Van Boxel et al. (1978) found that chronic schizo-affective psychoses had significant ventricular dilatation when compared with patients with chronic anxiety or obsessions. Standish-Barry et al. (1982) found significant ventricular enlargement in 50 cases of severe, chronic endogenous depressions. Rieder et al. (1983) established that, after age correction, there was pathological enlargement of the ventricular system in 15 chronic schizo-affective and 19 bipolar affective patients that was identical with that seen in 28 chronic schizophrenics. Similarly Nasrallah et al. (1982) reported an abnormal ventricular brain-ratio of 7.5 in 24 young manics, comparable to that of 55 chronic schizophrenics (8.7) and significantly different from age-matched controls (4.5). Several of the investigations briefly outlined formally demonstrated that the structural brain changes were independent of alcohol usage, prior electroconvulsive therapy, or neuroleptic administration.

Thus it is clear that in all forms of psychosis, be it schizophrenic, schizo-affective, manic or depressive, chronicity is correlated with structural brain damage. The probability of occurrence, of course, is different in the various psychoses. There are reasons to conclude that in psychosis the chronicity dimension is independent of the neural disregulation which determines the clinical form of the psychosis (see Flor-Henry, 1969, 1983c for discussion). A recent study (Reveley et al., 1984) confirms this view: the cerebral ventricular volume of 21 schizophrenics from 21 monozygotic twin-pairs was evaluated. There was a pronounced increase in cerebral ventricular size in schizophrenics without a family history of psychosis, while the ventricular size of the schizophrenics with familial psychosis was similar to that of the controls. In the normal controls, however, those twins with a history of birth complications had ventricular dilatation approaching that of the abnormal schizophrenic twins.

In a previous study (Reveley et al., 1982) it was shown that, although in normal monozygotic twins ventricular size was 'under a high degree of genetic control', in monozygotic twins discordant for schizophrenia, the schizophrenic twin had consistently larger ventricles than either his healthy co-twin or the control twins.

I have already reviewed the evidence which suggests that the topographic distribution of serotoninergic systems is bilaterally asymmetrical in its cortical projections and biased towards the non-dominant hemisphere. Gottfries et al. (1974) found a correlation between the amplitude of left hemispheric evoked potentials and CSF concentrations of homovanillic acid (HVA), a DA metabolite, this suggesting a dominant hemispheric bias for dopaminergic systems. A left hemispheric-DA interaction was also implied by the circadian-dependent variations in right ear acoustic threshold (i.e. left hemisphere) first observed by Gruzelier and Hammond (1976) in schizophrenia. The effect was abolished by chlorpromazine. The left ear (i.e. right hemisphere) showed no variations in acoustic threshold and no chlorpromazine interaction. This last study is consistent with earlier reports, such as that of Serafetinides (1973) who described how schizophrenics who recovered on chlorpromazine exhibited left hemispheric EEG alterations. In healthy normal subjects there is also evidence of a left hemispheric bias in the distribution of this neurotransmitter, since following a single intravenous injection of chlorpromazine predominantly left hemispheric changes occur in the power spectral EEG parameters (Laurian et al., 1981).

Von Knorring et al. (1983), administering imipramine to normal subjects, found a significant consequent increase in left frontal alpha power (i.e. corresponding to right hemisphere activation), which implies the presence of a right hemisphere bias for noradrenergic systems. Indeed, Oke et al. (1978) noted significant neurochemical asymmetries in NA distribution in the human thalamus: higher concentrations on the left side posteriorly and higher concentrations on the right side anteriorly. More recently Oke (1983) describes three variations on the above pattern, the first of a right lateralised distribution of NA throughout the mid-thalamus and pulvinar, the second of a diagonal pattern such as left ventral and right dorsal, and the third consisting of combinations of the above patterns. Because Rossor et al. (1980), in the neurochemical analysis of 3-5 neurotransmitters in 9 structures, both right and left sides, of 14 normal human brains, found only one significant asymmetry by a t-test analysis (of increased γ-aminobutyric acid [GABA] in the left substantia nigra), the authors concluded that there was 'no evidence for lateral asymmetry of neurotransmitters in post mortem human brain'. Glick et al. (1982; Glick, 1983), however, reanalysed the raw data of Rossor et al. by correlational analysis. The results showed the presence of lateral asymmetries in several brain regions and transmitter systems. Notably there was a left brain bias for cholinergic, GABAergic and dopaminergic systems. Importantly, the left-right asymmetries in glutamate decarboxylase (GAD) and GABA were positively correlated in all 9 brain regions studied. This was of particular importance since GABA and GAD reflect the same neurotransmitter system but were measured by different techniques. At the level of the globus pallidus the increased levels of choline acetyltransferase and DA on the left side with the higher concentration opposite to the side of motor lateral preference shows that in this respect humans and rats have a similar organisation, since in rats the side of lateral preference is also opposite to the striate with higher DA concentration (Glick, 1983).

With respect to the left-sided bias for cholinergic systems shown in the Rossor data as reanalysed by Glick et al., it is of interest that Gainotti et al. (1983) have also found a significant increase in cholinergic activity on the left side of the human brain, notably in the posterior parts of the first temporal gyrus, as measured by choline acetyltransferase activity.

Dramatically highlighting the importance of neurochemical asymmetries in the pathogenesis of psychosis is the study of Reynolds (1983) which, in two series of schizophrenic brains examined postmortem, reveals a specific increase of DA in the amygdalae of the left hemisphere (both compared to control brains and to the right brain of the schizophrenics). Modern neuropathological investigations are beginning to reveal lateralised structural changes, in the expected directions, in the endogenous psychoses. For example, Frith and his collaborators at the Medical Research Council Centre, Northwick Park Hospital, in comparing 40 schizophrenic and 30 affective psychotic brains (post-mortem), report the presence of thinning of the left parahippocampal cortex in schizophrenics and of the right in affectives. It was not a sex effect (Firth, 1984, personal communication). Examining the trends for catecholamine concentrations in the controls, it is noteworthy that NA values are higher in the right amygdala than in the left, whereas DA is higher in the left than in the right in the two regions analysed: the amygdaloid and caudate nuclei. These non-significant trends are consistent with the investigations reviewed above (data of Reynolds).

There is increasing evidence that alcohol, although of course it influences the whole central nervous system, has a specific effect on the right hemisphere in humans. Kostandov et al. (1982) reviewed this material. In their own investigations, Kostandov and his collaborators show that following a small amount of alcohol ingestion the perception time of visual stimuli presented to the left visual field (right hemisphere) is prolonged in normal subjects, thus resulting in the inversion of the normal hemispheric asymmetry of perception time to visual stimuli. Further, the late cortical evoked responses (visual) after alcohol have a significantly greater latency and reduced amplitude over the right hemisphere. Ciesielski et al. (1984) have replicated these results in 8 male alcoholics with a history of alcohol problems of 10-12 years' duration, tested after a period of 4 weeks' abstinence. Visual memory cognitive reaction time was longer after tachistoscopic projection to the right hemisphere, normals exhibiting the opposite relation with slower processing during left hemisphere and faster during right hemisphere presentation. In addition, visual potentials had significantly longer latency and reduced amplitude at N 200 (parietal) and P 300 (occipital) in the right hemisphere compared to the left, normals exhibiting the converse relationship. A state-dependent inhibition of right hemisphere function by alcohol in normals and a more prolonged (permanent?) right hemisphere hypofunction in alcoholics are therefore implied by these data.

Reciprocal relationships exist between the various neurotransmitter systems. The inverse functional reciprocity existing between cholinergic and noradrenergic systems is well known. Similar reciprocities link dopaminergic and GABAergic systems (Garbutt and van Kammen, 1983) and serotoninergic and noradrenergic neurotransmitters (Stone, 1983). The reciprocity of cholinergic and dopaminergic systems is illustrated by the acute dyskinesias induced by antidopaminergic agents and relieved by anticholinergic drugs (contrasted with tardive dyskinesias, the results of rebound hyperdopaminergic activity after neuroleptic withdrawal, which are relieved by cholinergic and aggravated by anticholinergic agents).

Figure I summarises the reciprocal relationships between the various neurotransmitter systems and their bilaterally asymmetrical cortico-limbic distribution.

The heuristic application of this model can be shown, for example, by taking the observation of Janowsky et al. (1973a,b) that intravenous injection of physostigmine transforms mania for some 90 minutes into a state of psychomotor retardation with depression. Thus, cholinergic activation in the left hemisphere will be correlated with a functional reduction of DA, this in turn leading to an increase in GABAergic inhibition. Consequently (left hemisphere) inhibition will be exaggerated by the increased cholinergic state. At the same time, the noradrenergic state will be reduced on account of the cholinergic-noradrenergic reciprocity, which will evoke a functional increase of serotoninergic inhibition (right hemisphere). Further, the left brain inhibition of right hemispheric systems will also be increased. The cholinergic state thus should be, theoretically, one of bilateral hemispheric neural inhibition. Conversely, keeping in mind that overall the left brain is inhibitory and the right brain is excitatory, an increase in functional right hemispheric noradrenergic state will be correlated with a fall in serotonin-mediated inhibition in that hemisphere, which will increase contralateral callosal excitatory pathways resulting in left hemisphere overactivation (i.e. mania or 'acute schizophrenia'). Similarly, a fall in noradrenergic function, producing an increase in right hemispheric inhibition, will decrease contralateral excitation (i.e. the left hemispheric inhibition of the bipolar syndrome). Again a functional increase in DA, correlated with a reduction of left hemispheric GABA, will weaken the left brain inhibition of right brain systems, inducing a secondary right hemispheric activation, a process that will be enhanced by the consequent noradrenergic state increase and corresponding decrease of right hemisphere serotonin inhibition (dopaminergic-cholinergic reciprocity, left, and cholinergic-noradrenergic reciprocity, bilateral). Antidopaminergic drugs will result in

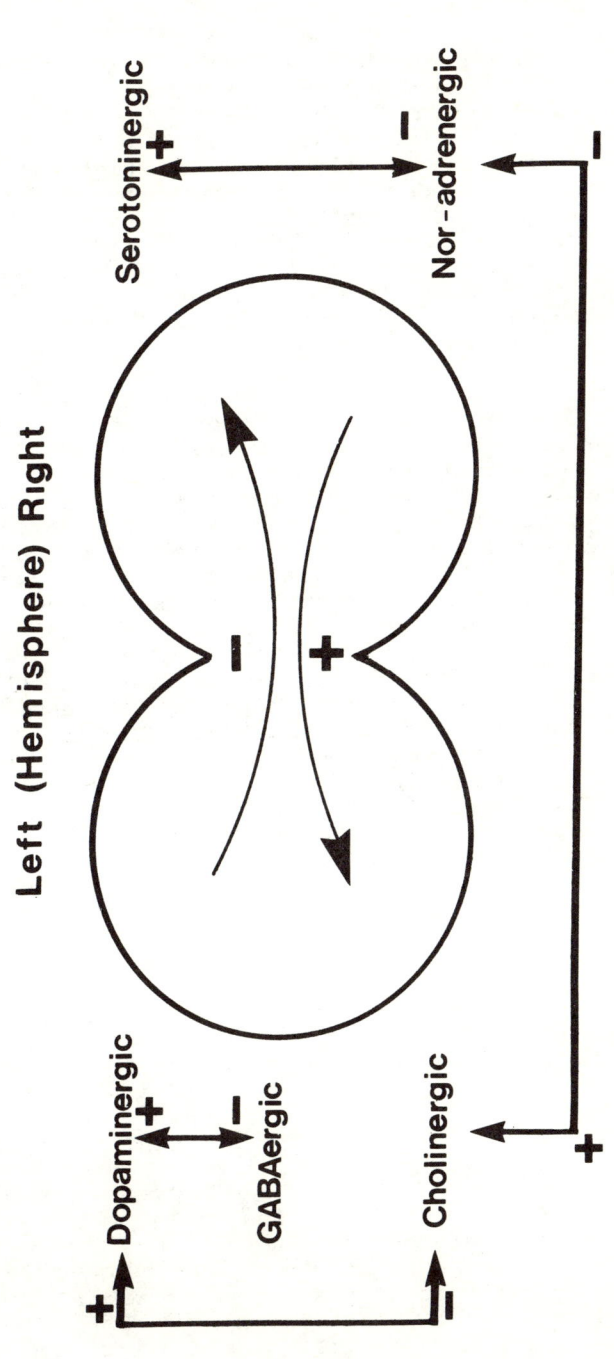

Fig. I. Reciprocal relationships between neurotransmitter systems and their bilaterally asymmetrical cortico-limbic distributions.

greater left hemisphere GABA inhibition; the associated increase in cholinergic functions correlated with a decrease in right hemisphere noradrenergic state, evoking a relative increase in right hemispheric serotonin, will also increase right brain inhibition (i.e. ? therapeutic effect on antidopaminergic drugs in schizophrenia and mania through bilateral increase of neural inhibition).

With regard to the effects of antidepressants on these interlocking, lateralised reciprocal interactions, noradrenergic potentiating agents will induce a relative decrement in right hemisphere serotonin inhibition, and hence activate the right hemisphere as well as the left through an increase of the contralateral right brain excitatory system. Simultaneously, the correlated decrease in left hemispheric cholinergic activity, leading to increased dopaminergic and decreased GABAergic tone, will activate the left hemisphere. Serotoninergic-potentiating antidepressants will increase right brain inhibition; the correlated fall in relative noradrenergic state (in the right) will be compensated by left brain cholinergic increase, dopaminergic decrease and GABAergic increase--hence increase in left brain inhibition of right brain systems. Finally, in the case of amphetamine, an increase in left hemisphere dopaminergic state, leading to reduced GABAergic state, will provoke left hemisphere activation and, by reducing the left brain inhibition of right brain sets, will also provoke right hemisphere activation. The correlated fall in cholinergic balance, by increasing noradrenergic and decreasing serotoninergic inhibition in the right brain, will further synergistically activate the right hemisphere.

In conclusion, the evidence is now substantial that, in the mood psychoses, depression is dependent on altered right hemispheric functions, and mania on a deeper disturbance of right hemispheric systems, producing a contralateral activation of the dominant hemisphere which is responsible for the salient symptomatology of mania and its frequent resemblance to the mental symptoms of 'acute schizophrenia'. Gender interactions are of fundamental importance. Bipolarity results from left hemisphere instability. According to the directionality of right hemisphere serotoninergic-noradrenergic balances, the induced right hemispheric shifts towards hyperfunctional or hypofunctional states determine excited or inhibited forms of bipolar syndromes.

The bilaterally asymmetrical distributions of

the major neurotransmitter systems and the reciprocal functional balances existing between them can be integrated with the brain model of mood, normal and abnormal, presented here and can also be related to the mental effects of psychotropic drugs and of amphetamine.

NOTES

1. I have discussed the implications of the differential hemispheric organisation of the male and female brain for psychopathology in detail elsewhere and will not repeat this here. The interested reader is referred to Flor-Henry (1974, 1978a, 1983d) and Flor-Henry and Koles (1982).

2. For those who for ideological or socio-politico-environmentalist convictions remain sceptical of the differential brain organisation of women and men, the result of genetically determined neurochemical interactions which occur in intrauterine life during critical developmental stages and which hinge principally on testosterone-left hemisphere interactions, I shall only cite one very recent study. Yeo et al. (1984) investigated the influence of sex and age on unilateral cerebral lesion sequellae. Lesion size and location were quantified by CAT scan and only equivalent lesions were compared in left and right lesion groups. A control group was included. Sex by group interactions were significant for left hemisphere variables: verbal-intellectual, right motor and sensory. In every interaction, the left brain-injured males performed worse than the left-injured females. However, the right-injured males were better than the right-injured females. There was no effect of age.

References

Adolfsson, R., Gottfries, C. J., Oreland, L., Roos, B. E., Wiberg, A., and Winbled, B. (1978) Monoamine oxidase activity and serotoninergic turnover in human brain. Prog. Neuro-Psychopharmacol. **2**, 225-230.

Boyd, J. and Weissman, M. (1981) Epidemiology of affective disorders: a reexamination and future directions. Arch. Gen. Psychiatry **38**, 1039-1046.

Brown, G. L., Goodwin, F. K., Ballenger, J. C., Goyer, P. R., and Major, L. F. (1979) Aggression in humans correlates with cerebrospinal fluid amine metabolites. Psychiatry Res. **1**, 131-139.

Bruder, G., Spring, B., Yozawitz, A., and Sutton, S. (1980) Auditory sensitivity in psychiatric patients and non-patients: monotic click detection. Psychological Med. **10**, 133-138.

Buchsbaum, M. S., Coursey, R. D., and Murphy, D. L. (1976) The biochemical high-risk paradigm: behavioral and familial correlates of low platelet monoamine oxidase activity. Science **194**, 339-341.

Buchsbaum, M. S. (1977) Psychophysiology and schizophrenia. Schizophrenia Bull. **3**, 7-14.

Buchsbaum, M. S., Coursey, R. D., and Murphy, D. L. (1980) Schizophrenia and platelet monoamine oxidase: research strategies. Schizophrenia Bull. **6**, 375-384.

Buck, R. and Duffy, R. J. (1980) Nonverbal communication of affect in brain-damaged patients. Cortex **XVI**, 351-362.

Chadwick, D., Hallett, M., Jenner, P., and Marsden, C. D. (1978) Serotonin and action myoclonus: a review. In: Neurotransmitter Systems and Their Clinical Disorders (Legg, N. J., ed.), Academic Press, London, New York, San Francisco, pp. 151-165.

Ciesielski, K. T., Madden, J. J., Blight, J., and Schopflocher, D. Electrophysiological and neuropsychological indicators of cortical-subcortical impairment in long term alcoholics. Int. J. Alc. Alcoholism (in press).

Cohen, M. R. and Niska, R. W. (1980) Localised right cerebral hemisphere dysfunction and recurrent mania. Am. J. Psychiatry **137**, 847-848.

Davidson, R. J. and Schaffer, C. E. (1983) Affect and disorders of affect: behavioral and electrophysiological studies. In: Laterality and Psychopathology (Flor-Henry, P. and Gruzelier, J., eds), Elsevier, North Holland, pp. 249-268.

Demisch, L., Georgi, K., Patzke, B., Demisch, K., and Bochnik, H. J. (1982) Correlation of platelet MAO activity with introversion: a study of a German rural population. Psychiatry Res. **6**, 303-311.

Denenberg, V. H. (1980) General systems theory, brain organisation and early experiences. Am. J. Physiol.: Regulatory, Integrative and Comparative Physiology **238**, R3-R13.

Denenberg, V. H. (1981) Hemispheric laterality in animals and the effects of early experience. Behav. Brain Sci. **4**, 1-21.

Diamond, M. C. (1980) New data supporting cortical asymmetry differences in males and females. Behav. Brain Sci. **3**, 233-234.

Fedora, O. and Fedora, S. (1983) Some neuropsychological and psychophysiological aspects of psychopathic and non-psychopathic criminals. In: Laterality and Psychopathology (Flor-Henry, P. and Gruzelier, J., eds), Elsevier, North Holland, pp. 41-58.

Finset, A. (1982) Depressive behavior, outburst of crying and emotional indifference in left hemiplegics. Presented at Second Annual Symposium of Models and Techniques of Cognitive Rehabilitation, March 27-31.

Frith, C. D. (1984) Personal communication.

Flor-Henry, P. (1969) Psychosis and temporal lobe epilepsy: a controlled investigation. Epilepsia **10**, 363-395.

Flor-Henry, P. (1973) Psychiatric syndromes considered as manifestations of lateralised temporal-limbic dysfunction. In: Surgical Approaches in Psychiatry (Laitinen, L. V. and Livingston, K. E., eds), Medical and Technical Publishing Co., Lancaster, England, pp. 22-26.

Flor-Henry, P. (1974) Psychosis, neurosis and epilepsy. Brit. J. Psychiatry **124**, 144-150.

Flor-Henry, P. (1976) Lateralised temporal-limbic dysfunction and psychopathology. Ann. N.Y. Acad. Sci. **280**, 777-795.

Flor-Henry, P. (1978a) Gender, hemispheric specialisation and psychopathology. Social Science & Medicine **12B**, 155-162.

Flor-Henry, P. (1978b) The endogenous psychoses: a reflection of lateralised dysfunction of the anterior limbic system. In: Limbic Mechanisms (Livingston, K. E. and Hornykiewicz, O., eds), Plenum Publishing Corp., New York and London, pp. 389-404.

Flor-Henry, P. (1979) On certain aspects of the localisation of the cerebral systems regulating and determining emotion. Biol. Psychiatry 14, 677-698.
Flor-Henry, P. and Koles, Z. J. (1980) EEG studies in depression, mania and normals: evidence for partial shifts of laterality in the affective disorders. Adv. Biol. Psychiatry 4, 21-43.
Flor-Henry, P. (1982) EEG characteristics of normal subjects: a comparison of men and women and of dextrals and sinistrals. Res. Commun. Psychol. Psychiat. Behav. 7, 21-38.
Flor-Henry, P. (1983a) Psychopathological implications of hemispheric laterality studies in animals. The Behavioral and Brain Sciences 1, 173-174.
Flor-Henry, P. (1983b) Mood, the right hemisphere and the implications of spatial information perceiving systems. Res. Commun. Psychol. Psychiat. Behav. 8, 143-170.
Flor-Henry, P. (1983c) Classification of the endogenous psychoses: modern evidence in a historical perspective. In: Cerebral Basis of Psychopathology, Wright-PSG, Littleton, Mass., pp. 17-38.
Flor-Henry, P. (1983d) The influence of gender on psychopathology. In: Cerebral Basis of Psychopathology, Wright-PSG, Littleton, Mass., pp. 97-116.
Flor-Henry, P. (1983e) Neurophysiological contributions to the study of psychotic states. In: Cerebral Basis of Psychopathology, Wright-PSG, Littleton, Mass., pp. 183-223.
Flor-Henry, P. (1983f) Hemispheric laterality and disorders of affect. In: Neurobiology of Mood Disorders (Post, R. M. and Ballenger, J. C., eds), Williams and Wilkins, Baltimore, pp. 467-480.
Flor-Henry, P., Fromm-Auch, D., and Schopflocher, D. (1983g) Neuropsychological dimensions in psychopathology. In: Laterality and Psychopathology (Flor-Henry, P. and Gruzelier, J., eds), Elsevier, North Holland, pp. 59-82.
Flor-Henry, P., Koles, Z. J., and Sussman, P. S. (1983h) Multivariate EEG analysis of the endogenous psychoses. Adv. Biol. Psychiatry 13, 196-210.
Flor-Henry, P., Koles, Z. J., and Reddon, J. R. EEG studies of psychosis: principal component and discriminant function analyses, in preparation.

Fromm-Auch, D. (1983) Neuropsychological assessment of depressed patients before and after drug therapy: clinical profile interpretation. In: Laterality and Psychopathology (Flor-Henry, P. and Gruzelier, J., eds), Elsevier, North Holland, pp. 83-102.

Gainotti, G. (1983) Laterality and affect: the emotional behavior of right and left brain-damaged patients. In: Hemisyndromes: Psychology, Neurology, Psychiatry (Myslobodsky, M., ed.), Academic Press, London, New York, San Francisco, pp. 175-192.

Garbutt, J. C. and van Kammen, D. P. (1983) The interaction between GABA and dopamine: implications for schizophrenia. Schizophrenia Bull. 9, 336-353.

Geschwind, N. and Behan, P. (1982) Left-handedness: association with immune disease, migraine and developmental learning disorder. Proc. Nat. Acad. Sci., U.S.A. 79, 5097-5100.

Glick, S. D., Ross, A. R., and Hough, L. B. (1982) Lateral asymmetry of neurotransmitters in human brain. Brain Res. 234, 53-63.

Glick, S. D. (1983) Cerebral lateralisation in the rat and tentative extrapolations to man. In: Hemisyndromes: Psychology, Neurology, Psychiatry (Myslobodsky, M., ed.), Academic Press, New York, London, San Francisco, pp. 7-26.

Gottfries, C. G., Perris, C., and Roos, B. E. (1974) Visual averaged evoked responses (AER) and monoamine metabolites in cerebrospinal fluid (CSF). Acta psychiatrica scand. Suppl. 255, 135-157.

Gruzelier, J. H. and Hammond, N. (1976) Schizophrenia: a dominant hemisphere temporal-limbic disorder? Res. Commun. Psychol. Psychiat. Behav. 1, 33-72.

Gruzelier, J. H. (1981) Hemispheric imbalances masquerading as paranoid and non-paranoid syndromes. Schizophrenia Bull. 7, 662-673.

Gupta, A. K., Jeavons, P. M., Hughes, R. C., and Covanis, A. (1983) Aura in temporal lobe epilepsy: clinical and electroencephalographic correlation. J. Neurol. Neurosurg. Psychiat. 46, 1079-1083.

Hawkins, R. A., Mazziotta, J. C., Phelps, M. E., Huang, S. C., Kuhl, D. E., Carson, R. E., Metter, M. J., and Riege, W. H. (1983) Cerebral glucose metabolism as a function of age in man: influence of the rate constants in the fluorodeoxyglucose method. J. Cerebral Blood Flow Metab. 3, 250-253.

Hicks, R. A. and Pellegrini, R. J. (1978) Handedness and anxiety. Cortex 14, 119-121.
Hommes, O. R. and Panhuysen, L. H. H. M. (1970) Bilateral intracarotid amytal injection. Psychiatr. Neurol. Neurochir. 73, 447-459.
Janowsky, D. S., El-Yousef, M. K., Davis, J. M., and Sekerke, H. J. (1973a) Parasympathetic suppression of manic symptoms by physostigmine. Arch. Gen. Psychiatry 28, 542-547.
Janowksy, D. S. (1973b) Antagonistic effects of physostigmine and methylphenidate in man. Am. J. Psychiatry 130, 1370-1376.
Kostandov, E. A., Arsumanov, Y. L., Genkina, O. A., Restchikova, T. N., and Shostakovitch, G. S. (1982) The effects of alcohol on hemispheric functional asymmetry. J. Studies on Alcohol 43, 411-426.
Laurian, S., Le, P. K., Baumana, P., Percy, M., and Gaillard, J.-M. (1981) Relationship between plasma levels of chlorpromazine and effects on EEG and evoked potentials in healthy volunteers. Pharmacopsychiatrica 14, 199-204.
Laurian, S., Gaillard, J.-M., Le, P. K., and Schopf, J. (1983) Topographic aspects of EEG profile of some psychotropic drugs. Adv. Biological Psychiatry 13, 165-171, and in: Neurophysiological Correlates of Normal Cognition and Psychopathology (Perris, C., Kemali, D., and Koukkou-Lehman, M., eds), Karger, Basel.
Levy, J. (1983) Commentary on P. Flor-Henry's functional hemispheric asymmetry and psychopathology. Integrative Psychiatry, July-August, 52-53.
Lipsey, J. R., Robinson, R. G., Pearlson, G. D., Rao, K., and Price, T. R. (1983) Mood change following bilateral hemisphere brain injury. Brit. J. Psychiatry 143, 266-273.
Lishman, W. A. and McMeekan, E. R. L. (1976) Hand preference patterns in psychiatric patients. Brit. J. Psychiatry 129, 158-166.
Mintz, M. and Myslobodsky, M. S. (1983) Two types of hemisphere imbalance in hemiparkinsonism coded by brain electrical activity and electrodermal activity. In: Hemisyndromes: Psychology, Neurology, Psychiatry (Myslobodsky, M. S., ed.), Academic Press, London, New York, San Francisco, pp. 213-238.
Moscovitch, M., Strauss, E., and Olds, J. (1981) Handedness in patients with unipolar endogenous depression who require electroconvulsive therapy. Am. J. Psychiatry 138, 988-990.

Nachshon, I. (1983) Hemisphere dysfunction in psychopathy and behavior disorders. In: Hemisyndromes: Psychology, Neurology, Psychiatry (Myslobodsky, M. S., ed.), Academic Press, London, New York, San Francisco, pp. 389-414.

Nasrallah, H. A., McGilley-Lolitters, M., and Jacoby, C. G. (1982) Cerebral ventricular enlargement in young manic males. J. Affec. Disorders **4**, 15-19.

Nordeen, E. J. and Yahr, P. (1982) Hemispheric asymmetries in the behavioral and hormonal effects of sexually differentiating mammalian brain. Science **218**, 391-393.

Oke, A., Keller, R., Mefford, J., and Adams, R. N. (1978) Lateralisation of norepinephrine in human thalamus. Science **200**, 1411-1413.

Oke, A. (1983) Norepinephrine distribution patterns in human thalamus. Int. J. Psychophysiology **1**, 109.

Oreland, L., Niberg, A., Asberg, M., Traskman, L., Sjoskand, L., Thoren, P., Bertilsson, L., and Tybring, G. (1981) Platelet MAO activity and monoamine metabolites in cerebrospinal fluid in depressed and suicidal patients and in healthy controls. Psychiatry Res. **4**, 21-29.

Orme, J. E. (1970) Left-handedness, ability and emotional disability. Br. J. Soc. Clin. Psychol. **9**, 87-88.

Pearlson, G. O. and Veroff, A. E. (1981) Computerised tomographic scan changes in manic-depressive illness. Lancet **ii**, 470.

Reuter-Lorenz, P. A., Givis, R. P., and Moscovitch, M. (1983) Hemispheric specialisation and the perception of emotion: evidence from right-handers and from inverted and non-inverted left-handers. Neuropsychologia **21**, 687-692.

Reveley, A. M., Reveley, M. A., Clifford, C., and Murray, R. M. (1982) Cerebral ventricular size in twins discordant for schizophrenia. Lancet **i**, 540-541.

Reveley, A. M., Reveley, M. A., and Murray, R. M. (1984) Cerebral ventricular enlargement in non-genetic schizophrenia: a controlled twin study. Brit. J. Psychiatry **144**, 89-93.

Reynolds, G. P. (1983) Increased concentrations and lateral asymmetry of amygdala dopamine in schizophrenia. Nature (Lond.) **305**, 527-529.

Rieder, R. O., Mann, L. S., Weinberger, D. R., van Kammen, D. P., and Post, R. M. (1983) Computed tomographic scans in patients with schizophrenia, schizo-affective and bipolar affective disorder.

Arch. Gen. Psychiatry **40**, 735-739.
Risberg, J. (1980) Regional cerebral blood flow measurements by 133 Xe-inhalation: methodology and applications in neuropsychology and psychiatry. Brain and Language **9**, 9-34.
Robinson, R. G. (1979) Differential behavioral and biochemical effects of right and left hemispheric cerebral infarction in the rat. Science **205**, 707-710.
Robinson, R. G. and Price, T. R. (1982) Post-stroke depressive disorders: a follow-up study of 103 patients. Stroke **13**, 635-641.
Robinson, R. G., Kubos, K. L., Starr, L. B., Rao, K., and Price, T. R. (1983) Mood changes in stroke patients: relationship to lesion location. Comp. Psychiatry **24**, 55-556.
Ross, E. and Rush, J. (1981) Diagnosis and neuroanatomical correlates of depression in brain-damaged patients. Arch. Gen. Psychiatry **38**, 1344-1354.
Rossor, M., Garett, N., and Iversen, L. (1980) No evidence for lateral asymmetry of neurotransmitters in post-mortem human brain. J. Neurochem. **35**, 743-745.
Sackeim, H. A., Greenberg, M. S., Weiman, A. L., Gur, R. C., Hungerbuhler, J. P., and Geschwind, N. (1982) Hemispheric asymmetry in the expression of positive and negative emotions: neurological evidence. Arch. Neurol. **39**, 210-218.
Sackeim, H. A. and Decina, P. (1983) Lateralised neuropsychological abnormalities in bipolar adults and in children of bipolar probands. In: Laterality and Psychopathology (Flor-Henry, P. and Gruzelier, J., eds), Elsevier, North Holland, pp. 103-128.
Sackeim, H. A., Epstein, D., Decina, P., Malitz, S., and Bruder, G. E. (1983) Auditory measures of lateralised activation imbalance in depression and effects of ECT. Presented at the VII World Congress of Psychiatry, Vienna, abstract no. **1124**, 243.
Sackeim, H. A. (1984) Personal communication.
Sai-Halasz, A., Brunecker, G., and Szera, S. (1958) Dimethyltryptamin: ein neues psychoticum. Psychiatria et Neurologia **135**, 285-301.
Schaffer, C. E., Davidson, R. J., and Saron, C. (1983) Frontal and parietal electroencephalogram asymmetry in depressed and nondepressed subjects. Biol. Psychiatry **18**, 753-762.
Serafetinides, E. A. (1973) Voltage laterality in the EEG of psychiatric patients. Dis. Nerv. Sys. **34**, 190-191.

Shaw, D. A. (1978) L-5-Hydroxytryptophan and depression. In: *Neurotransmitter Systems and Their Clinical Disorders* (Legg, N. J., ed.), Academic Press, London, New York, San Francisco, pp. 201-206.

Silberman, E. K., Weingartner, H., Stillman, R., Chen, H.-J., and Post, R. M. (1983) Altered lateralisation of cognitive processes in depressed women. *Am. J. Psychiatry* **140**, 1340-1344.

Standish-Barry, H. M. A. S., Bouras, N., Bridges, P. K., and Bartlett, J. R. (1982) Pneumo-encephalographic and computerised axial tomography scan changes in affective disorder. *Brit. J. Psychiatry* **141**, 614-617.

Stone, E. A. (1983) Problems with current catecholamine hypotheses of antidepressant agents. *Behav. Brain Sci.* **6**, 535-577.

Tucker, D. M., Stenslie, C. E., Roth, R. S., and Shearer, S. L. (1981) Right frontal lobe activation and right hemisphere performance: decrement during a depressed mood. *Arch. Gen. Psychiatry* **38**, 169-174.

Uytdenhoef, P., Portelange, P., Jacquy, J., Charles, G., Linkowski, P., and Mendlewicz, J. (1983) Regional cerebral blood flow and lateralised hemispheric dysfunction in depression. *Brit. J. Psychiatry* **143**, 128-132.

Van Boxel, P., Bridges, P. K., Bartlett, J. R., and Traver, T. (1978) Size of cerebral ventricles in 66 psychiatric patients. *Brit. J. Psychiatry* **133**, 500-506.

Van Praag, H. M. (1984) Depression, suicide and serotonin metabolism in the brain. In: *Neurobiology of Mood Disorders, Volume 1 of Frontiers of Clinical Neuroscience* (Post, R. M. and Ballenger, J. C., eds), Williams and Wilkins, Baltimore, London, pp. 601-618.

Vom Saal, F. S., Grant, W. M., McMullen, C. W., and Laves, K. S. (1983) High fetal estrogen concentrations: correlation with increased adult sexual activity and decreased aggression in male mice. *Science* **220**, 1306-1309.

Von Knorring, L. (1983) Interhemispheric EEG differences in affective disorders. In: *Laterality and Psychopathology* (Flor-Henry, P. and Gruzelier, J., eds), Elsevier, North Holland, pp. 315-338.

Von Knorring, L. and Oreland, L. (1983) Personality traits related to platelet monoamine oxidase (MAO) activity. *Unpublished paper presented at International Conference on Individual Differences*, London, July 6-9.

Von Knorring, L. (1984) Personal communication.
Von Nagy, K. (1963) Pneumoencephalgraphische befunde bei endogenen psychosen. Der Nervenarzt **34**, 543-548.
Winokur, G. and Crowe, R. R. (1983) Bipolar illness. Arch. Gen. Psychiatry **40**, 57-58.
Yeo, R. A., Turkheimer, E., and Bigler, E. D. (1984) The influence of sex and age on unilateral cerebral lesion sequelae. Presented at 12th Annual Meeting of the International Neuropsychology Society, Houston, Texas, February.
Yeudall, L. T., Fedora, O., Fedora, S., and Wardell, D. (1981) Neurosocial perspective on the assessment and etiology of persistent criminality. Australian J. Forensic Sci. **13**, 131-159; **14**, 20-44.

5.

CLINICAL FEATURES OF AFFECTIVE DISORDERS I: DIAGNOSIS, CLASSIFICATION, RATING SCALES, OUTCOME AND EPIDEMIOLOGY

R. C. Bland

Diagnosis

Introduction

Historical and literary references to depression, such as the accounts of Saul, who suffered episodes of sadness, hopelessness and guilt, Hippocratic references to melancholia, Burton's Anatomy of Melancholy in 1624, and Shakespeare's description of Hamlet's cyclic mood changes, are numerous.
During the nineteenth century Falret and Baillarger described 'folie circulaire' and 'folie a double forme', a disorder with acute onset, exacerbations and remissions, with relative normality between episodes, higher frequency of occurrence in women, and with a hereditary contribution.
Kraepelin (1921) clearly stated his views on manic-depressive insanity when he wrote 'manic depressive insanity--includes on the one hand the whole domain of so-called periodic and circular insanity, on the other hand simple mania, the greater part of the morbid states termed melancholia, and also a not inconsiderable number of cases of amentia.' (Amentia referred to confusional or delirious insanity.)
It is apparent that many of Kraepelin's concepts are embodied in current diagnostic and classification systems.

Concepts

Delineation from Normality. There is no difficulty in recognising that feelings of sadness and unhappiness are a normal response to setbacks in life or to sad and unhappy events. Clinicians, however, consider depression to be an illness, quite unlike the normal experience of unhappiness.

Unhappiness from time to time is an almost universal phenomenon, but incapacitating depression is relatively uncommon, and yet there are infinite gradations between the two extremes. It is obvious that a broad diagnostic scheme will include many more persons than a much narrower and restrictive system.

Unfortunately there are no universally accepted cut-off points for what constitutes normality and what constitutes illness.

Comparisons of self-reports on depressive symptoms and results of a structured interview on the same sample of the general adult population have been reported recently (Myers and Weissman, 1980; Boyd et al., 1982). The self-report questionnaire was the Center for Epidemiologic Studies-Depression Scale (CES-D), and the diagnostic assessment was made using the SADS-L interview (Schedule for Affective Disorders and Schizophrenia, Spitzer and Endicott, 1978) and RDC criteria (Research Diagnostic Criteria, Spitzer et al., 1978). Of the persons scoring above the cut-off score on the CES-D, only one-third had a current major depression based on the RDC criteria.

Recent efforts to define diagnostic criteria, which establish symptom duration, minimum numbers of symptoms present, severity of symptoms and degree of incapacity, attempt to delineate a depressive illness from feelings of unhappiness or sadness (Wing et al., 1974; Feighner et al., 1972, Spitzer et al., 1975).

Mania, which is far less common than depression, poses fewer problems in making the distinction from a variant of the normal. Relatively mild hypomanic states, however, give the same delineation problems as depression.

Classification Systems. There have been numerous attempts and systems for classifying affective disorders in the last 50 years (Kendell, 1976), and these have included from one to thirteen categories.

Kendell (1976) describes three basic classification systems. The first is simple typologies, where depressions are divided into a variable number of discrete entities. This categorical approach, familiar throughout medicine, identifies discrete disease entities frequently useful in etiological studies. The current (9th) and previous editions of the International Classification of Diseases use

this approach (WHO, 1978).
   The second type of classification system uses tiered typologies. The St. Louis criteria (Feighner et al., 1972; Feighner, 1981) introduced the concept of a distinction between primary and secondary disorders. The disorder is primary when there is no pre-existing psychiatric condition such as schizophrenia, anxiety neuroses, phobia, neurosis, obsessive compulsive neurosis, hysteria, alcoholism, drug dependency, antisocial personality, homosexuality or other sexual deviations, mental retardation or organic brain syndrome. Also patients with life threatening or incapacitating medical illness preceding and paralleling the depression do not receive the diagnosis of primary depression. A similar approach is followed in the RDC (Spitzer et al., 1978) and in DSM III (Diagnostic and Statistical Manual of Mental Disorders, 3rd edition; American Psychiatric Association, 1980), although with somewhat different criteria. All of these systems also incorporate the bipolar-unipolar distinction to classify primary affective disorders (see below).
   The third type of classification system is dimensional rather than typological, and Kendell (1976) uses the psychotic/neurotic continuum to illustrate this, having failed to demonstrate clear differentiation of the more severe (psychotic) from the less severe. He points out that 'psychotic' and 'neurotic' are terms which are difficult to define with precision, and has regarded psychotic/neurotic as synonymous to endogenous/reactive and equivalent to severe/mild (thus disregarding the dubious etiological implications of endogenous and reactive). While the system may be statistically satisfactory, few clinicians would regard the patient with acute onset, unvarying depressed mood, marked retardation, severe insomnia, significant weight loss and guilt and suicidal ideas as differing only in degree of severity from the patient with anxiety, depressed mood varying from day to day, initial insomnia, emotional outbursts and no weight loss.

Unipolar and Bipolar Illnesses. Kraepelin (1921), in writing about manic-depressive psychoses, had a broad concept of the illness and included patients who had both manic and depressive episodes, or either alone, in the same group. He also included involutional melancholia, which he had earlier regarded as distinct.
   Leonhard (1959) differentiated two large groups within the affective psychoses based on course of

the illness variables. This depended on the presence of both manic and depressive episodes in the same patient (bipolar) or the occurrence of only manic or depressive episodes (monopolar, now called unipolar). Subsequent investigations suggested that the hereditary factor was more marked in the bipolar patients than in the unipolar, and that personality characteristics of cyclothymia were more likely to be found in the bipolars.

Leonhard's work was developed further by Angst (1966) in Switzerland and Perris (1966) in Sweden, who later compared findings (Angst and Perris, 1968), and by Winokur et al. (1969) in the United States. The bipolar-unipolar distinction is now almost universally accepted and is implicit in classification systems.

Apart from the course of the illness, much of the validation of the unipolar-bipolar distinction rests on studies of first degree relatives of unipolar and bipolar probands.

Perris (1966) achieved almost a complete separation.

Morbid risk in first degree relatives

Relatives %

Perris (1966)
Patients	Bipolar	Unipolar
Unipolar	0.35	7.4
Bipolar	10.8	0.58

Angst (1966)
Unipolar	0.29	9.1
Bipolar	3.7	11.2

A large part of the differences between Angst's and Perris' findings result from Perris not including relatives with one or two episodes of depression in the unipolar relatives, but of classing them as uncertain. If this is taken into account, the findings are very similar. In all cases, the risk to relatives is higher than that found in the general population.

What emerges from these results and those from many subsequent studies is that, with few exceptions, bipolar illness is found much more frequently in relatives of bipolar probands than in relatives of unipolar probands. Unipolar illnesses are found in relatives of both bipolar and unipolar probands, but perhaps with a somewhat higher frequency in the

Clinical Features of Affective Disorders I

unipolar proband relatives. Thus, although the two illnesses may be distinguished, there is overlap (Gershon, 1983).

Currently there are efforts to subdivide bipolar disorders. Fieve and Dunner (1975) and Dunner (1983) proposed the following:

Bipolar I - hospitalised for mania at least once

Bipolar II - hospitalised for depression, symptoms of mania not resulting in hospitalisation

Bipolar other (Cyclothymic disorder) - symptoms of depression and mania resulting in treatment but not hospitalisation

Cyclothymic personality - symptoms of depression and mania not resulting in treatment

Unipolar - outpatient treatment or hospitalisation for depression: no history of mania

Depressive personality - depressive symptoms not resulting in treatment

This classification resulted from a practical need to classify cases that were being reviewed and failed to meet the full requirements of hospitalised treatment for mania which had been used in the studies by Angst (1966), Perris (1966), or Winokur et al. (1969).

Akiskal (1981, 1983) proposed a slightly different classification, similar to that of Feighner (1978, 1981):

Recurrent mania - no evidence for clinical depression

Bipolar I - mania and depression

Bipolar II - depression and spontaneous hypomania

Unipolar II - recurrent depressions, bipolar family history; may switch to hypomania with pharmacologic challenge

Unipolar I - depressions with low frequency of episodes and no bipolar history

There is overlap between Akiskal's unipolar IIs and

Fieve and Dunner's (1975) bipolar IIs, and Akiskal (1983) considers that many recurrent depressions probably belong to the bipolar spectrum of disorders.

It is apparent that, while active work is proceeding with subclassification along these lines, all issues are far from resolved.

There have been efforts to subdivide primary unipolar depressives based on family history. Winokur et al. (1978) and Van Valkenburg et al. (1977) have attempted to define depressive spectrum disease (DSD) as those patients with a family history of alcoholism or antisocial personality, familial pure depressive disease (FPDD), those with a family history of depression only, and sporadic depressive disease (SDD) where there is no family history. Symptoms were found not to differ between DSD and FPDD (Andreason and Winokur, 1979). The status of these subdivisions remains a subject for further research.

Angst and colleagues (Angst, 1980; Angst et al., 1980; Angst et al., 1981) use a somewhat different approach. Patients are defined as:

Dm: preponderantly depressed with hypomania
MD: severely manic and severely depressed
Md: preponderantly manic with mild depression

M and D mean treatment was required in hospital; m and d mean ambulatory treatment or no treatment required.

In common with most studies, age of onset was lower in those patients (Md and MD) with severe mania.

In the family genetics, proband sex differences are quite marked, but with very small numbers, and the results are therefore inconclusive.

Secondary Affective Disorders. As mentioned above (Feighner et al., 1972; Robins and Guze, 1972), the St. Louis group distinguished between primary and secondary affective disorders, based on the evidence of another psychiatric disorder predating the affective disorder.

Others (Klerman and Barrett, 1973; Greist and Greist, 1979; Klerman and Hirschfield, 1979) have drawn attention to the associations between medical illnesses and drug reactions. Examples include a wide variety of endocrine disorders, vitamin and mineral disorders, infectious neurological conditions, collagen diseases, cardiovascular diseases, malignancies and metabolic disorders, and drugs such as estrogens, progesterone, antihypertensives, antiparkinsonian agents, anticancer and antituberculosis medications. Klerman (1983) recommends that the concept of secondary affective disorders be extended to include not only those affective disorders secondary (in time) to another psychiatric disorder, but also to include those which are secondary to or associated with significant medical disease or drug reactions. This would seem to be eminently sensible, since affective disorders secondary to various medical disorders would not only confound a study dealing with primary affective disorders, but should be the subject for separate investigations.

It should be emphasised that the primary/secondary distinctions made in this way are largely atheoretical, designed to collect 'uncontaminated' groups of patients. There is considerable debate about the usefulness of the distinction made in this way, and what the boundaries should be (see Roth, 1981).

Unipolar Mania. Whether this condition exists has been much debated. Winokur et al. (1969) found it to be a rare entity; Perris (1966) reported that 11% of his large group of bipolar patients had histories of manic episodes only. Bratfos and Haug (1968) followed up 207 patients, half of whom were first admissions; of these 80% were unipolar depressed, but of the 20% who were classed as bipolar, 10% (i.e. 2% of the total patient group) had only manic episodes. Mendlewicz and Fleiss (1974) found in 134 successive bipolar admissions no patients who had had manic episodes only. However, Nurnberger et al. (1979) found 15.7% of bipolar patients had mania only. Rennie (1942) found that 26% of his bipolar patients had mania only, Shobe and Brion (1971) found 33% in this category, Pfohl et al. (1982) 34%, Stenstedt (1952) 65%, Bland and Orn (1982) 65%, Abrams and Taylor (1974) 28%, and Chopra (1975) 85%. Thus there seems little doubt of the existence of unipolar mania although it is possible that some of these patients could be classified as Md using Angst's (1980) system, and they certainly would fit Fieve and Dunner's (1975) Bipolar I category.

There is more doubt, however, whether these patients differ in family history or any other respect from those patients who are bipolar and have both manic and depressed episodes, except that they appear to have less frequent episodes (Nurnberger et

al., 1979; Pfohl et al., 1982; Bland and Orn, 1982).
It is also significant that despite extensive periods of follow-up, many of the patients classed as unipolar manic patients did not have recurrences. Note that studies such as those of Rennie (1942), Carlson et al. (1974), and Angst et al. (1973), which did not limit patients included to first admission or first episodes, record much lower proportions of patients without recurrences, for obvious reasons.

	Follow-up	Bipolars without recurrences, i.e. single episode mania
Stenstedt (1952)	1-30 yrs	32%
Rennie (1942)	10-25 yrs	4%
Lundquist (1945)	10-20 yrs	55%
Bland & Orn (1982)	12-18 yrs	26%

Unipolar Depression. There has been little doubt that unipolar depressions are distinct from bipolar disorders, with a later age of onset, and a higher proportion of females to males than is found in bipolar disorders. Genetic aspects based on family studies have been mentioned above.
A person whose first episode of illness is manic is classed with the bipolars (perhaps somewhat confusing, but unipolar manias are also classed with the bipolars); however, persons having a first depressive episode may eventually prove to be unipolar (depressed) or have a subsequent manic episode and become bipolars. Dunner et al. (1976) retrospectively showed that 21% of 152 bipolars had a depressive episode prior to the first attack of mania, but only 2% had 3 successive depressive episodes before their initial manic attack. Winokur and Morrison (1973) followed 225 depressives for 20 years and found only 9 had subsequent manic attacks. On this basis and with the probability of a 1-5% error in classification, but needing to maintain sample sizes in studies, Dunner et al. (1976) suggest that patients be classed as unipolar after waiting 6 months following a single depression.
The recurrence or non-recurrence of depression is infrequently discussed. Studies of first admission depressed patients over long periods of time consistently show that a high proportion of the patients do not have a recurrence.

	Length of follow-up	Single episode depressions as a proportion of unipolars
Lundquist (1945)	10-20 yrs	61%
Stenstedt (1952)	1-30 yrs	58%
Bland & Orn (1982)	12-18 yrs	55%

In these examples, more than half of those hospitalised and treated for a first depressive episode did not have a recurrence. Little work has been done on distinguishing characteristics of recurrent and non-recurrent major depressive disorders.

Diagnosis and Diagnostic Criteria

The last decade has been highly significant for psychiatric diagnosis because of two major developments.

Criteria have been developed for establishing diagnostic validity, and the problem of low interrater reliability in diagnosis has been reduced by the development of clearly defined operational diagnostic criteria.

Criteria for establishing diagnostic validity have been divided into phases (Feighner et al., 1972; Woodruff et al., 1974; Feighner 1981):

1. Clinical description of the disease with delineation from other disorders, and delimitation allowing specific exclusion of doubtful cases.

2. Laboratory studies including psychological, chemical, radiological and physiological tests shown to be reliable and reproducible.

3. Family studies and examination of pedigrees enhance diagnostic validity, but also require combining with twin and adoptee data.

4. Longitudinal, follow-up, natural history studies, both prospective and retrospective, are required to validate original diagnoses.

Lack of operational definitions for psychiatric disorders has proved a major obstacle to progress in reaching agreement amongst clinicians and researchers. During the early 1950s, Robins, Guze and colleagues at Washington University in St. Louis started work on developing reliable structured interview schedules. This work was integrated into an article on diagnostic criteria for use in psychiatric research (Feighner et al., 1972) which gave detailed operational criteria for a number of disorders. This was later expanded in collaboration with Spitzer and Endicott of the New York State Psychiatric Institute (as part of the NIMH Collaborative Research Program) and included colleagues from Harvard and Iowa. The result was the production of the Research Diagnostic Criteria (RDC) (Spitzer et al., 1975). Structured interviews--the various versions of the Schedule for Affective Disorders and Schizophrenia (SADS)--were also published (Spitzer and Endicott, 1978). Other interviews were also produced and published (e.g. Helzer et al., 1981).

During this period, a number of important reliability studies were conducted (Helzer et al., 1977a,b; Spitzer et al., 1978). These showed that, using the standardised interviews and operational definitions, the level of reliability in psychiatric diagnosis was at least at the level of the best psychological tests, and vastly improved over the results in earlier studies without the benefit of such instruments (Matarazzo, 1983).

The DSM III (APA, 1980) was perhaps the logical outcome of the vastly increased awareness of the importance of diagnosis and the possibility of making reliable diagnoses. DSM I and DSM II produced lists of clinical disorders, associated with which were brief thumbnail descriptions of the condition. There were no diagnostic criteria suitable for resolution of diagnostic problems. Many of the researchers responsible for the development of the Feighner criteria and the Research Diagnostic criteria were also involved in developing DSM III, but whereas the former two sets of criteria were produced by small groups of researchers, with research use in mind, DSM III involved numerous committees and has to be used as an official national system of diagnosis and nomenclature. DSM III is probably the first official system of nomenclature to be exposed to extensive testing and field trials prior to its introduction.

It is also unique in its use of various axes. Axis I includes all psychiatric illnesses with the exception of personality disorders and specific developmental disorders of childhood, which constitute Axis II. Axis III is used to classify physical disorders and conditions which may coexist with Axis I and Axis II disorders.

Axes IV and V are new concepts introduced with DSM III and originally intended for use in research settings or to provide additional information of value in planning treatment or predicting outcome. Axis IV is used to judge the severity of psychosocial stressors on an 8 point rating scale; examples of each level of stress are given. The basic concept is similar to that in the Schedule of Recent Events (Holmes and Rahe, 1967) and other similar scales (e.g. Paykel et al., 1971). Axis V is used to assess on a single scale of 5 points from superior to poor the highest level of adaptive functioning in the past year, in three major areas: social relations, occupational functioning, and use of leisure time.

The most recent development is the NIMH Diagnostic Interview Schedule (DIS) (Robins et al., 1981), a highly structured interview schedule, allowing either lay interviewers or clinicians to make psychiatric diagnoses according to DSM III criteria, Feighner criteria and Research Diagnostic Criteria. The DIS, now in its third edition, does not include all of the DSM III diagnoses, but does have those likely to be of concern to researchers working with affective disorders. Each question is highly structured, and 'probing' (eliciting further information) is also conducted according to a structured format. The DIS was developed primarily as a research instrument. The option of using lay interviewers, and still achieving reliable diagnoses, enhances its ability to be used in community surveys and probably represents a significant advance in this area. Its advantages in the selection of patients for all types of studies, and particularly its applicability to patient selection for drug studies, have been quickly recognised.

Diagnosis has been a matter of concern not only in the United States. In Britain, working over a period of 25 years, Wing and associates (Wing et al., 1974; Wing, 1983) developed the Present State Examination (PSE), now in its ninth edition, as a system for reliably describing clinical phenomena. There is also a computer program CATEGO for classification, and an Index of Definition defining threshold points. CATEGO defines classes, and Wing does not regard this as the equivalent of clinical diagnoses. The PSE has been used in two large scale international studies, the US-UK diagnostic project (Cooper et al., 1972) and the International Pilot Study of Schizophrenia (WHO, 1973), and has now been translated into more than forty languages. Its use in North America has not been as widespread as the use of the Feighner criteria and the Research Diagnostic Criteria. A structured interview combination of PSE9 and DIS (the Composite Interview Schedule) is now being tested.

The International Classification of Diseases (ICD-9) (9th Revision, WHO, 1978) must be mentioned since in most countries it is the official classification system. For affective disorders it is not a system, and its classifications bear little resemblance to the research classification systems, except for the exclusion of involutional melancholia as a separate entity. No clear definitions or operational criteria are provided, merely brief descriptions of disorders. Overlap between categories is possible and schizoaffective disorder is included in schizophrenia rather than as a separate entity or with the affective disorders. It remains primarily a classification of diseases for coding morbidity and mortality data. In the United States, the National Center for Health Statistics was responsible for reviewing ICD-9 and the eventual production of ICD-9-CM (Clinical Modification) (Commission on Professional and Hospital Activities, 1978). It is generally compatible with its parent system ICD-9; however, in the affective disorders the numbering systems are not compatible. All of the terms in the DSM III were included in the ICD-9-CM or have been introduced since the original publication. Two additional codes are used in ICD-9-CM in the affective disorders which are not in DSM III. These are 296.0 Manic disorder, single episode, and 296.1 Manic disorder, recurrent episode.

The requirements of research are that patients studied must be as clearly defined (diagnosed) as is possible in the light of current knowledge. This requires the use of a set of established diagnostic criteria, and possibly reference to other aspects such as severity of the condition at the time of inclusion of the individual; and for affective disorders, where many issues are not resolved, it may require careful documentation of family history, selection of recurrent or non-recurrent disorders only, as well as selection decisions based on polarity and primary/secondary criteria.

It should be noted that using these systems the endogenous-reactive question is not addressed, and Nelson and Charney (1980) found that a considerable proportion of patients classed otherwise as 'reactive' met the criteria (RDC) for primary affective disorder, and consider that the criteria include a heterogeneous group of depressed patients which requires further refinement (which is part of DSM

III with the use and definition of melancholia).
The diagnostic combination of various states of anxiety with depression is unresolved (Roth, 1981; Roth and Mountjoy, 1982). This combination is probably the most common finding in outpatient practice, and therefore may pose considerable difficulties in selecting patients for studies.

What follows is an outline of some of the diagnostic systems and criteria currently being used in research in affective disorders. A more complete review and reprint of diagnostic criteria in current use for schizophrenia and the affective disorders is given by Berner et al. (1983).

Diagnostic Criteria

The Feighner or St. Louis Criteria (Feighner et al., 1972; Feighner, 1981). Diagnostic criteria are given for primary depression and for mania. They are 'episode' rather than 'illness' diagnoses, and include symptom duration and exclusion criteria.

Primary Depression

A through C are required.

A. Dysphoric mood characterised by symptoms such as the following: depressed, sad, blue, despondent, hopeless, 'down in the dumps', irritable, fearful, worried, or discouraged.
B. At least five of the following are required for 'definite' depression; four are required for 'probable' depression.
   1. Poor appetite or weight loss (positive if 2 pounds a week or 10 pounds or more a year when not dieting).
   2. Sleep difficulty (insomnia or hypersomnia).
   3. Loss of energy, e.g. fatigability or tiredness.
   4. Agitation or retardation.
   5. Loss of interest in normal activities, or decreased sex drive.
   6. Feelings of self-reproach or guilt (may be delusional).
   7. Complaints of or actual diminished ability to think or concentrate, such as slow-thinking or mixed up thoughts.
   8. Recurrent thoughts of death or suicide, including thoughts of wishing to be dead.
C. A psychiatric illness lasting at least one month with no pre-existing psychiatric condi-

tions such as schizophrenia, anxiety neurosis, phobic neurosis, obsessive-compulsive neurosis, hysteria, alcoholism, drug dependency, antisocial personality disorder, homosexuality and other sexual deviations, mental retardation, or organic brain syndrome. (Patients with life-threatening or incapacitating medical illness preceding and paralleling the depression do not receive the diagnosis of primary depression.)
D. There are patients who fulfill the above criteria, but who also have a massive or peculiar alteration of perception and thinking as a major manifestation of their illness. These patients are currently classified as having a schizoaffective psychosis.

Mania

A through C are required.

A. Euphoria or irritability.
B. At least three of the following must also be present:
   1. Hyperactivity (includes motor, social and sexual activity).
   2. Push of speech (pressure to keep talking).
   3. Flight of ideas (racing thoughts).
   4. Grandiosity (may be delusional).
   5. Decreased sleep.
   6. Distractibility.
C. A psychiatric illness <u>lasting at least two weeks</u> with no pre-existing psychiatric conditions such as schizophrenia, anxiety neurosis, phobic neurosis, obsessive compulsive neurosis, hysteria, alcoholism, drug dependency, antisocial personality disorder, homosexuality and other sexual deviations, mental retardation or organic brain syndrome.
D. There are patients who fulfill the above criteria, but who also have a massive or peculiar alteration of perception and thinking as a major manifestation of their illness. These patients are currently classified as having a schizoaffective psychosis.

Clinical Features of Affective Disorders I

Research Diagnostic Criteria (RDC) (Spitzer et al., 1975, 1978).

Subtypes of affective disorder

1. Manic disorder
2. Hypomanic disorder
3. Bipolar I (bipolar depression with mania)
4. Bipolar II (bipolar depression with hypomania)
5. Major depressive disorder
   a) primary   ) In all cases sub-
   b) secondary   ) jects must meet the
   c) recurrent unipolar) criteria for 'de-
   e) psychotic   ) finite' or 'proba-
   e) incapacitating) ble' major depres-
   f) endogenous   ) sive disorder.
   g) agitated   ) These subtypes have
   h) retarded   ) criteria which may
   i) situational   ) be of use in se-
   j) simple   ) lecting a particu-
) lar subgroup of pa-
) tients for study.
) An individual sub-
) ject may meet the
) criteria for more
) than one subtype.

There are also categories of minor and intermittent depressive disorder and generalised anxiety disorder with depression.
The diagnostic criteria are given below (from Spitzer, 1978). Note that there are inclusion, exclusion, duration and severity criteria (requires treatment or impairment of social functioning).

Manic Disorder

(May immediately precede or follow Major Depressive Disorder.)
A through E are required for the episode of illness being considered.

A. One or more distinct periods with a predominantly elevated, expansive, or irritable mood. The elevated, expansive, or irritable mood must be a prominent part of the illness and relatively persistent although it may alternate with depressive mood. Do not include if apparently due to alcohol or drug use.
B. If mood is elevated or expansive, at least three of the following symptom categories must

be definitely present to a significant degree, four if mood is only irritable. (For past episodes, because of memory difficulty, one less symptom is required.) Do not include if apparently due to alcohol or drug use.
  (1) More active than usual--either socially, at work, at home, sexually, or physically restless.
  (2) More talkative than usual or felt a pressure to keep talking.
  (3) Flight of ideas or subjective experience that thoughts are racing.
  (4) Inflated self-esteem (grandiosity, which may be delusional).
  (5) Decreased need for sleep.
  (6) Distractibility, i.e., attention is too easily drawn to unimportant or irrelevant external stimuli.
  (7) Excessive involvement in activities without recognizing the high potential for painful consequences, e.g., buying sprees, sexual indiscretions, foolish business investments, reckless driving.

C. Overall disturbance is so severe that at least one of the following is present:
  (1) Meaningful conversation is impossible.
  (2) Serious impairment socially, with family, at home, at school, or at work.
  (3) In the absence of (1) or (2), hospitalization.

D. Duration of manic features at least one week beginning with the first noticeable change in the subject's usual condition (or any duration if hospitalized). If became "manic" after hospitalization, the rater should differentiate between manic and hypomanic periods on the basis of apparent severity.

E. None of the following which suggest Schizophrenia is present. (Do not include if apparently due to alcohol or drug use.)
  (1) Delusions of being controlled (or influenced), or thought broadcasting, insertion, or withdrawal.
  (2) Non-affective hallucinations of any type throughout the day for several days or intermittently throughout a one week period.
  (3) Auditory hallucinations in which either a voice keeps up a running commentary on the subject's behaviors or thoughts as they occur, or two or more voices converse with

each other.
(4) At some time during the period of illness had more than one week when he exhibited no prominent depressive or manic symptoms but had delusions or hallucinations.
(5) At some time during the period of illness had more than one week when he exhibited no prominent manic symptoms but had several instances of marked formal thought disorder, accompanied by either blunted or inappropriate affect, delusions or hallucinations of any type, or grossly disorganized behavior.

Hypomanic Disorder

(May immediately precede or follow Major Depressive Disorder.)
  A through D are required.

A. Has had a distinct period with predominantly elevated, expansive, or irritable mood. The elevated, expansive, or irritable mood must be relatively persistent or occur frequently. It may alternate with depressive mood. Do not include if mood change is apparently due to alcohol or drug use.
B. If the mood is elevated or expansive, at least two of the symptoms noted in Manic Disorder B must be present, three symptoms if mood is only irritable.
C. Duration of mood disturbance at least two days. Definite if elevated, expansive, or irritable mood lasted for one week, probable if two to six days.
D. The episode being considered does not meet the criteria for Schizophrenia, Schizo-affective Disorder, or Manic Disorder.

Bipolar Depression with Mania (Bipolar 1)

At some time in his life has met the criteria for Manic Disorder and Major Depressive Disorder, Minor Depressive Disorder, or Intermittent Depressive Disorder. Probable if the Manic Disorder is only probable.

Bipolar Depression with Hypomania (Bipolar 2)

At some time in his life has met the criteria for both Hypomanic and Major Depressive Disorder, Minor

Clinical Features of Affective Disorders I

Depressive Disorder, or Intermittent Depressive Disorder, and has never met the criteria for Manic Disorder. Probable if the Hypomanic Disorder is only probable.

Major Depressive Disorder

(May immediately precede or follow Manic Disorder.)
A through F are required for the episode of illness being considered.

A. One or more distinct periods with dysphoric mood or pervasive loss of interest or pleasure. The disturbance is characterized by symptoms such as the following: depressed, sad, blue, hopeless, low, down in the dumps, "don't care anymore," or irritable. The disturbance must be prominent and relatively persistent but not necessarily the most dominant symptom. It does not include momentary shifts from one dysphoric mood to another dysphoric mood, e.g., anxiety to depression to anger, such as are seen in states of acute psychotic turmoil.

B. At least five of the following symptoms are required to have appeared as part of the episode for definite and four for probable (for past episodes, because of memory difficulty, one less symptom is required).
  (1) Poor appetite or weight loss or increased appetite or weight gain (change of 1 lb. a week over several weeks or ten lbs. a year when not dieting).
  (2) Sleep difficulty or sleeping too much.
  (3) Loss of energy, fatigability, or tiredness.
  (4) Psychomotor agitation or retardation (but not mere subjective feeling of restlessness or being slowed down).
  (5) Loss of interest or pleasure in usual activities, including social contact or sex (do not include if limited to a period when delusional or hallucinating). (The loss may or may not be pervasive.)
  (6) Feelings of self-reproach or excessive or inappropriate guilt (either may be delusional).
  (7) Complaints or evidence of diminished ability to think or concentrate, such as slowed thinking, or indecisiveness (do not include if associated with marked formal thought disorder).
  (8) Recurrent thoughts of death or suicide, or any suicidal behavior.

- C. Duration of dysphoric features at least one week beginning with the first noticeable change in the subject's usual condition (definite if lasted more than two weeks, probable if one to two weeks).
- D. Sought or was referred for help from someone during the dysphoric period, took medication, or had impairment in functioning with family, at home, at school, at work, or socially.
- E. None of the following which suggest Schizophrenia is present:
  - (1) Delusions of being controlled (or influenced), or of thought broadcasting, insertion, or withdrawal.
  - (2) Non-affective hallucinations of any type throughout the day for several days or intermittently throughout a one week period.
  - (3) Auditory hallucinations in which either a voice keeps up a running commentary on the subject's behaviors or thoughts as they occur, or two or more voices converse with each other.
  - (4) At some time during the period of illness had more than one month when he exhibited no prominent depressive symptoms but had delusions or hallucinations (although typical depressive delusions such as delusions of guilt, sin, poverty, nihilism, of self-deprecation, or hallucinations with similar content are not included).
  - (5) Preoccupation with a delusion or hallucination to the relative exclusion of other symptoms or concerns (other than typical depressive delusions of guilt, sin, poverty, nihilism, self-deprecation or hallucinations with similar content).
  - (6) Definite instances of marked formal thought disorder (as defined in this manual), accompanied by either blunted or inappropriate affect, delusions or hallucinations of any type, or grossly disorganized behavior.
- F. Does not meet the criteria for Schizophrenia, Residual Subtype.

Subtypes of major depressive disorder

This section is primarily for studies in which there is interest in one or more subtypes of Major Depressive Disorder. The diagnoses in this section describe different ways of categorizing such subjects who meet the criteria for Probable or Definite Major Depressive Disorder, and therefore many subjects will meet the criteria for several categories. Probable in this section refers to the subtype, not the certainty that the condition meets the criteria for Major Depressive Disorder.

a. Primary major depressive disorder

The first appearance of probable or definite Major Depressive Disorder was not preceded by any of the following (either probable or definite) although these conditions may have occurred afterwards:
Schizophrenia, Schizo-affective Disorder, Panic Disorder, Phobic Disorder, Obsessive Compulsive Disorder, Briquet's Disorder (Somatization Disorder), Antisocial Personality, Alcoholism, Drug Use Disorder, or Preferential Homosexuality.
Episodes of Manic Disorder or Hypomanic Disorder may or may not have been present.

b. Secondary major depressive disorder

A period of Major Depressive Disorder (either probable or definite) was preceded by any of the conditions listed below (either probable or definite). (Note: It is possible for a subject to have had both Primary and Secondary Major Depressive Disorders, for example, depression at age 20 and 40 and Alcoholism beginning at age 30 and another depressive episode later.) Another category, Depressive Syndrome Superimposed on Residual Schizophrenia, is also a type of Secondary Depression. Check the condition(s) which existed prior to the development of Secondary Major Depressive Disorder.

____ Schizophrenia (with full remission)
____ Obsessive Compulsive Disorder
____ Phobic Disorder
____ Antisocial Personality
____ Drug Use Disorder
____ Schizo-affective Disorder
____ Panic Disorder
____ Briquet's Disorder (Somatization Disorder)
____ Alcoholism
____ Preferential Homosexuality (not limited to discrete periods of life)
____ Anorexia
____ Transsexualism
____ Organic Brain Syndrome

The St. Louis group no longer makes a diagnosis of Secondary Depression because of a pre-existing life-threatening condition.

c. Recurrent unipolar major depressive disorder

This is for individuals who have never met the criteria for Manic Disorder, Hypomanic Disorder, or Schizo-affective Disorder, Manic Type but who have had two or more episodes that met the criteria for probable or definite Major Depressive Disorder each separated by at least two months of return to more or less usual functioning.

d. Psychotic major depressive disorder

This category is considered for all subjects who have had a Major Depressive Disorder (either probable or definite). Note: The term Psychotic Depressive Reaction in the standard nomenclature often involves the additional concepts of severity of functional impairment and endogenous phenomena which are not included in this category and are covered separately in other subtypes. This category here is not used in the sense of a psychotic-neurotic dichotomy and thus there is no implication that subjects not so classified thereby have a neurotic depression. (Note: The only delusional or hallucinating subjects who would be considered here are those who do not meet the criteria for Schizo-affective Disorder.)

Either A or B is required.
   A. Delusions
   B. Hallucinations

e. Incapacitating major depressive disorder

This category is considered for all subjects who have had a probable or definite Major Depressive Disorder. It is applied to subjects who might be classified as Psychotic Depressive Reaction in the standard nomenclature on the basis of extreme severity of functional impairment.

> Because of severity of depressive symptoms, the subject is unable to carry out any relatively complex goal-directed activity such as work, taking care of the house, or sustaining attention and participation in social or recreational activities, i.e., hobbies, reading,

going to the movies. Do not count if due to refusal or lack of motivation to do the tasks. (If hospitalized, the impairment in functioning should be such that the patient obviously could not carry out the activities if given a chance to do so.)

f. Endogenous major depressive disorder

This category is considered for all subjects with a current episode that meets the criteria for probable or definite Major Depressive Disorder. It is applied to those subjects who show a particular symptom picture that many research studies indicate is associated with good response to somatic therapy. Ignore the presence or absence of precipitating events even though this feature is often associated with the term "endogenous."

From groups A and B a total of at least four symptoms for probable, six for definite, including at least one symptom from group A.

A. (1) Distinct quality of depressed mood, i.e., depressed mood is perceived as distinctly different from the kind of feeling he would have or has had following the death of a loved one.
    (2) Lack of reactivity to environmental changes (once depressed doesn't feel better, even temporarily, when something good happens).
    (3) Mood is regularly worse in the morning.
    (4) Pervasive loss of interest or pleasure.
B. (1) Feelings of self-reproach or excessive or inappropriate guilt.
    (2) Early morning awakening or middle insomnia.
    (3) Psychomotor retardation or agitation (more than mere subjective feeling of being slowed down or restless).
    (4) Poor appetite.
    (5) Weight loss (two lbs. a week over several weeks or 20 lbs. in a year when not dieting).
    (6) Loss of interest or pleasure (may or may not be pervasive) in usual activities or decreased sexual drive.

g. Agitated major depressive disorder

This category is considered for all subjects with a current episode that meets the criteria for probable or definite Major Depressive Disorder. At least two of the following manifestations of psychomotor agitation (not mere subjective anxiety) are required for several days during the current episode:

(1) Pacing.
(2) Handwringing.
(3) Unable to sit still.
(4) Pulling or rubbing on hair, skin, clothing, or other objects.
(5) Outbursts of complaining or shouting.
(6) Talks on and on or can't seem to stop talking.

h. Retarded major depressive disorder

This category is considered for all subjects with a current episode that meets the criteria for probable or definite Major Depressive Disorder. At least two of the following manifestations of psychomotor retardation are required for at least one week during the current episode:

(1) Slowed speech.
(2) Increased pauses before answering.
(3) Low or monotonous speech.
(4) Mute or markedly decreased amount of speech.
(5) Slowed body movements.

i. Situational major depressive disorder

This category is considered for all subjects with a current episode that meets the criteria for a probable or definite Major Depressive Disorder. It is applied to those subjects in whom the depressive illness has developed after an event or in a situation that seems likely to have contributed to the appearance of the episode at that time. In making this judgment consider the amount of stress inherent in the event or situation, the cumulative effect of such stresses, and the closeness of the events to the onset or exacerbation of the depressive episode.

Definite is for situations in which the episode almost certainly would not have developed at that time, in the absence of the external events.

Example: Depressive episode immediately following the sudden death of a loved one. Probable is for situations in which the episode probably would not have developed at that time, in the absence of the external events.

Example: Depressive episode several months after increasing business difficulties.

j. Simple major depressive disorder

This category is considered for all subjects with a current episode that meets the criteria for probable or definite Major Depressive Disorder. It is applied to depressive episodes that develop in a person who has shown no significant signs of psychiatric disturbance in the year prior to the development of the current episode, with the exception of symptomatology associated with either Major or Minor Depressive Disorder, Manic or Hypomanic Disorder.

Often depressive episodes begin with symptoms other than those in the classic depressive syndrome, such as phobias, panic attacks, or excessive somatic concerns. In such instances, these symptoms should be regarded as part of the depressive episode unless the duration of the other symptoms is sufficient to warrant a separate diagnosis.

Note: The concept of Simple Major Depressive Disorder is not identical with the concept of Primary Major Depressive Disorder. An individual who had Alcoholism followed by more than one year of abstinence who then developed a depression would be categorized as having both a Simple and a Secondary Major Depressive Disorder.

DSM III Classification of Affective Disorders (APA, 1980)

Bipolar disorder

296.6x	mixed	Note: fifth digit codes for manic or mixed episode:
296.4x	manic	
296.5x	depressed	6 - in remission
		4 - with psychotic features
		7 - mood incongruent psychotic features
		2 - without psychotic features
		0 - unspecified

Major depression

296.2x	single episode	Note: fifth digit codes for depressive episode:
296.3x	recurrent	
		6 - in remission
		4 - with psychotic features
		7 - mood incongruent psychotic features
		3 - with melancholia
		2 - without melancholia
		0 - unspecified

Clinical Features of Affective Disorders I

Other specific affective disorders

301.13 Cyclothymic disorder
300.40 Dysthymic disorder (depressive neurosis)

Atypical affective disorders

296.70 Atypical bipolar disorder
296.82 Atypical depression

Psychotic disorders not elsewhere classified

295.70 Schizoaffective disorder

DSM III Diagnostic Criteria for Episodes (these have been abbreviated; for the full criteria see DSM III [APA, 1980]).

Major depressive episode

A. Essential - dysphoric mood or loss of interest or pleasure in all or almost all usual activities or pastimes.

B. At least four of the following present nearly every day for at least two weeks:
   1. Appetite or weight change (increase or decrease)
   2. Insomnia or hypersomnia
   3. Psychomotor agitation or retardation
   4. Loss of interest or pleasure in usual activities (including sex)
   5. Loss of energy, fatigue
   6. Worthlessness, self reproach or inappropriate guilt
   7. Diminished ability to think or concentrate
   8. Recurrent thoughts of death or suicide or suicidal behavior

C. Exclusions
   1. Patients with mood incongruent delusion(s) or hallucination(s) or bizarre behavior when an affective syndrome is not present.
   2. Patients whose affective syndrome is superimposed on schizophrenia, schizophreniform disorder or paranoid disorder.
   3. Patients whose disorder is due to any organic mental disorder (there is a diagnosis of organic affective syndrome), or due to uncomplicated bereavement.

Clinical Features of Affective Disorders I

Fifth digit subclassifications have been mentioned above, only melancholia will be given in more detail. This is used for additional classification of patients who meet the criteria for major depressive episode.
With melancholia.
A. Loss of pleasure in all or almost all activities.
B. Lack of reactivity, even temporary, to pleasurable stimuli.
C. At least three of:
   1. A different and distinct quality of depressed mood.
   2. Worse in the mornings.
   3. Early morning waking (at least 2 hours).
   4. Retardation or agitation.
   5. Anorexia or weight loss.
   6. Excessive or inappropriate guilt.

Manic episode

A. Essential: elevated, expansive or irritable mood.
B. Three of the following present and persistent for at least one week:
   1. Increased activity or restlessness.
   2. Pressure to talk or increased talkativeness.
   3. Flight of ideas or racing thoughts.
   4. Increased self-esteem (grandiosity).
   5. Decreased sleep.
   6. Distractibility.
   7. Involvement in reckless activities.
C. Exclusions
   As for major depressive episode.

DSM III Diagnostic Criteria for Major Affective Disorders (abbreviated)

296.6   Bipolar disorder, mixed.
        The current episode includes the full picture of manic and major depressive episodes, and the depressive symptoms must last at least a full day.

296.4   Bipolar disorder, manic.
        Currently in a manic episode.

296.5   Bipolar disorder, depressed.
        Has had at least one manic episode and is currently in a major depressive episode.

Clinical Features of Affective Disorders I

296.2   Major depression, single episode

296.3   Major depression, recurrent
One or more major depressive episodes and no history of manic or hypomanic episodes.

Detailed criteria are also given for cyclothymic and dysthymic disorders.
It should be noted that diagnosis is in two stages, episode diagnosis and illness diagnosis, and that episode diagnosis requires satisfying symptom, duration, and exclusion criteria.

Rating Scales Used for Measuring the Severity of Mania and Depression

Making the diagnosis, even if stringent criteria are used, does not measure the severity of the depression or mania, yet measurements of severity are essential, for example, in assessing the progress of a patient or the effect of treatment. Moreover it may be necessary to make frequent measures.

The usefulness of the brief global ratings, which were used extensively until the last decade, is highly questionable. Such scales frequently miss key changes in symptomatology induced by different treatments (Shopsin et al., 1975). Therefore more specific ratings are necessary.

For depression two types of scale exist, those based on statements of the patients and those based on interviewer judgement; for obvious reasons only the latter type are useful in assessing mania.

Hamilton (1982) outlines the requirements for scales: they should have validity, sensitivity and reliability. Validity means that scores accurately reflect different grades of severity; sensitivity signifies that changes in symptom intensity are reflected in changes in scores on the scale; and reliability is the extent to which random error interferes with scores, the most important in clinical trials being interrater reliability.

Recent reviews of rating scales for depression (Hamilton, 1982) and for mania (Shopsin, 1979; Tyrer and Shopsin, 1982) are available and most of the scales are readily accessible.

Mania

Tyrer and Shopsin (1982), in their review of rating scales for mania, conclude that the Manic

State Rating Scale (MS) (Beigel et al., 1971) or its modification (MMS) by Blackburn et al. (1977) are likely to be the scales of choice where experienced nurse raters are used. The MS consists of 26 items rated 0-5 for frequency and 0-5 for severity, the individual item score being the product of these ratings. This scale has been adequately assessed for reliability and validity. The MMS has 28 items and a glossary, but reliability and validity may not be as high as for the MS.

Briefer scales, which can be used for outpatients and are intended for use by trained clinician raters and which are reported to have high validity and reliability, are the Mania Rating Scale (MRS) (Young et al., 1978) and the Bech-Rafaelson Mania Rating Scale (BRMS or BRMAS) (Bech et al., 1978, 1979; Bech, 1981). Both scales consist of eleven items each rated 0-4 and thus total scores range from 0-44. Both have fairly detailed definitions for rating each item.

The items rated in the BRMAS are: activity (motor), activity (verbal), flight of thoughts, voice/noise level, hostility/destructiveness, mood, self-esteem, contact, sleep, sexual interest, and work.

The MRS items are: elevated mood, increased motor activity-energy, sexual interest, sleep, irritability, speech (rate and amount), language-thought disorder, content, disruptive-aggressive behavior, appearance, and insight.

Depression

Scales for depression have been more numerous than those for mania, but despite their regular appearance, few survive.

The most widely used observer-rated scale is that of Hamilton (1967) which consists of 17 items, 9 rated on 4 levels and 0 for absent, the remainder rated on only 2 levels for the presence of the symptom. Its purpose is to measure the severity of the illness in patients diagnosed as depressed. It also serves as the bench mark to which newer scales are compared; two of these will be mentioned.

The Bech-Rafaelson Melancholia Scale (BRMES) (Bech, 1981) consists of 11 items each rated from 0 (normal) to 4, and its structure is very similar to the same authors' mania scale. Clear and quite precise instructions are given, and its authors claim high interrater reliability, and, as a test of validity, high correlation with the Hamilton Rating

Scale.

Montgomery and Asberg (1979) developed a scale starting with 65 items on a comprehensive psychopathology scale, selecting the 17 items most commonly occurring in patients with primary depressive illness and then selecting the 10 items which showed the largest changes with treatment and the highest correlation to overall change. Interrater reliability was high and scores correlated significantly with the Hamilton Rating Scale, and it showed a greater sensitivity to change than the Hamilton, indicating perhaps greater usefulness in detecting responders and non-responders in therapeutic trials. The 10 items are: apparent sadness, reported sadness, inner tension, reduced sleep, reduced appetite, concentration difficulties, lassitude, inability to feel, pessimistic thoughts, suicidal thoughts. Each item is recorded on a scale from 0-6. Rating instructions are provided, and definitions for some points on the scale, but some intermediate points are left to the rater's judgement.

The Beck Depression Inventory (Beck et al., 1961) is by far the most widely used self-assessment scale and consists of 21 items each rated 0-3, and requires that the patient judges how he feels at the time. Moderately high correlations with the Hamilton scale (.72-.82) are reported (Hamilton, 1982). Other self-report scales do not seem to be very widely used in recent work.

Outcome

Recurrent and Non-recurrent Disorders

This has been discussed above under unipolar mania and unipolar depression and it is suggested that a considerable proportion of patients will not experience a second episode of illness. Some authors, e.g. Angst et al. (1973) and Carlson et al. (1974), find non-recurrent disorders a rarity. A possible explanation is the way in which patients are included in studies, i.e. including a high proportion of cases with illnesses already known to be recurrent. This may not be the whole explanation. Winokur (1975) demonstrated that in a mixed group of first episode and readmission patients, those who were in their first episode were more likely to have a recurrence than those who were in a repeat episode at the index admission.

Episode Duration

A few studies have reported the proportion of patients with chronic unremitting illnesses on follow-up.

		Bipolar	Unipolar
1.	Single unremitting illness episode (Rennie, 1942)	1/66 (2%)	14/142 (10%)
2.	Chronic outcome (Rennie, 1942)	7/66 (11%)	19/142 (13%)
	(Lundquist, 1945)	8/103 (8%)	44/216 (20%)
3.	Continuously ill (Bratfos & Haug, 1968)	19/42 (45%)	39/165 (24%)
	(but in total, of those followed more than 5 years, 23% were continuously ill)		
4.	Chronically ill (Carlson et al., 1974) (constant symptoms requiring treatment)	6/49 (12%)	

Length of follow-up is of importance, and with longer follow-up there is a tendency to show increasing proportions of patients recovering.

The mean duration of episodes of mania and depression has also been examined. Bratfos and Haug (1968) recorded a range of 2 months to over 6 years, with a median of 7 months and a mean of 13 months. Rennie (1942) reported an average length of first episode of 6.5 months. Lundquist (1945) reported medians of 6-8 months for both manic and depressive episodes, older patients having longer attacks. Angst et al. (1973) reviewing 2798 bipolar first episodes found means of 2.7 months and for 2074 unipolar first episodes, means of 3.3 months. These shorter durations are in keeping with those of less than 2 months found by Winokur et al. (1969). There is evidence that episode length remains stable for a given individual (Angst et al., 1973).

Episode Frequency

Few reports are available detailing the frequency of episodes, that is, the number of episodes in a given time period, or the intervals between episodes. Bratfos and Haug (1968) report a symptom-free interval after the first episode (in those patients who have a recurrence) of 32 months (2-7 years). Angst et al. (1973) found mean cycle lengths (interval between onset of one episode and the next episode) to be 33 months for bipolar patients, first episode, decreasing to 11 months after the fourth episode, and for unipolar patients 37 months for the first episode, decreasing to 13 months after the fourth. These authors report decreasing cycle length with increased number of episodes, stabilising after the fourth or fifth attack. Carlson et al. (1974) followed 53 bipolar patients after a mean of 14.7 years from the onset of illness and found the mean number of episodes to be 5.8, which would give an average of 30 months between episodes. Some patients who were rapid cyclers are excluded and the actual frequency of attack may therefore be greater. Bland and Orn (1982) followed 102 patients after 15 years. For the bipolar (mania and depression) patients the mean number of episodes was 7.4 for a mean cycle duration of 24 months; for the recurrent depressed patients the number of episodes was 3.4 for a cycle duration of 52 months.

From the above it seems likely that recurrent bipolar patients will have an episode every 2-3 years, and recurrent unipolars every 3-4 years. The question of decreasing cycle length with an increasing number of episodes is not resolved.

Long Term Outcome

There are far fewer studies of the outcome in affective disorders than there are of the outcome in schizophrenia.

As with schizophrenia, earlier studies categorised patients into 2 or 3 outcome groups, usually without specifying the criteria. Also for affective disorders there has been a commonly held assumption that, in accordance with Kraepelin's statements, there is fairly complete recovery between episodes.

More recently studies have used multidimensional outcome measures, either the same as, or with similar concepts to, those used in schizophrenia studies.

Strauss and Carpenter (1972) published some of the best known outcome assessment criteria (for schizophrenia). They separately rated: duration of non-hospitalisation, social contacts, employment, and absence of symptoms; the scores on each measure could then be combined for an overall outcome measure. The WHO (1979), as part of its international studies of schizophrenia (in which a number of patients with affective disorders were included), used factors of symptomatic outcome, length of the inclusion episode, percentage of time in a psychotic episode, pattern of course, type of subsequent episodes, degree of social impairment, and length of time out of hospital as individual measures and combined them as an estimate of overall outcome.

Bland and Orn (1978) used measures of psychiatric condition, social adjustment, and economic productivity as individual scales which could be combined. As a separate measure they also used loss of productive time. They later used these measures, which had been used for schizophrenics, on a group of patients with affective disorders (Bland and Orn, 1982; Bland, 1984). Tsuang et al. (1979) and Tsuang and Dempsey (1979) used measures covering marital, residential and occupational status and psychiatric symptoms, which could be added to give a combined overall outcome measure. The report of Carlson et al. (1974) was one of the earlier studies to use a variety of outcome measures, but it did not combine them.

The increasing complexity and sophistication of outcome measurement is to be welcomed since it has long been recognised that 'symptom free' does not necessarily mean that the patient will be able to resume normal social relations or take up former employment satisfactorily.

Welner et al. (1977) review the problems of outcome studies in bipolar disorders, including separation of bipolar and unipolar groups, the entry point of cases (i.e. from the first episode), and the definitions of remission; they also review the earlier studies.

The findings from various studies are shown below.

Rennie (1942)

37% (76/208) of patients with affective disorder were permanently recovered for 5 years or longer.
30% (20/66) of patients with manic depressive disorder were permanently recovered for 5 years or longer.
39% (56/142) of patients with depressive disorder were permanently recovered for 5 years or longer.

Bratfos and Haug (1968)

'Continuously ill'   Bipolar 45%   Unipolar 24%

Clinical Features of Affective Disorders I

Also stated 'about 20% of all patients followed 5 years or more--chronic course with varying degrees of social incapacity'.

Shobe and Brion (1971)

Recovered ('no or minimal residual symptoms')
    Bipolar 47% (7/15)   Unipolar 60% (58/96)
Not recovered ('unable to work or to function socially most of the time')
    Bipolar 53% (8/15)   Unipolar 15% (14/96)

Carlson et al. (1974)

Used four scales to rate job status, social functioning, family interaction and mental status. Each was scored 1 (worst) to 4 (best). Followed 47 bipolar patients, 5-10% rated in the lowest category on each scale, and 16-21% in the highest. Estimating global outcome (for 49 bipolar patients) (not from adding the scale scores): 12% were chronically ill and 57% had been well during the 3 years preceding follow-up.

Tsuang and Winokur (1975)

		Mania (N=55)	Depression (N=145)
psychiatric)	none	36.4%	46.2%
disability)	moderate	34.5%	27.6%
)	marked	29.1%	26.2%

Tsuang et al. (1979) assessed outcome on four scales each rated 1-3 and used the mean to give a global score. They also presented the proportion of patients scoring 'poor' (the lowest rating) on each scale.

	Marital	Residential	Occupational	Psychiatric	Global
Mania: (N=86)					
'poor' rating	22%	14%	24%	29%	
mean on 1-3 scale	2.46	2.54	2.42	2.20	2.38
Depression: (N=212)					
'poor' rating	9%	12%	17%	22%	
mean on 1-3 scale	2.46	2.56	2.46	2.35	2.42

Bland and Orn (1982) assessed outcome on three scales, each rated 0 (worst) to 3 (best), added to give a global score, from 0 (worst) to 9 (best). They separately reported on depressed patients (all were first admissions) who had no recurrence in a 15-year follow-up (single depression).

	Scale (mean scores)			
	Economic	Social	Psychiatric	Combined
Mania ± Depression (N=27)	2.41	2.22	1.74	6.37
Recurrent Depression (N=34)	2.21	2.18	1.76	6.15
Single Depression (N=41)	2.76	2.66	2.71	8.12

These results are very similar to those of Tsuang et al. (1979). Both groups found little difference between the bipolars and recurrent depressives. Both groups included schizophrenic patients and found the outcome for them was worse. Tsuang et al. included a control group, which had a much better outcome, whereas Bland and Orn reported the nonrecurrent depressives, who had a considerably better outcome than the bipolars or recurrent depressives.

The WHO (1979) give outcome results on a number of patients with affective disorders. Outcome was assessed using the multidimensional measures mentioned above. The patients were then divided into 5 outcome levels. Bland (1984) divided his patients into 5 outcome groups (the same patients and outcome measures given above, Bland and Orn, 1982) for comparison with the results of the WHO. The findings are shown in Table 1.

These studies both indicate a generally favorable outcome for recurrent depressions and bipolar patients, and Bland and Orn (1982) and Bland (1984) show that for single episode depressions the outcome is better than for those with repeat episodes.

A different method of analysis, using the life table (Fleiss et al., 1976; Keller et al., 1982a,b) is likely to be used more frequently in the future, particularly in following patients to estimate the prophylactic effect of treatments such as lithium. It offers significant advantages when patients are followed for varying lengths of time, and it is necessary to compare various forms of treatment.

Table 5.1: Percentage Distribution of Patients in Outcome Groups (WHO Terminology)

	(N)	Very favorable	Favorable	Intermediate	Unfavorable	Very unfavorable	
Psychotic depression							
WHO (1979)	(70)	39	31	19	4	7	100
Recurrent depression							
Bland (1984)	(34)	29.4	32.4	23.5	11.8	2.9	100
Single episode depression							
Bland (1984)	(41)	87.8	2.4	2.4	4.9	2.4	100
Mania and depression							
WHO (1979)	(51)	49	31	12	6	2	100
Bland (1984)	(27)	44.4	18.5	22.2	14.8	0	100

Clinical Features of Affective Disorders I

Epidemiology of Affective Disorders

Epidemiology is the study of the distribution of diseases in populations and of the factors which influence that distribution. Several types of data are produced which have a variety of uses: to study the illness to chart historical trends, to delineate new syndromes, to compute morbid risks, and to identify causal and contributory factors, and plan and evaluate health services. Some knowledge of the epidemiology of a disease is also necessary in selecting samples of patients for other study purposes, to determine whether such samples can be considered representative of the disorder or a particular subset of the disorder.

The type of information generated includes calculations of rates of the disease (usually incidence and prevalence), variations in the rates over time and by location, and the identification of risk factors (e.g. age, sex, social class, place of residence, race).

For a variety of reasons epidemiological studies in North America have changed dramatically in recent years (Weissman and Klerman, 1978). In the post-World War II period, most studies concentrated on 'mental illness' rather than on specific disorders. Obviously a requirement for studying specific disorders is that a diagnosis can be agreed upon. Scandinavian workers achieved this to a large extent in earlier studies; but in the United States, the development of research diagnostic criteria provided impetus to more specific studies, and the production of interview schedules using these criteria, which could be administered by lay interviewers, laid the groundwork for the more recent epidemiological work. It is of interest that the comprehensive data from one of the earlier surveys, in Stirling County, has been reanalysed in accordance with DSM III criteria, and the results found to be very similar to those from later studies (Murphy, 1980).

Comprehensive, up-to-date reviews of the epidemiology of affective disorders have been published (Boyd and Weissman, 1982; Weissman and Boyd, 1983) which discuss findings in three categories: depressive symptoms, non-bipolar depression, and bipolar disorders. These categories will be used in this summary.

Clinical Features of Affective Disorders I

Depressive Symptoms

The reason for inclusion of depressive symptoms as a separate category is that such symptoms are very common; they are detected on community surveys, but do not necessarily bear a close relationship to depressive illnesses defined by research diagnostic criteria.
   The findings from a number of studies have been summarised (Boyd and Weissman, 1982; Weissman and Boyd, 1983) and it has been found that the point prevalence (number of individuals affected at a point in time, compared to the total population) ranges from 13-20% (10-19% for men and 20-34% for women). Risk factors include lower socioeconomic status, increased life events, lack of social supports, divorce and separation, and older males and younger females. The last finding of increased risk in older males and younger females is consistent with results found from using mental health questionnaires such as the General Health Questionnaire (Goldberg, 1972) which largely tap depressive symptoms (D'Arcy, 1982).

Non-bipolar Depression

This term is used to cover what might be included in major depressive disorders and avoid the controversial aspects of their subclassifications.
   The point prevalence, from various studies limited to the newer diagnostic techniques, and for western countries, is 3.2% for males and 4.5-9.3% for females (Boyd and Weissman, 1982). These figures are rather higher than those produced from the earlier studies reviewed by Krauthammer and Klerman (1979), who suggest, for affective psychosis, a range of 0.005-0.3%. Dohrenwend et al. (1980) give a median prevalence rate for affective psychosis of 0.3%. These large differences are undoubtedly partly explained by different methodologies, but it is possible that some of the newer diagnostic techniques are not stringent enough and include too many cases.
   Boyd and Weissman (1982) review incidence data based on case registers (i.e. treated cases) and show annual rates for men of 130-201/100,000 and for women 320-500/100,000. Only about 20% of persons with such disorders actually get treatment (Weissman et al. 1981), so these figures showing treated cases are probably a considerable underestimate of the true incidence. Incidence figures based on hospi-

talisation data show much lower figures.
Risk factors include:
Sex: about twice as many women as men, with an even higher proportion of women in the milder, more neurotic and non-recurrent conditions.

Age: both sexes tend to show increasing rates with age; women may 'peak' from age 35-45 (there is little evidence to suggest any menopausal peak), and have a second peak after age 60 years. Mean age of onset (at about 40 years) tends to be younger in women than men.

Family history: a family history of affective disorder or alcoholism increases risk.

Childhood experiences and personality: disruption and hostility in childhood as well as early parental loss have been suggested as risk factors, but require further confirmation, as do various personality attributes which have been implicated.

Life events: various studies have shown that depressed patients compared to normals have experienced an excess of life events falling into the category of 'exits' (usually losses). Lack of an intimate relationship is also implicated. The post partum period carries an excess risk for a variety of disorders.

Bipolar Disorders

Epidemiologic studies generally include in this group' all patients who have ever had a manic episode. A few studies separate those with only manic episodes from those with both manic and depressive attacks.

The ratio of bipolar to unipolar patients in studies of treated first episode cases varies from 14-32% (Lundquist, 1945; Stenstedt, 1952; Bratfos and Haug, 1968; Shobe and Brion, 1971; Bland and Orn, 1982). Lower ratios tend to be found in community or out-patient studies, since manic episodes are more likely to lead to admission than are depressed episodes.

Incidence is reviewed by Boyd and Weissman (1982), who give a range of annual rates between 9-15.2 per 100,000 men, and 7.4-32 per 100,000 women. These figures are about 8-10% of those for unipolar disorders, but the studies are not directly comparable. Krauthammer and Klerman (1979) suggest (based on reviewing biographic studies) that if the more ill-defined depressions are removed the figures approach the 25% ratio of bipolar to unipolar found with hospitalisation data on first admissions.

Risk factors.
Sex: the female preponderance common to all affective disorders is not as pronounced in bipolar disorders, where the sex ratio more nearly approaches equality.
Age: onset is earlier than in unipolar disorders; there is little if any sex difference and the modal age of onset is about 30 years in most studies (although onset in old age is by no means unknown).
Social class: higher social classes are generally found to have a higher incidence (this is in marked contrast to schizophrenia).
Marital status: weak trends towards higher rates in the single and divorced have been noted. It is not certain whether this is a result of the illness rather than a risk factor.
Family history: marked, with both bipolar and unipolar relatives being found.

References

Abrams, R. and Taylor, M. A. (1974) Unipolar mania. A preliminary report. Arch. Gen. Psychiatry 30, 441-443.

Akiskal, H. S. (1983) The bipolar spectrum: new concepts in classification and diagnosis. In: Psychiatry Update (Grinspoon, L., ed.), American Psychiatric Press, Washington, D.C., pp. 271-292.

Akiskal, H. S. (1981) Clinical overview of depressive disorders and their pharmacological management. In: Neuropharmacology of Central Nervous System and Behavioral Disorders (Palmer, G. C., ed.), Academic Press, New York, pp. 37-72.

American Psychiatric Association (1980) Diagnostic and Statistical Manual of Mental Disorders (3rd ed.). APA, Washington, D.C.(Used with permission)

Andreason, N. and Winokur, G. (1979) Newer experimental methods for classifying depression. Arch. Gen. Psychiatry 36, 447-452.

Angst, J. (1966) Zur Ätiologie und Nosologie der endogener depressiver Psychosen. Springer, Berlin.

Angst J. (1980) Clinical typology of bipolar illness. In: Mania, an Evolving Concept (Belmaker, R. H. and Van Praag, H. M., eds), Spectrum, New York, pp. 61-76.

Angst, J., Baastrup, P., Grof, P., Hippius, H., Poeldinger, W., and Weis, P. (1973) The course of monopolar depression and bipolar psychoses. Psychiatr. Neurol. Neurochir. (Amst.) 76, 489-500.

Angst, J., Frey, R., Lohmeyer, B., and Zerbin-

Rudin, E. (1980) Bipolar manic-depressive psychoses: results of a genetic investigation. Human Genetics **55**, 237-254.

Angst, J., Grigo, H., and Lanz, M. (1981) Classification of depression. Acta psychiatr. scand. **63** (Suppl. 290), 23-28.

Angst, J. and Perris, C. (1968) Zur Nosologie endogener Depressionen. Vergleich der Ergebnisse zureier Untersuchungen. Arckiv fur Psychiatrie **210**, 373-386.

Bech, P. (1981) Rating scales for affective disorders: their validity and consistency. Acta psychiatr. scand. **64** (Suppl., 295).

Bech, P., Bolwig, T. G., Kramp, P., and Rafaelson, O. J. (1979) The Bech-Rafaelson Mania Scale and the Hamilton Depression Scale. Acta psychiatr. scand. **59**, 420-430.

Bech, P., Rafaelsen, O. J., Kramp, P., and Bolwig, T. G. (1978) The mania rating scale: scale construction and interobserver agreement. Neuropharmacology **17**, 430-431.

Beck, A. T., Ward, C. H., Mendelson, M., Mock, J., and Erbaugh, J. (1961) An inventory for measuring depression. Arch. Gen. Psychiatry **4**, 561-571.

Beigel, A., Murphy, D. L., and Bunney, W. E. (1971) The manic-state rating scale. Arch. Gen. Psychiatry **25**, 256-262.

Berner, P., Gabriel, E., Katschnig, H., Kieffer, W., Koehler, K., Lenz, G., and Simhandl, C. (1983) Diagnostic Criteria for Schizophrenic and Affective Psychoses. World Psychiatric Association.

Blackburn, I. M., Loudon, J. B., and Ashworth, C. M. (1977) A new scale for measuring mania. Psychol. Med. **7**, 453-458.

Bland, R. C. The long-term mentally ill: an epidemiological perspective. Can. J. Psychiatry (in press).

Bland, R. C. and Orn, H. (1978) 14-year outcome in early schizophrenia. Acta psychiatr. scand. **58**, 327-338.

Bland, R. C. and Orn, H. (1982) Course and outcome in affective disorders. Can. J. Psychiatry **27**, 573-578.

Boyd, J. H. and Weissman, M. M. (1982) Epidemiology. In: Handbook of Affective Disorders (Paykel, E. S., ed.), Guilford, New York, pp. 109-125.

Boyd, J. H., Weissman, M. M., Thompson, D., and Myers, J. K. (1982) Screening for depression in a community sample. Arch. Gen. Psychiatry **39**, 1195-2000.

Bratfos, C. and Haug, J. O. (1968) The course of manic depressive psychosis: a follow-up investigation of 215 patients. Acta psychiatr. scand. **44**, 89-112.

Carlson, G. A., Kotin, J., Davenport, Y. B., and Adland, M. (1974) Follow-up of 53 bipolar manic-depressive patients. Brit. J. Psychiatry **124**, 134-139.

Chopra, H. D. (1975) Family psychiatric morbidity, parental deprivation and socio-economic status in cases of mania. Brit. J. Psychiatry **126**, 191-192.

Commission on Professional and Hospital Activities (1978) The International Classification of Diseases, 9th Revision, Clinical Modification. Ann Arbor, Michigan.

Cooper, J. E., Kendell, R. E., Gurland, B. J., Sharp, L., Copeland, J. R. M., and Simon, R. J. (1972) Psychiatric Diagnosis in New York and London: A Comparative Study of Mental Hospital Admissions, Maudsley Monograph No. 20. Oxford University Press, London.

D'Arcy, C. (1982) Prevalence and correlates of non-psychotic psychiatric symptoms in the general population. Can. J. Psychiatry **27**, 316-324.

Dohrenwend, B. P., Dohrenwend, B. S., Gould, M. S., Link, B., Neugebauer, R., and Wunsch-Hitzig, R. (1980) Mental Illness in the United States: Epidemiological Estimates. Praeger, New York.

Dunner, D. L. (1983) Sub-types of bipolar affective disorder with particular regard to bipolar II. Psychiatric Developments **1**, 75-86.

Dunner, D. L., Fleiss, J. L., and Fieve R. R. (1976) The course of development of mania in patients with recurrent depression. Am. J. Psychiatry **133**, 905-908.

Feighner, J. P. (1978) The nosology and phenomenology of primary affective disorders. Proceedings of II World Congress of Biological Psychiatry, Barcelona, Spain.

Feighner, J. P. (1981) Nosology of primary affective disorders and application to clinical research. Acta psychiatr. scand. **63** Suppl. 290, 29-41.

Feighner, J. P., Robins, E., Guze, J. B., Woodruff, R. A., and Winokur, G. (1972) Diagnostic criteria for use in psychiatric research. Arch. Gen. Psychiatry **26**, 57-73.(Copyright 1972, Am. Med. Assoc.)

Fieve, R. R. and Dunner, D. L. (1975) Unipolar and bipolar affective states. In: The Nature and Treatment of Depression (Flach, F. F. and Draghi,

S. C., eds), John Wiley and Sons, New York, pp. 145-166.
Fleiss, J. L., Dunner, D. L., Stallone, F., and Fieve, R. R. (1976) The life table: a method for analyzing longitudinal studies. Arch. Gen. Psychiatry **33**, 107-112.
Gershon, E. S. (1983) The genetics of affective disorders. In: Psychiatry Update (Grinspoon, L., ed.), American Psychiatric Press, Washington, D.C., pp. 434-457.
Goldberg, D. (1972) The Detection of Psychiatric Illness by Questionnaire. Oxford University Press, London.
Greist, J. and Greist, T. (1979) Antidepressant Treatment: The Essentials. Williams and Wilkins, Baltimore.
Hamilton, M. (1967) Development of a rating scale for primary depressive illness. Brit. J. Soc. Clin. Psychology **6**, 278-296.
Hamilton, M. (1982) Symptoms and assessment of depression. In: Handbook of Affective Disorders (Paykel, E. S., ed.), Guilford, New York, pp. 3-11.
Helzer, J. E., Clayton, P. J., Pambakian, R., Reich, T., Woodruff, R. A., and Reveley, M. A. (1977a) Reliability of psychiatric diagnosis: II, the test/retest reliability of diagnostic classification. Arch. Gen. Psychiatry **34**, 136-141.
Helzer, J. E., Robins, L. N., Croughan, J. L., and Welner, A. (1981) Renard diagnostic interview. Arch. Gen. Psychiatry **38**, 393-398.
Helzer, J. E., Robins, L. N., Taibleson, M., Woodruff, R. A., Reich, T., and Wish, E. D. (1977b) Reliability of psychiatric diagnosis: I. A methodological review. Arch. Gen. Psychiatry **34**, 129-133.
Hirschfield, R. M. A. and Klerman, G. L. (1979) Treatment of depression in the elderly. Geriatrics **34**, 51-57.
Holmes, T. H. and Rahe, R. H. (1967) The social readjustment scale. J. Psychosom. Res. **11**, 213-218.
Keller, M. B., Shapiro, R. W., Lavori, P. W., and Wolfe, N. (1982a) Recovery in major depression: analysis with the life table and regression models. Arch. Gen. Psychiatry **39**, 905-910.
Keller, M. B., Shapiro, R. W., Lavori, P. W., and Wolfe, N. (1982b) Relapse in major depressive disorder: analysis with the life table. Arch. Gen. Psychiatry **39**, 911-915.
Kendell, R. E. (1976) The classification of depres-

sion: a review of contemporary confusion. Brit. J. Psychiatry 129, 15-28.

Klerman, G. L. (1983) Nosology and diagnosis of depressive disorders. In: Psychiatry Update (Grinspoon, L., ed.), American Psychiatric Press, Washington, D.C., pp. 356-382.

Klerman, G. L. and Barrett, J. (1973) The affective disorders: clinical and epidemiologic aspects. In: Lithium: Its Role in Psychiatric Research and Treatment (Gershon, S. and Shopsin, B., eds), Plenum Press, New York, pp. 201-232.

Kraepelin, E. (1921) Manic Depressive Insanity and Paranoia. E. and S. Livingstone, Edinburgh.

Krauthammer, C. and Klerman, G. (1979) The epidemiology of mania. In: Manic Illness (Shopsin, B., ed.), Raven Press, New York, pp. 11-28.

Leonhard, K. (1959) Aufteilung der Endogenen Psychosen. Springer, Berlin.

Lundquist, G. (1945) Prognosis and course in manic depressive psychoses: a follow-up study of 319 first admissions. Acta psychiatr. neurol. scand., Suppl. 35.

Matarazzo, J. D. (1983) The reliability of psychiatric and psychological diagnosis. Clin. Psychol. Rev. 3, 103-145.

Mendlewicz, J. and Fleiss, J. L. (1974) Linkage studies with X-chromosome markers in bipolar (manic-depressive) and unipolar (depressive) illnesses. Biol. Psychiatry 9, 261-294.

Montgomery, S. A. and Asberg, M. (1979) A new depression scale designed to be sensitive to change. Brit. J. Psychiatry 134, 382-389.

Murphy, J. (1980) Continuities in community-based psychiatric epidemiology. Arch. Gen. Psychiatry 37, 1215-1223.

Myers, J. K. and Weissman, M. M. (1980) Use of a self-report symptom scale to detect depression in a community sample. Am. J. Psychiatry 137, 1081-1084.

Nelson, J. C. and Charney, D. S. (1980) Primary affective disorder criteria and the endogenous-reactive distinction. Arch. Gen. Psychiatry 37, 787-793.

Nurnberger, J., Roose, S. P., Dunner, D. L., and Fieve, R. R. (1979) Unipolar mania: a distinct clinical entity? Am. J. Psychiatry 136, 1420-1423.

Paykel, E. S., Prusoff, B. A., and Uhlenhuth, E. H. (1971) Scaling of life events. Arch. Gen. Psychiatry 25, 340-347.

Perris, C. (1966) A study of bipolar (manic-depres-

sive) and unipolar recurrent depressive psychoses. Acta psychiatr. scand. **42**, Suppl. 194.
Pfohl, B., Vasquez, N., and Nasrallah, H. (1982) Unipolar vs bipolar mania: a review of 247 patients. Brit. J. Psychiatry **141**, 453-458.
Rennie, T. A. C. (1942) Prognosis in manic depressive psychoses. Am. J. Psychiatry **98**, 801-814.
Robins, E. and Guze S. (1972) Classification of affective disorders: The primary-secondary, the endogenous, and the neurotic-psychotic concepts. In: Recent Advances in the Psychobiology of Depressive Illness (Williams, T. A., Katz, M. M., and Shield, J. A., eds), Department of Health Education and Welfare, Washington, D.C.
Robins, L. N., Helzer, J. E., Croughan, J., and Ratcliff, K. S. (1981) The National Institute of Mental Health Diagnostic Interview Schedule. Arch. Gen. Psychiatry **38**, 381-389.
Roth, M. (1981) Problems in the classification of affective disorders. Acta psychiatr. scand. **63**, Suppl. 290, 42-51.
Roth, M. and Mountjoy, C. Q. (1982) The distinction between anxiety states and depressive disorders. In: Handbook of Affective Disorders (Paykel, E. S., ed.), Longman, New York, pp. 70-92.
Shobe, F. O. and Brion, P. (1971) Long-term prognosis in manic-depressive illness: a follow-up investigation of 111 patients. Arch. Gen. Psychiatry **24**, 334-337.
Shopsin, B. (1979) Part I: Mania: Clinical aspects, rating scales and incidence of manic depressive illness. In: Manic Illness (Shopsin, B., ed.), Raven Press, New York, pp. 57-74.
Shopsin B., Gershon S., Thompson, H., and Collins, P. (1975) Psychoactive drugs in mania: a controlled comparison of lithium carbonate, chlorpromazine, and haloperidol. Arch. Gen. Psychiatry **32**, 34-42.
Spitzer, R. L. and Endicott, J. (1978) NIMH Clinical Research Branch Collaborative Program on the Psychobiology of Depression: Schedule for Affective Disorders and Schizophrenia (3rd ed.), New York State Psychiatric Institute, Biometrics Research Division, New York.
Spitzer, R. L., Endicott, J., and Robins, E. (1975) Research Diagnostic Criteria (RDC) for a Selected Group of Functional Disorders (2nd ed.), New York State Psychiatric Institute, Biometrics Research Division, New York.
Spitzer, R. L., Endicott, J., and Robins, E. (1978) Research Diagnostic Criteria (3rd ed.), New York

State Psychiatric Institute, Biometrics Research Division, New York.
Spitzer, R. L., Endicott, J., and Robins, E. (1978) Research diagnostic criteria. Arch. Gen. Psychiatry 35, 773-782.
Stenstedt, A. (1952) A study in manic depressive psychosis. Acta psychiatr. scand., Suppl. 79.
Strauss, J. S. and Carpenter, W. T. (1972) The prediction of outcome in schizophrenia. I. Characteristics of outcome. Arch. Gen. Psychiatry 27, 739-746.
Tsuang, M. T. and Dempsey, M. (1979) Long term outcome of major psychoses. II. Schizoaffective disorder compared with schizophrenia affective disorders, and a surgical control group. Arch. Gen. Psychiatry 36, 1302-1304.
Tsuang, M. T. and Winokur, G. (1975) The Iowa 500: field work in a 35 year follow up of depression, mania and schizophrenia. Can. Psychiat. Assoc. J. 20, 359-365.
Tsuang, M. T., Woolson, R. F., and Fleming, J. A. (1979) Longterm outcome of major psychoses. I. Schizophrenia and affective disorders compared with psychiatrically symptom-free surgical conditions. Arch. Gen. Psychiatry 36, 1295-1301.
Tyrer, S. and Shopsin, B. (1982) Symptoms and assessment of mania. In: Handbook of Affective Disorders (Paykel, E. S., ed.), Guilford, New York.
Van Valkenburg, C., Lowry, M., Winokur, G., and Cadoret R. (1977) Depression spectrum disease vs. pure depressive disease. J. Nerv. Ment. Dis. 165, 341-347.
Weissman, M. M. and Boyd, J. H. (1983) The epidemiology of affective disorders: rates and risk factors. In: Psychiatry Update, Vol. II (Grinspoon, L., ed.), American Psychiatric Press, Washington, D.C.
Weissman, M. M. and Klerman, G. (1978) Epidemiology of mental disorders: emerging trends in the United States. Arch. Gen. Psychiatry 35, 705-712.
Weissman, M. M., Myers, J. K., and Thompson, D. (1981) Depression and its treatment in a U.S. urban community, 1975-1976. Arch. Gen. Psychiatry 38, 417-421.
Welner, A., Welner, Z., and Leonard M. A. (1977) Bipolar manic-depressive disorder: a reassessment of course and outcome. Comp. Psychiatry 18, 327-332.
Wing, J. K. (1983) The use and misuse of the PSE.

Brit. J. Psychiatry **143**, 111-117.

Wing, J. K., Cooper, J. E., and Sartorius, N. (1974) The Measurement and Classification of Psychiatric Symptoms. Cambridge University Press, London.

Winokur, G. (1975) The Iowa 500: heterogeneity and course in manic-depressive illness (bipolar). Comp. Psychiatry **16**, 125-131.

Winokur, G., Behar, D., Van Valkenburg, C., and Lowry, M. (1978) Is a familial definition of depression both feasible and valid? J. Nerv. Ment. Dis. **166**, 764-768.

Winokur, G., Clayton, P., and Reich, T. (1969) Manic Depressive Illness. C. V. Mosby, St. Louis.

Winokur, G. and Morrison, J. (1973) The Iowa 500: follow up of 225 depressives. Brit. J. Psychiatry **123**, 543-548.

Woodruff, R. A., Goodwin, D. W., and Guze, S. B. (1974) Psychiatric Diagnosis (1st ed.). Oxford University Press, New York.

World Health Organisation (1973) The International Pilot Study of Schizophrenia. WHO, Geneva.

World Health Organisation (1978) Mental Disorders: Glossary and Guide to Their Classification in Accordance with the Ninth Revision of the International Classification of Diseases, Vol. I. WHO, Geneva.

World Health Organisation (1979) Schizophrenia: an International Follow-up Study. John Wiley, New York.

Young, .R. C., Biggs, J. T., Ziegler, V. E., and Meyer, D. A. (1978) A rating scale for mania: reliability, validity and sensitivity. Brit. J. Psychiatry **133**, 429-435.

6.

CLINICAL FEATURES OF AFFECTIVE DISORDERS II: ENHANCING THE PRODUCTIVITY OF PHARMACOTHERAPEUTIC AND BIOCHEMICAL RESEARCH

P. Hays

It is very likely that one day we shall have a natural classification of the affective illnesses. We may expect that such a system will permit us to diagnose these illnesses in detail, to predict responses to particular drugs with a confidence bordering on certainty, and to designate the biochemical anomaly associated with the clinical diagnosis we make and the etiological factors that operated. It would thus resemble in its organization the current classification of the anemias, with the proviso that since the central nervous system is more complex than the hemopoietic system, the classification will presumably be correspondingly more complicated.

At present, as described in the previous chapter, we have several conflicting systems of classification, many of them of a simple, binary type. Where several systems are extant, and have been so for some time, it is likely that none is comprehensively correct, though this does not mean that none has any merit. Because of the range of factors we know can operate, and the variability of the syndromes we can already recognize, it is improbable that simple binary classifications can designate two disease entities or even, as a rule, one disease entity and an as yet unanalyzed remainder. Binary classifications must always be suspect because their convenience and ease of application make for an acceptability that may divert us from the task of more accurate categorizations. Nevertheless, a well-chosen binary classification, even though it does not isolate a pathological entity, may be advantageous if it greatly reduces the heterogeneity of one of the populations we examine after the whole group of affective patients have been divided into two moieties. The division of affective illnesses into unipolar and bipolar states, for example, was very helpful because, though neither unipolar nor bipolar affective illness is a homogeneous grouping, unipolar illnesses would seldom be mistakenly called bipolar illnesses and, because of the consequent exclusion of unipolars, the bipolar group is reduced to manageable and potentially analyzable proportions. Bipolar (that is, _potentially_ bipolar) illnesses starting with a depressive episode may be mistakenly included in the unipolar group unless special precautions are taken, this admixture meaning that the manageability of the unipolar group is not equally enhanced. This inequality is a predictable corollary of using preliminary binary divisions of this kind and is not disadvantageous as long as it is kept in mind when studies are done on patients designated as having unipolar illnesses. An analogous situation exists in relation to the classical and scientifically productive division of psychoses into organic and functional, which also accomplished a useful reduction in the heterogeneity of one moiety without a corresponding reduction in the other. Those patients with the syndromes regarded as organic will have organic etiologies operating, so that psychogenic psychoses are excluded and heterogeneity is reduced sharply, while those with the syndromes designated as functional may or may not have organic etiologies operating (for example, depression may be a prodrome of dementia or parkinsonism and may follow concussion, while a schizophreniform syndrome may herald general paresis, follow amphetamine abuse or mark temporal lobe lesion) and thus remain almost as heterogeneous as before.

We will all acknowledge that science is provisional, but our present classifications of the affective illnesses are very provisional indeed. It is unlikely that we can improve our present system merely by giving the matter more thought. It is likely that what we require is more information about the illnesses we see. Clinical observations are essential, of course, but are hard to use in developing further schemata, probably (at least in part) because we are not asking the right questions or are not attending to clues spontaneously offered by our patients. Clinical classifications, even those which will prove in time to have been correct, are also hard to confirm experimentally by extraneous means, as we are at an early stage of development in the field. In the same way, a nineteenth-century physician making a clinical distinction between typhoid and typhus, a distinction now regarded as easy and obvious, would have had a hard time to demonstrate the correctness of his views before microbiological developments permitted independent confirmation. Indeed, historically the matter was settled otherwise, clinical distinguishing features being clarified after the bacteriologists had enabled the physicians to work out what questions to ask and what manifestations selectively to observe.

In psychiatry, thanks to pharmacological and biochemical advances over the last thirty years, we do now have some independent guides to nosology. These measures are not so consistent as those provided in earlier days by the bacteriologists, but in those times pathological homogeneity was provided by epidemics rather than by skilled and sophisticated clinical diagnosis. In psychiatry we have few epidemics and those that happen, such as reserpine-induced depression and amphetamine-psychosis, are slow to develop, hard to recognize and, once recognized, are aborted.

It is well known that if an effective and established antidepressant is given to a well-selected group of patients, only about three-quarters will be relieved of symptoms (Cooper and Magnus, 1984). Similarly, failure of dexamethasone to suppress serum cortisol takes place at best in a bare majority of a well-selected series of patients (Carroll, 1982). One might suppose that what we need is a better drug or a better test, but this is not necessarily the most helpful way of expressing the deficiency. It is not that an effective antidepressant sometimes works and sometimes does not, in a truly hit-or-miss fashion. We know that a patient who has responded in the past to a given antidepressant will, in a second attack, be much more likely to respond to that drug than the three times out of four that we would expect if we calculated the odds on the basis of drug-trial results alone. With only slightly less confidence, we expect that an antidepressant which has proved effective in a patient's first-degree relative will be correspondingly more likely to relieve the patient's symptoms (Cooper and Magnus, 1984). Similarly, the dexamethasone suppression test, when positive, is so in a consistent manner; when it exists, the anomaly disappears as the patient improves and if he relapses it returns more regularly than might be expected if we based our assessment of the odds on the probabilities reported in the literature (Carroll, 1982).

It follows that there are some depressions, or some people with depressions, who are distinct, and thus potentially distinguishable in advance, from the others. This proposition helps to define the role of the clinician who is concerned with drug trials or biochemical research.

The clinician is needed for case-selection, in the first instance, and his function at this stage can be described in a few words. Patients must be selected according to criteria which are specified in easily accessible literature, generally accepted for these purposes, and widely used. In this way the results can be compared with those of other workers, and will add to the body of knowledge in a useful fashion. In the case of drug trials he will also be concerned in the assessment and reassessment of patients to determine what changes have taken place after therapy.

However, as indicated earlier, the clinician should anticipate that tests on these patients or drug trial results will produce the familiar division into two moieties, neither of them small. Both our knowledge that patients selected by criteria presently available are heterogeneous and the results of previous trials and investigations bolster this anticipation. The clinician is therefore to be presented, at the nominal close of one investigation, with an opportunity which in effect constitutes the start of another.

He finds himself with a group of patients whom he has assessed and found to fit the criteria in use, of whom one sub-group responded in one biological way, and the other in another. A hypothesis presents itself, namely that there are some clinical distinctions to be made between these sub-groups. If all he has done, which was probably what he was asked to do, was record data pertinent to the selection criteria, then his capacity to test this important hypothesis is impaired. Clearly, if one sub-group of patients responded to medication and one did not, then clinical differences between the two will now be dominated by features relating to current severity. Even in the case of biochemically stated distinctions, the passage of time since selection will introduce factors which, though they are not totally random, will cloud clinical distinctions which are intended to have predictive value. Finally, if he knows the allocation of individual patients to one sub-group or another, then any subsequent clinical reassessments will not be done "blind" and will suffer from that tendency to precipitate induction which makes psychiatry a graveyard of theories, and will bias his observations.

If these arguments are accepted, then the clinician who is interested in research, wishes to be involved in cooperative ventures which stand a chance of making real advances, and is jealous of his time, may draw certain conclusions.

First, he will allocate only a small proportion of his time to case-selection. Much of this, in practice, is often done by simple questionnaires and with the assistance of junior staff, but the existence of precise criteria does not relieve the clinician of the responsibility for ensuring that the information used in the checklists is of the first quality. Equal care needs to be taken with assessing alteration in patients after therapy, and any alterations which take place but are not allowed for in the protocols should be documented.

He will also note that published papers seldom include an account of a detailed clinical comparison of the two moieties that emerge when the experiments, whether pharmacological or biochemical, are completed; and that research proposals with which he may consider aligning himself are commonly similarly deficient. If he acknowledges that divisions will be disclosed by the work that is planned, he can forearm himself by recording detailed data in advance, and as the price of his involvement can insist that the necessary expenditure of time can be budgeted for. At first sight it may seem a forlorn endeavour to record a mass of information on a large number of patients without being certain that what is elicited and recorded will be needed. However, this feature of the activity, a feature which is anyway common to most original research, is ameliorated by our awareness that two or more groups are going to be identified so that the clinician may compare them, and by a justifiable expectation that, whatever the biochemical bases for the distinctions between the groups, it is overwhelmingly likely that these will be reflected in clinical observations. It is true that at the present moment it is hard to say what clinical observations.

Of course, if we knew what observations to make or to stress, our problems would already have been solved. It is therefore necessary to identify categories of information within which the useful data will probably lie. It can be said that some of those features which are possessed by some but not all of the patients will be useful in distinguishing, and that for obvious reasons of economy these should be selected from features which are known to have at least some relevance to some affective illnesses. It is also true that the syndromes of affective illnesses have been repeatedly analyzed, so that novel results may more hopefully be sought in the realm of antecedents rather than mental-state examinations. Nevertheless, when patients are selected and assessed at the outset of an experiment, a lot of detailed information is recorded. Patients who fit criteria are alike but far from identical, and it would be wasteful not to use this information when comparing the two groups.

In relation to clinical data of other kinds, and proceeding from the general to the particular, family histories should be taken in such a way that the numbers and sex of first- and second-degree family members are recorded. Where relatives have been ill, they should be interviewed or their case-notes obtained, or both. A family history of personality deviations as well as actual psychiatric illnesses should be sought, though it is not usually practical to undertake this in any but first-degree relatives.

Premorbid personalities are disordered more frequently in patients with affective illness than is the case in the rest of the population, but are not invariably disordered. Assessment of premorbid personalities is therefore suited to this type of prospective work. Some care is necessary to prevent affective symptoms from obscuring these accounts, but the clinician can take the obvious precautions, such as obtaining accounts from relatives as well as from the patients.

Many, though not the overwhelming majority, of patients with affective illnesses are under some kind of psychological stress at the time of onset, that is to say, when the first psychiatric symptoms appeared which were continuous in time with the ultimate development of the full syndrome. Because recurrences may occur with trivial stresses or as a consequence of medication changes, stresses for which a causative role is proposed are best assessed in relation to the first episode.

Information of the kind sketched in the past few paragraphs, together with other data which the clinician's own observations or theories suggest to him, renders possible a more important collaboration than is provided by mere case-selection. If, using new clinical criteria, we can successfully distinguish between biologically determined moieties, then we will have made the clinical role more reciprocal and productive, and edged nosology in the right direction by the application of one of the techniques of classical scientific method.

References

Carroll, B. J. (1982) The dexamethasone suppression test for melancholia. <u>Brit. J. Psychiatry</u> **140**, 292-304.

Cooper, A. J. and Magnus, R. V. (1984) Strategies for the drug treatment of depression. <u>Can. Med. Assoc. J.</u> **130**, 383-390.

7.

MONOAMINE OXIDASE INHIBITORS AS ANTIDEPRESSANTS

D. L. Murphy, T. Sunderland, I. Campbell, and R. M. Cohen

Introduction

The three monoamine oxidase (MAO) inhibitors currently most used, phenelzine, tranylcypromine, and isocarboxazid, are all first-generation antidepressants. They became available before the tricyclic antidepressants, over thirty years ago, but have never been as widely used as the tricyclics. In fact, they nearly became completely supplanted by the tricyclics on the basis of safety, partly due to concerns about the hepatotoxicity exhibited by some of the early hydrazine MAO inhibitors such as iproniazid, as well as the more general liability of this drug class to interact with certain foodstuffs and other drugs and occasionally produce hypertensive and central nervous system reactions.

Their continued usage is certainly a function of their efficacy as antidepressants, which has repeatedly been demonstrated in randomized, double-blind comparisons both with placebo and with tricyclics. The persistent suggestions that the MAO inhibitors might be therapeutically effective in some patients who were or might be tricyclic non-responders (for example, patients with atypical depression) have also contributed to their continued use.

This chapter will review the evidence on the efficacy of MAO inhibitors as antidepressants, especially the question of who MAO inhibitor-responsive patients might be. Recent studies using modern diagnostic criteria will be particularly emphasized, as will recent data on how MAO inhibitors compare to tricyclics, and whether the MAO inhibitors are all equivalent in their effects, or need to be considered separately in making treatment choices. It will also evaluate their safety, and their side effects. In addition, discoveries in the last decade concerning how they might act biochemically, and, in particular, their human pharmacology, will be highlighted.

It is discoveries from the basic science area and in clinical pharmacology that have been responsible to a large extent for the increased interest in development of new MAO-inhibiting antidepressants. After a hiatus of almost twenty years, at least four new MAO inhibitors have entered clinical study phases over the last several years. These new drugs all exhibit some biochemical features--substrate-selectivity and reversible inhibition of the enzyme--that are different from those of phenelzine, tranylcypromine, and isocarboxazid.

Are the MAO Inhibitors Effective as Antidepressants --and in which Patients?

The Drugs

Clinically studied MAO inhibitors are listed in Table 7.1. All of the original MAO inhibitors irreversibly inhibit the enzyme, although the nature of the interaction with the active site of MAO is different for the hydrazines (such as phenelzine and isocarboxazid, which contain an N-N group; see Figure 7.1) than for cyclopropylamines (such as tranyl-

Table 7.1: Monoamine oxidase inhibitors used clinically

Irreversible MAO inhibitors currently available:
    Phenelzine, tranylcypromine, isocarboxazid

Irreversible MAO inhibitors no longer available in the U.S.:
    Iproniazid, pheniprazine, nialamide

Irreversible, substrate-selective MAO inhibitors currently under study in the U.S.:
    MAO-A inhibitors: clorgyline, Lilly 51641
    MAO-B inhibitors: deprenyl, pargyline

Reversible, substrate-selective MAO-A inhibitors currently under study in Europe:
    Cimoxatone, amiflamine, moclobemide, CGP 11305 A

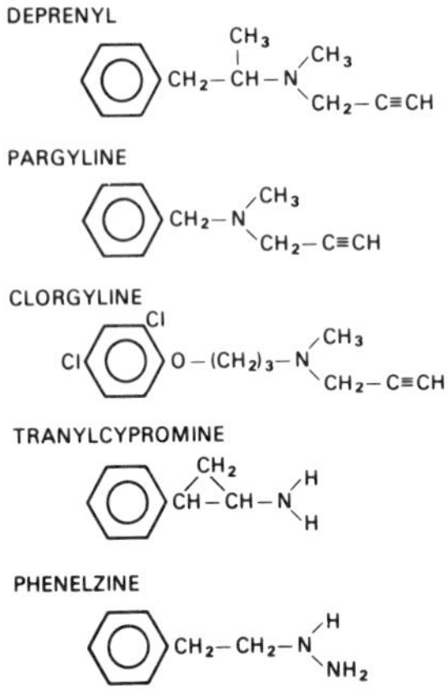

MAO Inhibitors

DEPRENYL

[structure: phenyl-CH₂-CH(CH₃)-N(CH₃)-CH₂-C≡CH]

PARGYLINE

[structure: phenyl-CH₂-N(CH₃)-CH₂-C≡CH]

CLORGYLINE

[structure: 2,4-dichlorophenyl-O-(CH₂)₃-N(CH₃)-CH₂-C≡CH]

TRANYLCYPROMINE

[structure: phenyl-cyclopropyl-CH-NH₂]

PHENELZINE

[structure: phenyl-CH₂-CH₂-NH-NH₂]

Figure 7.1: Structures of some representative acetylenic, cyclopropylamine, and hydrazine MAO inhibitors studied clinically for antidepressant effects

cypromine and Lilly 51641, which contain a three-carbon cyclic group) and the acetylenic inhibitors (such as clorgyline and deprenyl, which contain a C≡H group) (Kenney et al., 1979; Maycock et al., 1976; Paech et al., 1979).

A necessary consequence of this irreversible inactivation of the enzyme, of course, is that return of normal MAO function in a tissue depends on the rate of synthesis of new enzyme molecules or new cells, whichever occurs first. Enzyme resynthesis has been estimated to occur with a half-time of 3-4 days in the liver, but this is longer (10-12 days) in brain (Nelson et al., 1979). Human platelet MAO activity only recovers as these cell fragments are replaced in the circulation, which occurs with a half-time of 5 days. Intestinal MAO, at least in some cells, is thought to recover rapidly from the effects of MAO inhibitors because epithelial cell half-lives are only 1-2 days. The reversible MAO inhibitors (Table 7.1), which have recently begun to be studied in man, do not form covalent bonds with the enzyme, but only inactivate the enzyme in proportion to tissue and plasma concentrations of the drugs.

As discussed below, most of the older MAO inhibitors act non-selectively on all monoamines which are substrates for the enzyme. Clorgyline and most of the newer, reversible MAO inhibitors under clinical study preferentially inhibit MAO type A (MAO-A). Serotonin (5-hydroxytryptamine; 5-HT), and to a lesser extent noradrenaline (NA) and probably adrenaline, are more actively deaminated by MAO-A. Dopamine and phenylethylamine are examples of substrates which are more readily deaminated by MAO-B, and whose metabolism is consequently more inhibited by MAO-B inhibitors such as deprenyl than by MAO-A inhibitors such as clorgyline.

Antidepressant Efficacy of the MAO Inhibitors

Approximately 20-25 controlled studies of MAO inhibitors as antidepressants which meet minimum dosage criteria have been conducted. Most of these have been competently reviewed elsewhere (for example, see Quitkin et al., 1970; Klein et al., 1980; Nies, 1983). They have been supplemented recently by several additional controlled studies regarding isocarboxazid (Davidson and Turnbull, 1983), tranylcypromine (Himmelhoch et al., 1982), and phenelzine (Davidson et al., 1981; Rowan et al., 1982). All of these recent studies have served to confirm the efficacy of these drugs, and have supported the conclusions drawn that several of the initial large studies done with phenelzine, which were otherwise well-designed investigations (e.g., Medical Research Council, 1965; Raskin et al., 1974), may be misleading because they used either inadequate drug doses and/or patient populations including predominantly subgroups of patients least likely to respond to MAO inhibitors (Quitkin et al., 1979).

Overall, the largest number of studies of the MAO inhibitors, especially phenelzine, have evaluated their effects in the 'atypical' depressive subgroup. Although clinical characteristics of the 'atypical' patients chosen for treatment vary considerably from study to study, generally outpatients with non-endogenous, non-vegetative depressive symptoms and with prominent anxiety, often associated with panic and phobic symptoms, have been investigated.

Of approximately 10 controlled studies comparing phenelzine with placebo in mixed populations of depressed patients, all but one demonstrated phenelzine to be therapeutically more active (Klein et al., 1980; Quitkin et al., 1979; Sheehan et al., 1980). Fewer comparisons with placebo are available for tranylcypromine and isocarboxazid, but more recent studies comparing MAO inhibitors with tricyclic antidepressants suggest similar results; of interest, responses in different clusters of symptoms may occur with the MAO inhibitors compared to the tricyclics (Klein et al., 1980; Nies, 1983; Quitkin et al., 1979). Also of note is that six-week efficacy studies of phenelzine generally have shown greater drug-placebo differences compared to four-week studies, suggesting a fairly long delay in onset of action for this drug, and the consequent need for longer trials at full therapeutic doses before declaring a patient unresponsive.

MAO inhibitors have also been investigated in patients with anxiety-related disorders. There are some indications that patients who experience panic disorder and related anxiety associated with atypical depression constitute the group most consistently responsive to MAO inhibitor treatment (Quitkin et al., 1979; Sheehan et al., 1980). Changing nomenclature and diagnostic classification schemes present problems in evaluating exactly what types of patients were included in earlier studies. Several double-blind trials have demonstrated the efficacy of MAO inhibitors in the treatment of patients with anxiety and mixed phobias, as well as patients with agoraphobia (Klein et al., 1980; Nies, 1983; Quitkin et al., 1979; Sheehan et al., 1980). A recent trial of phenelzine compared to imipramine and placebo in patients with agoraphobia and panic disorder showed both drugs significantly more effective than placebo, with some suggestions of a superiority of the MAO inhibitor over the tricyclic (Sheehan et al., 1980).

There are fewer controlled studies available of MAO inhibitors in severely depressed inpatients. Nonetheless, tranylcypromine, phenelzine, isocarboxazid, and clorygline have all been reported as effective in the majority of these studies, including several recently completed investigations (Davidson et al., 1981; Lipper et al., 1979). Two of the exceptions (Medical Research Council, 1965; Raskin et al., 1974) were noted above as large investigations whose interpretation is handicapped by inadequate phenelzine doses (45 mg/day) and other problems.

Which Patients Respond to MAO Inhibitors?

A continuing focus of clinical speculation and study is the question of defining and ultimately predicting which patients might be MAO inhibitor-responsive. A symptom profile published by West and Dally

(1959) on the basis of their impressions that patients with 'atypical depression' responded best to iproniazid stimulated many attempts to better delineate who should be included in an atypical depression subgroup (Paykel et al., 1983) and to develop predictive criteria for therapeutic responsiveness to MAO inhibitors (Robinson et al., 1978; Paykel et al., 1979; Giller et al., 1982; Nies, 1983).

The current status of this controversial area can be summarized as follows. A recent report by one group with over five years of continuous work on this question involving over 150 patients indicated that highly statistically significant symptom differences can be defined for patients divided into responders or non-responders to phenelzine versus amitriptyline (Robinson et al., 1983). The MAO inhibitor responders included patients with more somatic anxiety, hyperphagia and/or hypersomnia, self-rated panic symptoms and hysterical personality traits. However, these are patient group differences only; attempts to identify individual patient symptom characteristics have not been successful, and response prediction for a given patient prior to treatment is not yet possible. Other recent reports by another major group in England have indicated less current success than that previously reported in identifying characteristics of phenelzine responders (Paykel et al., 1979, 1982).

Thus, the predictive status remains clouded for the frequently cited characteristics typifying MAO inhibitor-responsive, atypically depressed patients: outpatients with non-endogenous, more 'neurotic' symptoms, including greater anxiety, phobias, reactivity of mood, and initial insomnia. The coexistence of panic symptoms with depression seemed the strongest single predictor of therapeutic responsiveness in the most recent compilation of the studies of Robinson and coworkers (Robinson et al., 1983).

It should be noted here that most of the recent work on defining MAO inhibitor-responsive depressed patients has been done using phenelzine. Our group reported that patients who responded most strikingly to the selective MAO-A inhibitor clorgyline were severely depressed inpatients with high Hamilton depression scale scores and endogenous features (Lipper et al., 1979; Murphy et al., 1981), while an earlier study in the same treatment setting found almost no responders to phenelzine in a similar group of patients (Murphy, 1975). Recently, another group has described isocarboxazid-responsive patients as being significantly different from those patients who did not improve in having greater pretreatment psychomotor retardation (Giller et al., 1982). This is in contrast to other studies with phenelzine showing least improvement with this drug in retarded depression, while outpatients with greater hostility, agitation, anxiety and atypical, neurotic depressive symptoms showed the greatest improvement (Paykel et al., 1979). As we have suggested elsewhere (Murphy et al., 1983, 1984), all the MAO inhibitors may not have the same clinical effects, and extrapolation from one MAO inhibitor to another may not be justified.

Studies comparing the efficacy of MAO inhibitors to a tricyclic might be expected to provide some hints regarding which patients might be more responsive to which type of drug. While there have been numerous attempts to compare tricyclics and MAO inhibitors, many earlier studies are flawed by mixed, inadequately described patient populations, by low, probably sub-therapeutic, doses of one or the other drug, and by inadequate post-hoc description of which patients responded to which drug. A recent study examining depressed outpatients compared phenelzine, 60 mg/day, with amitriptyline, 150 mg/day (Nies, 1983). The two drugs were equally effective as antidepressants, with a similar range of side-effects. Interestingly, phenelzine had a significantly greater effect than the tricyclic on both self-ratings and observer-ratings of anxiety (Nies, 1983). This finding is consistent with several other reports indicating that anxiety subscores in depressed populations correlate with a successful outcome following treatment with phenelzine. In our group's studies with clorgyline, significant antianxiety and antidysphoric effects on an array of both self and observed ratings equalled and in some cases exceeded in magnitude the changes in depression ratings (Murphy et al., 1981, 1984). It might well be that the 'atypical' depressives originally proposed as peculiarly responsive to MAO inhibitors were in fact those with significant anxiety.

Side Effects of the MAO Inhibitors
=================================

The most common side effects generally encountered with the MAO inhibitors are summarized in Table 7.2. Postural hypotension with dizziness, due to the sympatholytic effects of some of the MAO inhibitors, is most often a problem in patients with lower pretreatment blood pressure. MAO inhibitor-related orthostatic hypotension needs to be differentiated from anxiety-related dizziness or light-headedness, and from the hypotension observed in some depressed patients related to poor appetite and inadequate fluid intake. In elderly depressed patients, hypotension may pose a dose-limiting problem, as it does with many of the tricyclics. Tranylcypromine and deprenyl appear to have less blood pressure-lowering effects than some of the other MAO inhibitors. The absence of direct anticholinergic effects makes the MAO inhibitors, like some of the newer heterocyclic antidepressants, more tolerable agents for use in the elderly (Georgotas et al., 1983).

Table 7.2: Side effects of the MAO inhibitors

Most frequent major side effects:
    Orthostatic hypotension with dizziness
    Weight gain
    Sexual dysfunction
    Edema

Other frequent side effects:
    Insomnia
    Daytime sedation
    Myoclonus
    Dry mouth

Uncommon, dangerous toxicities:
    Dietary pressor amine interaction -
        the tyramine ('cheese') hypertensive
        response[a]
    Drug interactions resulting in the MAO
        inhibitor CNS syndrome[b]

---

a. Most frequently reported with aged, unpasteurized cheeses; pickled or smoked fish or meat such as herring, sausage, pate, and chicken liver; yeast or meat extracts; red wine; and fava beans (which contain L-dopa).
b. Dangerous interactions possible with stimulants, sympathomimetics and decongestants (e.g. amphetamine, cocaine, ephedrine, phenylephrine, phenylpropanolamine); tricyclic antidepressants; some antihypertensives (methyl-dopa, reserpine, guanethidine); and some narcotics (e.g. meperidine).

Among other side effects, attention has been drawn to behavioral toxicities such as restlessness, agitation, insomnia, and, in bipolar patients, switches into mania (Murphy, 1977). Drug-related changes in sexual dysfunction generally involve retarded ejaculation and anorgasmia with intact sexual interest and erectile function. Sexual dysfunction may be another manifestation of the reduction in sympathetic nervous system outflow which results in hypotension, and hence principally represent an MAO-A inhibitor-related consequence; the selective MAO-B inhibitor deprenyl does not appear to cause these problems (Knoll, 1981). Anorgasmia is also noted in some case reports of female patients, but its frequency and basis in women has not yet been studied. Other possible contributions to sexual dysfunction associated with MAO inhibitors may result from neuroendocrine changes.

Careful clinical assessment of these problems may permit the continued use of effective MAO inhibitor doses. Division of dosage times may minimize some of these side effects, but opinion remains divided about choice of regimens, and individualization often is necessary. For example, patients with symptomatic hypotension often do best with drug doses distributed over four nearly equal time periods, while patients with complaints of insomnia during tranylcypromine treatment may do better receiving more of their drug earlier in the day.

The two most hazardous side effects which may occur during MAO inhibitor treatment are hypertensive responses resulting from dietary amines or sympathomimetic drug ingestion, and the central nervous system (CNS) MAO inhibitor interaction syndrome. Chronic treatment with MAO inhibitors increases pressor response to oral or intravenous tyramine ten to thirty-fold. Normally, 400 to 800 mg of tyramine ingested orally in a fasting state will raise systolic blood pressure 300 mm Hg. During MAO inhibitor treatment, the same blood pressure response can be observed with tyramine concentrations as low as 10 mg (Dollery et al., 1983). As a point of reference, three ounce servings of different aged cheese and pickled herring have been measured and found to contain tyramine concentrations over the broad range of < 1 to 180 mg (Blackwell et al., 1967). Such amounts could clearly present a risk of a hypertensive response. The large variations in actual amount of tyramine found in different types of cheeses and other foods depend upon their age, time of non-refrigerated storage and related circum-

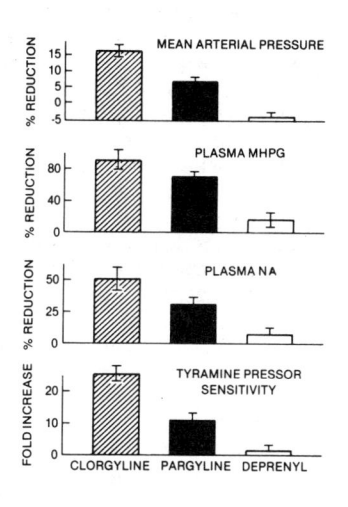

Figure 7.2: Alterations in blood pressure, noradrenaline metabolism, and tyramine pressor sensitivity during chronic treatment with clorgyline, pargyline, and deprenyl.

stances. Fortunately, with the dietary and drug precautions indicated in Table 7.2, hypertensive responses due to foods containing tyramine or other pressor amines or due to sympathomimetic drugs are rare, according to large studies involving several hundred patients (Nies, 1983; Raskin, 1972). In fact, the overall incidence of side effects of all types is no higher than for the tricyclics in several studies comparing these drugs (Robinson et al., 1978; Nies, 1983).

While hypertensive reactions are generally thought to result from an impairment of tyramine metabolism together with an enhanced amount of NA stored in sympathetic nerve terminals available for release by tyramine, it now appears that the increased amount of stored NA resulting from MAO-A inhibition is most responsible for the altered sensitivity to tyramine (Murphy et al., in press; Murphy et al., 1983; Pickar et al., 1981a). The magnitude of inhibition of NA metabolism, as reflected in reduced plasma 3-methoxy,4-hydroxyphenylglycol (MHPG) concentrations, is highly correlated with the enhanced blood pressure response to tyramine (Pickar et al., 1981a; Figure 7.2). Use of the selective MAO-B inhibitor deprenyl, which in low doses has only minimal effects on NA metabolism, leads to lesser tyramine potentiation (Figure 7.2).

In contrast to tyramine hypertensive responses, which are mediated by the peripheral sympathetic nervous system, another syndrome with prominent CNS involvement may occur when certain CNS-active drugs are taken after MAO inhibition is established (see Table 7.2). This syndrome is characterized by delirium often progressing to coma, seizures and other neurologic abnormalities, including hyperreflexia, dilated and fixed pupils, severe hyperthermia (with temperatures to 108°F), hypotension, and acute renal failure. Unlike the tyramine hypertensive crisis which responds to adrenergic blocking agents such as phentolamine, reversal of the central syndrome follows treatment with chlorpromazine, barbiturates, possibly dantrolene, and massive support measures (Goekapp and Carbaat, 1982; White and Simpson, 1981).

Possible Mechanisms Involved in the Antidepressant Effects of MAO Inhibitors

MAO Inhibitors in Man: Clinical Pharmacology

Possible associations between the biological consequences of MAO inhibitor administration and the behavioral responses to these drugs have been explored in a number of ways. Unlike the situation for many drugs, including the tricyclic antidepressants, little useful information can be obtained from measurement of plasma concentrations of currently available MAO inhibitors. The hydrazines, cyclopropylamines, and acetylenic inhibitors are quite rapidly cleared from plasma, with half-lives measured in hours (Campbell et al., 1979; Robinson et al., 1980), while their actions as irreversible inhibitors of MAO produce effects lasting for days or weeks. Thus, there is no necessary association between the concentrations of the irreversible MAO inhibitors in plasma and the amount of MAO inhibitor present in tissues.

Measurement of platelet MAO inhibition has been used to estimate tissue MAO activity changes in patients receiving MAO inhibitors, and has provided evidence that higher phenelzine doses, on the order of 60-75 mg/day (or 1 mg/kg), yield greater than 80-85% enzyme inhibition (Nies, 1983). This level of inhibition is associated with significantly greater antidepressant and antianxiety efficacy than lesser amounts of platelet MAO inhibition (Nies, 1983; Raft et al., 1981). No general association between pretreatment platelet MAO activity and response to phenelzine has been observed.

It should be noted that the association between reductions in platelet MAO activity and clinical response has only been validated for phenelzine. This relationship does not hold for a selective MAO-A inhibitor with antidepressant properties like clorgyline. We have reported negligible reductions of platelet MAO-B activity during clorgyline-induced clinical improvement, which was associated with greater than 85% selective inhibition of MAO-A as reflected in changes of urinary amine metabolites (Murphy et al., 1979, 1981). Similarly, very low doses (5-10 mg/day) of the partially selective MAO-B inhibitors pargyline and deprenyl inhibit over 95% of platelet MAO activity in a matter of a few hours, while not consistently producing antidepressant effects. Tranylcypromine, and to a lesser extent isocarboxazid, also yield marked platelet MAO inhibition at clinically sub-therapeutic doses (Giller and Lieb, 1980).

Some individual pharmacologic properties of these drugs may contribute to differences in their clinical consequences, such as the reportedly greater stimulant properties of tranylcypromine, which seems related to its amphetamine-like amine releasing properties. However, neither this effect, nor the NA uptake-inhibiting effect of the (-)-isomer of tranylcypromine, are as important as MAO inhibition for the antidepressant action of the clinically available, racemic ($\pm$)-tranylcypromine, since the (+)-isomer, which is a better MAO inhibitor but poorer uptake inhibitor, is the more effective antidepressant (Reynolds et al., 1980; Moises and Beckmann, 1981; Gorenstein and Gentil, 1981).

Biological Changes Produced by MAO Inhibition: Their Relationship to Antidepressant Effects

There is good evidence that the clinical responses to MAO inhibitors result primarily from delayed biochemical consequences of reduced oxidative deamination of biogenic amines, rather than some other property of these drugs. Numerous animal studies have demonstrated rapid changes in brain noradrenergic and serotonergic functional activity in response to MAO inhibitor antidepressants. The ability to inhibit oxidative deamination and produce elevations in cellular biogenic amine concentrations corresponds most closely to the behavioral changes produced by those drugs which are active clinically (Squires, 1978; Murphy et al., 1983).

For many years, the pharmacological and behavioral effects of MAO inhibitors in animals were studied almost exclusively following acute, high-dosage drug administration. A delay of two or more weeks, however, has generally been observed before the onset of both antidepressant efficacy as well as some prominent side effects such as orthostatic hypotension when these drugs are administered chronically (Roy et al., in press). These temporal discrepancies have led to studies of the adaptive changes that take place in the noradrenergic, serotonergic, and other physiologic systems during the continued administration of MAO inhibitors in animals and man.

In rats, the daily administration of the selective MAO-A inhibiting antidepressant clorgyline, as well as the non-selective inhibitors phenelzine and tranylcypromine, leads to a rapid, sustained increase in brain NA and serotonin concentrations (Campbell et al., in press). After several weeks' treatment with MAO inhibitors, reductions in brain alpha$_2$-adrenoreceptor numbers and in beta-adrenoreceptors and their functional activity--as measured by NA-stimulated cyclic-AMP formation--as well as in serotonin receptor numbers, have been observed (Cohen et al., 1982; Kellar et al., 1981; Murphy et al., 1983). These changes occur at low doses of both nonselective MAO inhibitors (nialamide and phenelzine) and the selective MAO-A inhibitor clorgyline, but occur only at high, probably nonselective doses of the partially selective MAO-B inhibitor pargyline (Murphy et al., in press). These neurochemical alterations induced by MAO-A inhibition are accompanied by a decrease in the firing rate of noradrenergic neurons in the locus ceruleus and a reduction in the sensitivity of cortical neurons to iontophoretically-applied NA and serotonin, presumably reflecting the changes in amine receptor numbers and function (Table 7.3; Campbell et al., in press; Olpe et al., 1980, 1981).

These adaptive neurochemical changes are also reflected in behavioral changes in animals, as chronic but not acute clorgyline treatment attentuates the reductions in locomotor activity produced by the alpha$_2$-adrenergic agonist clonidine and the serotonin agonist m-chlorophenylpiperazine (Cohen et al., 1982, 1983). Clonidine's effects under these circumstances are believed to be mediated through an alpha$_2$-adrenoreceptor presynaptic system. These latter results in rodents are in agreement with findings from a recent clinical study indicating that clonidine's hypotensive effects, also believed to involve alpha$_2$-adrenoreceptors, are significantly reduced after treatment with clorgyline for 21 days (but not 3 days) in depressed patients (Siever et al., 1982).

The question of which of the amines affected by MAO inhibition is most likely to be involved in therapeutic response has recently been approached in comparative studies using clorgyline, pargyline, and deprenyl for their substrate-selective actions (Lipper et al., 1979; Murphy et al., 1981). The largest aggregation of evidence from these studies suggests that reductions in depressive symptoms during treatment with MAO inhibitors are most closely correlated with NA neurotransmitter system changes, as based on direct measurements of the plasma and cerebrospinal fluid concentration of NA and its metabolites, and on a series of indirect measures of changes in noradrenergic function, such as blood pressure alterations, during MAO inhibitor treatment

Table 7.3: Some effects of chronic MAO inhibitor administration on brain monoamine metabolism and related functions

---

Early changes:
    Reduced monoamine deamination
    Increased noradrenaline, dopamine and serotonin

Adaptive changes:
    Reduced locus ceruleus and raphe neuronal firing rates
    Reduced alpha$_2$- and beta-adrenoceptors and reduced serotonin receptor density

Persisting functional changes:
    Decreased central sympathetic outflow with reduced plasma noradrenaline and orthostatic hypotension
    Increased vesicular noradrenaline in peripheral sympathetic neurons, with susceptibility to hypertensive episodes from tyramine

---

(Murphy et al., 1983; Roy et al., in press). The data suggest that a reduction in central noradrenergic output, dependent upon longer-term drug administration (rather than an acutely-produced NA increase), is most closely associated with clinical improvement (Major et al., 1979; Murphy et al., 1984).

Our group's comparisons of the biological and clinical consequences of treatment with clorgyline, pargyline, and deprenyl have led to some additional tentative conclusions. As pargyline (and, from preliminary evidence, deprenyl) had minimal antidepressant activity, the fifty-fold elevations in phenylethylamine excretion observed in patients treated with pargyline and deprenyl would not seem to be relevant to clinical efficacy (Murphy et al., 1981). Changes in tyramine sensitivity which are associated with clinical effectiveness do not seem to be directly related to clinical changes via any selective alterations in tyramine metabolism. Rather, the enhanced sensitivity to tyramine found with MAO inhibition seems to depend upon changes in the amount of increased NA stored in neurons available for release by tyramine (Pickar et al., 1981b). The positive association between clinical antidepressant responses and changes in tyramine sensitivity thus serve to reinforce the conclusion that NA changes are most likely connected with clinical response (Murphy et al., 1983, 1984).

Some Practical Considerations in the Clinical Use of MAO Inhibitors

Before beginning treatment with an MAO inhibitor, some drug education for the patient is necessary with regard to diet and the use of other drugs. Although as indicated above, large scale study experience indicates that reactions have become rare, evaluation of possible compliance problems prior to beginning treatment is useful. The list of foods and drugs to be avoided needs to be followed at all times during treatment and for two weeks after treatment is discontinued. Should the rare but hazardous explosive headache associated with elevated blood pressure, flushing, heart pounding, perspiration, and nausea occur, the patient needs to seek emergency room treatment immediately. Examples of patient instructions regarding MAO inhibitors and sample lists of dietary restrictions have been provided elsewhere (Folks, 1983).

General experience is that therapeutic effects may be delayed, taking three to six weeks to become maximal, although some symptomatic changes and some side effects may occur early in treatment. Some side effects (e.g. sedation) that appear early in treatment can be expected to diminish over time, while others may require dosage adjustment (e.g. dizziness from postural hypotension).

With regard to beginning treatment, delay in reaching adequate therapeutic doses will prolong the time to clinical recovery, but rapid increases in dosage may occasionally produce more early side effects. On the other hand, holding a healthy, normotensive patient for two or three weeks at a subtherapeutic dosage (i.e., 30-45 mg/day of phenelzine rather than the generally required 60-75 mg/day) will neither avoid possible postural hypotension (which in some patients does not occur until after several weeks at full treatment doses), nor constitute an adequate drug trial until three to six weeks' treatment of full dosage is completed. Titration of drug dosage against side effects is often necessary, and small increments or decrements in dosage can be very meaningful.

Although the irreversible MAO inhibitors (see Table 7.1) remain bound for the lifespan of the enzyme molecule, some information suggests that different physiologic functions are affected by different degrees of enzyme inhibition, or the secondary consequences of this inhibition (Murphy et al., in press; Murphy et al., 1983). Some clinical implications of these differences include the following: temporarily withholding a dose or two of an MAO inhibitor can result in rapid recovery (within a period of 6 to 10 hours) from severe postural hypotension with dizziness so severe that sitting or standing was not possible (Roy et al., in press). Similarly, dietary tolerance for tyramine-containing foods or tyramine administered in oral test doses can occur more rapidly (e.g. in a week) than the usually recommended 'safe' time of two weeks. This may be the result of a more rapid turnover of intestinal barrier cells, and the possibility that normal function returns more rapidly in the liver and in the sympathetic nervous system than in the brain. The return of REM sleep and dreaming, which we have found to take approximately a week, is sometimes associated with a rebound increase in REM sleep associated with vivid dreams and, rarely, muscular disinhibition at night (Cohen et al., 1983). Some indications of the slow return to normal function in the brain include exaggerated neuroendocrine and hypertensive responses to amphetamine observed weeks after MAO-inhibitor discontinuation, and muscular spasms, clonus, hypertension, and autonomic symptoms reported in two patients following a single dose of the tricyclic antidepressant clomipramine, administered one month after discontinuation of clorgyline (Insel et al., 1983).

MAO Inhibitors Combined with Tricyclic Antidepressants

A series of reviews have indicated that, if used judiciously, MAO inhibitors and tricyclics can be safely combined (White and Simpson, 1981). Early, non-controlled studies had provided some evidence that combined treatment was effective in individual patients non-responsive to either class of drugs alone, and recently several controlled studies have supported the efficacy of combined use. These recent controlled trials, however, do not demonstrate any increase in efficacy for combined treatment vs. the MAO inhibitor or tricyclic alone in unselected depressed patient populations (Razani et al., 1983; White and Simpson, 1981; Young et al., 1979), and controlled studies of combined treatment and of MAO inhibitor-tricyclic crossover treatment in tricyclic or MAO inhibitor non-responding patients remain to be done. Thus, while it seems clear that MAO inhibitors and tricyclics can be used safely in combination if the two are started concurrently (or an MAO inhibitor added to a tricyclic in low, gradually increasing doses), if parenteral use is avoided, if imipramine is avoided, and if dosage is kept at relatively modest levels, it would seem that combination treatment still requires further study and should generally be reserved for patients who are non-responders to MAO inhibitors and one or more tricyclic-related drugs given alone.

MAO Inhibitors Combined with Lithium and Other Drugs

Preliminary findings suggest that lithium combined with MAO inhibitors may be an effective treatment. In one study, 21 tricyclic-unresponsive depressed patients were treated with lithium carbonate followed by tranylcypromine; 11 had a complete remission, 5 were substantially better, and the remaining 5 improved initially but developed hypomania (Himmelhoch et al., 1982). To date this has not been followed up with a double-blind study, and, of course, it is not known what the outcome would have been if either lithium or tranylcypromine had been used alone. Case reports have also suggested that the addition of lithium to phenelzine in phenelzine non-responsive patients can lead to rapid improvement (Nelson and Byck, 1982).

A small, unusually treatment-resistant bipolar patient group whose manic episodes were controlled by lithium and other drugs but who had recurrent, disabling depressions responded well to the addition of very low doses of the selective MAO-A inhibitor clorgyline, with more prolonged intervals of euthymia and decreased severity of depressive cycles (Potter et al., 1982). Three earlier, double-blind studies demonstrated that tryptophan, when combined with an MAO inhibitor, was superior to the MAO inhibitor and placebo, but this combination has not become widely used (Nies, 1983; Quitkin et al., 1979).

Summary
======

There is substantial evidence that MAO inhibitors with different chemical structures are all effective antidepressant drugs. The question of whether specific MAO inhibitor-responsive subgroups of depressed patients exist remains controversial. Although some retrospective analyses have identified some depressive symptoms which are more common in responders to MAO inhibitors than in non-responders, most recent studies have failed to find consistent clinical symptom patterns which predict antidepressant response, or which discriminate between responders to tricyclic antidepressants and responders to MAO inhibitors. However, investigations using newer types of MAO inhibitors suggest that these drugs, as well as some standard MAO inhibitors, may possess not only different biochemical effects but also may differ in their clinical effects on different patient populations. Recent research on the clinical pharmacology and biochemical pharmacology of MAO inhibition has led to the development of some substrate-selective MAO inhibitors which are now undergoing early clinical trials, and have also led to refinements in clinical use which should permit more exact study of the clinical efficacy and mechanism of action of the different MAO inhibitors in man.

References

Blackwell, B., Marley, E., Price, J., and Taylor, D. (1967) Hypertensive interactions between monoamine oxidase inhibitors and foodstuffs. Brit. J. Psychiatry 113, 349-365.

Campbell, I. C., Robinson, D. S., Lovenberg, W., and Murphy, D. L. (1979) The effects of chronic regimens of clorgyline and pargyline on monoamine metabolism in the rat brain. J. Neurochem. 32, 49-55.

Campbell, I. C., Shilling, D. J., Lipper, S., Slater, S., and Murphy, D. L. (1979) A biochemical measure of monoamine oxidase type A and type B inhibitor effects in man. J. Psychiatr. Res. 15, 77-84.

Campbell, I. C., Gallager, D. W., Hamburg, M. A., Tallman, J. F., and Murphy, D. L. Electrophysiological and receptor studies in rat brain: effects of clorgyline. Eur. J. Pharmacol. (in press).

Cohen, R. M., Aulakh, C. S., Campbell, J. C., and Murphy, D. L. (1982) Functional subsensitivity of alpha$_2$ adrenoreceptors accompanying reductions in yohimbine binding after clorgyline treatment. Eur. J. Pharmacol. 81, 145-148.

Cohen, R. M., Aulakh, C. S., and Murphy, D. L. (1983) Long-term clorgyline treatment antagonizes the eating and motor function responses to m-chlorophenylpiperazine. Eur. J. Pharmacol. 94, 175-179.

Cohen, R. M., Ebstein, R. P., Daly, J. W., and Murphy, D. L. (1982) Chronic effects of a monoamine oxidase-inhibiting antidepressant: decreases in functional alpha-adrenergic autoreceptors precede the decrease in norepinephrine-stimulated cyclic adenosine 3':5'-monophosphate systems in rat brain. J. Neurosci. 2, 1588-1595.

Davidson, J., McLeod, M. N., Turnbull, C. D., and Miller, R. D. (1981) Psychopharmacology. A comparison of phenelzine and imipramine in depressed inpatients. J. Clin. Psychiatry 42, 395-397.

Davidson, J. and Turnbull, C. (1983) Isocarboxazid. J. Affec. Disorders 5, 183-189.

Dollery, C. T., Brown, M. J., Davies, D. S., Lewis, P. J., and Strolin-Benedetti, M. (1983) Oral absorption and concentration-effect relationship of tyramine with and without cimoxatone, a type-A specific inhibitor of monoamine oxidase. Clin. Pharmacol. Ther. 34, 651-662.

Folks, D. G. (1983) Monoamine oxidase inhibitors: reappraisal of dietary considerations. J. Clin. Psychopharmacol. 3, 249-252.

Georgotas, A., Friedman, E., McCarthy, M., Mann, J., Krakowski, M., Siegel, R., and Ferris, S. (1983) Resistant geriatric depressions and therapeutic response to monoamine oxidase inhibitors. Biol. Psychiatry 18, 195-205.

Giller, E., Bialos, D., Riddle, M., Sholomskas, O., and Harkness, L. (1982) Monoamine oxidase inhibitor-responsive depression. Psychiatr. Res. 6, 41-48.

Giller, E. and Lieb, J. (1980) MAO inhibitors and platelet MAO inhibition. Commun. Psychopharmacol. 4, 79-82.

Goekopp, J. G. and Carbaat, P. A. (1982) Treatment of neuroleptic malignant syndrome with dantrolene. Lancet ii, 49-50.

Gorenstein, C. and Gentil, V. (1981) Tranylcypromine isomers: single-dose effects in normal human subjects. Psychopharmacology 75, 400-403.

Himmelhoch, J. M., Fuchs, C. Z., and Symons, B. J. (1982) A double-blind study of tranylcypromine treatment of major anergic depression. J. Nerv. Ment. Dis. 170, 628-634.

Insel, T. R., Roy, B. F., Cohen, R. M., and Murphy, D. L. (1982) Possible development of the serotonin syndrome in man. Am. J. Psychiatry 139, 954-955.

Kellar, K. T., Cascio, C. S., and Butler, T. A. (1981) Differential effects of electroconvulsive shock and antidepressant drugs on serotonin-2-receptors in rat brain. Eur. J. Pharmacol. 69, 515-518.

Kenney, W. C., Nagy, J., Salach, J. I., and Singer, T. P. (1979) Structure of the covalent phenylhydrazine adduct of monoamine oxidase. In: Monoamine Oxidase: Structure, Functions, and Altered Functions (Singer, T. P., Von Korff, R. W., and Murphy, D. L., eds), Academic Press, New York, pp. 25-38.

Klein, D. F., Gittelman, R., and Quitkin, F., eds. (1980) Diagnosis and Drug Treatment of Psychiatric Disorders: Adults and Children, 2nd ed. Williams and Wilkins, Baltimore.

Knoll, J. (1981) The pharmacology of selective MAO inhibitors. In: Monoamine Oxidase Inhibitors: The State of the Art (Youdim, M. B. H. and Paykel, E. S., eds), John Wiley and Sons, New York, pp. 45-61.

Lipper, S., Murphy, D. L., Slater, S., and Buchsbaum, M. S. (1979) Comparative behavioral effects of clorgyline and pargyline in man: a preliminary evaluation. Psychopharmacology 62, 12-128.

Major, L. F., Murphy, D. L., Lipper, S., and Gordon, E. (1979) Effects of clorgyline and pargyline on deaminated metabolites of norepinephrine, dopamine and serotonin in human cerebrospinal fluid. J. Neurochem. 32, 229-231.

Maycock, A. L., Abeles, R. H., Salach, J. I., and Singer, T. P. (1976) The structure of the covalent adduct formed by the interaction of 3-dimethylamino-1-propyne and the flavine of mitochondrial amine oxidase. Biochemistry 15, 114-125.

Medical Research Council (1965) Clinical trial of the treatment of depressive illness. Br. Med. J. 1, 881-886.

Moises, H.-W. and Beckmann, H. (1981) Antidepressant efficacy of tranylcypromine isomers: a controlled study. J. Neural Transm. 50, 185-192.

Murphy, D. L. (1977) The behavioral toxicity of monoamine oxidase inhibiting antidepressants. Adv. Pharmacol. Chemother. 14, 71-105.

Murphy, D. L., Garrick, N. A., and Cohen, R. M. (1983) Monoamine oxidase inhibitors and monoamine oxidase: biochemical and physiological aspects relevant to human psychopharmacology. In: Drugs in Psychiatry - Vol. 1 - Antidepressants (Burrows, G. D., Norman, T. R., and Davies, E., eds), Elsevier/North Holland Biomedical Press, Amsterdam, pp. 209-227.

Murphy, D. L., Brand, E., Baker, M., van Kammen, D., and Gordon, E. (1975) Phenelzine effects in hospitalized unipolar and bipolar depressed patients: behavioral and biochemical relationships. In: Neuropharmacology, vol. X (Boissier, J. R., Hippius, H., and Pichot, P., eds), Elsevier, New York, pp. 788-799.

Murphy, D. L., Lipper, S., Slater, S., and Shiling, D. (1979) Selectivity of clorgyline and pargyline as inhibitors of monoamine oxidases A and B in vivo in man. Psychopharmacology 62, 129-132.

Murphy, D. L., Pickar, D., Jimerson, D., Cohen, R. M., Garrick, N. A., Karoum, F., and Wyatt, R. J. (1981) Biochemical indices of the effects of selective MAO inhibitors (clorgyline, pargyline and deprenyl) in man. In: Clinical Pharmacology in Psychiatry (Usdin, E., Dahl, S., Gram, L. F., and Lingjaerde, O., eds), Macmillan Press, London, pp. 307-316.

Nelson, J. C. and Byck, R. (1982) Rapid response to lithium in phenelzine non-responders. Brit. J. Psychiatry 141, 85-86.
Nies, A. (1983) Clinical applications of MAOI's. In: Drugs in Psychiatry, vol. 1 (Burrows, G. D., Norman, T. R., and Davies, B., eds), Elsevier, Amsterdam, pp. 229-247.
Olpe, H.-R. (1981) Differential effects of clomipramine and clorgyline on the sensitivity of cortical neurons to serotonin: effect of chronic treatment. Eur. J. Pharmacol. 69, 375-377.
Olpe, H.-R. and Schellenberg, A. (1980) Reduced sensitivity of neurons to noradrenaline after chronic treatment with antidepressant drugs. Eur. J. Pharmacol. 63, 7-13.
Paech, C., Salach, J. I., and Singer, T. P. (1979) Suicide inactivation of monoamine oxidase by transphenylcyclopropylamine. In: Monoamine Oxidase: Structure, Functions, and Altered Functions (Singer, T. P., Von Korff, R. W., and Murphy, D. L., eds), Academic Press, New York, pp. 39-50.
Paykel, E. S., Parker, R. R., Rowan, P. R., Rao, B. M., and Taylor, C. N. (1983) Nosology of atypical depression. Psychol. Med. 13, 131-139.
Paykel, E. S., Parker, R. R., Penrose, R. J. J., and Rassaby, E. R. (1979) Depressive classification and prediction of response to phenelzine. Brit. J. Psychiatry 134, 572-581.
Paykel, E. S., Rowan, P. R., Parker, R. R., and Bhat, A. V. (1982) Response to phenelzine and amitriptyline in subtypes of outpatient depression. Arch. Gen. Psychiatry 39, 1041-1049.
Pickar, D., Cohen, R. M., Jimerson, D. C., Lake, R. L., and Murphy, D. L. (1981) Tyramine infusions and selective MAO inhibitor treatment. II. Interrelationships among pressor sensitivity changes, platelet MAO inhibition and plasma MHPG reduction. Psychopharmacology 74, 8-12.
Pickar, D., Lake, C. R., Cohen, R. M., Jimerson, D. C., and Murphy, D. L. (1980) Alterations in noradrenergic function during clorgyline treatment. Commun. Psychopharmacol. 4, 379-386.
Potter, W. Z., Murphy, D. L., Wehr, T. A., Linnoila, M., and Goodwin, F. K. (1982) Clorgyline. A new treatment of patients with refractory rapid-cycling disorder. Arch. Gen. Psychiatry 39, 505-510.
Quitkin, F., Rifkin, A., and Klein, D. F. (1979) Monoamine oxidase inhibitors. A review of antidepressant effectiveness. Arch. Gen. Psychiatry 36, 749-760.

Raft, D., Davidson, J., Wasik, J., and Mattox, A. (1981) Relationship between response to phenelzine and MAO inhibition in a clinical trial of phenelzine, amitriptyline and placebo. Neuropsychobiology 7, 122-126.

Raskin, A. (1972) Adverse reactions to phenelzine: results of a nine-hospital depression study. J. Clin. Pharmacol. 12, 22-25.

Raskin, A., Schulterbrandt, J. G., Reatig, N., Crook, T. H., and Olde, D. (1974) Depression subtypes and response to phenelzine, diazepam, and a placebo. Arch. Gen. Psychiatry 30, 66-75.

Razani, J., White, K. L., White, J., Simpson, G., Sloane, R. B., Rebal, R., and Palmer, R. (1983) The safety and efficacy of combined amitriptyline and tranylcypromine antidepressant treatment. A controlled trial. Arch. Gen. Psychiatry 40, 657-661.

Reynolds, G. P., Rausch, W.-D., and Riederer, P. (1980) Effects of tranylcypromine stereoisomers on monoamine oxidation in man. Brit. J. Pharmacol. 9, 521-523.

Robinson, D. S., Kayser, A., Corcella, J., Howard, D., and Nies, A. (1983) Hyperphagia, hypersomnia, panic attacks, hysterical traits, and somatic anxiety predict phenelzine response in depressed outpatients. Abstracts of the Annual Meeting of the American College of Neuropsychopharmacology 83, 103.

Robinson, D. S., Nies, A., and Cooper, T. B. (1980) Relationships of plasma phenelzine levels to platelet MAO inhibition, acetylator phenotype, and clinical outcome in depressed outpatients. Clin. Pharmacol. Ther. 20, 180.

Robinson, D. S., Nies, A., Ravaris, C. L., Ives, J. O., and Bartlett, D. (1978) Clinical psychopharmacology of phenelzine: MAO activity and clinical response. In: Psychopharmacology: A Generation of Progress (Lipton, M. A., Dimascio, A., and Killam, K. F., eds), Raven Press, New York, pp. 961-973.

Rowan, P. R., Paykel, E. S., and Parker, R. R. (1982) Phenelzine and amitriptyline: effects on symptoms of neurotic depression. Brit. J. Psychiatry 140, 475-483.

Roy, B. F., Murphy, D. L., Lipper, S., Siever, L., Alterman, I. S., Jimerson, D., Lake, C. R., and Cohen, R. M. Cardiovascular effects of the selective monoamine oxidase-inhibiting antidepressant clorgyline: correlations with clinical responses and changes in catecholamine metabolism. J. Clin. Psychopharmacol. (in press).

Sheehan, D. V., Ballenger, J., and Jacobsen, G. (1980) Treatment of endogenous anxiety with phobic, hysterical, and hypochrondriacal symptoms. Arch. Gen. Psychiatry 37, 51-59.

Siever, L. J., Uhde, T. W., and Murphy, D. L. (1982) Possible sensitization of alpha$_2$-adrenergic receptors by chronic monoamine oxidase inhibitor treatment in psychiatric patients. Psychiatry Res. 6, 293-302.

Squires, R. F. (1978) Monoamine oxidase inhibitors: animal pharmacology. In: Handbook of Psychopharmacology, Affective Disorders: Drug Actions in Animals and Man, vol. 14 (Iversen, L. L., Iversen, S. D., and Snyder, S. H., eds), Plenum Press, New York, pp. 1-58.

West, E. D. and Dally, P. J. (1959) Effects of iproniazid in depressive syndromes. Brit. Med. J. 1, 1491-1494.

White, K. and Simpson, G. (1981) Combined MAOI-tricyclic antidepressant treatment: a reevaluation. J. Clin. Psychopharmacol. 1, 264-282.

8.

TRICYCLIC ANTIDEPRESSANTS

J. M. Baker and W. G. Dewhurst

Introduction and History
========================

Although monoamine oxidase inhibitors, specifically iproniazid, had been found to be effective antidepressants, the toxic effects were considered to be too great. Liver damage was frequent and clinicians became cautious in their use of these compounds. Kuhn, working in close collaboration with the firm of Geigy, considered variations on the chlorpromazine model and eventually found that the compound G22355 had antidepressant effects. This product is now known as imipramine (Kuhn, 1957), the first tricyclic antidepressant (TCA) and still the standard against which other antidepressants are measured. Just as chlorpromazine and its phenothiazine congeners had a tremendous effect on the treatment of schizophrenia, imipramine was destined to provide similar dramatic improvement in the treatment of depressive disorders.

Clinical Usefulness
===================

The proper management of a patient with depressive illness must always begin with accurate diagnosis. From time to time the consultant may see patients who may be suffering from myxoedema, parkinsonism, or some other unrelated condition and have been treated rigorously with TCAs. A detailed history and physical examination are the only way of ensuring the nosological status of a patient.

The second important distinction to be made is between bipolar and unipolar illnesses. A bipolar illness is defined in DSM III as occurring in a patient who, at any time, has had a manic episode irrespective of episodes of depression. This author (W.G.D.) would go further and regard an illness as bipolar whenever parents or close relatives have had a manic episode. The importance of making the distinction is simple. In patients with bipolar illness the administration of TCAs may precipitate a manic attack whereas this adverse effect does not occur in unipolar disease.

The next step in the proper management of such a patient is to decide whether or not the patient should be in hospital. Consideration should be given to physical symptoms (for example, signs of cardiac, thyroid, or kidney disease) which necessitate close monitoring. Secondly, psychological variables, especially suicidal intent, must be assessed. Since the TCAs take some time to be effective, strict nursing care in hospital is mandatory for suicidal patients. Finally, if the patient's social environment is so intolerable that geographical isolation from such stresses is important, admission to hospital should be considered.

The next step is to identify all possible causes of the depressive episode. Certain hypotensive agents, for example, are notorious in producing depression and obviously should be withdrawn (in consultation with the internist looking after the patient). Unfortunately, depression so induced, for example by reserpine, may run an autonomous course of its own, and even removing the cause does not absolve the doctor from treating the depression.

When these various decisions have been made, the treatment of depression can be considered complete only if attention is paid to physical, psychological and sociological factors.

In severe depression reassurance is the most important watchword although certain psychological treatments such as cognitive therapy have won acceptance. Attention to social matters may also be necessary but a word of caution is required here. Some of the troubles of which depressed patients complain, such as being a bad husband or a poor workman, are often 'the depression speaking' and it is nearly always best to defer alteration of the social environment until the patient's mood has improved.

Next the clinician must choose an antidepressant drug. Initial therapy of uncomplicated depression usually involves the use of a TCA. In practice the author has found it useful to divide the TCAs into two broad groups: those which are sedating and those which are alerting. Amitriptyline is the prototype of the first group and imipramine of the second (see section on sedation). However, because of the cardiotoxicity known to occur with amitriptyline the authors routinely use doxepin as the preferred sedative type of antidepressant.

The choice of which type of antidepressant to give depends on the patient's clinical state. A patient who shows a syndrome of depression with considerable agitation, anxiety, sleeplessness, or lack of appetite is best suited to the doxepin type of antidepressant. Conversely, the patient who exhibits a syndrome of depression with apathy, anergia, and at times overeating is best suited to imipramine.

Various therapeutic tests or laboratory procedures have also been suggested to aid the clinician in his choice of antidepressants. It has been suggested that patients excreting low amounts of MHPG respond best to the imipramine type of antidepressant whereas those excreting high amounts of MHPG respond better to amitriptyline (for details, see Chapter 2 by Huang and Maas in this book). Another simple test suggested is to give amphetamine for a 24-hour period; those responding will probably be best treated with imipramine, whereas those showing little response are presumed to do best with amitriptyline (Maas and Huang, 1980). To date the evidence concerning these predictive tests is somewhat inconclusive (see Chapter 2 for a more complete discussion).

As to dosage, for the average adult 150 to 200 mg a day, usually in divided doses, is nearly always satisfactory. In most laboratories blood levels may be obtained to ensure that the drug is being adequately absorbed. In the case of one particular antidepressant, nortriptyline, a suggestion of a therapeutic window has been made. This means simply that below and above a certain therapeutic range beneficial effects fall off. For nortriptyline the range has been estimated at between 50 and 140 ng/ml. Such an effect, however, has not really been firmly established for other antidepressants and the commonest mistake of nonpsychiatric practitioners is to give too little. Because of the sedative effects of doxepin the major dose is most conveniently given at night and in the case of imipramine the reverse is true.

A bare minimum of two weeks is usually considered necessary as an adequate trial of treatment, and three or four weeks will usually be required before improvement occurs. One must base duration of therapy on the natural history of most unipolar depressions which last a minimum of three months. There is no such thing as a lower maintenance dose. Full therapeutic doses must be given throughout the whole of the treatment period. If, at the end of three months, the patient seems well then it is worthwhile halving the dose and waiting another two to three weeks to see if symptoms return. If they do not then the drug may be terminated.

Failure to Respond

Again, at the risk of being repetitious, the most common failure of a patient to respond to a tricyclic antidepressant is a misdiagnosis. Assuming the diagnosis is correct a second problem is patient compliance. The more frequently a drug is to be taken, the less likely is the patient to follow instructions. A third problem is absorption. Many antidepressant products are coated and certain brands may not provide adequate bioavailability. Yet another problem is liver metabolism; patients who have ingested a variety of drugs previously may have increased liver oxidases to metabolize antidepressants. Barbiturates are particularly notorious in inducing liver enzymes. Yet another cause of failure to respond may be a dosage which results in blood levels outside the therapeutic window mentioned for certain compounds in a later section of this chapter.

Consideration of the reasons for failure to respond (including lack of patient compliance) indicate that in these cases blood levels of TCAs are essential in order to assess therapy fairly.

Intravenous Antidepressants

Although intravenous administration of the first introduced TCAs such as amitriptyline has been used, undesirable side effects such as sedation were frequent. However, with the introduction of clomipramine, intravenous administration has been increasingly used. A more rapid response may be seen, often within the first week of treatment. Other indications for this route of administration are patients who are refractory to oral antidepressants or who may be suspected of not taking the dose orally. Kielholz (Kielholz et al., 1979), in particular, has been an enthusiastic advocate of this method of treatment and also includes maprotiline in the list of antidepressants which may be so administered. A collaborative research project under the auspices of the World Health Organization has already been started and one must await more definitive evidence for the safety and proper indications for this type of approach.

Comparison and Combinations with other Treatments for Depression

It is the author's view that adequate administration for three to four weeks of either an imipramine-type or a doxepin-type antidepressant sufficiently covers the spectrum of TCAs. If the patient does not respond, assuming the reasons cited in the last section are excluded, then it is best to switch either to another form of treatment or to a combination with another type of antidepressant. Combinations with monoamine oxidase inhibitors (MAOIs), which initially were viewed with great caution by clinicians, are now not unusual. The second drug, however, should be added gradually and in the author's view this should be done only in hospital where monitoring of vital signs, including blood pressure, is available.

The most authoritative report on the combination of MAOIs and TCAs is that given in the position paper of the American College of Neuropsychopharmacology in 1981 (Ayd, 1981). The combination is regarded as useful in patients who are resistant to ordinary trials of standard antidepressants as long as certain guidelines are followed.

> The two types of drugs can pose special hazards if combined in certain ways, particularly if the tricyclic is added to treatment with an MAOI begun a week or more prior. We would advise the clinician to avoid such practice and probably also to avoid the addition of an MAOI to an established course of a tricyclic. Rather, the safest course would take the patient off either type of drug for at least one week, then begin both types together within the same day or two, starting with low dosages and gradually increasing dosage of both drugs together, depending on the individual patient's tolerance and clinical improvement.

Whilst tricyclic antidepressants have proved a boon to patients with many depressive disorders, there is still little doubt that for the severe depression ECT may be required and is still regarded as more efficacious. This procedure, however, requires an anaesthetic and hospital conditions which may preclude its use.

Structures of the Tricyclic Antidepressants: The Relationship of Structure to Therapeutic Activity and Occurrence of Side Effects

The chemical structures of the tricyclic antidepressants (TCAs) are illustrated in Figure 8.1.

Many of the TCAs are structurally related to neuroleptic compounds and share similar side effects. For example, imipramine and desipramine are analogs of the phenothiazines, amitriptyline and nortriptyline resemble the thioxanthene neuroleptics, and amoxapine is a metabolite of loxapine.

As can be seen from Figure 8.1, desipramine, nortriptyline, protriptyline and amoxapine are secondary amines, while imipramine, amitriptyline, doxepin, clomipramine and trimipramine are tertiary amines. A very simplified approach to the differences between these two groups has stated that the secondary amines primarily block the reuptake of noradrenaline (NA), and the tertiary amines that of 5-hydroxytryptamine (5-HT; serotonin) (Klein et al., 1980). Therefore the secondary amines would be most useful in depressions thought to be due to a deficiency of NA while the tertiary compounds could be used when a deficiency of 5-HT appears to be the problem. This distinction, however, becomes less clear when one considers that the tertiary amines are metabolized to secondary amines and thus both classes of TCA are present after administration of the tertiary compounds. Furthermore, Klein et al. (1980) state that there has never been a report of a depression which does not respond to a secondary compound but will respond to a tertiary amine.

Significant differences between the secondary and tertiary compounds are found in their side effect profiles. The tertiary compounds, especially amitriptyline, trimipramine and doxepin, cause more sedation than the secondary amines (Klein et al., 1980). Anticholinergic side effects seem to be more prominent with administration of the tertiary compounds (Ananth, 1983), with amitriptyline and doxepin showing the greatest incidence of these effects. Of the secondary compounds, desipramine appears to have the lowest anticholinergic effect. Another difference is blockade of the α-adrenergic receptor, thought to be the cause of postural hypo-

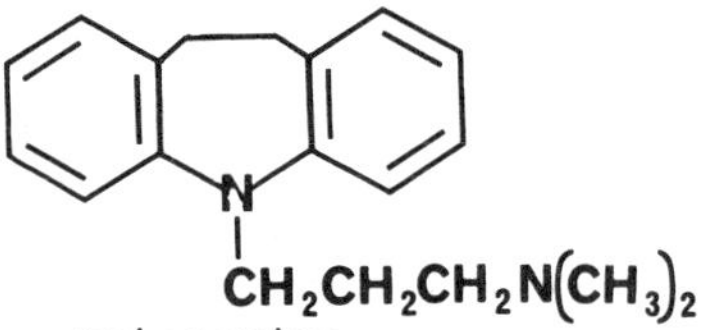

Imipramine

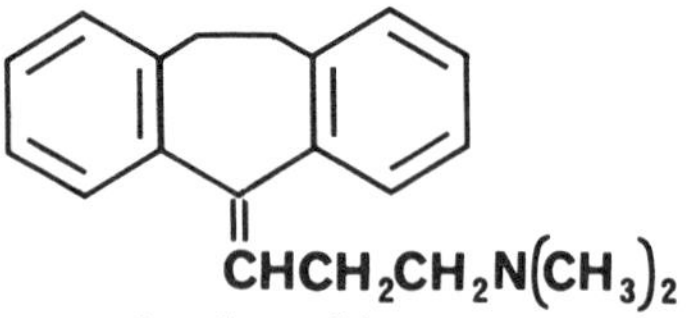

Amitriptyline

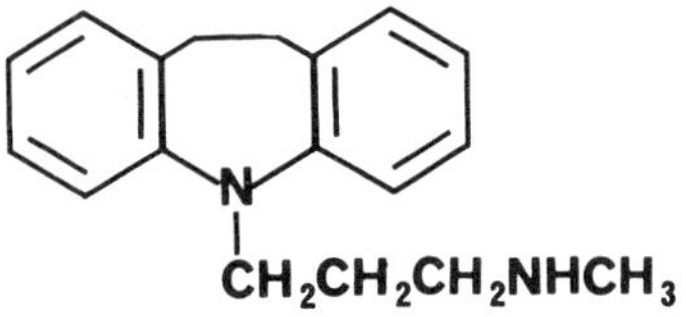

Desipramine
(Desmethylimipramine)

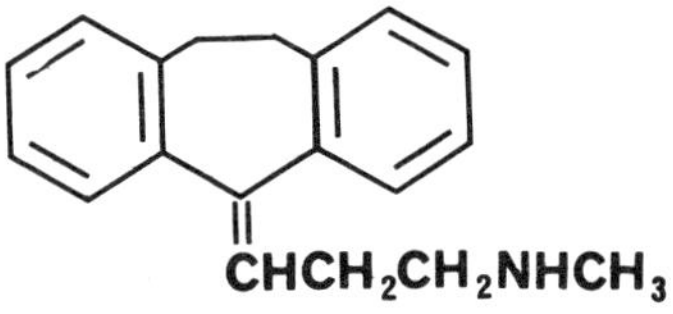

Nortriptyline

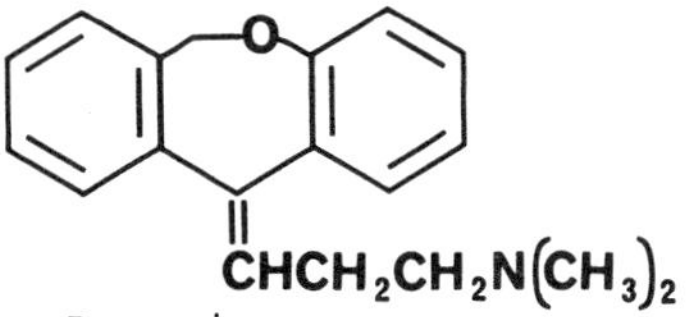

Doxepin

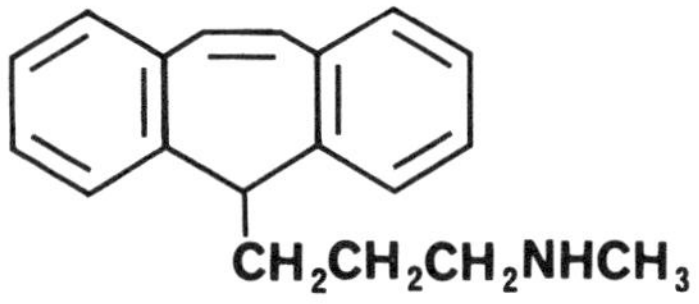

Protriptyline

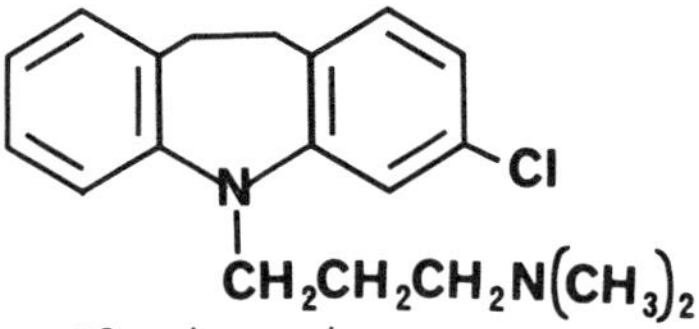

Clomipramine

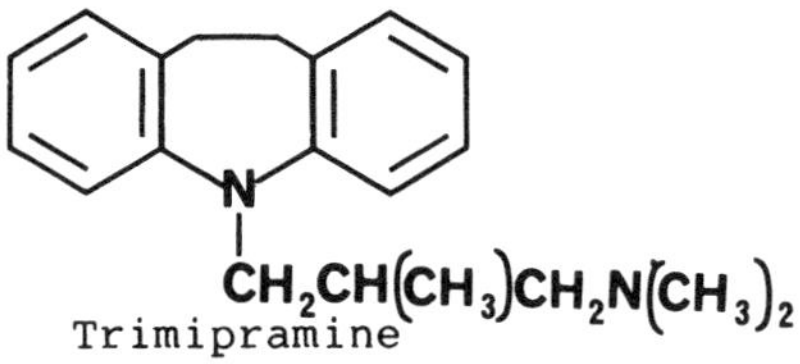

Trimipramine

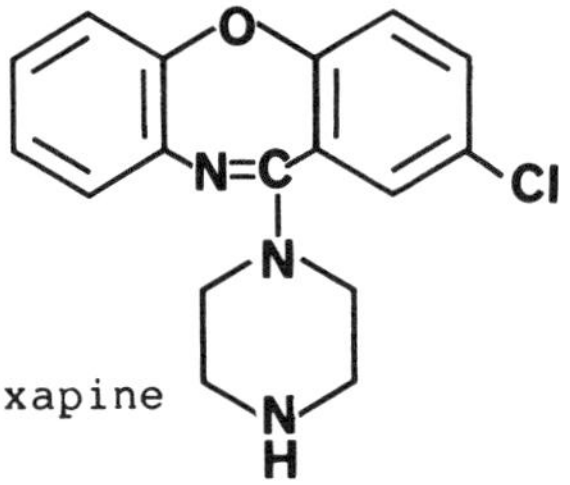

Amoxapine

Figure 8.1: The structures of the tricyclic antidepressants

tension. Since this effect is more predominant with the tertiary amines, these compounds should be avoided in patients troubled by this side effect and the secondary amines, protriptyline or desipramine, tried instead (Ananth, 1983). Finally, the secondary and tertiary compounds differ in their ability to block the central histamine H_2 receptor. The tertiary compounds block the H_2 receptor to a greater extent than the secondary tricyclics (amitriptyline has a greater affinity for this receptor than cimetidine). Since the blockade of central H_2 receptors may result in hallucinations, confusion, depression and delirium, it is suggested that the use of amitriptyline and doxepin be avoided in psychotic depression (Ananth, 1983).

Side Effects and Their Management

The major side effects associated with the TCAs are classified by The Medical Letter (Abramowicz, 1980b) in the following manner: **frequent** - anticholinergic actions, hypotension, drowsiness, weight gain; **occasional** - mania, tremor, first-degree heart block, tachycardia, other arrhythmias, skin rash, facial sweating, confusion; **rare** - cholestatic jaundice, bone marrow depression, seizures, peripheral neuropathy, severe cardiovascular effects in patients with cardiac disease, photosensitivity, dysarthria, withdrawal symptoms.

Anticholinergic Effects.
The most common anticholinergic effects experienced are dry mouth, blurred vision, constipation, urinary retention, tachycardia and exacerbation of narrow-angle glaucoma. These effects are particularly troublesome in the elderly and may necessitate the use of another type of drug in this patient group. In general, anticholinergic side effects are more severe during therapy with the tertiary amines than with the secondary amines (Ananth, 1983). Table 8.1 gives a schematic representation of the degree of cholinergic blockade experienced with some of the TCAs.

If these side effects are particularly troublesome, the patient may be given a once-daily dose at bedtime or switched to a drug with less anticholinergic potency. Dry mouth may be managed by suggesting that the patient chew sugarless gum or candy and brush his teeth more often. Oral pilocarpine or bethanechol chloride (25 mg, three times daily) have also been used (Klein et al., 1980). Constipation is a very common side effect occurring in up to 30%

Tricyclic Antidepressants

Table 8.1: Relative anticholinergic effects of some tricyclic antidepressants (Baldessarini, 1980; Ananth, 1983; Glenn and Taska, 1984)

Amitriptyline	
Doxepin = Nortriptyline	Decreasing
Imipramine	Anticholinergic
Desipramine = Protriptyline	Side Effects ↓

of patients (Klein et al., 1980) and can be overcome by the use of fiber laxatives (Metamucil®, Fibyrax®) or water-retaining laxatives (e.g. Milk of Magnesia). Urinary retention is more uncommon, occurring most often in men over 45 years old. For more severe cases it may be necessary to stop the TCA for 24 hours and restart at a lower dose with concurrent bethanechol chloride administration. Blurred vision may be treated by use of pilocarpine eyedrops. Patients should be cautioned against driving or operating machinery if their vision is affected. Klein et al. (1980) have suggested that TCAs can often be used in patients suffering from glaucoma if local cholinergic agents are used, concurrent tonometry is employed, and ophthalmological consultation is sought.

One unusual side effect, seen particularly with imipramine, is paradoxical sweating, especially about the head and neck in the area of distribution of the superior cervical ganglion. This effect is temperature-dependent, and while it may be very annoying for patients there appears to be very little that can be done to overcome it. A change to another tricyclic compound might be tried.

The tricyclic antidepressants may also trigger an anticholinergic psychosis, manifested as delusion, confusion and disorientation (Glenn and Taska, 1984). The risk of developing such an effect is increased if other anticholinergic drugs are used (e.g. phenothiazines). Physostigmine may be effective in treating some cases of toxic confusional state, and diazepam may be used if sedation is required (Baldessarini, 1980). Estimates on the incidence of this side effect vary. Baldessarini (1980) claims that it is common, occurring in 10% of all patients and in more than 30% of patients over 50 years of age, while Klein et al. (1980) suggest

5%. Preskorn and Simpson (1982) have demonstrated that the effect is related to the total plasma concentration of amitriptyline and nortriptyline. Out of 100 patients studied, 14 developed plasma concentrations above 300 ng/ml. Of these 14 patients, 6 out of 7 with levels above 450 ng/ml experienced delirium, while none of the 6 with levels between 300 and 450 ng/ml showed this effect. These results suggest that delirium may best be treated by lowering the dosage and monitoring plasma levels. Ananth (1983) has referred to the possibility of a toxic confusional state arising from central blockade of histamine H_2 receptors. Since H_2 blockade is highest with amitriptyline and doxepin, compounds which also have strong anticholinergic effects, it is difficult to clarify the mechanism underlying the occurrence of toxic confusional states.

Orthostatic Hypotension. Postural hypotension is a common problem during treatment with TCAs, especially in the elderly. The effect appears to be greater with the tertiary amines than with the secondary compounds and is probably due to α-adrenergic blockade (Snyder and Peroutka, 1984). Ananth (1983) suggests that when postural hypotension is a problem the tertiary amines and trazadone should be avoided, and protriptyline, desipramine or maprotiline used instead. Reports have suggested that 14% of patients on imipramine had falls or ataxia and another 7% had treatment stopped or modified due to severe dizziness (Glenn and Taska, 1984). Unfortunately, tolerance does not develop to orthostatic hypotension as it does to sedation and anticholinergic effects. Patients should be cautioned against sudden postural changes.

Sedation. Mechanisms for causing sedation could include central inhibition of the reuptake of 5-HT, central inhibition of NA activity at the $α_1$ receptor, or central antihistamine (H_1) activity. Since TCAs have been shown to possess all these properties, it is no surprise that they all can result in some sedation. When sedation is a desirable effect Ananth (1983) has suggested the use of doxepin, trimipramine or amitriptyline; when alertness is required protriptyline, desipramine and imipramine may be used. Amoxapine is reported to be less sedating than amitriptyline (Abramowicz, 1981). Once-daily dosing at bedtime may help to confine sedative effects to the night when they are more appropriate and result in increased alertness during the day.

Cardiotoxicity. The most serious cardiovascular complications reported with administration of tricyclics result from a direct quinidine-like myocardial depression resulting in widening of the QRS complex and P-R interval and some flattening of the T wave. In addition these compounds can suppress premature atrial and ventricular contractions and produce all types of cardiac arrhythmias (Glenn and Taska, 1984).

The most extensively studied compound is nortriptyline. With this drug it appears that there is little risk in young or middle-aged patients with no previous history of heart disease. Adverse effects increase if doses above the therapeutic window (> 200 ng/ml) are employed (Klein et al., 1980). There have been reports of an increased incidence of sudden unexplained deaths in patients over 70 years old treated with amitriptyline. Tachycardia which persists even after 13 months of treatment has been reported (Klein et al., 1980). In addition imipramine has been implicated in the occurrence of myocardial infarction and congestive heart failure (Baldessarini, 1980). The development of high plasma 10-hydroxynortriptyline levels after administration of moderate doses of nortriptyline has also been linked to development of congestive heart failure (Young et al., 1984). Doxepin appears to be less cardiotoxic than other tricyclic compounds from human data but not from animal studies. This result may be due to the fact that doxepin is less bioavailable than the other compounds (Klein et al., 1980). Amoxapine appears to be quite safe as well, but at this time not enough data exists to make a true assessment of its cardiotoxic potential. For patients with impaired cardiovascular function the best recommendation appears to be that they be treated jointly by a psychiatrist and an internist and followed with serial ECGs (Klein et al., 1980). Amitriptyline should be avoided in these patients.

Weight Gain. Weight gain associated with the administration of TCAs has been attributed to central histamine H_1 receptor blockade (Ananth, 1983), although this effect could also be due to increased availability of central 5-hydroxytryptamine. The Medical Letter (Abramowicz, 1980b) lists weight gain as a frequently occurring side effect. It may manifest as a craving for sweets and is not necessarily related to the alleviation of depression. It may become so severe that patients will refuse the drug in order to control their weight (Klein et al.,

1980). Lowering the drug dose may help the problem. Ananth (1983) states that all the tricyclics cause weight gain and no one drug is better than another. Conversely, he also suggests that in patients where weight gain is desirable, tertiary amines are preferable to secondary compounds due to their higher antihistaminic potency.

Allergic Reactions. Skin reactions, appearing as a patchy erythematous flush, occur occasionally during treatment with tricyclic antidepressants, usually early in treatment. These reactions may subside if the drug dosage is decreased. Photosensitivity is rare and may be managed by wearing protective clothing or using a sunscreen which protects against UVA radiation (Klein et al., 1980). It has been reported that the incidence of skin rashes with amoxapine (3-5%) is greater than with other tricyclics (Robinson, 1984).

Cholestatic jaundice has been reported to occur rarely, usually in the first few months of therapy, and responds to drug withdrawal. Agranulocytosis (occurring only in weeks 2 to 8 of therapy), leukocytosis, leukopenia, eosinophilia, and Loeffler's syndrome have been observed infrequently (Klein et al., 1980).

Disorders of Movement. A fine rapid tremor, usually of the upper extremities and occasionally the tongue, occurs in 10% of younger patients and more frequently in the elderly (Baldessarini, 1980; Klein et al., 1980). Also occurring rarely are twitching, convulsions, dysarthria, paresthesia, peroneal palsies, sudden falls, and ataxia. These latter two side effects may be especially important in the elderly since they may result in serious injuries (Klein et al., 1980). The fine tremor has been reported to respond to low doses of propranolol (Baldessarini, 1980) or diazepam (Klein et al., 1980). The tremor does not respond to anti-Parkinsonian therapy.

True extrapyramidal side effects occur only very rarely with all the tricyclics except amoxapine. This compound possesses significant dopaminergic receptor-blocking activity. The in vivo neuroleptic activity as measured by radioreceptor assay after an average daily dose of 234 mg of amoxapine was equivalent to that of haloperidol, trifluoperazine, fluphenazine or loxapine (Robinson, 1984). The extrapyramidal effects of amoxapine appear to be manifested most commonly as akathesia.

Tardive dyskinesia also occurs during amoxapine therapy, with incidence being greatest in women over 60 years old. Complete recovery has been reported after the drug has been discontinued for several months (Robinson, 1984). While tardive dyskinesias have not been reported to be caused by the other tricyclic compounds, they may worsen this effect if it is already present.

A paradoxical agitation has been reported to occur occasionally during initiation of therapy with imipramine (Klein et al., 1980). This effect is manifested by a sudden increase in anxiety, agitation, restlessness, and insomnia when the dose is increased too rapidly and may last for several hours after drug administration. Klein has further observed that this effect occurs frequently in patients suffering from panic disorder. Diazepam is recommended as an antidote. He also states that these same patients develop a very marked antipanic therapeutic effect if the drug is restarted at a lower dose and gradually increased.

Sexual Dysfunction. A loss of libido has been reported to occur occasionally during tricyclic therapy, with a more pronounced effect due to the agents with a higher anticholinergic potency, e.g. amitriptyline (Klein et al., 1980). Other sexual problems reported include slowness in achieving erection, delayed ejaculation, nonejaculation, retrograde ejaculation, and painful ejaculation.

Effects on Sleep. As would be expected of compounds which have a sedative effect, TCAs modify the type as well as the duration of sleep the patient experiences. Baldessarini (1980) states that these compounds decrease the number of awakenings, decrease REM (rapid-eye-movement) sleep, and increase stage 4 sleep. He further states that these drugs should not be used as hypnotics since their administration will result in a hangover if they are given in adequate dosage.

For patients experiencing insomnia as a symptom of their depression, antidepressants are often given as a single bedtime dose. This method of administration results in fewer daytime side effects and often improves the quality of sleep. Unfortunately some patients experience night terrors while on this regimen and should be changed to a multiple dosing schedule (Glenn and Taska, 1984).

Withdrawal. A withdrawal syndrome has been described after sudden cessation of administration (especially at doses above 150 mg per day for longer than two months) consisting of: nausea, vomiting, headache, malaise, myalgia, coryza, chills, cold sweats, dizziness, abdominal pain, diarrhea, anorexia, insomnia, anxiety, restlessness, and irritability (Klein et al., 1980; Baldessarini, 1980; Glenn and Taska, 1984). Such symptoms could easily be mistaken for the 'flu'. It has been suggested that the syndrome is primarily one of cholinergic overdrive and could be treated by administration of atropine (Glenn and Taska, 1984). Klein et al. (1980) suggest restarting the tricyclic antidepressant at about 150 mg per day and slowly weaning over one to two weeks.

Overdose. Deliberate overdosage with tricyclic antidepressants is a life-threatening situation. Death has occurred from 2000 mg (or less in children) of imipramine or the equivalent and severe intoxication has occurred at doses above 1000 mg. Patients who are suicidal or severely depressed should not be given prescriptions for more than 2000 mg at a time (Baldessarini, 1980; Glenn and Taska, 1984).

The presenting signs of overdose are primarily those of cholinergic blockade, including: dry mouth, urinary retention, absent bowel sounds, mydriasis, agitation, restlessness, pressured speech, and seizures. Further deterioration may lead to coma with a variety of cardiac arrhythmias and hypotension (Klein et al., 1980; Baldessarini, 1980). By far the most dangerous complication of overdosage is the occurrence of cardiac arrhythmias, which may reappear for several days after the initial critical period.

Initial treatment should include gastric lavage, administration of activated charcoal, and supportive measures. Peritoneal lavage and hemodialysis are not beneficial. Forced diuresis is ineffective and may be dangerous due to increased circulatory load (Klein et al., 1980). Physostigmine has been used to alleviate the antimuscarinic, cardiotoxic and neurotoxic features, but can itself cause bronchospasm, increased respiratory secretion, muscle weakness, bradycardia, hypotension, and seizures (Abramowicz, 1980a). Baldessarini (1980) has suggested that it might best be used in cases of mild intoxication where vital signs are stable and coma is absent; The Medical Letter (Abramowicz, 1980a), on the other hand, suggests that physostigmine be reserved for life-threatening situations, for example, coma with respiratory depression, uncontrollable seizures, or severe hypotension. Whatever the situation, it seems that extreme caution and careful monitoring should accompany physostigmine use.

Cardiotoxicity, hypotension, and the maintenance of intravascular volume may be difficult to manage since the effects of α-adrenergic agonists may be blocked, and the digitalis glycosides, quinidine and procainamide are contraindicated. Phenytoin may be given and will also help to control seizures. Propranolol may also be used. Diazepam may provide further seizure control. In addition, the physician may have to contend with hypoxia, hypo- or hypertension and metabolic acidosis (Baldessarini, 1980).

Drug Interactions. Drugs and drug groups interacting with TCAs are listed for quick reference in Table 8.2.

Table 8.2: Drugs and drug classes reported to interact with tricyclic antidepressants (see the text for a detailed discussion of mechanisms) (Abramowicz, 1980b; Baldessarini, 1980; DeVane, 1980; Klein et al., 1980; Miller and Macklin, 1983; Glenn and Taska, 1984).

---

alcohol	methylphenidate
amphetamine	monoamine oxidase inhibitors
aspirin	oral contraceptives
barbiturates	phenothiazines (especially
chloral hydrate	thioridazine)
chloramphenicol	phenylbutazone
cigarettes	phenytoin
cimetidine	scopalamine
clonidine	sympathomimetic amines
L-DOPA	(e.g. noradrenaline and
guanethidine	adrenaline)
haloperidol	trihexyphenidyl

A number of drugs have been reported to displace TCAs from plasma albumin binding sites. This displacement may result in increased therapeutic effect or in development of toxicity. Drugs reported to have this property include: phenytoin, phenylbutazone, aspirin, scopalamine, and phenothiazines (Baldessarini, 1980). Patients started on one of these substances after stabilization on a TCA should be carefully monitored for signs of toxicity and the dose of the antidepressant should be lowered if necessary.

A number of substances may alter liver metabolism of the tricyclics. Usually the hydroxylation reaction is the one affected. Since the hydroxylated metabolites are more water soluble, they are excreted more rapidly than the parent compounds; however these metabolites may also be active therapeutically and in producing toxicity, so the results of a change in metabolism are not always clear-cut. Patients should be closely monitored to assess whether a change in dosage is necessary. Substances and conditions reported to increase liver metabolism of tricyclics include: barbiturates, cigarette smoking and alcoholism (during the times when alcohol is not present). Liver metabolism may be decreased by cimetidine, phenothiazines, some steroids (e.g. oral contraceptives), haloperidol, methylphenidate, amphetamine, and alcoholism (during acute intoxication) (Baldessarini, 1980; DeVane, 1980; Glenn and Taska, 1984; Miller and Macklin, 1983). In addition DeVane (1980) lists the following compounds which affect plasma concentration of tricyclics by an unspecified mechanism (benzodiazepines, fluphenazine, and L-triiodothyronine were found to have no effect):

  decreased - chloral hydrate, trihexyphenidyl
  increased - chloramphenicol

A potentially serious interaction between tricyclics and exogenously administered biogenic amines (NA and adrenaline) has been reported (Abramowicz, 1980b; Baldessarini, 1980; Klein et al., 1980). Patients given these biogenic amines while also taking TCAs show larger than expected increases in blood pressure and a greater incidence of arrhythmias. Antidepressants should be discontinued prior to surgery where biogenic amines may be given. In addition, the use of NA with local anesthetic for dental procedures has been associated with a syndrome of throbbing headache which may progress to a loss of consciousness; this effect has occurred more often in patients taking tricyclic compounds. Patients should be told to inform their dentist about their medication before they undergo treatment (Klein et al., 1980).

Additive sedative effects will occur when tricyclics are given with other sedatives (e.g. alcohol), and additive anticholinergic effects are seen with such drugs as phenothiazines and antiparkinson drugs. Tricyclics have been shown to decrease the effect of L-DOPA and block the effects of clonidine and guanethidine. This latter interaction with guanethidine may occur to a lesser extent with doxepin since this drug reportedly does not block noradrenaline reuptake to the same extent as other tricyclic antidepressants (Baldessarini, 1980). In addition, one of us (J.M.B.) has observed a patient who experienced anticholinergic side effects but no therapeutic effect from desipramine during concurrent α-methyl-DOPA therapy. It is not known whether this lack of effect was due to a drug interaction or some other cause.

The risk of central toxicity of MAOIs increases when concomitant therapy with tricyclic compounds is undertaken. This effect may be manifested as hyperpyrexia, convulsions and coma. Extreme caution should be used when initiating this type of therapy and patients should be carefully monitored (Abramowicz, 1980b; Baldessarini, 1980). An increased incidence in the cardiotoxicity associated with thioridazine during tricyclic therapy has also been reported (Abramowicz, 1980b).

Metabolism, Significance of Plasma Levels and Use in Specific Patient Groups

Metabolism. The main metabolic routes for degradation of tricyclic antidepressants include desalkylation and hydroxylation followed by glucuronide conjugation and excretion in urine. The hydroxylated metabolites may be active, but are often more water soluble than the parent compounds and are more rapidly excreted (Glenn and Taska, 1984). The metabolism of imipramine is illustrated in Figure 8.2.

Amitriptyline is demethylated to its active metabolite nortriptyline, and amitriptyline, nortriptyline and protriptyline undergo aliphatic hydroxylation at the 10 position, followed by glucuronide conjugation and excretion. Doxepin is demethylated to a secondary amine, nordoxepin, which is an active metabolite; further degradation is similar to that for desmethylimipramine shown in Figure 8.2 (DeVane et al., 1980; Baldessarini, 1980).

The main metabolite of amoxapine is 8-hydroxyamoxapine which is a potent inhibitor of NA reuptake and has a biological half-life (30 h) which is longer than that of the parent compound. The 7-hydroxy

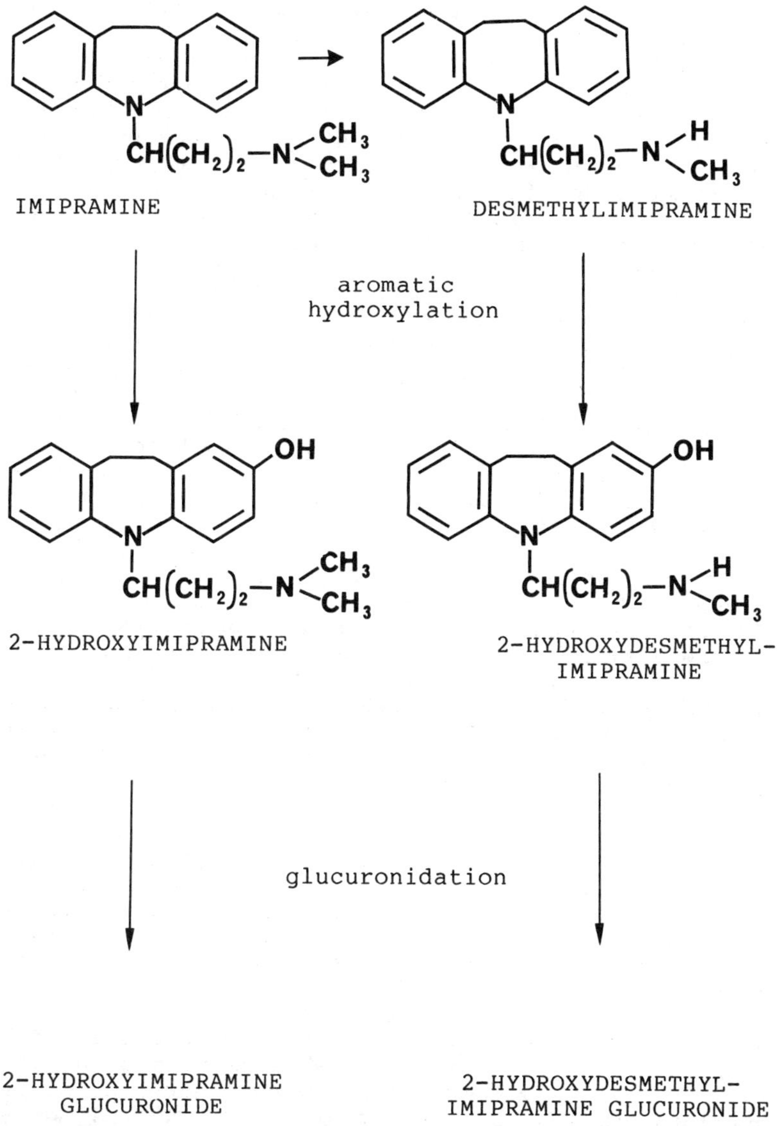

Tricyclic Antidepressants

IMIPRAMINE → DESMETHYLIMIPRAMINE

aromatic hydroxylation

2-HYDROXYIMIPRAMINE

2-HYDROXYDESMETHYL-IMIPRAMINE

glucuronidation

2-HYDROXYIMIPRAMINE GLUCURONIDE

2-HYDROXYDESMETHYL-IMIPRAMINE GLUCURONIDE

Figure 8.2: Metabolism of imipramine and desmethylimipramine.

metabolite also occurs and is a potent dopamine antagonist, showing significant neuroleptic activity. The development of extrapyramidal effects and possibly tardive dyskinesia may be due in part to this metabolite (Glenn and Taska, 1984).

Metabolism of the tricyclic compounds occurs exclusively in the liver by the cytochrome P450 enzyme system. Demethylation, N-oxidation and aromatic hydroxylation are all independent pathways and therefore variations in metabolic rate may occur at several different steps. Large interpatient variation in metabolism has been noted, with up to a 30-fold difference in plasma concentration after a particular drug dose being noted between certain patients. Furthermore, a large variability in the ratio of parent compound to active metabolite has been noted (e.g. 0.07-5.5 for imipramine:desipramine). It is probable that some variation in pharmacological effect and occurrence of side-effects from patient to patient could depend on the pattern and extent of metabolic conversion (DeVane, 1980). For a further discussion of the metabolism of tricyclics, see Chapter 12 (Rudorfer and Potter) of this book.

Pharmacokinetics and the Significance of Plasma Levels. The TCAs are all aliphatic amines, having pKa's of 8.4 or greater and are therefore highly ionized at body pH. They are lipophilic and are widely distributed in body tissues with volumes of distribution ranging from 8 to 34 l/kg (Baldessarini, 1980). Especially high tissue concentrations are found in cerebral tissue, cardiac tissue, and, in the case of doxepin, in the eye as well (DeVane, 1980). These tricyclic compounds are highly bound to plasma proteins (greater than 90%) (Baldessarini, 1980) and may be displaced by a variety of other drugs as discussed previously. Half-lives ($t_{1/2}$) are reported to be: amoxapine, 8 h; amitriptyline, 15 h; desipramine, 18 h; doxepin, 17 h; imipramine, 13 h; nortriptyline, 31 h; protriptyline, 78 h; trimipramine, 8 h (Baldessarini, 1980; Glenn and Taska, 1984; Abramowicz, 1981).

The TCAs are rapidly absorbed after oral administration with peak plasma concentrations occurring in 2 to 6 h (12 h for protriptyline). Absorption is complete in the fasting state but has not been studied in the presence of food. The availability after an oral dose is low (30% as compared with 70% by the intravenous route) due to an extensive 'first pass' effect from liver metabolism (DeVane, 1980).

Because of this effect, ratios of metabolites to parent compounds may vary, depending on the route of administration, and this result may alter the development of side effects or the eventual therapeutic effect.

A number of other factors have been reported to influence plasma tricyclic levels (DeVane, 1980). Aging results in an increase in plasma concentration after a particular oral dose, especially for imipramine and amitriptyline. Black patients may exhibit higher plasma concentrations and a more rapid therapeutic effect than Caucasians. Females show a different response from males, but this effect does not appear to be due to pharmacokinetic factors. For example, females are reported to show improvement when thyroid hormone is added during tricyclic therapy. Smoking is reported to decrease the plasma concentration of imipramine and desipramine but has no effect on nortriptyline levels. Hepatic disease results in a decrease in metabolism. Plasma protein binding has been shown to be higher in patients with hyperlipoproteinemia and has been correlated with plasma cholesterol and triglyceride concentrations. Free imipramine has been shown to be negatively correlated with α-1-acid glycoprotein and since this substance may vary in inflammation, malignancy, and hepatic and renal disease, tricyclic binding may be altered in these conditions. Finally, depression itself may change plasma concentration. Depressed patients are reported to show a higher steady-state concentration and slower clearance of nortriptyline than normal subjects. This effect has been suggested to be due to a decrease in hepatic blood flow and therefore metabolism in 'retarded' depression (DeVane, 1980).

Many studies have attempted to define the relationship between tricyclic plasma levels and therapeutic response (see Chapter 14 by Montgomery in this book). It appears that a linear relationship exists between concentration of imipramine plus desmethylimipramine (effective concentration > 225 ng/ml) and between amitriptyline plus nortriptyline (effective concentration 160-240 ng/ml) and clinical response (Risch et al., 1981; Baldessarini, 1980). Low plasma levels of imipramine and desmethylimipramine may inhibit recovery as compared with placebo treatment (Matuzas et al., 1982). This result may be due to the presence of side effects with little accompanying therapeutic effect.

Nortriptyline appears to show a curvilinear relationship between concentration and effect with a 'therapeutic window' between 50 and 140 ng/ml (Risch et al., 1981; Baldessarini, 1980). Desipramine, protriptyline, and doxepin probably exhibit a relationship between plasma level and therapeutic effect but the details have not been clearly defined (Risch et al., 1981).

Not only may plasma levels reflect therapeutic effect, they may also be correlated with the development of side effects. Adverse effects such as increased perspiration, dry mouth, changes in visual accommodation and decreased salivary flow are weakly related to plasma tricyclic concentration. On the other hand, cardiovascular effects such as orthostatic hypotension and tachycardia are not related to plasma levels (DeVane, 1980).

Measurement of plasma levels may be used to hasten or improve therapeutic effect, decrease toxicity, assess compliance with the medication regimen, and investigate drug-drug interactions or bioequivalence of pharmaceutical preparations (Risch et al., 1981). Only measurements taken at 'steady-state' are meaningful, that is, when elimination equals intake. The time necessary to reach steady-state is four to five times the half-life; therefore at least one to two weeks must be allowed after initiation of therapy or a change in dosage before plasma levels may be taken. For protriptyline, one must wait three to four weeks. Sampling should be done during the elimination phase of the plasma concentration vs time curve, a minimum of 8 h after the last dose. The most convenient time will therefore be in the morning before the first dose of the day. Plasma levels obtained in this way are comparable if the patient is on a single or multiple dosing schedule (DeVane, 1980).

A number of authors have reported that it is possible to predict eventual steady-state levels of tricyclics from plasma levels achieved after a single test dose of the drug (Perel, 1983; Braithwaite et al., 1982; Madakasira et al., 1982). Various intervals between the test dose and plasma collection have been employed (e.g. 18, 24, 36 and 48 h). Such a test must be calibrated in each laboratory due to large variations in assay methods. Once the appropriate conditions have been established, this type of determination could be used to optimize the dosage given to a particular patient and thus decrease the time required to achieve a therapeutic effect.

<u>Use in Specific Patient Groups</u>. Special care must

be taken when using tricyclic antidepressants to treat children and the elderly. The Medical Letter recommends that low initial doses be used in both these groups with gradual increases to achieve the desired effect (Abramowicz, 1980b). The same blood levels as mentioned previously for adult patients are appropriate when treating children for depression or enuresis. Smaller doses and lower blood levels may be appropriate for the hyperkinetic child (25-100 mg/day; 56 ng/ml) (DeVane, 1980). Tricyclic compounds are less highly protein-bound in children, and young patients are more susceptible to cardiotoxicity and seizure-induction by these drugs (DeVane, 1980; Baldessarini, 1980). In addition, the lethal dose in children is much lower than in adults, so intentional or accidental overdose should be treated with great caution.

Elderly patients have a decreased ability to hydroxylate the tricyclic antidepressants, resulting in higher than expected blood levels. These patients may require one-half to two-thirds of the dose needed for younger adults. In addition the decrease in body fat which occurs in aging may result in a more rapid accumulation of tricyclic compounds in plasma (Glenn and Taska, 1984). Elderly patients may experience more dizziness, orthostatic hypotension, constipation, urinary retention, edema, and muscle tremor (Baldessarini, 1980); they may have pre-existing heart disease; and they may be more susceptible to toxic psychosis at usual doses (Abramowicz, 1980a). For these reasons, careful dosage adjustment and drug selection are necessary in these patients.

Conclusion
==========

There is no doubt that TCAs, despite their side effects, have proven a boon to many patients who suffered in misery through depressive illnesses. Under sensible conditions many patients can be treated as outpatients, and an illness that might have gone on for many months can be terminated rapidly to restore the patient to good health. It can be stated unequivocally that the TCAs have revolutionized the treatment of one of the major illnesses in psychiatry.

References

Abramowicz, M. (ed.) (1980a) Physostigmine for tricyclic antidepressant overdosage. *The Medical Letter* 22, 55.

Abramowicz, M. (ed.) (1980b) Drugs for psychiatric disorders. *The Medical Letter* 22, 77-83.

Abramowicz, M. (ed.) (1981) Amoxapine (Asendin)—a new antidepressant. *The Medical Letter* 23, 39-40.

Ananth, J. (1983) Choosing the right antidepressant. *Psychiatric J. Univ. of Ottawa* 8, 20-26.

Ayd, F. J. Jr. (1981) Combined MAOI-tricyclic antidepressant treatment: a reevaluation. *Int. Drug Ther. Newsletter* 16, 23-24.

Baldessarini, R. J. (1980) Drugs and the treatment of psychiatric disorders. In: *Goodman and Gilman's The Pharmacological Basis of Therapeutics*, 6th ed. (Gilman, A. G., Goodman, L. S., and Gilman, A., eds), MacMillan, New York, pp. 418-427.

Braithwaite, R., Dawling, S., and Montgomery, S. (1982) Prediction of steady-state plasma concentrations and individual dosage regimens of tricyclic antidepressants from a single test dose. *Ther. Drug Monitoring* 4, 27-31.

DeVane, C. L. (1980) Tricyclic antidepressants. In: *Applied Pharmacokinetics: Principles of Therapeutic Drug Monitoring* (Evans, W. E., Shentag, J. J., and Jusko, W. J., eds), Applied Therapeutics Inc., Spokane, WA, pp. 549-585.

Glassman, A. H. (1984) The newer antidepressant drugs and their cardiovascular effects. *Psychopharmacol. Bull.* 20, 272-279.

Glenn, M. and Taska, R. J. (1984) Antidepressants and lithium. In: *The Psychiatric Therapies*, Amer. Psychiatric Assoc., Washington, D.C., pp. 85-118.

Kielholz, P., Terzani, S., and Gastpar, M. (1979) Treatment for therapy-resistant depression. *Int. Pharmacopsychiatry* 14, 94-100.

Klein, D. F., Gittelman, R., Quitkin, F., and Rifkin, A. (eds) (1980) Review of the literature on mood-stabilizing drugs. In: *Diagnosis and Drug Treatment of Psychiatric Disorders: Adults and Children*, 2nd ed., Williams & Wilkins, Baltimore, pp. 268-303.

Kuhn, R. (1957) Uber die behandlung depressiver zustande mit einem iminodibenzylderivat (G 22355). *Schweiz. Med. Wschr.* 87, 1135-1140.

Lydiard, R. B., Pottash, A. L. C., and Gold, M. S. (1984) Speed of onset of action of the newer antidepressants. Psychopharmacol. Bull. 20, 258-271.

Maas, J. W. and Huang, Y. (1980) Noradrenergic function and depression, too much or too little? Can. J. Neurol. Sci. 7, 267-268.

Madakasira, S., Preskorn, S., Weller, R., and Pardo, M. (1982) Single dose prediction of steady-state plasma levels of amitriptyline. J. Clin. Psychopharmacol. 2, 136-139.

Matuzas, W., Javaid, J., Glass, R., Davis, J., Ross, J., and Uhlenhuth, E. (1982) Plasma concentrations of imipramine and clinical response among depressed outpatients. J. Clin. Psychopharmacol. 2, 140-142.

Miller, D. and Macklin, M. (1983) Cimetidine-imipramine interaction: a case report. Am. J. Psychiatry 140, 351-352.

Perel, J. (1983) Tricyclic antidepressant plasma levels, pharmacokinetics and clinical outcome. Psychiatric Update, vol. II, American Psychiatric Press, Inc., Washington, D.C., pp. 491-511.

Preskorn, S. and Simpson, S. (1982) Tricyclic-antidepressant-induced delirium and plasma drug concentration. Am. J. Psychiatry 139, 822-823.

Risch, S. C., Janowsky, D. S., and Huey, L. Y. (1981) Plasma levels of tricyclic antidepressants and clinical efficacy. In: Antidepressants: Neurochemical, Behavioral and Clinical Perspectives (Enna, S. J., Malick, J. B., and Richelson, E., eds), Raven Press, New York, pp. 183-217.

Robinson, D. S. (1984) Adverse reactions, toxicities and drug interactions of newer antidepressants: anticholinergic, sedative and other side effects. Psychopharmacol. Bull. 20, 280-290.

Snyder, S. H. and Peroutka, S. J. (1984) Antidepressants and neurotransmitter receptors. In: Neurobiology of Mood Disorders (Post, R. M. and Ballenger, J. C., eds), Williams & Wilkins, Baltimore, pp. 686-697.

Young, R., Alexopoulos, G., Shamoian, C., Dhar, A., and Kutt, H. (1984) Heart failure associated with high plasma 10-hydroxynortriptyline levels. Am. J. Psychiat. 141, 432-433.

9.

RECENT ADVANCES IN ANTIDEPRESSANTS

N. F. Damlouji, J. P. Feighner and M. H. Rosenthal

For the past 30 years tricyclic antidepressants (TCAs) and monoamine oxidase inhibitors (MAOIs) have been the standard pharmacological agents used for the treatment of depression. Although both classes of drugs are generally successful in 65-75% of patients, they have significant and untoward side effects, are potentially lethal when used for suicide attempts, and are generally slow in their onset of therapeutic action. These properties have prompted research for newer compounds that are safer, have a more rapid onset of action, and have a wider therapeutic spectrum and a higher efficacy. Currently, research in the development and clinical testing of new antidepressants is very active throughout the world, with as many as 60-70 compounds in various stages of development. Over the next few years, quite a few of these antidepressant agents will be available on the market for the treatment of depression.

The first-generation antidepressants include the tricyclics imipramine and amitriptyline, their congeners and metabolites. The term 'second-generation antidepressants' refers to new tricyclics which are variations of the tricyclic structure. The third-generation antidepressants are the newest compounds in development and have chemical structures that are unique, or atypical. It is difficult to find a functional system to classify the newer and older antidepressant compounds. Although it is popular to classify antidepressants by function, and as to which neurotransmitter system they have the most affinity for (Lapierre, 1983), Richelson (1984) classifies antidepressants by the number of rings in the molecule. There is, however, no clear relationship between the ring structure and antidepressant activity of the drugs.

New Antidepressants

This article reviews 18 of the new antidepressant compounds that are at one stage or another of development. Using Richelson's classification, we present them according to their chemical structure, which is the number of rings in the molecule. We have used the category of novel antidepressants for compounds such as nomifensine and paroxetine which are structurally unique or unrelated to the conventional antidepressants (Tables 9.1 and 9.2).

New Antidepressants

Monocyclics

Bupropion. Bupropion is a chloropropriophenone and the first of the unique class of monocyclic aminoketone antidepressants (Soroko et al., 1977). The drug appears to have mild dopaminergic activity, demonstrated by its ability to reverse tetrabenazine sedation and its potentiation of L-Dopa. Its lack of significant effect on noradrenaline (NA) and 5-hydroxytryptamine (5-HT; serotonin) activity in the central nervous system (CNS), as well as the absence of anticholinergic and antihistaminic effects, makes its exact mode of action in the CNS unclear (Ferris et al., 1983). Although more stimulating than the traditional antidepressants, no direct stimulant effect nor MAO inhibitory effect has been found in vivo. It does not enhance the impairment of psychomotor performance in the presence of ethanol or benzodiazepines (Burroughs Wellcome, 1982). When administered in combination with a variety of commonly prescribed drugs, including antipsychotics, antihypertensives, antiarrhythmics, and analgesics, no significant drug-drug interactions have been demonstrated (Maxwell et al., 1981). Repeated clinical studies in a variety of outpatient protocols have shown bupropion to be lacking in adverse cardiovascular effects, including abnormalities in conduction time, blood pressure, pulse, or the production of orthostatic hypotension (Fleet et al., 1983). Overdose attempts with bupropion have failed to demonstrate any direct cardiotoxic effect or lethality. Seizure activity has been noted with rapid escalation of drug dosage during the initial phase of treatment and at doses of 600 mg or greater (Ferris et al., 1983). Antidepressant activity in both inpatient and outpatient settings have shown bupropion to be a safe and effective broad-spectrum antidepressant. In a double-blind placebo-controlled four-center study comparing bupropion to a placebo, the bupropion group had a 60-70% response compared to 20-30% for the placebo control. The side effects in the treatment group included dry mouth, agitation, insomnia, tremor, constipation, nausea and vomiting; however, the side-effect profile was generally low, and there were no significant differences between the complaints of the placebo and bupropion treatment groups (Burroughs Wellcome, 1982).

Our group and others have described other areas where bupropion may be useful in addition to its antidepressant activity. The clinical observations that this drug tends to cause weight loss (Harto-Traux et al., 1983) and stimulate libidinal drive (Crenshaw et al., unpublished data) are being studied at the present time. Bupropion may also be helpful in a selective group of bipolar patients because of its apparent lack of induction of manic or psychotic symptoms in this population. Nonresponders to TCAs generally respond well to bupropion.

Because of its low side-effect profile, nonsedating properties, and lack of apparent cardiotoxicity, this compound may be well suited for the geriatric population, as well as those with cardiovascular illness. The average daily dose for outpatients appears to be 300-450 mg per day in divided doses. For inpatients, it is 400-600 mg per day in divided doses.

Clovoxamine. Clovoxamine is an aralkyl ketone and a monocyclic which has been demonstrated to be a powerful inhibitor of neuronal NA and serotonin reuptake. Its metabolism results in metabolites which are virtually inactive on the neuronal inhibition of serotonin or NA reuptake (Claassen et al., 1978). This is in clear contrast to other antidepressants, which have been shown to have a series of active metabolites which later go on to be developed as independent compounds. Clovoxamine is also lacking in MAO inhibitory properties, has no ganglionic blocking effect, possesses neither sedative nor amphetamine-like properties, and fails to demonstrate any significant anticholinergic effects in animal test models. There appear to be some cardiovascular effects from the drug, but these seem to be minimal. For instance, when a 10 mg/kg dose of clovoxamine was compared to the same amount of amitriptyline in dogs, the electrocardiograms did not show any significant changes with clovoxamine, in contrast to the situation with amitriptyline. However, at a 25 mg/kg dose of clovoxamine, AV block occurred in some animals. Clovoxamine does block the antihypertensive effect of clonidine as well as the neuronal blocking effects of guanethadine (Robinson et al., 1982).

Double-blind studies have been conducted comparing clovoxamine with imipramine, clomipramine, amitriptyline, and placebo. Overall response rates to clovoxamine were comparable to those seen with the reference compounds. Mild cardiovascular changes were noted. There was a rise in the mean heart rate (5-10 beats/min) in 4 of the double-blind studies and some lowering of the mean blood pressure in 2 of the studies. The electrocardiograms in all of the studies failed to demonstrate any clinically significant changes attributable to clovoxamine. There were some mild effects in 2 hepatic enzymes in 3 patients; however, this was not significantly different from effects observed with the reference drug. The most frequent complaints with clovoxamine were dry mouth, nausea, headache, constipation, hypotension, somnolence, and tremor. Fewer anticholinergic side effects were reported compared to the reference drug, amitriptyline (Clanca et al., 1983).

Fezolamine. Fezolamine is a unicyclic compound which acts biochemically as a typical amine uptake blocker, primarily affecting the accumulation of NA. It appears not to have dopaminergic or serotonergic CNS effects. It has no antihistaminergic activity, but is mildly anticholinergic. Reported adverse effects have been mild in severity and commonly described as lightheadedness, nausea, drowsiness, headache, and gastrointestinal disturbances. Its relatively short half-life allows it to be given in divided doses during the day in a range of 100 mg to 400 mg. Preliminary open-label trials in our research clinic indicate potent antidepressant effects with a low side-effect profile.

Fluvoxamine. This unicyclic compound belongs to the class of aralkyl ketone oxime ethers. Fluvoxamine has been demonstrated as a potent and specific inhibitor of serotonin reuptake without demonstrable dopamine (DA), NA, antihistamine, or anticholinergic activity (Claassen et al., 1978). It is a stimulating compound which potentiates serotonin and has no MAO inhibitory effects. While its clinical profile is similar to the bicyclic compounds zimelidine and fluoxetine, there are remarkably few metabolites of fluvoxamine and its sole excretory organ is the kidney (Feighner, 1983).

We conducted at our center a double-blind, placebo-controlled study comparing fluvoxamine with imipramine in hospitalized patients meeting DSM III criteria for major affective illness: depressed, recurrent, single, unipolar, and bipolar. Significantly, there were fewer patients in the fluvoxamine-treated group reporting moderate or severe cardiovascular complaints than in the imipramine- or placebo-treated groups. There were no systematic differences in the fluvoxamine-treated group with regard to biochemical or hematological variables. The most common side effects in the fluvoxamine group were: nausea, vomiting, somnolence, headache, agitation, tremor, dry mouth, and constipation. Fluvoxamine was not only tolerated better than imipramine, but its anticholinergic activity was indistinguishable from that of the placebo. Results showed that, at day 28, 57% of fluvoxamine-treated patients improved compared to 38.3% in the imipramine and 6.8% in the placebo groups. At the end of the 6-week study, fluvoxamine-treated patients showed even more improvement (62%) compared to imipramine (40%) and placebo (4%) (Feighner et al., unpublished). The therapeutic dose range of fluvoxamine is 150-300 mg as a single or divided dose, given early in the day (Doogan, 1980).

Bicyclics

Citalopram. This drug is a bicyclic phthalone derivative which has been shown to be extremely potent and selective as an inhibitor of neuronal serotonin, with no demonstrable effect either in vivo or in vitro on the uptake of NA or DA (Hyttel, 1982). Receptor binding studies fail to demonstrate antagonistic activity toward DA, NA, serotonin, histamine, or gamma-aminobutyric acid (GABA) by citalopram. The drug is unusual compared to many older and newer-generation antidepressants in that both parent compound and its metabolites seem to be purely serotonergic in their activity (Oyehaug et al., 1984).

During Phase II studies, Pedersen et al. (1982) followed 19 patients for 6 weeks of treatment on citalopram. Eleven of 16 endogenously depressed patients responded and were maintained 8-113 weeks. After discontinuation of treatment, 7 of those 16 patients relapsed and were treated again with citalopram. Six responded completely to the retreatment. Of significance in this open-label study was the lack of cardiovascular effects produced by the drug: there were no effects on blood pressure, pulse rate, orthostasis, or the electrocardiograms. One patient in the study overdosed on citalopram and had a plasma level 6-fold greater than the therapeutic level, but survived with no signs of toxicity or sequelae. The drug has a 33-h half-life with peak concentration 2-4 h after a single daily dose, and is excreted by both hepatic and renal routes (Overo, 1982). Therapeutic dose ranges between 40 to 100 mg daily. Because of its long serum half-life and low side-effect profile, citalopram is well suited for once-a-day dosage commencing with full therapeutic dose on day 1 of treatment.

Fluoxetine. Fluoxetine is a bicyclic antidepressant of the phenylpropylamine class of antidepressant compounds. This drug is a potent inhibitor of serotonin reuptake in the CNS (Wong et al., 1974) and is highly selective and specific for that neurotransmitter. It lacks CNS activity on the dopaminergic or noradrenergic systems (Wong, 1982). Both pharmacologic and clinical studies demonstrated the drug's lack of anticholinergic and antihistaminic side effects. The drug has been shown to have no appreciable cardiotoxicity in overdose situations.

We have recently completed a double-blind study comparing fluoxetine to doxepin in a geriatric population. While our sample size was relatively small (N = 44), fluoxetine and doxepin compared favorably in their efficacy for the treatment of depression in this population. Outpatients in the study ranged in age from 64 to 90 years of age, and all met RDC criteria for major affective disorder, depressed. Improvement from baseline to endpoint was statistically significant for both groups, and the major difference between the two drugs in this study was the reported lower incidence of side effects in the fluoxetine-treated group, with 3 out of 24 fluoxetine-treated patients and 6 out of 23 doxepin-treated patients reporting significant side effects. Compliance was also more of a problem in the doxepin group, with a higher dropout rate than in the fluoxetine-treated group being observed (Feighner et al., unpublished data).

We have also completed a double-blind, randomly assigned comparison of fluoxetine and amitriptyline in a nongeriatric adult outpatient population. Both treatment groups demonstrated statistically significant improvement from baseline to the endpoint; however, fluoxetine patients demonstrated greater improvement with fewer side effects than did the amitriptyline patients. Only 3 out of 22 fluoxetine patients discontinued the study because of adverse effects, whereas 9 out of 22 amitriptyline patients dropped out of the study because of an inability to tolerate the drug. Common side effects with amitriptyline were anticholinergic effects. Fluoxetine patients complained of nausea, diarrhea, and restlessness. There were no drug-related laboratory abnormalities noted; however, the fluoxetine group was noted to have lost an average of 3 pounds versus a nonsignificant weight gain in the amitriptyline group (Feighner et al., in press). Because of its activating properties, fluoxetine is best given in a single or divided dose during the day. The therapeutic range appears to be from 20-80 mg daily (Eli Lilly Research Laboratories, 1983). Because of its long serum half-life and low side-effect profile, this compound is well suited for once-a-day dosing starting with a full therapeutic dose on day 1.

Also, because of consistent sustained weight loss noted in our earlier studies, pilot studies in exogenous obesity and bulimorexic disorders are in progress. Preliminary data indicate the potential usefulness of fluoxetine in these disorders.

Tomoxetine. This compound is structurally related to fluoxetine, differing only in the 2-methyl substitution which confers on tomoxetine its propensity as a potent and selective inhibitor of NA uptake. Preclinical pharmacological studies showed the drug to have no CNS serotonergic, anticholinergic, or antihistaminic activity (Wong et al., 1982). Cardiotoxicity was studied over a variety of doses and compared to that of amitriptyline. Like its parent compound fluoxetine, this drug had no significant effect on QRS duration over a 2-10 mg/kg i.v. dose range. The QRS duration varied directly with increasing doses of amitriptyline (Eli Lilly Co., 1983a).

Open-label clinical trials have been conducted on 37 patients to whom tomoxetine was administered in divided doses of 40 to 90 mg. Seventeen of 36 patients showed 'much to very much' improvement, with 6 of 36 experiencing no change or worsening. Major side effects included insomnia, dry mouth, headache, and nervousness (Eli Lilly Co., 1983b). More extensive double-blind comparison trials with placebo are now in progress.

Viloxazine. Viloxazine is a bicyclic compound chemically related to propranolol. It is a catecholamine reuptake-inhibitor with little antihistamine and anticholinergic effects (Ban, 1982). In many studies viloxazine has been found to be equal in efficacy to imipramine and amitriptyline, with some studies showing a more rapid onset of action than imipramine (Mindhom, 1979). Common side effects reported with viloxazine include nausea, vomiting, dizziness, headaches, and dry mouth. The nausea and vomiting are diminished with the use of enteric-coated tablets (Murphy, 1975). The drug seems to have less cardiovascular toxic effects than the standard tricyclics and seems to have some anticonvulsant properties (Mindhom, 1979). The therapeutic dose range is 150-300 mg daily.

BW647U. BW647U is a chemically novel bicyclic compound which is an aminomethyl phenylthiobenzyl alcohol. In vitro neurochemical studies indicate that this compound is a weak inhibitor of serotonin and NA reuptake in the synaptosomes of rat hypothalamus, and a weak inhibitor of DA uptake into striatal synaptosomes. In vivo studies, however, indicate that there is no significant inhibition of uptake of serotonin, NA, or DA in the CNS, and no anticholinergic, antihistaminergic, MAO inhibitory, or direct-stimulant activity. The mode of action of this drug is unknown.

Initial double-blind clinical field trials in a limited number of patients showed the drug to be efficacious when compared to placebo; however, side effects and adverse reactions have appeared and include minor EKG alterations (ST-T wave changes) and puritic rashes at higher doses. More extensive clinical field trials are underway to ascertain whether the side effects will outweigh the potential benefits of this compound. The dose range appears to be 300-900 mg in daily divided doses.

Tricyclic Compounds

Dothiepin. Dothiepin hydrochloride is a second-generation tricyclic antidepressant which is structurally similar to amitriptyline. This compound has been used for 10 years in Europe as an antidepressant which is also anxiolytic (Goldstein and Claghorn, 1980). Dothiepin appears to affect the CNS in a way similar to amitriptyline, in that it inhibits both serotonin and NA reuptake in the CNS, but has less anticholinergic effects. There is no apparent antihistaminic activity or MAO inhibition (Marrion Laboratories, 1983). Cardiovascular changes seem to be less with dothiepin, but it still requires the same caution as traditional tricyclics because of its atropine-like action and potential for cardiotoxicity (Kazetska et al., 1978).

Dothiepin has been compared to amitriptyline, imipramine, and anxiolytics in a variety of studies and has been shown to be as effective as the traditional antidepressants with regard to its efficacy. It has also been shown to be equally efficacious to chlordiazepoxide in double-blind comparisons and hence its reported usefulness in treating highly agitated depressive states (Johnson et al., 1973). It has a relatively long half-life of 22 h and can be given as a single-bedtime dose in the range of 100-300 mg.

Tetracyclics

Mianserin. Mianserin is a tetracyclic antidepressant and has a unique profile of activity compared to the more traditional drugs. It provides a presynaptic alpha-adrenergic blocking activity, with strong antihistaminic properties and weak CNS anticholinergic effects. There is no in vivo neurochemical evidence that mianserin has an effect on the uptake or turnover of serotonin in the CNS (Leonard, 1984). Mianserin does not decrease the antihypertensive action of drugs such as guanethadine. It has been used extensively in European and other industrialized countries and is considered to be safe and efficacious (Brogden et al., 1978), having low cardiovascular toxicity even in overdose cases, and has shown little in the way of drug-drug interactions with cardiovascular or psychotropic drugs (Conti et al., 1979).

In our center we completed a 6-week double-blind study comparing mianserin with amitriptyline in 81 outpatients (Feighner et al., 1983). The mean daily dose of mianserin was 105 mg at bedtime, and for amitriptyline 154 mg at bedtime. Both groups showed statistically significant improvement from baseline on all parameters, and both drugs were similar on all efficacy parameters. At the endpoint, 57% of the mianserin patients and 54% of the amitriptyline patients achieved a 50% or greater reduction on the HAM-D scale. There were also significant differences on the side effect profiles of these two drugs. Twenty-six of 41 mianserin patients reported side effects, while 39 of the 40 amitriptyline patients reported drug-related side effects. The common side effects for amitriptyline were anticholinergic, while the most common side effect for mianserin was drowsiness.

Because of its efficacy and low incidence of significant side effects, the drug should be particularly well suited for the geriatric population. Its relatively long half-life allows it to be given once daily at bedtime, and the dose range is 30-150 mg daily.

ORG3770 (6-AZAmianserin). ORG3770 is a 6-AZA analogue of mianserin and has been developed as one of a series of piperazinoazepines which were synthesized and evaluated for their potential as psychotropic agents. Its pharmacological profile is slightly different than that of the parent compound mianserin. It shows no activity on the adrenergic beta-1 receptor, is weakly antiserotonergic, moderately anticholinergic and anti-alpha-adrenergic, and is strongly antihistaminergic. Its potency is equal to that of mianserin with regard to its activity on the postsynaptic alpha receptor and the ability to evoke NA release by blocking presynaptic alpha receptor activity (Pharmaceutical Research Institute, 1982).

This compound is still in the early stages of clinical testing. Preliminary data demonstrated an efficacy similar to mianserin's but with less sedation. The reported effective daily dose is in the range of 20 to 40 mg daily, which can be given as a single h.s. dose.

Oxaprotiline. Oxaprotiline is a hydroxy analogue of maprotiline, a tetracyclic antidepressant, which in animal studies appears to be a more potent NA reuptake inhibitor than maprotiline, with less atropine-like side effects. The drug lacks CNS serotonergic and dopaminergic activity. It has approximately the same antihistaminic and cardiovascular toxicity in therapeutic doses as maprotiline, but approximately half the anticholinergic side effects (Ciba Geigy, 1982).

Results from a large double-blind, multicentered study comparing oxaprotiline with amitriptyline and placebo in 278 outpatients with major depressive disorder indicate equal efficacy for the two drugs and statistical superiority for both over placebo. Oxaprotiline had a superior side effect profile, with far fewer sedative and anticholinergic side effects. Fewer patients dropped out because of adverse effects with oxaprotiline, and overall it was much better tolerated than amitriptyline (Roffman et al., 1982).

Oxaprotiline has a sufficiently long serum half-life that once-a-day dosage at bedtime is sufficient, and the dose range appears to be 25-200 mg (Feighner et al., 1983).

Novel Antidepressants

Adinazolam. Adinazolam is an amino alkyl derivative of alprazolam, a triazolobenzodiazepine discovered to possess potential as the first benzodiazepine with antidepressant activity (Fabre, 1976; Feighner et al., 1983). The attractive properties of this class of drugs--i.e., less cardiotoxicity, lower overall incidence of serious adverse effects, lack of anticholinergic effects, and increased margin of safety in overdosage--have added to the enthusiasm for exploring these compounds for greater antidepressant activity. While initially adinazolam appeared to be less potent than alprazolam in animal studies, it does cause some inhibition of NA reuptake and potentiates noradrenergic transmission (Lahti et al., 1983).

An open-label study of adinazolam (Pyke et al., 1983) was conducted at several centers, using 42 patients with severe depression. Up to 90 mg in divided daily doses were used, and the drug appeared to be reasonably well tolerated, with the usual benzodiazepine side effects. Several bipolar patients became hypomanic on the drug. Significantly, by day 7, 21 of 37 patients had a HAM-D which declined by 50% or more. The rapid onset was sustained over the 42-day trial. A multicentered double-blind study comparing adinazolam to imipramine in outpatients for long-term treatment is currently in progress. While the drug appears to compare favorably, long-term studies suggest a need for slow withdrawal to avoid the usual reaction from abrupt cessation of benzodiazepines, with the risk of seizures and other withdrawal symptoms.

Indalpine. Indalpine has a chemical structure totally unrelated to the tricyclic antidepressants --it is a 4-alkyl piperidine. Its primary effect on the CNS is that of a potent and selective inhibitor of serotonin reuptake. In radioligand studies, it is second only to citalopram in its potency to inhibit serotonin reuptake. There appear to be no CNS effects on NA or DA. The drug has no significant antihistaminic effects, but does have mild, but not clinically significant, anticholinergic effects, and there is no MAO inhibition (Gueremy et al., 1980). There is a suggestion that this drug may have anxiolytic-like properties due to its potentiation of morphine-induced analgesia (Groupe Pharmuka, 1984).

Several Phase I as well as open-label clinical trials have been completed. Compared to imipramine, indalpine appears to be much better tolerated, especially regarding anticholinergic and cardiovascular effects. In a 5-center study of 100 patients, the dropout rate in the indalpine group was slightly less than half that of the imipramine group. Another study comparing indalpine to placebo showed statistically significant improvement in HAM-D scores by day 8, suggesting that this drug may have a more rapid onset of activity than older generation compounds. Most frequently reported side effects included gastrointestinal disturbances such as nausea and vomiting, drowsiness, and tremor.

The drug has a relatively short half-life of approximately 9 h, and is given in a therapeutic range of 100-250 mg in divided doses daily.

Nafasadone. Nafasadone belongs to the class of triazolopyridine compounds which have shown potential as antidepressants. Trazodone, the parent compound of this class, was the first novel antidepressant marketed in the United States. Trazodone is primarily serotonergic in activity, less lethal with an overdose, lacks anticholinergic effects, and is overall less cardiotoxic than the standard tricyclics (Ayd, 1979). Initial studies of nafasadone indicated that it is pharmacologically similar to trazodone except that it has significantly less alpha adrenolytic effects. The side-effect profile for nafasadone is similar to that of trazodone, but overall nafasadone is much better tolerated, with less sedation.

Our center is currently conducting an open-label inpatient evaluation of nafasadone and, to date, 18 patients have been evaluated, with preliminary results indicating an antidepressant effect. The therapeutic dose is from 100-400 mg in divided doses.

Nomifensine. Nomifensine is distinctly different from the tricyclic antidepressants, and is a tetrahydroisoquinoline which actively blocks the reuptake of DA and NA *in vivo* (Brogden et al., 1979). There appears to be no clinically significant CNS effect on serotonin, and it is clinically devoid of anticholinergic side effects and histaminic receptor activity (Hoffman, 1977). While equally efficacious to reference drugs, including imipramine and amitriptyline, nomifensine appears to be relatively more stimulating and especially useful in depression with psychomotor retardation. Such stimulation has been noted clinically to exacerbate manic and psychotic symptoms, requiring the cautious use of nomifensine in these conditions.

Although not a stimulant, the self-administration of this compound in certain animal studies has raised concern about its abuse potential. Thus far, in carefully controlled clinical studies, the problem of patient abuse has not been reported, nor has such abuse been reported on a worldwide basis, although the drug has been available since 1977 (Taeuber et al., 1979).

Of all the compounds currently in use, or being screened for antidepressant effects, nomifensine is unique in that it has substantial anticonvulsive activity in man (Trimble and Robertson, 1984). As a result, this is the compound of first choice in Europe for treating depressed epileptic patients.

Studies conducted in our research center in severely depressed patients show this drug to be safe, effective, and well tolerated in adults and by the elderly. The drug's relative lack of sedation, low cardiotoxicity compared to the TCAs (Burrows et al., 1978), rapid absorption and renal excretion make it especially useful in geriatric and medically ill patients.

The dose range is from 50-200 mg per day given in divided doses. Side effects include dry mouth, tremulousness, restlessness, insomnia, and, infrequently, drug fever (Poldinger and Gammel, 1978).

Paroxetine. This potent inhibitor of serotonin uptake is a drug of the phenylpiperidine class and has been demonstrated to exert weak effects upon NA, DA and anticholinergic activity in vitro, and appears to have little in vivo effect on these neurotransmitters (Squires, 1974). It does appear to be weakly antihistaminic, but contains no MAO-inhibiting activity. Paroxetine, when compared to a variety of antidepressants, was shown to have the greatest selectivity of all for serotonin inhibition and comparatively little effect on NA uptake (Buus Lassen et al., 1980).

During animal and early clinical studies, paroxetine appeared to be well tolerated by the cardiovascular system, with little direct or indirect effect via the peripheral NA system. The traditional interaction seen between TCAs and antihypertensive agents such as guanethadine (Petersen, 1979), presumably through inhibition of neuronal uptake, is significantly reduced in paroxetine-treated animals. This is further reflected in an LD_{50} (in dogs) which is twice as great as those observed for amitriptyline or imipramine.

Currently under Phase II investigation, the drug has been observed to be well tolerated in open-label study (Dorup et al., 1982), with 15 of 19 patients reporting a modest to good response. It has a long half-life, and could be given in a single daily dose that ranges from 20-60 mg. Major side effects reported have been insomnia, nausea, and drowsiness.

Conclusions

The new generation of antidepressants show a marked departure from the older generation of drugs in use. The series of new compounds offer highly selective actions on the neurotransmitters. Their selective activity, and understanding of the sites of actions of these compounds, will enhance our understanding of the biochemical and neurophysiological changes in depression.

The newer agents have less anticholinergic side effects, are less cardiotoxic, and less dangerous with overdosage than the traditional antidepressants in current use. Some specific antidepressants, such as nomifensine, offer an additional safety property, an anticonvulsive effect. The newer-generation antidepressants reduce the unwanted side effects seen with tricyclics and have greater compliance with a lower side-effect profile. The newer compounds seem to offer the same percentage of improvement as the older antidepressants, but they give us an alternative with which to treat those patients with treatment-resistant depressions.

Although there have been several claims for the new antidepressants having an early onset of therapeutic action, this effect has yet to be substantiated (Gelenberg, 1984). In our search for a therapeutic breakthrough in the treatment of depression, it remains important for us to evaluate carefully the newer generation of antidepressants and caution ourselves on premature claims in comparing them to the older compounds.

In summary, the newer compounds do offer new options for patients with intractable depressions who may fail to respond to the standard drugs in use. These new compounds are more specific with less anticholinergic and cardiovascular side effects and are less lethal with overdose. It is important for the clinician to keep abreast of the rapid technological changes now taking place in the antidepressant field.

Table 9.1: Pharmacologic profile

DRUG	CNS ACTIVITY 5-HT	CNS ACTIVITY NA	CNS ACTIVITY DA	ANTI-ACh	ANTI-HIST	CARDIO-TOXICITY	OTHER PROPERTIES
MONOCYCLIC							
Bupropion	0	0	+1	0	0	0	Mechanism of CNS activity unknown
Clovoxamine	+3	+2	0	0	0	+1	Selective serotonin reuptake inhibitor
Fezolamine	0	+2	0	0	0	+1	Serotonin and NA reuptake inhibitor
Fluvoxamine	+4	0	0	0	0	0	Selective serotonin reuptake inhibitor
BICYCLIC							
Citalopram	+4	0	0	0	0	0	Selective serotonin reuptake inhibitor
Fluoxetine	+4	0	0	0	0	0	Selective serotonin reuptake inhibitor
Tomoxetine	0	+3	0	0	0	+1	Selective NA reuptake inhibitor
Viloxazine	+2	+2	+1	0	0	0	Chemically related to beta-adrenergic receptor blockers. Anticonvulsant properties.
TRICYCLIC							
Dothiepin	+3	+3	0	+2	0	+2	

Table 9.1 (cont'd)

DRUG	CNS ACTIVITY 5-HT	NA	DA	ANTI-ACh	ANTI-HIST	CARDIO-TOXICITY	OTHER PROPERTIES
TETRACYCLIC							
Mianserin	+1	+2	0	0	+4	0	Alpha-2 antagonist
ORG-3770 (6-AZAmianserin)	+1	+2	0	+2	+3	0	Mianserin analogue
Oxaprotiline	0	+4	0	+1	+2	+2	Analogue of maprotiline
NOVEL ANTIDEPRESSANTS							
Adinazolam	0	+1	0	0	0	0	GABAergic, slight NA effect
Indalpine	+4	0	0	+1	0	+1	No MAO-inhibiting effect
Nafasadone	+3	0	0	0	0	+1	Trazodone analogue, weak alpha-1 antagonist
Nomifensine	0	+3	+2	0	0	+1	Amphetamine-like properties seen in animals; anticonvulsant effects
Paroxetine	+3	+1	0	0	+1	+1	Minimal blockade of guanethidine

Table 9.2: Clinical profile

DRUG	CHEMICAL CLASS	EFFICACY	SIDE EFFECTS	DAILY DOSE
MONOCYCLIC				
Bupropion	Chlorpropiophenone	Similar to TCAs. Low propensity to excerbate mania. Useful in bipolar disorders.	Restlessness, insomnia, diaphoresis, seizures	300-600 mg; divided daytime dose
Clovoxamine	2-Aminoethyl oxime ether (unicyclic)	Similar to TCAs.	Dry mouth, nausea, headache, diarrhea, hypotension, somnolence, insomnia, tremor	75-400 mg in divided dose
Fezolamine	Diphenylpyrazole	Similar to TCAs.	Lightheadedness, nausea, drowsiness, headache	400 mg in single or divided dose
Fluvoxamine	Aralkylketone oxime ether	Similar to TCAs. Effective in eating disorders.	Diarrhea, weight loss, restlessness, tremulousness, nausea	150-300 mg single a.m. dose (half-life 33 h)

Table 9.2 (cont'd)

DRUG	CHEMICAL CLASS	EFFICACY	SIDE EFFECTS	DAILY DOSE
BICYCLIC				
Citalopram	Bicyclic phthalone	Similar to TCAs in onset of activity	Dyspepsia, nausea, sweating (during first 2 weeks tested)	40-100 mg single or divided daytime dose
Tomoxetine	Phenylpropylamine	Similar to TCAs	Insomnia, headache, nervousness, dry mouth, palpitations	40-90 mg divided dose
Viloxazine	Tetrahydroxazine	Similar to TCAs	Nausea, vomiting, headache	100-300 mg daily
BW647U	Phenylthiobenzyl alcohol	Similar to TCAs	Headache, mild sedation, incoordination, dizziness, nausea, skin rash	300-900 mg divided dose
TRICYCLIC				
Dothiepin	Thiepin derivative	Similar to amitriptyline	Dry mouth, sedation, headache, blurred vision, constipation, dizziness, weight gain	150-300 mg h.s. or divided

Table 9.2 (cont'd)

DRUG	CHEMICAL CLASS	EFFICACY	SIDE EFFECTS	DAILY DOSE
TETRACYCLIC				
Mianserin	Tetracyclic	Similar to TCAs	Sedation, weight gain	30-150 mg single h.s. dose
6-AZAmianserin	Tetracyclic	Similar to mianserin	Drowsiness, weight gain	20-40 mg h.s.
Oxaprotiline	Tetracyclic (bridged tricyclic)	Similar to TCAs	Dry mouth, constipation, blurred vision, orthostatic faintness	25-200 mg single h.s. dose or divided dose with major portion h.s.
NOVEL				
Adinazolam	Aminoalkyl-triazolobenzodiazepine	Similar to TCAs	Sedation, cognitive slowing, withdrawal	30-90 mg divided dose
Indalpine	4-Alkylpiperidine	Similar to TCAs	Nausea, dyspepsia, diarrhea, sedation, tremor, insomnia	75-250 mg divided dose
Nafasadone	Triazolopyridine	Similar to trazodone	Dizziness, headache, nausea, hypotension	100-400 mg divided dose

Table 9.2 (cont'd)

DRUG	CHEMICAL CLASS	EFFICACY	SIDE EFFECTS	DAILY DOSE
Nomifensine	Tetrahydroiso-quinoline	Greatest effect in psychomotor retarded depression. Significant propensity to exacerbate mania and psychotic symptoms; has anticonvulsant effect and useful in depressed epileptics.	Tremulousness, insomnia, dry mouth	50-200 mg single or divided daytime dose
Paroxetine	Phenylpiperidine	Similar to TCAs	Insomnia, drowsiness, nausea	20-60 mg single daily dose

References

Ayd, F. (1979) Trazodone: a unique new broad-spectrum antidepressant. Int. Drug. Ther. Newsletter 14, 33-40.

Ban, T. (1982) Monoamine uptake inhibitors. In: Non-Tricyclic and Non-Monoamine Oxidase Inhibitors (Lehmann, H. E., ed.), Karger, Basel, pp. 1-16.

Brogden, R. N., Heel, R. C., Speight, T. M., and Avery, G. S. (1978) Mianserin: a review of its pharmacological properties and therapeutic efficacy in depressive illness. Drugs 16, 273-301.

Brogden, R. N., Heel, R. C., Speight, T. M., and Avery G. S. (1979) Nomifensine: a review of its pharmacological properties and therapeutic efficacy in depressive illness. Drugs 18, 1-24.

Burroughs Wellcome Company (1982) Data on file. Research Triangle Park, North Carolina.

Burrows, G. D., Vohra, J., Dumovic, P., Scoggins, B. A., and Davies, B. (1978) Cardiological effects of nomifensine, a new antidepressant. Med. J. Aust. 1, 341-343.

Buus Lassen, J., Lund, J., and Sondergaard, I. (1980) Central and peripheral 5-HT uptake in rats treated chronically with femoxetine, paroxetine, and chlorimipramine. Psychopharmacology 68, 229-233.

Ciba-Geigy (1982) Summary for Investigation: Oxaprotiline. Pharmaceutical Research Division, Summit, N.J.

Clanca, A., Freeman, H. L., Hole, G., and Wakelin, J. (1983) Clovoxamine, a new nontricyclic antidepressant: a European multicenter initial study. Comp. Psychiatry 24, 179-182.

Claassen, V., Boschman, Th. A. C., Dhasmana, K. M., Hillen, F. C., Vaatstra, W. J., and Zwagemakers, J. M. A. (1978) Pharmacology of clovoxamine, a new non-tricyclic antidepressant. Arzneim.-Forsch. 28, 1756-1766.

Claassen, V., Davies, J. E., Hertting, G., and Placheta, P. (1977) Fluvoxamine, a specific 5-hydroxytryptamine uptake inhibitor. Brit. J. Pharmacol. 60, 505-516.

Conti, L., Cassano, G. B., and Sarteschi, P. (1979) Clinical experience with mianserin. In: Mianserin Hydrochloride: Progress in the Pharmacotherapy of Depression (Rees, W. L., Drykonigen, G., and Ogara, R. C., eds), Excerpta Medica, Amsterdam.

Doogan, D. P. (1980) Fluvoxamine as an antidepressant drug. Neuropharmacology 19, 1215-1216.

Dorup, C., Meidahl, B., Petersen, I.-M. et al. (1982) Pharmacopsychiatry **15**, 183-186.

Eli Lilly & Co. (1983a) Tomoxetine: A Clinical Investigational Manual, August.

Eli Lilly & Co. (1983b) Clinical Field Trials Reports.

Eli Lilly Research Laboratories (1983) Fluoxetine Hydrochloride: Clinical Investigation Manual, May.

Fabre, L. F. (1976) Pilot open label study with alprazolam (U31,889) in outpatients with neurotic depression. Curr. Ther. Res. **19**, 661-668.

Feighner, J. P. (1983) The new generation of antidepressants. J. Clin. Psychiatry **44** (sec. 2), 49-55.

Feighner, J. P., Aden, G. C., Fabre, L. F., Rickels, K., and Smith, W. T. (1983) Comparison of alprazolam, imipramine, and placebo in the treatment of depression. J. Am. Med. Assoc. **249**, 3057-3064.

Feighner, J. P., Frost, N. R., Merideth, C. H., Hendrickson, G., and Jacobs, R. S. A comparative trial of fluoxetine and amitriptyline in outpatients with major depressive disorder. J. Clin. Psychiatry (to be published).

Feighner, J. P., Jacobs, R. S., Jackson, R. E., Hendrickson, G., Merideth, C. H., and O'Meara, P. D. (1983) A double-blind comparative trial with mianserin and amitriptyline in outpatients with major depressive disorders. Brit. J. Clin. Pharmacol. **15**, 227S-237S.

Feighner, J. P., Roffman, M., and Dixon, R. B. (1981) An early clinical trial of oxaprotiline in hospitalized patients with primary depression. Curr. Ther. Res. **29**, 363-369.

Ferris, R. M., Cooper, B. R., and Maxwell, R. A. (1983) Studies of bupropion's mechanism of antidepressant activity. J. Clin. Psychiatry **44** (sec. 2), 74-78.

Fleet, J. V. W., Manberg, P. J., Miller, L. L., Harto-Truax, N., Sato, T., Fleck, R. J., Stern, W. C., and Cato, A. E. (1983) Overview of clinically significant adverse reactions to bupropion. J. Clin. Psychiatry **44** (sec. 2), 191-196.

Gelenberg, A. J. (1984) New antidepressant drugs: a clinical perspective. Psychopharmacol. Bull. **20**, 291-294.

Goldstein, B. J. and Claghorn, J. L. (1980) An overview of seventeen years of experience with dothiepin in the treatment of depression in Europe. J. Clin. Psychiatry **41** (sec. 2), 64-70.

Gueremy, C., Audiau, F., and Champseix, A. (1980) 3-(4-Piperidinylalkyl)indoles, selective inhibitors of neuronal 5-hydroxytryptamine uptake. J. Med. Chem. 23, 1306-1310.

Groupe Pharmuka (1984) Indalpin: Investigator's Brochure.

Harto-Traux, N., Stern, W. C., Miller, L. L., Soto, T. L., and Cato, A. E. (1983) Effects of bupropion on body weight. J. Clin. Psychiatry 44 (sec. 2), 183-186.

Hoffmann, I. (1977) A comparative review of the pharmacology of nomifensine. Brit. J. Clin. Pharmacol. 4, 69S-79S.

Hyttel, J. (1982) Citalopram--pharmacological profile of a specific serotonin uptake inhibitor with antidepressant activity. Prog. Neuro-Psychopharmacol. & Biol. Psychiatry 6, 277-295.

Johnson, F., Sacco, F. A., and Yellowley, T. W. (1973) Chlordiazepoxide and dothiepin compared in anxiety/depression in general practice. Practitioner 211, 362-364.

Kazetska, V., Zimanova, J., and Vojtechovsky, M. (1978) Cardiotoxicity of prothiadene in clinical trials. Agressologie 19D, 203-209.

Lahti, R. A., Sethy, V. H., Barshun, C., and Hester, J. B. (1983) Pharmacological profile of the antidepressant adinazolam, a triazolobenzodiazepine. Neuropharmacology 22, 1277-1282.

LaPierre, Y. D. (1983) New antidepressant drugs. J. Clin. Psychiatry 44 (sec. 2), 41-44.

Leonard, B. E. (1984) Pharmacology of new antidepressants. Prog. Neuro-Psychopharmacol. & Biol. Psychiatry 8, 97-108.

Marrion Laboratories, Inc. (1983) Dothiepin Hydrochloride: A Clinical Brochure for Investigators, rev. Jan. 1983.

Maxwell, R. A., Mehta, W. B., Tucker, W. E. et al. (1981) In: Pharmacological and Biochemical Properties of Drug Substances, vol. 3 (Goldberg, M. E., ed.), American Pharmaceutical Association, Washington, D.C., p. 1055.

Mindhom, R. H. (1979) Tricyclic antidepressants and amine precursors. In: Psychopharmacology of Affective Disorders (Paykel, E. S. and Coppen, A., eds), Oxford University Press, Oxford, pp. 123-158.

Murphy, J. E. (1975) Vivalan: drug profile. J. Int. Med. Res. 3, 122-125.

Overo, K. F. (1982) Kinetics of citalopram in man: plasma levels in patients. Prog. Neuro-Psychopharmacol. & Biol. Psychiatry 6, 311-318.

Oyehaug, E., Ostensen, E. T., and Salvesen, B. (1984) High performance liquid chromatographic determination of citalopram and four of its metabolites in plasma and urine samples from psychiatric patients. J. Chromatogr. 308, 199-208.

Pedersen, O. L., Kragh-Sorensen, P., Bjerre, M., Overo, K. F., and Gram, L. F. (1982) Citalopram, a selective serotonin reuptake inhibitor: clinical antidepressive and long-term effect--a Phase II study. Psychopharmacology 77, 199-204.

Petersen, E. N. (1979) The interaction of desipramine and the 5-HT uptake inhibitors femoxetine and paroxetine with the acute hypotensive effect of guanethidine in conscious spontaneously hypertensive rats. J. Pharm. Pharmacol. 31, 638-640.

Pharmaceutical Research Institute (1982) Investigator's Brochure: ORG3770, pp. 1-9.

Poldinger, W. and Gammel, G. (1978) Differences in effect between nomifensine and nortriptyline. Intl. Pharmacopsychiatry 13, 58-68.

Pyke, R., Coh, J. B., Feighner, J. P. et al. (1983) Open-label studies of adinazolam in severe depression. Psychopharmacol. Bull. 19, 96-98.

Richelson, E. (1984) The newer antidepressants: structures, pharmacokinetic, pharmacodynamics, and proposed mechanisms of action. Psychopharmacol. Bull. 20, 213-223.

Robinson, J. F. and Doogan, D. P. (1982) A placebo controlled study of the cardiovascular effects of fluvoxamine and clovoxamine in human volunteers. Brit. J. Clin. Pharmacol. 14, 805-808.

Roffman, M., Gould, E. E., Brewer, S. J., Lau, H., Sachais, B., Dixon, R. B., Kaczmarek, L., and LeSher, A. (1982) A double-blind comparative study of oxaprotiline with amitriptyline and placebo in moderate depression. Curr. Ther. Res. 32, 247-256.

Soroko, F. E., Mehta, N. B., Maxwell, R. A., Ferris, R. M., and Schroeder, D. H. (1977) Bupropion hydrochloride (±-t-butylamino-3-chloropropiophenone HCl): a novel antidepressant agent. J. Pharm. Pharmacol. 29, 767-770.

Squires, R. F. (1974) Effects of noradrenaline pump blockers on its uptake by synaptosomes from several brain regions: additional evidence of dopamine terminals in the frontal cortex. J. Pharm. Pharmacol. 26, 364-366.

Taeuber, K., Zapf, R., Rupp, W., and Badian, M. (1979) Pharmacodynamic comparison of the acute effects of nomifensine, amphetamine and placebo in healthy volunteers. Intl. J. Clin. Pharm.

Biopharm. **17,** 32-37.
Trimble, M. and Robertson, M. (1984) <u>Antidepressant Drugs, Seizures and Epilepsy</u>. Hoechst-Roussel Pharmaceuticals, Inc.
Wong, D. T., Horng, J. S., Bymaster, F. P., Hauser, K. L., and Molloy, B. B. (1974) A selective inhibitor of serotonin uptake: Lilly 110140, 3-(p-trifluoromethylphenoxy)-N-methyl-3-phenylpropylamine. <u>Life Sci.</u> **15,** 471-479.
Wong, D. T., Threlkeld, P. G., Best, K. L., and Bymaster, F. P. (1982) A new inhibitor of norepinephrine uptake devoid of affinity for receptors in rat brain. <u>J. Pharmacol. Exp. Ther.</u> **222,** 61-65.
Wong, D. T. (1982) Neurotransmitter receptor profiles of fluoxetine and other antidepressant drugs. <u>Fed. Proc.</u> **41,** 1636.

10.

PHARMACOLOGICAL APPROACHES TO MANIA

Y. D. Lapierre and J. Telner

Introduction
============

The introduction of lithium in the treatment of manic-depressive illness by Cade in 1949 revolutionized the conceptualization of this illness. The previously elaborated psychodynamic formulations as well as the consequent psychotherapeutic approaches had been essentially unsuccessful in controlling this disorder. Subsequently, the introduction of antidepressants led to the formulation of amine hypotheses of affective disorders (Coppen, 1967; Schildkraut, 1969). The possibility of relating clinical findings and pharmacological mechanisms of certain psychotropic agents with successful therapy opened a number of vistas of investigation, on the rationale of the amine hypotheses as well as treatment modalities based on hypothetical constructs derived from neurochemical functions. These included neurotransmitter systems involving noradrenaline, dopamine, acetylcholine, gamma-aminobutyric acid (GABA) as well as other neurochemical hypotheses involving endocrine systems and cellular membranes of the central nervous system.

In this chapter an attempt is made to review the treatment strategies of mania and to relate them to pharmacological findings and mechanisms of action.

Treatment Approaches Based on Biogenic Amine Hypotheses

The original hypothesis put forward by Schildkraut (1965) proposed that mania was associated with an excess of catecholamines, more particularly, noradrenaline (NA; norepinephrine) at functionally important receptor sites in the brain. This hypothesis was based on clinical observations of patients developing hypomania while on imipramine treatment for depression. These patients simultaneously developed higher levels of normetanephrine secretion during these episodes.

Subsequently, Coppen (1967) suggested that an excess of serotonin (5-hydroxytryptamine; 5-HT) could be associated with the production of mania. This arose from observations that depression could occur after treatment with reserpine, a depletor of CNS 5-HT, while the administration of tryptophan, a precursor amino acid of 5-HT, helped improve depression.

The close biochemical relationship of dopamine (DA) to NA led to a further hypothesis that central DA over-activity may be a significant factor in the development of mania (Goodwin et al., 1970). This hypothesis was suggested by observations that neuroleptic DA receptor blockers improved patients in a manic state while L-Dopa, a DA precursor, occasionally produced manic symptomatology.

The treatment strategies capitalized on these three hypotheses, with a number of chemicals being tested based on these theoretical constructs and clinical observations. These will be reviewed, using the model of the metabolic pathways of these biogenic amines.

Inhibition of tyrosine hydroxylase, the rate-limiting enzyme in catecholamine synthesis, may be accomplished by the administration of alpha-methyl-para-tyrosine (AMPT). This has resulted in control of manic symptoms in a few reported cases (Brodie et al., 1971; Bunney et al., 1971). The drug has not been consistent in controlling mania, suggesting that this may be a treatment applicable to a subgroup of patients which at this time is not easily identifiable. Para-chlorophenylalanine (PCPA) inhibits tryptophan hydroxylase (the enzyme which converts tryptophan to 5-HT), thus leading to a depletion of 5-HT, which should theoretically decrease manic symptoms. This remains to be demonstrated. Reserpine, a depletor of catecholamines and 5-HT, has contributed to bringing manic symptoms under control in selected cases (Lapierre et al., unpublished results). This treatment is still under investigation. Alpha-methyldopa, an antihypertensive agent, is metabolized to alpha-methylnoradrenaline which acts as a false neurotransmitter, thus decreasing the functional availability of NA at receptor sites. This unfortunately has not resulted in control of mania and is mentioned for the sake of completeness. In the same way, inhibition of dopamine beta-hydroxylase by fusaric acid inhibits the production of NA but does not result in control of mania (Sack and Goodwin, 1974). Methysergide, an anti-serotonin agent, was found to be beneficial in the treatment of mania (Dewhurst, 1968). These findings could not be replicated consistently in followup studies (Coppen et al., 1969; Fieve et al., 1969). Cinanserin, another anti-serotonin agent, was also found to be useful in certain manic patients but again, results were not consistently positive (Itil et al., 1971; Kane, 1970).

Treatment Approaches Based on Dopamine Blockade

As mentioned earlier, the original catecholamine hypothesis of Schildkraut (1965) suggested that mania was associated with an excess of catecholamines and particularly NA. Another catecholamine, DA, has also been implicated as being over-active (Goodwin et al., 1970). The evidence for this is indirect but nevertheless should still be entertained. L-Dopa, the precursor of DA, has not only been shown to exert some antidepressant effects in retarded depressions but, more importantly, has induced hypomania in some bipolar patients (Butcher and Engle, 1969; Murphy et al., 1971). However, L-Dopa is also a precursor of NA, which suggests that DA may be involved minimally or not at all in these changes. More convincing evidence for a role of DA in affective illness has been demonstrated more recently with the use of somewhat selective DA receptor agonists. For example, Post et al. (1978) showed antidepressant effects as well as manic episodes with piribedil in one patient. This was reversed with pimozide, a DA receptor antagonist. Furthermore, in the same study the authors were able to show a correlation between CSF levels of the DA metabolite homovanillic acid and degree of clinical improvement, suggesting a relationship between the antidepressant effect of the DA receptor agonist and deficiency in the DA system. The finding that DA receptor alteration by neuroleptics is blocked by the antimanic drug lithium further suggests a role for DA receptors in mania and may partially explain the biological basis for treatment of mania with neuroleptics (Gerner et al., 1976).

The standard neuroleptic utilized in the treatment of mania is chlorpromazine. This drug, being the first phenothiazine to be widely used as a neuroleptic, came into use as a non-specific antimanic agent and subsequently served as the standard drug for comparison of therapeutic effect with lithium. Aside from chlorpromazine's pharmacological activity on DA receptors, this drug has effects on other systems, including blockade of adrenergic alpha receptors (Peroutka et al., 1977), histamine H-1 receptors (Richelson, 1978), as well as muscarinic cholinergic receptors (Iversen, 1975). Other actions of this agent include blockade of peripheral 5-HT receptors and neuronal reuptake mechanisms (Byck, 1975; Gordon, 1967) as well as binding to central 5-HT receptors (Peroutka and Snyder, 1980).

Whether the effects observed with chlorpromazine are specific or secondary to its sedating properties in the acute manic patient is not clear. However, in a large collaborative study of 255 acutely manic patients, Prien et al. (1972) reported that chlorpromazine was effective in reducing manic symptomatology and compared well with lithium carbonate. The superiority of chlorpromazine appeared mainly in the highly active patients where the patient was more easily brought under control with the neuroleptic than with lithium. However, in mild to moderate mania, these differences were less pronounced and lithium may have been the treatment of choice. Shopsin et al. (1975) observed that chlorpromazine, although it did produce considerable sedation, did not significantly alter the underlying mania qualitatively and the patients did not show consistent improvement. Another feature of chlorpromazine treatment of mania relates to its side effects, these being sedation and the neurovegetative side effects of cholinergic and noradrenergic blockade (Platman, 1970).

Haloperidol, a butyrophenone neuroleptic, has been widely used in the treatment of acute mania (Baastrup, 1968; Shopsin and Gershon, 1971). Schou (1968) recommended haloperidol as an effective form of treatment in acute mania. It has been demonstrated as more rapidly effective in the control of acute mania symptoms than lithium. It also has the added advantage of producing fewer neurovegetative side effects, although it may be associated with a higher incidence of acute extrapyramidal symptoms (Shopsin et al., 1975). It has been effectively utilized in combination with lithium in the treatment of acute manic patients. Isolated reports of encephalopathy with this combination (Cohen and Cohen, 1974) have not been replicated in the review of larger numbers of cases (Juhl et al., 1977). The advantage of combining these two treatments lies in the fact that haloperidol brings the manic condition under more rapid control while lithium has a latency period for effectiveness (Krishna et al., 1978).

Whereas chlorpromazine has a number of neurotransmitter systems as target systems and haloperidol is possibly more specifically a DA blocker, a third class of neuroleptic, the diphenylbutylpiperidines, with pimozide as its prototype, is more specifically a DA receptor blocker (Seeman et al., 1976). Pimozide has been shown to have a lower affinity than chlorpromazine for both NA alpha receptors and histamine H-1 receptors in the brain (Peroutka and Snyder, 1980), which indirectly suggests that it is a more specific DA receptor blocker. Since the sedative properties of neuroleptics are related to their affinity for NA alpha receptors (Peroutka and Snyder, 1980), it has been suggested that these agents exert their antimanic effect on central DA systems rather than simply sedating the patient.

The antimanic activity of pimozide was clearly demonstrated by Cookson et al. (1981). Although its sedative effect is less pronounced than that of chlorpromazine initially, its control of manic symptomatology is equivalent and possibly superior after two weeks of treatment.

Control of the acute manic state can be effectively attained with neuroleptic medication. However, once the acute episode has subsided, prophylactic or maintenance treatment with neuroleptics has its limitations. These limitations are mainly related to the side effect profile of these drugs, which includes sedation, neurovegetative symptoms and the side effects related to DA receptor blockade in the extrapyramidal system, the most troublesome and serious of these being the high risk of tardive dyskinesia, a risk which may be greater in patients with affective disorders (Rosenbaum et al., 1977). There are at present insufficient controlled long-term studies of neuroleptics in the prophylactic treatment of manic-depressive illness to conclusively recommend such an approach.

Approaches Based on Cholinergic Mechanisms

The bases of using methods of modifying cholinergic mechanisms in affective disorders were clinical observations dating back to 1950 when Rowntree (1950) administered cholinesterase inhibitors to normal and manic-depressive subjects. Both groups developed apathy, lassitude, psychomotor retardation and depression. One of the manic patients relapsed upon withdrawal of the inhibitor. Subsequently, Gershon and Shaw (1961) observed depression occurring in individuals poisoned with cholinesterase inhibitor insecticides, while more recently Risch et al. (1981) showed that intravenous administration of physostigmine (an agent which increases central cholinergic activity by inhibiting cholinesterase, the enzyme that metabolizes acetylcholine) to normal volunteers free of personal or family history of affective disorder caused depression as well as confusion.

From these clinical observations, Janowsky et al. (1972), as well as Davis and Berger (1978), hypothesized that mania may be the result of decreased acetylcholine with or without changes in NA. Janowsky et al. (1973) subsequently reported a reduction in manic symptoms after physostigmine administration. This improvement of manic symptomatology persisted for up to 90 minutes. Although not a clinically useful method, it did lead to further investigation of acetylcholine mechanisms.

It is noteworthy that improvement in mania via physostigmine has been shown to be partially reversed by methylphenidate, which increases central catecholamine activity. This finding lends support to the idea of an 'imbalance' between acetylcholine and catecholamine systems in mania (Janowsky et al., 1970).

Janowsky et al. (1972) have shown that enhancing cholinergic activity with lecithin can induce or worsen depression in susceptible individuals. Lecithin has been shown to raise serum-free choline levels (Wurtman et al., 1977) and, presumably through transport and metabolism, the level of acetylcholine at neuronal synapses (Hirsch and Wurtman, 1978). Cohen et al. (1980) administered lecithin to 8 manic patients. Their preliminary results suggested that lecithin may improve the response to neuroleptics and lithium in certain refractory patients. Subsequently, Schreier (1982) reported on a single case of bipolar illness who, although refractory to lithium and haloperidol, did respond to long-term administration of lecithin in doses reaching 23 g daily. Cohen et al. (1982) did a small double-blind comparison of placebo and lecithin and observed improvement in 5 of 6 patients while on lecithin, in doses of 30 mg daily, within one week. These sparse results available on the use of lecithin suggest that it is relatively non-toxic and possibly effective, especially in patients refractory to standard methods of treatment.

Approaches Based on GABA Mechanisms

A role for gamma-aminobutyric acid (GABA) in mania has been suspected since the demonstration that the GABA antagonist bicuculline injected into the mesencephalic ventral tegmental area of cats modified behaviour (Stevens et al., 1974). The further observation that GABA changes modified behaviour led to its evaluation in manic-depressive illness. Lambert et al. (1975) observed that a derivative of valproate, dipropylacetamide, improved patients with mania. It was thus hypothesized that GABA, a presynaptic neuromodulator, could have some antimanic properties.

Valproate has been shown to raise brain levels of GABA as well as decrease GABA turnover in a dose-dependent manner (Bernasconi and Martin, 1974; Pinder et al., 1977). A double-blind placebo-controlled trial by Emrich et al. (1980), using an ABA design, provided interesting evidence in 5 cases that valproate did indeed have antimanic properties. The dosage utilized ranged from 1800 to 3000 mg daily. Follow-up for 2-3 years in a small number of patients supported the suggested evidence that GABA-ergic mechanisms, as modified by sodium valproate, could have antimanic properties. At this time, however, the evidence is still sparse and must be duplicated.

Chouinard et al. (1983), in a study using clonazepam, invoked mechanisms other than GABA to explain their findings that clonazepam may have some antimanic properties. The rationale for attempting to control mania with clonazepam was based on the following: 5-HT is decreased both in mania and depression (Prange et al., 1974) while the antimanic lithium has been shown to increase the synthesis of 5-HT, amongst numerous other actions (Bowers and Henninger, 1977; Fyro et al., 1975). The anticonvulsants carbamazepine and valproic acid are efficacious in acute mania (Ballenger and Post, 1980; Folks et al., 1982). Taken together, it was hypothesized that an agent with both 5-HT-potentiating and anticonvulsant properties might be beneficial in the treatment of mania. Clonazepam appears to have these properties and thus may have antimanic potential which cannot be attributed to dopaminergic blockade since it does not produce an elevation of plasma prolactin levels (Chouinard et al., 1983).

If any such antimanic action does exist for clonazepam, it is more likely due to the GABA-ergic effect which it shares with other benzodiazepines. The findings are preliminary and yet to be duplicated.

The GABA-ergic agents are treated separately from the anticonvulsants because of their particular interest from a theoretical viewpoint which is more in keeping with modern conceptualization of brain function. Anticonvulsants will be considered separately.

Treatment Modalities Using Anticonvulsants

Carbamazepine. Carbamazepine exerts a variety of actions on various brain systems. It resembles imipramine more closely than the neuroleptics in that it has a tricyclic structure. However, compared to imipramine, its blockade of NA reuptake is relatively weak. Post et al. (1984) have suggested that the finding by Purdy et al. (1977) that carbamazepine partially blocked release of ^{3}H-NA and inhibited isometric contraction in the rabbit ear artery could indicate a possible mode of action for this agent in both phases of manic-depression. Thus, during the depressive phase, carbamazepine may function like other tricyclic antidepressants and block NA reuptake, while during mania, where there may be a hyperactivity of NA, the drug may inhibit NA release and thus return levels of this amine to normal. However, the effects of carbamazepine on NA metabolism are not clear, and whether the few noted effects are related to its antimanic action has not yet been determined (Post et al., 1984).

In a similar vein, data accumulated so far do not suggest that the antimanic effects of carbamazepine are mediated through DA or 5-HT mechanisms. For example, while neuroleptics can cause parkinsonian side effects as well as tardive dyskinesia, these effects have not been induced with carbamazepine treatment, suggesting that the direct blockade of post-synaptic DA receptors is not involved in carbamazepine's mechanism of action (Reynolds, 1975). As well, animal studies where the effects of carbamazepine are studied after manipulation of brain 5-HT levels show that the drug's anticonvulsant properties are not lessened (Crunelli et al., 1979; Quattrone et al., 1978). As GABA mechanisms have been recently postulated to play a role in affective disorders (Berrettini and Post, 1984), the effects of carbamazepine on GABA have been investigated. Preliminary studies, however, have failed to show effects of carbamazepine on brain GABA levels in animals or CSF levels in clinical studies (Post et al., 1980), although GABA turnover is decreased by this agent (Bernasconi and Martin, 1979).

A recent innovative hypothesis for the mechanism of action of carbamazepine involves its dampening of the kindling process. This process, originally observed by Goddard et al. (1969), describes increases in electrophysiologic and convulsive response to a previously subthreshold stimulus in the limbic area after daily stimulation. Carbamazepine has been shown in several studies to be most effective, compared to other anticonvulsants, in inhibiting discharges from this area (Wada et al., 1976; Ashton and Wauquier, 1979). Based on the hypothesis that pathological activation of one or more areas in the limbic system could be one mechanism involved in manic-depressive illness, it has been proposed that carbamazepine may act psychotropically by dampening limbic system excitability as well as inhibiting the spread of after-discharges.

Carbamazepine was initially introduced in medicine for a number of neurological-related problems including trigeminal neuralgia, pain syndromes and temporal lobe epilepsy. During treatment of these conditions, it was observed that behaviour was also modified. This led to the initial observation by Okuma et al. (1973) that carbamazepine was therapeutic in mania. This was followed by other observations by the same authors (Okuma et al., 1977) as well as by Ballenger and Post (1980). From these observations, it can be suggested that carbamazepine is a viable alternative to lithium in the treatment of mania. Dosage is regulated by plasma levels, which appear to be therapeutic at levels of 8.0 to 12.0 µg/ml. The drug is generally well tolerated within this blood level range. Neurological side effects include dizziness, nausea, drowsiness and mild tremor. The main toxicity relates to white blood count which tends to be depressed in the early stages of treatment. There have been a few cases of aplastic anemia reported in carbamazepine-treated patients. The use of carbamazepine as a long-term prophylactic agent in bipolar affective disorder is gradually becoming an accepted alternative to lithium. Although there still have not been adequate double-blind controlled longitudinal studies, the observations of Kishimoto et al. (1983) certainly are supportive of this suggestion. Carbamazepine appears well tolerated in conjunction with lithium in partially responsive patients (Lipinski and Pope,

1982; Post et al., 1984). There has been a case report of possible neurotoxicity related to this combination (Chaudhry and Waters, 1983).

Diphenylhydantoin. Diphenylhydantoin (DPH) was reported on one occasion (Kubanek and Rowell, 1946) to improve manic psychosis. This was based on a case observation of improvement in 5 of 7 manic psychotics. These observations have not been followed up and the putative mechanisms remain unexplained.

Treatment with Propranolol

Propranolol has been reported to exert some antimanic effects (Atsmon et al., 1972) and these actions were initially observed as more pronounced in schizoaffective patients. A subsequent study supported the possibility of antimanic effects of d-propranolol (Emrich et al., 1979). Unfortunately, the dosage required to bring about control of mania is at such a high level that its generalized use in mania is unlikely. The mechanism of action for this potential antimanic agent is unclear. Propranolol has been shown to be a suppressor of noradrenergic transmission (Whitelock and Evans, 1978), but could also exert its possible anti-manic effects by inhibiting central serotonergic transmission, since animal studies have shown that this agent inhibits the hyperactivity syndrome induced by increasing the functional activity of 5-HT but does not inhibit the hyperactivity produced by increasing DA activity (Green and Grahame-Smith, 1976).

Treatment Based on Electrolyte Disturbances

The initial observations of loss of sodium and water following treatment with lithium (Baer et al., 1970) suggested that this may be a contributing factor in lithium's therapeutic action. This, coupled with the observation that carbonic anhydrase inhibitors in high doses could have an antimanic effect, opened up the possibility of the use of a carbonic anhydrase inhibitor such as benanilamide in high doses (1,000-2,000 mg daily) to control mania (Tanimukai et al., 1970). However, these observations have not been explored further and are included for completeness. It is unlikely that this will be an effective venue of therapy. A similar conclusion for other electrolytes including potassium, magnesium and calcium must be made at this time, especially since disturbances in peripheral electrolyte metabolism are not necessarily accompanied by psychopathological symptoms and brain electrolyte metabolism may be regulated independent of its counterpart in the periphery.

Treatment Approaches Based on Opioid Mechanisms

The use of naloxone as a specific opiate blocker has been investigated in two double-blind studies of manic patients. No therapeutic effect was obtained to support further investigation of opioid mechanisms (Pickar et al., 1982; Davis et al., 1980).

Treatment Based on Neuroendocrine Concepts

A preliminary observation by Horrobin et al. (1976) suggested that high levels of prolactin could be a contributing factor to the manic syndrome, and sudden improvement in 2 patients treated with bromocriptine led to further exploration by Smith et al. (1980). These investigators completed a double-blind study of 23 manic females and found no evidence of therapeutic benefits to be derived from bromocriptine although the drug did lower prolactin levels.

Treatment Based on Calcium Metabolism

A single case report on the use of a calcium channel blocker, verapamil, lends further support to some of the invoked mechanisms in lithium action and also has heuristic value in the further exploration of mania (Dubovsky et al., 1982). Of course, this is but a single case report and must be considered within these limitations.

Treatment of Mania with Lithium

Most review articles on the use of lithium in psychiatry refer to the original report by Cade in 1949 who related his findings in the treatment of manic excitement with lithium carbonate (Cade, 1949). Subsequently, the drug gradually gained acceptance in Australia and Europe. The focus of research in lithium therapy of manic-depressive illness centered on Denmark and was promulgated by Mogens Schou (Schou, 1959). Since then there has been an exponential increase of publications on lithium as it relates to psychiatric conditions.

The treatment of manic disorders is intrinsically related to manic-depression and other affective disorders. This section will deal with the treatment of acute mania and the prophylaxis of manic episodes in manic-depressive illness.

Lithium has been dmonstrated to be active against both manifestations of manic-depressive disorder and can serve as a prophylactic against both manias and depressions. It would appear that it does not simply stimulate or suppress, but rather stabilizes cerebral processes that are out of balance. Because of this unique action, lithium differs from the conventional antidepressant and antimanic drugs (Baastrup and Schou, 1967; Schou, 1976). Numerous investigations of lithium's actions have shown a variety of metabolic effects including interactions with the cations sodium, potassium, magnesium and calcium, membrane transport systems, with various neurotransmitter systems including uptake, synthesis, release and reuptake, and with cyclic AMP.

Rather than outline the manifest effects of lithium on the systems mentioned above (these are well described in recent reviews such as those by Cooper et al., 1978; Schou, 1981; Ahuwali and Singhal, 1983; Bunney and Garland, 1983), several hypotheses for lithium's psychotropic effects will be described.

Taking into consideration the physiochemical properties of lithium, Eigen (1976) speculated on the ways in which lithium may exert its therapeutic and prophylactic actions. One plausible hypothesis involves the repairing of a biological defect which could be a lack of substrate or a genetically biased alteration of a receptor. Bunney and Murphy (1976a) have suggested that lithium may act on the presynaptic membrane regulating neurotransmitter release. An alternative hypothesis put forth by the same investigators involves the stabilization of postsynaptic receptor site transitional processes. Bunney et al. (1977, 1979) have suggested that the switch from a retarded depression into mania may be associated with the release of neurotransmitter that is amplified by a supersensitive neuronal receptor. They hypothesized that lithium might counteract the manic-depressive process by blocking the development of supersensitive neuronal receptors since withdrawal of long-term lithium treatment does not affect DA receptors (although it does prevent the increase in receptor number induced by haloperidol; Pert, 1978). Harrison-Read (1981) suggested that lithium may increase and/or stabilize release of DA. Huey et al. (1981) have produced results suggesting a balance between presynaptic alpha-adrenergic and post-synaptic beta-adrenergic mechanisms which could prevent the emotional changes in both depression and mania. Other researchers, notably Ebstein and Belmaker (1979) as well as Forn and Valdecasas (1971), have suggested that lithium may exert its therapeutic actions through inhibition of adenylate cyclases within the central nervous system.

Sen et al. (1976) proposed that lithium may correct a sodium pump deficiency noted to occur in both phases of manic depression. Byck (1976) suggested that lithium may exert its therapeutic effect through the modification of receptor affinity for enkephalin, which may function as a transmitter. Schou et al. (1981) have more recently offered a hypothesis which differs from most other suggested mechanisms of action in that it does not involve a direct, etiologically-based mechanism but rather the indirect and peripheral effects of lithium. These authors suggest that since the constancy of calcium and magnesium in serum is all-important in symptoms in general, including mental changes, lithium may produce its effects indirectly by increasing magnesium and calcium concentration.

Numerous investigations have shown that lithium affects many systems, and various hypotheses for its mechanism of action have been espoused. At present, it is difficult to favor any one hypothesis and the mechanism(s) of action in this ion's therapeutic and prophylactic effects therefore remains an enigma.

There is now little doubt that lithium is an effective antimanic agent. The successful outcome in the treatment of manic patients rates from 60-100%, with a general consensus placing the average improvement rate at 70-80% (Gershon, 1970; Tupin, 1970; Schou, 1968b). Lithium has been compared to chlorpromazine in open and double-blind studies. The former drug resulted in superior amelioration of core manic symptomatology related to mood and ideation whereas the latter improved psychomotor agitation more effectively (Johnson et al., 1968). Lithium has also been compared to haloperidol, with similar results (Schou, 1968a).

Studies on lithium have emphasized primarily the treatment of acute mania in a general adult population. However, there is evidence that it is also effective in juvenile manic-depressive illness (Kelly et al., 1976) as well as in patients with manic-depressive illness following brain damage (Oyewumi and Lapierre, 1981).

Pharmacological Approaches to Mania

The therapeutic index of lithium is low because of the narrow range within which therapeutic levels can safely be maintained. For this reason, patient selection is of utmost importance. In addition to selecting patients who are reliably compliant, the physical status of the patient must be taken into consideration with regard to the metabolism and toxicology of lithium. Lithium is completely absorbed through the gastrointestinal tract and is excreted primarily (over 95%) through the kidneys. Being a water-soluble ion, it penetrates most body compartments. Endocrine, cardiovascular and kidney functions should be assessed prior to initiating lithium therapy. The careful monitoring of serum levels throughout the period of treatment as well as the monitoring of the same body functions mentioned above is essential to avoid lithium intoxication as well as to facilitate an early detection of side effects. To avoid lithium intoxication, serum lithium levels should be kept below 2.0 mEq/l. The generally indicated levels for control of acute mania range from 1.0 to 1.5 mEq/l, whereas in the prophylactic treatment of manic-depression, the generally required levels are 0.6 to 1.2 mEq/l (Prien et al., 1971). There may be a higher risk of relapse below 0.6 mEq/l, although a substantial number of patients may have their illness controlled at levels as low as 0.4 mEq/l (Waters et al., 1982). To achieve these serum levels, dosage requirements may range from 600 to 2,500 mg. of lithium carbonate daily. After initiation of treatment with lithium, there is usually a latency period of 10-14 days to obtain full therapeutic effect. It is not uncommon to cover this period with a neuroleptic in order to accelerate the therapeutic process.

The toxicology of lithium is complex because of the ubiquitous distribution of the lithium ion. The endocrine systems which may be involved are the thyroid- and insulin-producing systems. Nontoxic goiter and hypothyroidism are not uncommon side effects, with elevated levels of TSH appearing quite regularly with lithium therapy. Patients with pre-diabetes may have elevated glucose tolerance and may become overtly diabetic. Electrocardiographic anomalies usually include conduction defects and rarely the 'sick sinus syndrome'. Central nervous system complications include seizures. These are generally restricted to near-toxic levels. Neuromuscular side effects are not uncommon, with tremor being the most frequent. This is generally well controlled with mild to moderate doses of propranolol, a beta-adrenergic blocker (Lapierre, 1976).

Adequate renal function is essential to treatment with lithium. There have been reports of interstitial glomerulosclerosis and decreased creatinine clearance in patients undergoing lithium treatment. These were reviewed extensively by Schou et al. (1981), and he concluded that these are rarely of clinically significant degree to require cessation of treatment. There is also evidence suggesting that a fractionation of dosage during the day sufficient to avoid high peak levels following absorption reduces the risk of these kidney lesions (Grof et al., 1980).

The prophylactic effect of lithium is maintained indefinitely. The mechanism by which this prophylaxis occurs is unknown, although several hypotheses have been formulated. The problem which arises for the clinician is the decision on cessation of treatment. This is a clinical decision based on the patient's genetic predisposition, past history of recurrence of mania, and his response to treatment. The prediction of response to lithium involves the consideration of a number of variables, including a clear diagnosis of primary affective disorder, fewer than four episodes of mania and/or depression within one year (i.e. slow cycler), euphoria and elation during the manic episode, and a family history of primary affective disorder (Ananth and Pecknold, 1978).

It was generally believed that upon discontinuation of lithium, the manic depressive process would continue in its previously cyclical manner with recurrence of illness occurring according to the normal cycle of the illness (Baastrup and Schou, 1967). However, recent reports suggest that the abrupt discontinuation of lithium therapy may result in a rapid recurrence of a rebound type of mania and destabilization of the illness (Small et al., 1971; Lapierre et al., 1980).

Summary and Conclusion
========================

Although the understanding of the biochemical substrate(s) of manic-depressive illness, and more particularly mania, is still incomplete, there is sufficient evidence to suggest that such a substrate does indeed exist. The amine hypotheses of manic-depressive illness have had heuristic value and have laid the framework for developing therapeutic strategies. Based on clinical observations of therapeutic efficacy of a variety of pharmacological agents, it may be surmised that although defects of catecholamine and indoleamine mechanisms may not be the ultimate biochemical abnormality, they may be an important link in a chain of events leading to the full-blown illness. Whether or not they are the result of other neurotransmitter defects remains unclear. There is sufficient evidence to suspect that this may be the case.

Lithium remains the mainstay of treatment of manic-depression, manic type. However, for the 15-25% of patients who are unresponsive to this agent, modulation of other neurotransmitter systems such as GABA, acetylcholine or DA may supplement or replace the use of lithium in the control of this illness.

It can be expected that in the future there will be developed more strategies involving other neurotransmitter systems which will help to clarify further the role of these complex neurotransmitter interactions in the etiopathogenesis of mania and manic-depressive illness.

Acknowledgements

The authors acknowledge the assistance of Ms. Marie Robertson and Dianna Hensel in the preparation of this chapter.

References

Ahluwalia, P. and Singhal, R. L. (1983) Lithium and central monoamine neurotransmitter systems. Drug Dev. Res. 3, 111-122.

Ananth, J. and Pecknold, J. C. (1978) Prediction of lithium response in affective disorders. J. Clin. Psychiatry 39, 95-100.

Ashton, D. and Wauquier, A. (1979) Behavioral analysis of the effects of 15 anticonvulsants in the amygdaloid kindled rat. Psychopharmacology 65, 7-13.

Atsmon, A., Blum, J., Steiner, M., Latz, A., and Wijsenbeek, H. (1972) Further studies with propranolol in psychotic patients. Psychopharmacologia (Berl.) 27, 249-254.

Baastrup, P. C. (1967) Supplementary information about lithium treatment of manic-depressive disorders. Acta psychiatr. scand. 203, 149-152.

Baastrup, P. C. and Schou, M. (1968) Lithium as a prophylactic agent: its effect against recurrent depressions and manic-depressive psychosis. Arch. Gen. Psychiatry 16, 162-172.

Baer, L., Platman, S. R., and Fieve, R. R. (1970) The role of electrolytes in affective disorders, NA, K and Li ions. Arch. Gen. Psychiatry 22, 108-113.

Ballenger, J. and Post, R. (1980) Carbamazepine in manic depressive illness: a new treatment. Am. J. Psychiatry 137, 782-789.

Bernasconi, R. and Martin, P. (1979) Effects of antiepileptic drugs on the GABA turnover rate. Abstract, Naunyn-Schmiedeberg's Arch. Pharmacol. 307, ref. 251.

Berrettini, W. H. and Post, R. M. (1984) GABA in affective illness. In: Neurobiology of Mood Disorders (Post, R. M. and Ballenger, J. C., eds), Williams & Wilkins, Baltimore, pp. 673-685.

Bowers, M. B. and Heninger, G. R. (1977) Lithium: clinical effects and cerebral spinal fluid acid monoamine metabolites. Commun. Psychopharmacol. 1, 135-145.

Brodie, H. K. H., Murphy, D. L., Goodwin, F. K., and Bunney, W. E. (1971) Catecholamines and mania. The effect of alpha-methyl-para-tyrosine on manic behavior and catecholamine metabolism. Clin. Pharmacol. Ther. 12, 218-224.

Bunney, W. E., Brodie, H. K. H., Murphy, D. L., and Goodwin, F. K. (1971) Studies of alpha-methyl-para-tyrosine, L-dopa and L-tryptophan in depression and mania. Am. J. Psychiatry 127, 872-881.

Bunney, W. E. and Garland, B. L. (1983) Possible receptor effects of chronic lithium administration. Neuropharmacology 22, 367-372.

Bunney, W. E. and Garland, B. L. (1984) Lithium and its possible modes of action. In: Neurobiology of Mood Disorders (Post, R. M. and Ballenger, J. C., eds), Williams & Wilkins, Baltimore, pp. 731-743.

Bunney, W. E. and Murphy, D. L. (1976) Neurobiological considerations on mode of action of lithium carbonate in the treatment of affective disorders. Pharmacopsychiatry 9, 142-147.

Bunney, W. E., Pert, A., Rosenblatt, J., Pert, C. B., and Gallager, D. (1979) Mode of action of lithium: some biological considerations. Arch. Gen. Psychiatry 36, 898-901.

Bunney, W. E., Post, R. M., Andersen, A. E., and Kopanada, R. T. (1977) A hypothesized neuronal receptor sensitivity mechanism in affective illness. Commun. Psychopharmacol. 1, 393-405.

Butcher, L. L. and Engel, J. (1969) Behavioral and biochemical effects of L-dopa after peripheral decarboxylase inhibition. Brain Res. 15, 233-241.

Byck, R. (1975) Drugs and the treatment of psychiatric disorders. In: The Pharmacological Basis of Therapeutics, 5th ed. (Goodman, L. S. and Gilman, A., eds), MacMillan, New York, pp. 152-200.

Byck, R. (1976) Peptide transmitters. A unifying hypothesis for euphoria, respiration, sleep, and the action of lithium. Lancet ii, 72-73.

Cade, J. F. (1949) Lithium salts in the treatment of psychotic excitement. Med. J. Aust. 2, 349-352.

Chaudhry, R. P. and Waters, B. G. (1983) Lithium and carbamazepine interaction: possible neurotoxicity. J. Clin. Psychiatry 44, 30-31.

Chouinard, G., Young, S. N., and Annabel, L. (1983) Antimanic effect of clonazepam. Biol. Psychiatry 18, 451-466.

Cohen, B. M., Lipinski, J. F., and Altesman, R. I. (1982) Lecithin in the treatment of mania: double-blind, placebo-controlled trials. Am. J. Psychiatry 139, 1162-1164.

Cohen, B. M., Miller, A. L., Lipinski, J. F., and Pope, H. G. (1980) Lecithin in mania: a preliminary report. Am. J. Psychiatry 137, 242-243.

Cohen, W. J. and Cohen, N. H. (1974) Lithium carbonate, haloperidol, and irreversible brain damage. J. Am. Med. Assoc. 230, 1283-1287.

Cookson, J., Silverstone, T., and Wells, B. (1981) Double blind comparative clinical trial of pimozide and chlorpromazine in mania--a test of the dopamine hypothesis. Acta psychiatr. scand. **64**, 381-397.

Cooper, T. B., Gershon, S., Kline, N. S., and Schou, M. (1978) Lithium: Controversies and Unresolved Issues. Excerpta Medica, Amsterdam, International Congresses, Series no. 478.

Coppen, A. (1967) The biochemistry of affective disorders. Brit. J. Psychiatry **113**, 1237-1264.

Coppen, A., Montgomery, A. S., Gupta, R. K., and Bailey, J. E. (1976) A double-blind comparison of lithium carbonate and maprotiline in the prophylaxis of the affective disorders. Brit. J. Psychiatry **128**, 479-485.

Coppen, A., Prange, A. J. Jr., Whybrow, P. C., Nogivera, R., and Paez, J. M. (1969) Methysergide in mania. A controlled trial. Lancet **ii**, 338-340.

Crunelli, V., Bernasconi, S., and Samanin, R. (1979) Evidence against serotonin involvement in the tonic component of electrically-induced convulsions and in carbamazepine anticonvulsant activity. Psychopharmacology **66**, 79-85.

Cundall, R. L., Brooks, P. W., and Murray, L. G. (1972) Controlled evaluation of lithium prophylaxis in affective disorders. Psychol. Med. **2**, 308-311.

Davis, G. C., Extein, I., Reus, V. I., Hamilton, W., Post, R. M., Goodwin, F. K., and Bunney, W. E. (1980) Failure of naloxone to reduce manic symptoms. Am. J. Psychiatry **137**, 1583-1585.

Davis, K. L. and Berger, P. A. (1978) Pharmacological investigations of the cholinergic imbalance hypothesis of movement disorders and psychosis. Biol. Psychiatry **13**, 23-49.

Dewhurst, W. G. (1968) Methysergide in mania. Nature (Lond.) **219**, 500-507.

Dubovsky, S. L., Franks, R. D., Lifschitz, M., and Coen, P. (1982) Effectiveness of verapamil in the treatment of a manic patient. Am. J. Psychiatry **139**, 502-504.

Ebstein, R. P. and Belmaker, R. H. (1979) Lithium and brain adenylate cyclase. In: Lithium: Controversies and Unresolved Issues (Cooper, T. B., Gershon, S., Kline, N. S., and Schou, M., eds), Excerpta Medica, Amsterdam, pp. 703-729.

Eigen, M. (1976) Possible mechanisms of action of lithium from the perspective of 'receptor' Li$^+$ interaction. In: The Neurobiology of Lithium (Bunney, W. E. and Murphy, D. L., eds), Neurosciences Research Program, Bolton, Boston, vol. 14, no. 2, pp. 142-144.

Emrich, H. M., Zerssen, D. V., Kissling, W., Moller, H. J., and Windorfer, A. (1980) Effect of sodium valproate on mania--the GABA-hypothesis of affective disorders. Arch. Psychiat. Nervenkr. 229, 1-16.

Emrich, H. M., Zerssen, D. V., Moller, H. J., Kissling, W., Cording, C., Schietsch, H. F., and Riedel, E. (1979) Action of propranolol in mania: comparison of effects of the d- and the l-stereoisomer. Pharmakopsychiatry 12, 295-304.

Fieve, R. R., Platman, S. R., and Fleiss, J. L. (1969) A controlled trial: methysergide and lithium in mania. Psychopharmacologia (Berl.) 15, 425-429.

Gerner, R. H., Post, R. M., and Bunney, W. E. (1976) A dopaminergic mechanism in mania. Am. J. Psychiatry 133, 1177-1180.

Gershon, S. (1970) Lithium in mania. Clin. Pharmacol. Ther. 11, 168-187.

Gershon, S. and Shaw, F. H. (1961) Psychiatric sequelae of chronic exposure to organophosphorous insecticides. Lancet i, 1371-1374.

Goddard, G. V., McIntyre, D. C., and Leech, C. K. (1969) A permanent change in brain function resulting from daily electrical stimulation. Exp. Neurol. 25, 295-330.

Goodwin, F. K., Brodie, H. K. H., Murphy, D., and Bunney, W. E. Jr. (1970) L-dopa, catecholamines and behaviour: a clinical and biochemical study in depressed patients. Biol. Psychiatry 2, 341-366.

Gordon, M. (1967) Pharmacological Agents, vol. II, Academic Press, New York.

Green, A. R. and Grahame-Smith, D. G. (1976) (-)-Propranolol inhibits the behavioral response of rats to increased 5-HT in the nervous system. Nature (Lond.) 260, 487-491.

Grof, P., MacCrimmon, D. J., Smith, E. K. M., Daigle, L., Saxena, B., Varma, R., Grof, E., Keitner, G., and Kenny, J. (1980) Long term lithium treatment and the kidney. Can. J. Psychiatry 25, 535-543.

Harrison-Read, P. E. (1981) Behavioral studies with lithium in rats: implications for animal models of mania and depression. In: *Neuroendocrine Regulation of Altered Behavior* (Hrdina, P. D. and Singhal, R. L., eds), Croom Helm, London, pp. 224-262.

Hirsch, M. J. and Wurtman, R. J. (1978) Lecithin consumption increases acetylcholine concentrations in rat brain and adrenal gland. *Science* **202**, 223-225.

Horrobin, D. F., Mtabaji, J. P., Karmali, R. A., Manku, M. S., and Nassar, B. A. (1976) Prolactin and mental illness. *Postgrad. Med. J.* **52**, suppl., 79-85.

Huey, Y., Janowsky, S., and Judd, L. (1981) Effects of lithium carbonate on methylphenidate-induced mood, behavior and cognitive processes. *Psychopharmacology* **73**, 161-167.

Itil, T. M., Polvan, N., and Holden, J. M. C. (1971) Clinical and electroencephalographic effects of cinanserin in schizophrenic and manic patients. *Dis. Nerv. Sys.* **32**, 193-200.

Iversen, L. L. (1975) Dopamine receptors in the brain. *Science* **188**, 1084-1089.

Janowsky, D. S., El-Yousef, M. K., Davis, J. M., and Sekerke, H. J. (1970) Antagonistic effects of physostigmine and methylphenidate in man. *Am. J. Psychiatry* **130**, 1370-1376.

Janowsky, D. S., El-Yousef, M. K., Davis, J. M., and Sekerke, H. J. (1972) A cholinergic-adrenergic hypothesis of mania and depression. *Lancet* **ii**, 632-635.

Janowsky, D. S., El-Yousef, M. K., Davis, J. M., and Sekerke, H. J. (1973) Parasympathetic suppression of manic symptoms by physostigmine. *Arch. Gen. Psychiatry* **28**, 542-547.

Johnson, G., Gershon, S., Burdock, E., Floyd, A., and Hekimian, L. Comparative effects of lithium and chlorpromazine in the treatment of acute manic states. *Brit. J. Psychiatry* (in press).

Johnson, G., Gershon, S., and Hekimian, L. (1968) Controlled evaluation of lithium and chlorpromazine in the treatment of manic states: an interim report. *Comp. Psychiatry* **9**, 563-573.

Juhl, R. P., Tsuang, M. T., and Perry, P. J. (1977) Concomitant administration of haloperidol and lithium carbonate in acute mania. *Dis. Nerv. Sys.* **38**, 675-676.

Kane, F. (1970) Treatment of mania with cinanserin, an antiserotonin agent. *Am. J. Psychiatry* **126**, 1020-1023.

Kelly, J. T., Koch, M., and Buegel, D. (1976) Lithium carbonate in juvenile manic depressive illness. Dis. Nerv. Sys. 37, 90-92.
Kishimoto, A., Ogura, C., Hazama, H., and Inoue, K. (1983) Long-term prophylactic effects of carbamazepine in affective disorder. Brit. J. Psychiatry 143, 327-331.
Krishna, R. N., Taylor, M. A., and Abrams, R. (1978) Combined haloperidol and lithium carbonate in treating manic patients. Comp. Psychiatry 119, 119-120.
Kubanek, J. L. and Rowell, R. C. (1946) The use of dilantin in the treatment of psychotic patients unresponsive to other treatment. Dis. Nerv. Sys. 7, 1-4.
Lambert, P.-A., Carraz, G., Borselli, S., and Bouchardy, M. (1975) Le dipropylacetamide dans le traitement de la psychose maniaco-depressive. L'Encephale I, 25-31.
Lapierre, Y. D. (1976) Control of lithium tremor with propranolol. Can. Med. Assoc. J. 114, 619-620.
Lapierre, Y. D., Gagnon, A., and Kokkinidis, L. (1980) Rapid recurrence of mania following lithium withdrawal. Biol. Psychiatry 15, 859-864.
Lipinski, J. F. and Pope, H. G. Jr. (1982) Possible synergistic action between carbamazepine and lithium carbonate in the treatment of three acutely manic patients. Am. J. Psychiatry 139, 948-949.
Miller, F. T. and Libman, H. (1979) Lithium carbonate in the treatment of schizophrenia and schizoaffective disorder: review and hypothesis. Biol. Psychiatry 14, 705-711.
Murphy, D. L., Brodie, H. K., Goodwin, F. K., and Bunney, W. E. (1971) L-dopa: regular induction of hypomania in 'bipolar' manic depressive patients. Nature (Lond.) 229, 135-136.
Okuma, T. and Kishimoto, A. (1977) Antimanic and prophylactic effects of tegretol (abstract). In: Proceedings of the 6th World Congress of Psychiatry, Honolulu, Hawaii, 1977, CIBA-GEIGY, Summit, N.J.
Okuma, T., Kishimoto, A., Inoue, K., et al. (1973) Antimanic and prophylactic effects of carbamazepine on manic-depressive psychosis. Folia Psychiatr. Neurol. Jpn. 27, 283-297.
Oyewumi, L. K. and Lapierre, Y. D. (1981) Efficacy of lithium in treating mood disorder after brain stem injury. Am. J. Psychiatry 183, 110-112.

Peroutka, S. J. and Snyder, S. H. (1980) Relationship of neuroleptic drug effects at brain dopamine, sertonin, α-adrenergic and histamine receptors to clinical potency. Am. J. Psychiatry **137**, 1518-1522.

Peroutka, S. J., U'Prichard, D. C., Greenberg, D. A., and Snyder, S. H. (1977) Neuroleptic drug interactions with norepinephrine alpha receptor binding sites in rat brain. Neuropharmacology **16**, 549-556.

Pert, A., Rosenblatt, J. E., Sivit, C., Pert, C. B., and Bunney, W. E. (1978) Long-term treatment with lithium prevents the development of dopamine receptors supersensitivity. Science **201**, 171-173.

Pickar, D., Vartanian, F., Bunney, W. E. Jr., Maier, H. P., Gastpar, M. T., Prakash, R., Sethi, B. B., Lideman, R., Belyaev, B. S., Tsytsulkooskaja, M. V. A., Jungkeinz, G., Nedopel, N., Verhoeven, W., and Van Praag, H. (1982) Short term naloxone administration in schizophrenic and manic patients—a World Health Organization collaborative study. Arch. Gen. Psychiatry **39**, 313-319.

Pinder, R. M., Brogden, R. N., Speight, T. M., and Avery, G. S. (1977) Sodium valproate: a review of its pharmacological properties and therapy efficacy in epilepsy. Drugs **13**, 81-123.

Platman, S. R. (1970) A comparison of lithium carbonate and chlorpromazine in mania. Am. J. Psychiatry **127**, 351-353.

Post, R. M., Ballenger, J. C., Hare, T. A., and Bunney, W. E. (1980) Lack of effect of carbamazepine on gamma-aminobutyric acid levels in cerebral spinal fluid. Neurology **30**, 1008-1111.

Post, R. M., Ballenger, J. C., Uhde, T. W., and Bunney, W. (1984) Efficacy of carbamazepine in manic depressive illness: implications for underlying mechanisms. In: Neurobiology of Mood Disorders (Post, R. M. and Ballenger, J. C., eds), Williams & Wilkins, Baltimore, pp. 777-816.

Post, R. M., Gerner, R. H., Carman, J. S., Gillin, J. C., Jimerson, D. C., Goodwin, F. K., and Bunney, W. E. (1978) Effects of a dopamine agonist piribedil in depressed patients: relationship of pre-treatment homovanillic acid to antidepressant response. Arch. Gen. Psychiatry **35**, 609-615.

Post, R. M. and Uhde, T. W. (1984) Carbamazepine and lithium carbonate synergism in mania. Arch. Gen. Psychiatry **41**, 210.

Prange, A. J., Wilson, I. C., Lynn, C. W., Alltop, L. B., and Stikeleather, R. A. (1974) L-Tryptophan in mania: contribution to a permissive hypothesis of affective disorders. Arch. Gen. Psychiatry 30, 56-62.

Prien, R. F., Caffey, E. M. Jr., and Klett, J. C. (1971) Lithium carbonate: a survey of the history and current status of lithium in treating mood disorders. Dis. Nerv. Sys. 32, 521-531.

Prien, R. F., Caffey, E. M., and Klett, J. C. (1972) Comparison of lithium carbonate and chlorpromazine in the treatment of mania. Arch. Gen. Psychiatry 26, 146-153.

Purdy, R. E., Julien, R. M., Fairhurst, A. S., and Terry, M. D. (1977) Effect of carbamazepine on the in vitro uptake and release of norepinephrine in adrenergic nerves of rabbit aorta and in whole brain synaptosomes. Epilepsia 18, 251-257.

Quattrone, A., Crunelli, V., and Samanin, R. (1978) Seizure susceptibility and anticonvulsant activity of carbamazepine, diphenylhydantoin and phenobarbital in rats with selective depletions of brain monoamines. Neuropharmacology 17, 643-647.

Reynolds, E. H. (1975) Neurotoxicity of carbamazepine. Adv. Neurol. 11, 345-353.

Richelson, E. (1978) Psychotropic drug blockade of histamine H_1 receptors, Abstract 349, Proceedings of Second World Congress of Biological Psychiatry, Barcelona.

Risch, S. C., Cohen, R. M., Janowsky, D. S., Kalin, N. H., Sitaram, N., Gillin, J. C., and Murphy, D. L. (1981) Physostigmine induction of depressive symptomatology in normal human subjects. Psychiat. Res. 4, 89-94.

Rosenbaum, A. H., Nien, R. G., Hanson, N. P., and Swanson, D. W. (1977) Tardive dyskinesia: relationship with a primary affective disorder. Dis. Nerv. Sys. 38, 423-427.

Rowntree, D. W., Neven, S., and Wilson, A. (1950) The effects of diisoprophylfluorophosphonate in schizophrenic and manic depressive psychosis. J. Neurol. Neurosurg. Psychiat. 13, 47-62.

Sack, R. L. and Goodwin, F. K. (1974) Inhibition of dopamine-β-hydroxylase in manic patients. A clinical trial with fusaric acid. Arch. Gen. Psychiatry 31, 649-654.

Schildkraut, J. J. (1965) The catecholamine hypothesis of affective disorders, a review of supporting evidence. Am. J. Psychiatry 122, 509-522.

Schildkraut, J. J. (1969) Neuropsychopharmacology and the affective disorders. New Engl. J. Med. 281, 302-308.

Schou, M. (1959) Lithium in psychiatric therapy: stock-taking after ten years. Psychopharmacologia (Berl.) 1, 65-78.

Schou, M. (1968a) Lithium in psychiatry: a review. In: Psychopharmacology - A Review of Progress, 1957-1967 (Efron, D. H., ed.), U.S. Government Printing Office, Washington, D.C., pp. 701-718.

Schou, M. (1968b) Special review: lithium in psychiatric therapy and prophylaxis. J. Psychiat. Res. 6, 67-95.

Schou, M. (1976) Current status of lithium therapy in affective disorders and other diseases. In: Lithium in Psychiatry: A Synopsis (Villeneuve, A., ed.), Press Universite Laval, Quebec, pp. 49-77.

Schou, M., Mellerup, E. T., and Rafaelsen, O. J. (1981) Mode of action of lithium. In: Handbook of Biological Psychiatry, Part IV (Van Praag, H. M., ed.), Marcel Dekker, New York, pp. 805-824.

Schou, M. and Vestergaard, P. (1981) Lithium and the kidney score. Psychosomatics 22, 92-94.

Seeman, P., Lee, T., Chau-Wong, M., and Wong, K. (1976) Antipsychotic drug doses and neuroleptic/dopamine receptors. Nature (Lond.) 261, 717-719.

Sen, A. K., Murthy, R., Stancer, H. C., Awad, A. G., Godse, D. D., and Grof, P. (1976) The mechanism of action of lithium ion in affective disorders, a new hypothesis. In: Membranes and Disease (Bolis, L., Hoffman, J. G., and Leaf, A., eds), Raven Press, New York, pp. 109-122.

Shopsin, B. and Gershon, S. (1971) Chemotherapy of manic-depressive disorder. In: Brain Chemistry and Mental Disease (Ho, B. T. and McIsaac, W. M., eds), Plenum Press, New York, pp. 319-377.

Shopsin, B., Gershon, S., Thompson, H., and Collins, P. (1975) Psychoactive drugs in mania--a controlled comparison of lithium carbonate, chlorpromazine and haloperidol. Arch. Gen. Psychiatry 32, 34-42.

Small, J. G., Small, I. F., and Moore, D. F. (1971) Experimental withdrawal of lithium in recovered manic-depressive patients: a report of five cases. Am. J. Psychiatry 127, 1555-1558.

Smith, A., Chambers, C., and Naylor, G. J. (1980) Bromocriptine in mania--a placebo controlled double blind trial. Brit. Med. J. 280, 86.

Stevens, J., Wilson, K., and Foote, W. (1974) GABA blockade, dopamine and schizophrenia: experimental studies in the cat. Psychopharmacologia (Berl.) 39, 105-119.

Tanimukai, H., Invi, M., and Kaneko, Z. (1970) Treatment and prophylaxis of manic states with a carbonic anhydrase inhibitor. Int. Pharmacopsychiatry 5, 35-43.

Tupin, J. (1970) The use of lithium for manic-depressive psychosis. Hosp. Comm. Psychiatry 21, 73-80.

Wada, J. A., Sato, M., Wake, A., Green, J. R., and Troupin, A. F. (1976) Prophylactic effects of phenytoin, phenobarbital and carbamazepine examined in kindling cat preparations. Arch. Neurol. 33, 426-434.

Waters, B., Lapierre, Y., Gagnon, A., Chaudhry, R., Tremblay, A., Sarantidis, D., and Gray, R. (1982) Determination of the optimal concentration of lithium for the prophylaxis of manic dperessive disorder. Biol. Psychiatry 17, 1323-1329.

Whitlock, F. A. and Evans, L. E. (1978) Drugs and depression. Drugs 15, 53-71.

Wurtman, R. J., Hirsch, M. J., and Growdln, J. H. (1977) Lecithin consumption raises serum free choline levels. Lancet ii, 68-69.

11.

NEUROBIOLOGICAL BASIS OF ANTIDEPRESSANT TREATMENTS

P. Blier and C. de Montigny

Introduction
============

The somatic treatments of major affective illnesses did not evolve from laboratory studies and deductive reasoning but rather from fortuitous clinical observations. They were first introduced in the 1930s with the use of electroconvulsive treatment (ECT), a therapy initially meant for schizophrenia. Subsequently, the antidepressant properties of monoamine oxidase inhibitors (MAOIs) and of tricyclic antidepressant (TCA) drugs, the two major classes of psychopharmacological agents most widely used in the treatment of these disorders, were also discovered entirely by serendipity. Selikoff et al. (1952) and Bloch et al. (1954) noticed mood elevation in pulmonary tuberculosis patients treated with the MAOI iproniazid. Although the MAO-inhibiting properties of iproniazid were already known, it was not hypothesized that MAOIs exerted their antidepressant effect by increasing the availability of monoamines until their therapeutic action was confirmed in depressed patients (Crane, 1957; Kline, 1958). In search of better antipsychotic drugs, Kuhn (1958) observed that the experimental tricyclic G-22355 (later called imipramine) made schizophrenics less depressed. It was not until 1964, however, that Glowinski and Axelrod proposed that noradrenaline (NA) reuptake blockade may contribute to the therapeutic effect of TCA drugs. The clinical efficacy of MAOI and TCA drugs, two classes of substances which increase the synaptic availability of monoamines, and the depressive state produced in some patients by the monoamine depleter reserpine largely served as the basis for the catecholamine hypothesis formulated in 1965 by Schildkraut. It stated that a functional deficit of NA in CNS regions involved in the control of emotion may be responsible for depression in man. Shortly after this theory was proposed, Coppen (1967) presented a similar hypothesis of a functional deficit of 5-hydroxytryptamine (5-HT, serotonin) in endogenous depression. This indoleamine hypothesis was derived from the pharmacological data mentioned above, and from the similar time course of the antidepressant effect of MAOIs and of the increase of human cerebral 5-HT produced by MAOI therapy.

Researchers then began trying to identify an anomaly of monoamine presynaptic functions in depressed patients. Unequivocal evidence for such an anomaly has not emerged. However, Asberg et al. (1976) reported a lower level of cerebrospinal fluid 5-hydroxyindoleacetic acid (5-HIAA), the main metabolite of 5-HT, in a subgroup of depressed patients. Nevertheless, neither changes of 5-HIAA levels nor levels of 3-methoxy-4-hydroxyphenylethylene glycol, the main metabolite of NA in the CNS, are correlated to therapeutic response or spontaneous remission (Goodwin and Post, 1975).

In recent years, therapeutic rather than etiological hypotheses have received more attention. Unfortunately, the distinction between these two has not often been clearly made; many investigators have concluded the involvement of a neuronal system in the genesis of the depressive syndrome from its modification by an antidepressant treatment.

Before reviewing and evaluating animal experiments, it must be stressed that a neurobiological modification produced by an antidepressant treatment can only be considered relevant to therapeutics if it meets the following criteria: specificity, dose congruence, time of onset and, finally, site of action.

As regards the first of these criteria, a modification, if it is to reach therapeutic significance, should not be produced by other types of drugs which do not have an antidepressant activity. For example, Kanof and Greengard (1978) reported that various TCA drugs can block the activity of histamine-2 sensitive adenylate cyclase in a cell-free preparation of mammalian brain. However, it is difficult to conceive that this neurobiological action of TCA drugs could be involved in their therapeutic effect since antipsychotic drugs are as effective as TCA drugs in this model.

A second requirement to be fulfilled is that of dose congruence. When choosing an optimal regimen for animal experiments, brain or plasma levels of a drug should approximate those that are obtained in man with therapeutic regimens. In the case of TCA drugs, a one-week dosage taken at one time (about 1.2 g or 18 mg/kg for an adult of average weight) can be lethal. This raises some doubts concerning the clinical relevance of the numerous animal studies in which a daily dose of 20 mg/kg has been used, even when pharmacokinetics are taken into account.

The third requirement that must be fulfilled is time-course congruence. The therapeutic effects of antidepressant drugs are usually not discernible within the first week of treatment whereas the side effects usually appear much more rapidly. It is thus difficult to attribute the antidepressant response to a neurobiological modification which occurs within a few days. For example, the $5-HT_2$ binding site labelled with $[^3H]$-spiroperidol has been thought to play a role in the clinical efficacy of antidepressant drugs. However, Blackshear and Sanders-Bush (1982) have shown that mianserin, a clinically effective tetracyclic substance, decreases the number of $5-HT_2$ binding sites upon both acute and chronic administrations. Similarly, indoleamine reuptake blockade, which occurs at most within a few hours, cannot account per se for the therapeutic response of several drugs presently available. Modifications in neuronal responsiveness induced only by repeated administration of these drugs would be better candidates.

Finally, a modification should occur in those regions of the brain which are involved in the control of mood, if clinical extrapolation is to be made from animal experiments. For instance, an increased α_1 adrenergic responsiveness of rat facial motoneurons and dorsal lateral geniculate nucleus (dLGN) has been reported following chronic treatment with TCA drugs (Menkes and Aghajanian, 1980; Menkes et al., 1981). This modification may well account for reversal of the typical motor retardation of depressed patients. However, such investigations should be undertaken in regions of the limbic system where NA exerts its effect via an α_1 receptor to ascertain whether this phenomenon is also involved in mood elevation.

Once a neurobiological modification produced by an antidepressant treatment reaches clinical relevance by fulfilling all four of these criteria, it should undergo clinical verification. This is the most difficult feat to achieve since there exist very few means of directly assessing the efficacy of neuronal systems in the human brain.

Down-Regulation of the Central β-Adrenergic System

In recent years, the role of cyclic nucleotides in synaptic transmission has been extensively investigated. Cyclic adenosine 3',5'-monophosphate (cAMP) is produced from ATP by the enzyme adenylate cyclase and most likely serves as a second messenger mediating the biological response to activation of a primary receptor site on postsynaptic membranes (for review, see Greengard, 1976). This model of noradrenergic transmission has been used by several groups who study brain slices of animals following long-term antidepressant treatments. All major classes of antidepressant treatments administered chronically to rats share the common property of reducing the accumulation of NA- and/or isoproterenol-stimulated cAMP, following a long- but not short-term treatment. This modification in biological response is often coupled with a decreased number of β-adrenergic binding sites evaluated by using the antagonist dihydroalprenolol (DHA) as a ligand. The affinity of these sites is not modified by any of the treatments thus far studied (Sulser, 1983). Table 11.1 presents the results of the radioligand binding studies for the rat cerebral cortex following long-term administration of a great variety of antidepressant treatments.

This β-adrenergic desensitization probably results from the modification of factors that modulate monoaminergic neurotransmission. These factors, illustrated in Figure 11.1, can be ascribed to the presynaptic system (A) or to the postsynaptic neuron (B). Using this model, it can be readily conceived how the various treatments presented in Table 11.1 may result in β-deamplification, either via a sustained NA signal input or via a decreased efficacy of postsynaptic transducing systems. Among the presynaptic factors, an enhanced release of NA could result from an increased firing rate of NA neurons. Welch et al. (1980) and Scuvee-Moreau et al. (1983) have found that trazodone, administered intravenously to rats, increases the firing rate of NA neurons which give rise to the NA innervation of forebrain regions (Jones and Moore, 1975). Even though this effect is not mediated by the somatic α_2 autoreceptor of NA neurons, the decreased number of β-sites observed following repeated administration of trazodone (Clemens-Jewery, 1978) could be attri-

Table 11.1: Effects of long-term antidepressant treatments on the number of β-adrenergic binding sites and cAMP formation in response to β-agonists in the rat cerebral cortex

ANTIDEPRESSANT TREATMENTS	NUMBER OF β ADRENERGIC SITES	cAMP FORMATION†	REFERENCES
TCA DRUGS			
Amitriptyline	↓	—	Sellinger-Barnette et al., 1980
Chlorimipramine	↓	—	Sellinger-Barnette et al., 1980
Desipramine	↓	↓	Frazer et al., 1974; Mishra et al., 1980; Sellinger-Barnette et al., 1980
Doxepin	↓	—	Clements-Jewery, 1978
Imipramine	↓	↓	Frazer et al., 1974; Schultz et al., 1981
Iprindole	↓	↓	Sellinger-Barnette et al., 1980; Wolfe et al., 1978
Nortriptyline	↓	—	Sellinger-Barnette et al., 1980
ATYPICAL DRUGS			
Bupropion	↓	—	Gandolfi et al., 1983; Sellinger-Barnette et al., 1980
Citalopram	0	—	Hyttel et al., 1983
Clenbuterol	↓	—	Hall et al., 1980
Fluvoxamine	↓	↓	Classen, 1983
Mianserin	0	↓	Clements-Jewery, 1978; Mishra et al., 1980
Nisoxetine	0	—	Mishra et al., 1979
Salbutamol	0	—	Hall et al., 1980
Trazodone	↓	—	Clements-Jewery, 1978
Zimelidine	0, ↓	↓	Mishra et al., 1980; Ross et al., 1981

Table 11.1 (cont'd)

ANTIDEPRESSANT TREATMENTS	NUMBER OF β ADRENERGIC SITES	cAMP FORMATION[†]	REFERENCES
MONOAMINE OXIDASE INHIBITORS			
Clorgyline	↓	↓	Campbell et al., 1979; Cohen et al., 1982
Deprenyl	0, ↓	0, ↓	Mishra et al., 1982; Youdim and Finberg, 1983; Zsilla et al., 1983
Nialamide	↓	—	Sellinger-Barnette et al., 1980
Pargyline[††]	0, ↓	↓	Campbell et al., 1979; Wolfe et al., 1978
Phenelzine	↓	—	Campbell et al., 1979
Tranylcypromine	↓	—	Sellinger-Barnette et al., 1980
OTHERS			
ECT	↓	↓	Gillespie et al., 1979; Vetulani and Sulser, 1975
REM sleep deprivation	↓	—	Mogilnicka et al., 1980

[†] cAMP stands for cyclic adenosine 3',5'-monophosphate, stimulated by isoproterenol and/or NA.
[††] The antidepressant efficacy of pargyline has been questioned in a recent placebo-controlled study (Murphy et al., 1981).
↓ signifies a reduction, 0 no modification, ↑ an increase.
ECT stands for electroconvulsive therapy and REM for rapid eye movement.

butable to an increased firing rate leading to increased release.

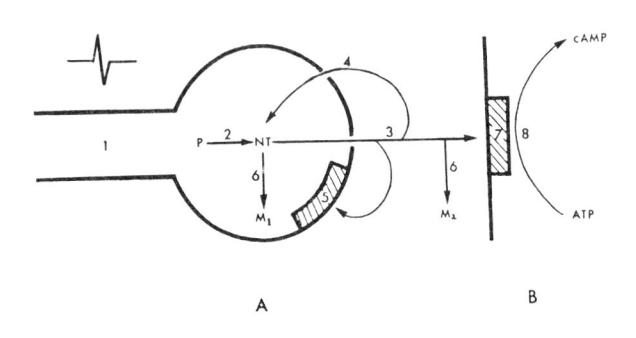

Figure 11.1: Factors regulating synaptic efficacy. 1) Firing rate of the presynaptic neuron; 2) neurotransmitter (NT) synthesis from precursor (P); 3) NT release; 4) NT reuptake; 5) Presynaptic receptor sensitive to NT; 6) Intra- and extracellular catabolism; 7) Postsynaptic receptor; 8) Postmembranal mechanisms following receptor site activation.

An increased release of NA can also be obtained by the blockade of terminal α_2 receptors which exert a negative feedback regulation (Langer, 1977). The two atypical antidepressant drugs mianserin and iprindole both reduce the NA-stimulated response in cAMP formation (Wolfe et al., 1978; Mishra et al., 1980). Given the well-documented α_2 blocking property of mianserin (Bauman and Maitre, 1977; Svensson et al., 1981), it is conceivable that desensitization of the β-adrenergic system could result from an increased release of NA by mianserin. Long-term administration of iprindole, a TCA drug which does not affect 5-HT or NA reuptake (Ross and Renyi, 1975a,b), increases the number of clonidine-labelled binding sites in cerebral cortex, suggesting that, in vivo, iprindole blocks the α_2 site (Reisine et al., 1980). Preliminary electrophysiological results from our laboratory also suggest that iprindole can block, at least acutely, the somatic α_2 receptor of NA neurons in the locus coeruleus. That iprindole exerts its postsynaptic effect via its presynaptic action on the NA system is corroborated by the failure of animals to develop subsensitivity in the ipsi- but not contralateral cortex after a unilateral locus coeruleus lesion (Sulser and Janowsky, 1982). Therefore, mianserin and iprindole may produce subsensitivity of the β adrenergic system by increasing the release of NA through blockade of the α_2 autoreceptor.

An increased NA signal input can also result from repeated administration of secondary amine antidepressant drugs, such as desipramine (Vetulani and Sulser, 1975), which potently impede the reuptake of NA (Ross and Renyi, 1975a,b). Similarly, tertiary amine antidepressant drugs, such as imipramine, become more potent NA reuptake agents after demethylation (Ross and Renyi, 1975a,b; Nagy and Johansson, 1977). As is the case for iprindole, a presynaptic mechanism for the down-regulation of the number of binding sites by desipramine is indicated by its failure to do so in the cerebral cortex contralateral to a lesion of the locus coeruleus (Sulser and Janowsky, 1982). Similarly, zimelidine could act on the postsynaptic β system via a presynaptic action, since its demethylated metabolite, norzimelidine, is a quite potent NA reuptake blocker (Hyttel, 1981).

MAO catalyzes the deamination of many monoamines, including NA (Blaschko, 1974). Blockade of intra- and/or extracellular MAO thus increases the availability of NA in the synaptic cleft, thereby inducing a desensitization of β target neurons (Vetulani and Sulser, 1975).

β Down-regulation could therefore be obtained by a heightened agonist supply resulting from increased firing rate, α_2 autoreceptor blockade, reuptake inhibition, or decreased catabolism. This notion is supported by the intensification and acceleration of β down-regulation produced by combining α_2 autoreceptor blockade with reuptake inhibition or decreased catabolism (Reisine et al., 1980; Johnson et al., 1980; Crews et al., 1981).

Down-regulation of the β-adrenergic system could also be obtained independently of the NA presynaptic element by manipulating factors affecting only the postsynaptic moiety. An interesting example is provided by the β_2 agonist clenbuterol, which induces a decrease in β receptor density (Hall et al., 1980). Another example is ECT which induces a rapid β subsensitivity (Gillespie et al., 1979). ECT can produce a subsensitivity of the β adrenergic system even in NA-denervated animals (Vetulani et al., 1976), as opposed to desipramine which is ineffective in the same paradigm (Sulser and Janowsky, 1982).

It is quite remarkable that such a great variety of antidepressant treatments exert this effect. Even rapid eye movement sleep deprivation, which can produce a marked antidepressant effect (Vogel et al., 1980), decreases β-receptor binding (Mogilnicka et al., 1980). The facts that most chronically administered antidepressant treatments produce β subsensitivity and that an elevation of β adrenergic binding has been found in the cerebral cortex of drug-free suicide victims (Zanko and Biegon, 1983) suggest that the NA system may be involved both in the therapy and etiology of major affective disorders. However, there are four lines of evidence that do not support the therapeutic hypothesis.

1. The decrease in β adrenergic function is not entirely specific to antidepressant treatment: amphetamine and chlorpromazine, which are not effective antidepressant drugs, have been reported to down-regulate the system in the rat cerebral cortex (Baudry et al., 1976; Schultz, 1976). Given the different factors that modulate NA neurotransmission, it is not surprising that long-term amphetamine also results in a β down-regulation since it releases NA from terminals and inhibits NA reuptake (Moore et al., 1970).

2. The subsensitivity of β receptor responses following an antidepressant treatment might represent a negative feedback mechanism, compensating for an increased quantity of synaptic NA, with no net change of the gain. Two groups of investigators undertook the task of verifying the net effect of antidepressant treatments on NA neurotransmission in vivo. They used as a model the production of melatonin in the rat pineal gland since its secretion is dependent upon a β activation of the catalyzing enzyme. Melatonin secretion can be stimulated by exogenously-administered β agonists, thereby assessing postsynaptic responsiveness, or by endogenously-released NA produced during the dark-phase of nighttime, thereby permitting the evaluation of overall synaptic efficacy. Following repeated administration of desipramine, Heydorn et al. (1982) observed a blunted elevation of melatonin in response to isoproterenol and also to the dark-phase period. On the other hand, Cowen et al. (1983), using the same TCA drug, did not observe any changes in the usual increase in melatonin produced by darkness whereas the isoproterenol-induced release was decreased,

thereby confirming that their treatment was effective in producing postsynaptic β desensitization. The discrepancy between these results may stem from the regimens of desipramine used. The former study, which suggests a deamplification of the NA signal as a net effect, was done with a dose of 10 mg/kg twice daily for 7 days whereas the latter, which points to an unmodified overall synaptic NA function, used a more clinically relevant dosage of 10 mg/kg once daily for ten days. Such results underscore the notion that clinically relevant doses should be utilized in order to permit valid extrapolation of the results of animal experiments to human therapeutics.

3. Another objection to the contention that a β down-regulation is responsible for the antidepressant response is the report that the β antagonist propanolol produces in some patients a depression which is reversed by the discontinuation of this drug (Waal, 1967; Petrie et al., 1982). By impeding the access of NA to the postsynaptic receptors, the efficacy of the system should be immediately decreased and depressed patients should feel better. Conversely, upon withdrawal, patients should see their condition worsen since supersensitivity develops during chronic β receptor blockade with propanolol (Tsukamoto et al., 1982).

4. Some antidepressant drugs, such as mianserin and zimelidine, can produce a decrease in cAMP formation without a concomitant reduction in the number of β sites (Mishra et al., 1980). This would suggest that the biological response, cAMP generation, is the critical effect that must be obtained in humans during antidepressant therapy. A reversal of the therapeutic effect produced by an antidepressant treatment should therefore be obtained by a pharmacological manipulation that increases cAMP formation. Shopsin et al. (1975, 1976) have shown that para-chlorophenylalanine (PCPA), a 5-HT synthesis inhibitor, produces a relapse of the depressive syndrome in patients successfully treated with a TCA drug or an MAOI. However, PCPA does not reverse the reduction of the NA-stimulated cAMP formation obtained in desipramine-pretreated rats (Gillespie et al., 1983).

In summary, most antidepressant treatments administered chronically thus far have been shown to cause a desensitization of the cAMP response to NA and/or a decreased number of β sites in brain slices of rat cerebral cortex. The direct therapeutic relevance can be questioned, but the results obtained with this biochemical approach have provided invaluable information on NA neurotransmission.

Electrophysiological Single-Cell Studies

The advantage of evaluating neuronal responsiveness by measuring changes of firing activity in intact animals is that it permits direct assessment of the effect of a neurotransmitter on an identified neuronal population. Indeed, neurons located within a given structure may not all use the same neurotransmitter. In the dorsal raphe, for example, only one out of three neurons is serotoninergic (Descarries et al., 1982). Therefore, a modification of binding parameters within a nucleus would not necessarily reflect a corresponding change in its output. Certainly, the firing activity of a monoamine neuron is not the only factor controlling its output, but it has nevertheless been demonstrated to play a critical role (for review, see Aghajanian, 1978).

In this section, antidepressant treatments will be discussed according to their probable post- or presynaptic sites of action according to the scheme of Figure 11.1. A summary of modifications of neuronal responsiveness to 5-HT and NA following long-term administration of various antidepressant treatments is presented in Table 11.2.

Postsynaptic Site of Action

TCA Drugs. The first single-cell study examining modifications of neuronal responsiveness to monoamines following repeated administration of various TCA drugs (de Montigny and Aghajanian, 1978) was published several years after the acute effects of these drugs on monoamine neurons were reported (Sheard et al., 1972). An increased responsiveness to microiontophoretically-applied 5-HT, but not to NA or γ-aminobutyric acid (GABA), was observed in the rat hippocampus and ventral lateral geniculate nucleus (vLGN) following chronic TCA drug administration (de Montigny and Aghajanian, 1978).

The development of this phenomenon was independent of the monoamine reuptake properties of the drugs tested; the doses administered were within the range of clinical regimens; and finally, this sensitization was not obtained following chronic administration of chlorpromazine, a tricyclic antipsychotic drug. Since then, four studies have confirmed this enhanced responsiveness to 5-HT in the hippo-

Table 11.2: Modifications of neuronal responsiveness to 5-HT and NA in various regions of the rat brain following long-term administration of antidepressant treatments

BRAIN STRUCTURES	TREATMENT	5-HT	NA	REFERENCES
Presynaptic neurons			α_1	
RAPHE DORSALIS	Desipramine	0	–	Blier and de Montigny, 1980
	Imipramine	0	–	Blier and de Montigny, 1980
	Iprindole	0	–	Blier and de Montigny, 1980
	Zimelidine	→	–	Blier and de Montigny, 1983
	Indalpine	→	–	Blier et al., 1984
	Femoxetine†	0	–	Blier and de Montigny, 1980
	Clorgyline	→	–	Blier and de Montigny, 1984
	Deprenyl††	0	–	Blier and de Montigny, 1984
	Phenelzine	→	–	Blier and de Montigny, 1984
			α_2	
LOCUS COERULEUS	Chloroimipramine	–	0	Scuvee-Moreau and Svensson, 1982
	Desipramine	–	→	Scuvee-Moreau and Svensson, 1982
	Imipramine	–	→	Scuvee-Moreau and Svensson, 1982; Sulser, 1983
	Iprindole	–	0	Scuvee-Moreau and Svensson, 1982
	Mianserin	–	→	Scuvee-Moreau and Svensson, 1982
	Zimelidine	–	→	Scuvee-Moreau and Svensson, 1982
	Clorgyline	–	0	Blier and de Montigny, 1984
	Deprenyl	–	0	Blier and de Montigny, 1984
	Phenelzine	–	0	Blier and de Montigny, 1984

Table 11.2 (cont'd)

BRAIN STRUCTURES	TREATMENT	5-HT	NA α1	REFERENCES
Postsynaptic regions				
DORSAL LATERAL GENICULATE NUCLEUS	Amitriptyline	↑	↑	Menkes and Aghajanian, 1981
	Chloroimipramine	↑	↑	Menkes and Aghajanian, 1981
	Desipramine	↑	↑	Menkes and Aghajanian, 1981
	Imipramine	↑	↑	Menkes and Aghajanian, 1981
	Iprindole	↑	↑	Menkes and Aghajanian, 1981
	Adinazolam	0	↑	Turmel and de Montigny, 1984
	Zimelidine	0	0	Turmel and de Montigny, 1984
VENTRAL LATERAL GENICULATE NUCLEUS	Amitriptyline	↑	—	de Montigny and Aghajanian, 1978
	Chloroimipramine	↑	—	de Montigny and Aghajanian, 1978
	Desipramine	↑	—	de Montigny and Aghajanian, 1978
	Imipramine	↑	—	de Montigny and Aghajanian, 1978
	Iprindole	↑	—	de Montigny and Aghajanian, 1978
	Femoxetine†	0	—	de Montigny and Aghajanian, 1978
FACIAL MOTOR NUCLEUS	Imipramine	↑	↑	Menkes et al., 1980
	Amitriptyline	↑	↑	Menkes et al., 1980
	Desipramine	↑	↑	Menkes et al., 1980
	Iprindole	↑	↑	Menkes et al., 1980

Table 11.2 (cont'd)

BRAIN STRUCTURES	TREATMENT	5-HT	NA	REFERENCES
Postsynaptic regions			$\underline{\beta}$	
CINGULATE CORTEX	Chloroimipramine	0	↓	Olpe and Schellenberg, 1980, 1981
	Desipramine	0	↓	Olpe and Schellenberg, 1980, 1981
	Iprindole	—	0	Olpe et al., 1981
	Maprotiline	—	↓	Olpe and Schellenberg, 1980
	Mianserin	—	0	Olpe et al., 1981
	Clorgyline	↓	—	Olpe and Schellenberg, 1980
	Deprenyl††	0	—	Olpe and Schellenberg, 1981
	Tranylcypromine	—	↓	Olpe and Schellenberg, 1980
ROSTRAL CORTEX	Chloroimipramine	0	—	Olpe and Schellenberg, 1981
	Desipramine	0	—	Olpe and Schellenberg, 1981
	Clorgyline	↓	—	Olpe and Schellenberg, 1981
	Deprenyl††	0	—	Olpe and Schellenberg, 1981
SOMATOSENSORY CORTEX	Imipramine	↑	—	Jones, 1980
CEREBELLUM	Desipramine	—	↓	Schultz et al., 1981

Table 11.2 (cont'd)

BRAIN STRUCTURES	TREATMENT	5-HT	NA	β?†††	REFERENCES
Postsynaptic regions					
HIPPOCAMPUS	Amitriptyline	↑		0	de Montigny and Aghajanian, 1978; Gravel and de Montigny, 1983
	Desipramine	↑	0		de Montigny and Aghajanian, 1978
	Chloroimipramine	↑	0		de Montigny and Aghajanian, 1978; de Montigny et al., 1981a; Gallager and Bunney, 1979
	Imipramine	↑		0	Blier et al., 1984; de Montigny and Aghajanian, 1978; Gallager and Bunney, 1979
	Iprindole	↑	0		de Montigny and Aghajanian, 1978
	Mianserin	↑	0		Blier et al., 1984
	Adinazolam	↑	0		Turmel and de Montigny, 1984
	Zimelidine	0	0		Blier and de Montigny, 1983; de Montigny et al., 1981a
	Indalpine	0	0		Blier and de Montigny, 1983
	Femoxetine†	0	0		Dahl et al., 1982
	Clorgyline	→	0		This chapter
	Phenelzine	0	0		
	Deprenyl††	0	0		
	ECT	↑	0		de Montigny, 1984

Table 11.2 (cont'd)

BRAIN STRUCTURES	TREATMENT	5-HT	NA	REFERENCES
Postsynaptic regions			?††††	
AMYGDALA	Desipramine	↑	↑	Wang and Aghajanian, 1980
	Imipramine	↑	↑	Wang and Aghajanian, 1980
	Iprindole	↑	↑	Wang and Aghajanian, 1980

Abbreviations and symbols are given in Table 11.1.
†Femoxetine has been shown to be an effective antidepressant drug. However, due to its rapid elimination (Mengel and Lund, 1982), femoxetine has been used in these electrophysiological experiments at a regimen insufficient to produce a sustained 5-HT reuptake blockade.
††Deprenyl was used at a regimen which produced a selective inhibition of type B MAO, as opposed to non-selective clinical regimens.
†††The electrophysiological response of hippocampal pyramidal neurons to NA has been suggested (Segal and Bloom, 1974), but not conclusively shown, to be mediated by β receptors.
††††This response possesses neither α_1 nor β characteristics (Wang and Aghajanian, 1980).

campus following repeated administration of TCA drugs (Gallager and Bunney, 1979; de Montigny et al., 1981a; Gravel and de Montigny, 1983; Blier et al., 1984). Other investigators have reported a similar enhancement of response to 5-HT applied microiontophoretically in the dLGN, the amygdala and the facial motor nucleus using similar regimens of various TCA drugs (Menkes and Aghajanian, 1980; Menkes et al., 1981; Wang and Aghajanian, 1981). Cingulate and rostral cortex are the only two regions which do not present an enhanced 5-HT responsiveness following chronic TCA drug administration (Olpe, 1981). However, not all regions of cerebral cortex maintain a normal response to 5-HT after chronic TCA drug administration as Jones (1980) observed an increased responsiveness in the somatosensory cortex.

The functional significance of this enhanced responsiveness to microiontophoretically-applied 5-HT is corroborated by three lines of experimental data. Firstly, the enhanced responsiveness to 5-HT of postsynaptic regions could have conceivably been dampened or cancelled out by a negative feedback loop terminating on presynaptic 5-HT neurons; this has been ruled out by the demonstration that neither the firing activity nor the sensitivity of presynaptic 5-HT neurons are modified following a 14-day treatment with various TCA drugs (Blier and de Montigny, 1980). Secondly, Wang and Aghajanian (1980) observed that the suppression of firing activity produced by the electrical stimulation of the ascending 5-HT pathway to the amygdala was prolonged following chronic TCA drug treatment. Activating the innervating pathway in such a manner produces a release of endogenous 5-HT and thus determines the overall efficacy of synaptic transmission. Thirdly, Menkes et al. (1980) demonstrated that the intravenous administration of the direct postsynaptic receptor agonist 5-methoxy-N,N-dimethyltryptamine (5-MeODMT) also reveals the TCA-induced modification of 5-HT sensitivity detectable by microiontophoretic application of 5-HT. In accordance with this effect of TCA drugs, Friedman et al. (1983) observed an enhanced head-twitch response, a behavior mediated by activation of 5-HT receptors on motoneurons (Jacobs and Klemfuss, 1975), following a challenge dose of 5-MeODMT in rats chronically treated with the same TCA drugs.

As opposed to the generally enhanced response to 5-HT seen following repeated administration of TCA drugs, the responsiveness to NA varies with the region investigated. Where the response to NA is mediated by a β receptor, as in the cerebellum and cingulate cortex, it is decreased by TCA drug administration (Olpe and Schellenberg, 1980; Schultz et al., 1981). The absence of any modification to microiontophoretically-applied NA onto hippocampal pyramidal neurons is not entirely discordant with the binding studies discussed earlier. Although the electrophysiological response to NA in that region has been reported to be β in nature (Segal and Bloom, 1974), we have not been able to obtain a good blockade of the NA suppression of firing using the β antagonist sotalol (de Montigny, unpublished observations). Unfortunately, there exists no behavioral paradigm that would permit functional assessment of central β-adrenergic function.

In the facial motor nucleus and dLGN, where NA exerts its effects via an α_1 receptor, TCA drugs enhance in parallel both NA and 5-HT responses during the course of a chronic treatment (Menkes and Aghajanian, 1980; Menkes et al., 1981). These single-cell data are in agreement with other studies evaluating established α_1 function in the spinal cord following repeated TCA drug administration: firstly, an increase in the intensity of the startle reflex; secondly, an enhanced flexor reflex in the hind limb of spinal rats; and finally, an increase in postdecapitation convulsions (Menkes et al., 1983; Vetulani et al., 1983; Maj et al., 1983). These last two α_1 responses are paired with an increased number of α_1 receptors whereas the first is not attributable to such a modification of membranal receptors. It would be essential to assess α_1 responsiveness in regions of the limbic forebrain in which NA mediates its effect via this receptor in order to link this modification to the antidepressant effect.

The responsiveness of locus coeruleus neurons to clonidine, which is mediated by an α_2 receptor (Cedarbaum and Aghajanian, 1977), is not altered consistently by all TCA drugs following repeated administration (Svensson and Usdin, 1978; Scuvee-Moreau and Svensson, 1982). Consequently, modulation of the sensitivity of somatic α_2 receptors cannot account per se for the therapeutic effectiveness of TCA drugs. Since α_2 receptors are located both pre- and postsynaptically (see Timmermans and van Zwieten, 1982 for a review), modifications of α_2 binding parameters should be interpreted with great caution. Similarly, changes in blood pressure and plasma MHPG, a NA metabolite, in humans induced by a challenge dose of clonidine may reflect somatic, terminal as well as postsynaptic α_2 responsiveness.

Electroconvulsive Therapy. ECT is generally recognized as more effective than TCA drugs in the treatment of affective disorders (Royal College of Psychiatrists, 1977). De Montigny (1984) reported a selective increase in the responsiveness of forebrain neurons to 5-HT and 5-MeODMT, but not to NA or GABA, following repeated ECT (de Montigny, 1984). A single shock or repeated subconvulsive shocks were ineffective in producing this effect. An enhanced responsiveness of postsynaptic neurons has also been demonstrated by the group of Grahame-Smith using the 5-HT syndrome behavioral model (Costain et al., 1979). It is striking that two completely different treatments, such as TCA drugs and ECT, exert the same neurobiological effect. However, this unity in their mode of action may be less surprising given the following clinical observations: firstly, the symptomatic profile of TCA and ECT responders is quite similar (American Psychiatric Association, 1978); secondly, a favorable response to a TCA drug is a good predictor of a future response to ECT; and, finally, TCA drugs are effective in the prophylaxis of relapses in ECT responders (Seager and Bird, 1962; Kay et al., 1970; American Psychiatric Association, 1978).

Mianserin and Adinazolam. Mianserin, a tetracyclic compound, has been shown to enhance selectively the response of hippocampal pyramidal neurons to 5-HT following repeated, but not acute, administration (Blier et al., 1984). Using behavioral paradigms that assess 5-HT responsiveness, two groups have also shown a postsynaptic sensitization by mianserin (Mogilnicka and Klimek, 1979; Friedman et al., 1983).

Adinazolam, a triazolobenzodiazepine that exerts a rapid antidepressant effect (Pike et al., 1983), also enhances the responsiveness of hippocampal neurons to 5-HT following a 14-day treatment (Turmel and de Montigny, 1984). As is the case with TCA drugs, the responsiveness to 5-HT and NA in the dLGN was increased after 14 days of treatment whereas only that to 5-HT was augmented after 5 days of treatment (de Montigny and Turmel, 1984). This stands in contrast to the parallel enhancement of 5-HT and NA responses by repeated administration of TCA drugs in the facial motor nucleus (Menkes and Aghajanian, 1981). Given the early onset of therapeutic action of adinazolam, the clear dissociation between the time courses of sensitizations to 5-HT and to NA makes 5-HT a more probable candidate than NA for mediating the antidepressant response to adinazolam.

Nature and Therapeutic Significance of the Enhanced Postsynaptic Responsiveness to 5-HT. The results of electrophysiological and behavioral studies show that an increased 5-HT responsiveness of postsynaptic neurons, whether they are located in the spinal cord or in the forebrain, is produced by TCA drugs, ECT, mianserin or adinazolam. Activation of 5-HT receptors on motoneurons, denoted S_1 by Aghajanian (1981), results in facilitation of firing, whereas activation of diencephalic and proencephalic 5-HT receptors, denoted S_3 according to the same classification, produces a suppression of firing. It is striking that TCA drugs enhance the response to 5-HT of neurons bearing these two types of receptors mediating different responses, and which have different pharmacological properties (Haigler and Aghajanian, 1975). It is unlikely that this modification results from a simple alteration of membranal receptors since studies examining the number of tritiated 5-HT-labelled sites (5-HT_1) have yielded contradictory results for the same drug (for a review, see Anderson, 1983). The number of spiroperidol-labelled sites (5-HT_2) varies in opposite directions following TCA drugs and ECT (Kellar et al., 1981), whereas both treatments enhance the 5-HT responses of postsynaptic neurons. An increase in the efficacy of the postreceptor transducing system, common to the S_1 and S_3 receptors, might then appear a more plausible mechanism of action for these treatments.

A first clinical verification of the notion that TCA drugs exert their effect via the 5-HT system was provided by the study of Shopsin et al. (1975). They observed that the administration of a small dose of PCPA, a 5-HT synthesis inhibitor, to formerly depressed patients improved by imipramine treatment induced a relapse of depression. Discontinuation of PCPA treatment rapidly reinstated therapeutic remission. On the other hand, the administration of a NA synthesis inhibitor, α-methyl-p-tyrosine (α-MPT) was without effect when administered to some of the same patients.

Recently, two other clinical studies supported the notion that TCA drugs exert their therapeutic effect via an increased postsynaptic 5-HT responsiveness. Firstly, there is the rapid antidepressant effect of lithium in TCA-refractory patients. Within 48 hours of lithium addition to the regimen of patients treated with, but not responding to, a TCA drug, there is a marked alleviation of the depressive syndrome in most patients (de Montigny et al., 1981b; de Montigny et al., 1983; Cournoyer et al., 1984). The efficacy of this combination treatment has been confirmed by other groups (Joyce et al., 1982; Price et al., 1983; Heninger et al., 1983). The choice of lithium therapy was based on the fact that a 48-hour treatment in animal experiments enhances the activity of 5-HT neurons without affecting postsynaptic 5-HT responsiveness (Grahame-Smith and Green, 1974; Sangdee and Franz, 1978; Blier and de Montigny, 1983). Therefore, the greater amount of 5-HT reaching already sensitized forebrain neurons may well account for the rapid antidepressant effect of lithium in TCA-resistant patients.

Heninger and Charney (1983) provided a third piece of clinical evidence supporting the hypothesis. They used as a paradigm the increase in plasma prolactin (PRL) levels produced by acute intravenous injection of L-tryptophan. Long-term treatments with amitriptyline or desipramine increased PRL response. These results provide strong evidence that in humans, as well as in rats, long-term treatment with TCA drugs enhances the overall function of the central 5-HT system.

Presynaptic Site of Action

5-HT Reuptake Blocker. Another line of evidence supporting the notion that the 5-HT system plays a major role in antidepressant therapy is the efficacy of 5-HT reuptake blockers in major depression. Five such compounds have been shown to exert a definite antidepressant effect. They are: citalopram (Gastpar and Gastpar, 1982; Lindegaard-Pedersen et al., 1982; Ofsti, 1982), indalpine (Chazot et al., 1978; Guelfi et al., 1981; Shopsin et al., 1983), femoxetine (Dahl et al., 1982; Reebye et al., 1982), fluvoxamine (Saletu et al., 1977; Guelfi et al., 1983), and zimelidine (Coppen et al., 1979; Gershon et al., 1982). It is generally assumed that these compounds exert their therapeutic effect by increasing the availability of 5-HT in the synaptic cleft, thus enhancing 5-HT neurotransmission. Two possible objections to this assumption required electrophysiological investigation: firstly, the rapid action of these drugs on 5-HT reuptake appeared irreconciliable with their delayed therapeutic efficacy and, secondly, a sustained increase of 5-HT availability could produce a desensitization of postsynaptic neurons, cancelling out the increased 5-HT signal input. The net effect of zimelidine and indalpine on 5-HT neurotransmission was studied by assessing: (1) depression of firing rate of 5-HT neurons upon acute administration; (2) the responsiveness of forebrain neurons to microiontophoretically-applied 5-HT and (3) the response of these same neurons to electrical stimulation of the 5-HT ascending pathway after chronic administration; (4) the firing activity of 5-HT neurons during the course of repeated administration; and (5) the sensitivity of the 5-HT autoreceptor following long-term administration (de Montigny et al., 1981a; Blier and de Montigny, 1983; Blier et al., 1984).

Scuvee-Moreau et al. (1981) have demonstrated the close correlation between the ability of TCA drugs to depress in vivo the firing rate of dorsal raphe 5-HT neurons and their ability to block in vitro 5-HT reuptake in synaptosomal preparations. As is the case with TCA drugs, zimelidine, its demethylated metabolite norzimelidine, and indalpine reduced the firing rate of 5-HT neurons in close correlation with in vitro 5-HT reuptake measures (de Montigny et al., 1981a; Ross et al., 1977; Le Fur et al., 1978; Blier et al., 1984).

The responsiveness of hippocampal pyramidal neurons to microiontophoretically applied 5-HT, NA, and GABA was not modified following long-term zimelidine or indalpine treatments. These electrophysiological results are in agreement with the report of Fuxe et al. (1983), which showed no modifications of $5-HT_1$ binding characteristics in the hippocampus following a similar regimen of zimelidine. The period of suppression of firing of these neurons produced by the electrical stimulation of the 5-HT pathway in zimelidine-treated rats was enhanced. Since the response of postsynaptic neurons to iontophoretically-applied 5-HT is unchanged and the response to activation of the endogenous 5-HT pathway is increased, the enhanced 5-HT synaptic transmission must then be ascribed to a modification of the properties of the 5-HT neuron itself, presumably by 5-HT reuptake blockade. Nevertheless, the delay of about two weeks for the therapeutic onset of these drugs had to be reconciled with their ability to block 5-HT reuptake within minutes.

In an attempt to unravel this apparent discrepancy, we assessed the activity of dorsal raphe 5-HT neurons during the course of repeated administration of 5-HT reuptake blockers. Following two days of zimelidine or indalpine administration, the firing activity of 5-HT neurons was markedly decreased. After seven days of treatment, their firing activity had considerably recovered but was still lower than in controls. By day 14, however, 5-HT neurons exhibited a normal firing rate. The initial decrease was not unexpected, given the great potency of these 5-HT reuptake blockers in reducing the firing rate of 5-HT neurons upon acute administration; it was rather the restoration of firing activity which called for an explanation. The responsiveness of 5-HT neurons to the selective 5-HT autoreceptor agonist LSD (Haigler and Aghajanian, 1974) was determined at the end of the treatment. A greater than 50% decrease in responsiveness of these neurons to intravenous LSD suggested that desensitization of the 5-HT autoreceptor might account for the slow adaptation of 5-HT neurons during sustained 5-HT reuptake blockade. We have recently brought direct evidence, using microiontophoretic applications of 5-HT onto 5-HT neurons, for a desensitization of the 5-HT autoreceptor following long-term treatment with a 5-HT reuptake blocker (Blier et al., 1984).

In conclusion, a sustained blockade of 5-HT reuptake will not result in an increased 5-HT neurotransmission until 5-HT neurons resume their normal electrical activity.

<u>Monoamine Oxidase Inhibitors</u>. Brain MAO exists in two forms, A and B. 5-HT and NA are catabolized by the A enzyme whereas dopamine (DA) is deaminated by both forms. Thus, the fact that clorgyline, a selective MAOI-A, is an effective antidepressant drug (Herd, 1965; Wheatley, 1970; Lippec et al., 1979; Murphy et al., 1981) strongly suggests that an enhanced availability of 5-HT and/or NA might underlie the therapeutic effect of MAOIs in major depression. Both positive (Mann et al., 1982; Mendlewicz and Youdim, 1983) and negative (Mendis et al., 1981) results have been reported in placebo-controlled studies of the antidepressant effect of deprenyl, a preferential MAOI-B, in major depression. However, a definite conclusion concerning the possible involvement of MAO-B in the therapeutic effect of MAOI drugs awaits studies using a dose of deprenyl selective for MAO-B. Indeed, in the studies mentioned the dose of deprenyl administered was certainly impeding both forms of the enzyme, as indicated by the post-mortem study of Riederer et al.

(1981) who found a marked inhibition of MAO-A in Parkinsonian patients treated with an even smaller dose of deprenyl.

All MAOIs tested thus far have been shown to decrease the firing rate of 5-HT neurons (Aghajanian and Haigler, 1972; Scuvee-Moreau, 1981). This reduction of firing activity is attributable to an accumulation of 5-HT since a PCPA pretreatment prevents the MAOI-induced inhibition of 5-HT neurons. The firing rate of locus coeruleus NA neurons can also be depressed by acute administration of MAOI (Scuvee-Moreau, 1981). These results are consistent with the negative feedback role played by monoamine autoreceptors located on the soma of these neurons.

As far as the respective implication of 5-HT and NA systems in mediating the therapeutic effect of MAOI drugs is concerned, no electrophysiological study had ever compared the effect of long-term administration of these drugs on these systems. We recently undertook such a systematic study, using the same paradigm as for 5-HT reuptake blockers, of three MAOI drugs: phenelzine, clorgyline and deprenyl. Phenelzine is a non-selective MAOI. Clorgyline and deprenyl were administered at doses selective for the A and B forms of the enzyme, respectively.

Two daily administrations of phenelzine and clorgyline, at clinically relevant doses, markedly decreased the firing rate of dorsal raphe 5-HT neurons; after 7 days of treatment, a partial recovery of firing activity was evident; and, after 21 days, 5-HT neurons were firing at their normal level. At this time, the responsiveness of the 5-HT autoreceptor was assessed; the ED_{50} values of intravenous LSD were increased two-fold in phenelzine- and clorgyline-treated animals as compared to controls. The restoration of firing activity and the decreased response to LSD indicate that the 5-HT autoreceptor had desensitized during repeated administration of clorgyline and phenelzine. This modification of responsiveness must be due to inhibition of type A MAO since the deprenyl treatment failed to modify either the firing rate of 5-HT neurons or their response to LSD (Blier and de Montigny, 1984).

These data concerning the 5-HT neurons stand in contrast to those obtained for NA neurons. The firing rate of locus coeruleus NA neurons was markedly decreased after phenelzine and clorgyline treatments, with no evidence of restoration by day 21. The unmodified firing rate of NA neurons following long-term treatment with deprenyl suggests that this drug did not inhibit type A MAO to a degree sufficient to alter this index of presynaptic function. The ED_{50} value for clonidine, a specific agonist of the α_2 somatic autoreceptor (Cedarbaum and Aghajanian, 1977), was not significantly modified in any of the treatment groups. Cohen et al. (1982) reported a decrease in the number and affinity of clonidine-labelled α_2 sites in the brainstem of rats following the same clorgyline treatment as used here. There are two possible explanations for the discrepancy with our results. Firstly, the same population of α_2 receptors may not have been assessed by the two methods: α_2 receptors are also present in high concentrations in other brainstem nuclei (Young and Kuhar, 1978) which do not give rise to forebrain projections as does the locus coeruleus (Jones and Moore, 1975). Secondly, membrane characteristics can sometimes be changed without affecting biological responses. Our electrophysiological data indicate that 5-HT, but not NA, neurons modify their properties under chronic antidepressant MAOI treatments. As opposed to treatment with MAOIs, chronic imipramine treatment decreases α_2 autoreceptor responsiveness and increases the firing of NA neurons, whereas other TCA drugs are devoid of such effects (Svensson and Usdin, 1978; Scuvee-Moreau and Svensson, 1982). Since various antidepressant drugs exert differential effects on NA neurons, it is unlikely that the functional state of these neurons is directly implicated in the therapeutic effects of MAOI and TCA drugs. In keeping with this notion, α-MPT, an NA synthesis inhibitor, did not affect the MAOI- or TCA-induced remission of depressed patients (Shopsin et al., 1975, 1976).

In order to determine whether those presynaptic modifications resulted in altered synaptic efficacy at postsynaptic sites, we have studied in chronically treated rats the responses of hippocampal pyramidal neurons to exogenous 5-HT and NA, applied by microiontophoresis, and to endogenously released 5-HT and NA by electrical activation of the respective afferent pathways.

The responsiveness of hippocampal pyramidal neurons to microiontophoretically-applied NA was not modified by any of the pretreatments, whereas that to 5-HT was decreased only in the clorgyline-treated animals. This selective change may be attributable to the great potency of clorgyline to inhibit MAO-A at the regimen used (Campbell et al., 1979). Such a decreased responsiveness to 5-HT induced by clorgyline at postsynaptic sites has also been shown in the cerebral cortex using microiontophoretic techniques (Olpe and Schellenberg, 1980). Lucki and Frazer (1982) have demonstrated a decreased responsiveness of motoneurons using the behavioral 5-HT syndrome in phenelzine-treated rats. This discrepancy with our results might be attributed to differences in the regimen of phenelzine: they injected 10 mg/kg/day of phenelzine whereas we used 2.5 mg/kg/day, which is more likely to produce MAO inhibition resembling that which is produced by regimens used in depressed patients (Robinson et al., 1978; Raft et al., 1981). Similarly, decreases in the number of 5-HT$_1$, 5-HT$_2$ and β binding sites following repeated MAOI administration have been reported but, again, the doses used were higher than those utilized in our study (Savage et al., 1979; Lucki and Frazer, 1982).

Experiments aimed at determining the <u>net</u> effect of long-term MAOI treatment on monoaminergic neurotransmission are in progress in our laboratory. To this end, we compare the effects in MAOI-treated and control rats of electrical stimulation of the ascending 5-HT and NA pathways on the firing activity of dorsal hippocampus pyramidal neurons using peristimulus time histograms.

Preliminary results indicate that the effect of the stimulation of the NA pathway is unmodified by long-term MAOI treatment. The availability of NA being increased by clorgyline and phenelzine, one could have expected these drugs to enhance the effectiveness of the stimulation of the NA pathway. Their lack of effect might be due to the unmodified sensitivity of the α$_2$ autoreceptors at the level of the terminals (as documented for their somatic counterpart; see above). If this were the case, the enhanced availability of NA at the terminals, activating normosensitive α$_2$ autoreceptors, would result in a compensatory reduction of the amount of NA released per impulse.

On the other hand, inhibition of MAO-A by clorgyline or phenelzine potentiates the effect of stimulating the ascending 5-HT pathway. Given the decreased responsiveness of the postsynaptic neuron to microiontophoretically-applied 5-HT in clorgyline-treated rats (see above), the results of the stimulation experiments demonstrate that the enhancing presynaptic effect of clorgyline on 5-HT neurons overcomes the attenuation of responsiveness to 5-HT of the target neurons. These results underscore the necessity of assessing overall synaptic efficacy for a valid estimation of the net modification of a neurotransmission.

Two sets of clinical data support the notion that MAOIs exert their effect via the 5-HT system. Firstly, Shopsin et al. (1976), whose work with TCA drugs has already been mentioned, also observed a rapid relapse in depressed patients successfully treated with an MAOI when PCPA was added to their regimen. A marked improvement was observed shortly after discontinuation of the 5-HT synthesis inhibitor. Secondly, Nelson and Byck (1982) observed a very rapid amelioration of the depressive syndrome following lithium addition to the regimen of patients treated with, but not responding to, phenelzine. A heightened 5-HT neurotransmission most likely accounts for this effect: the increased synaptic availability of 5-HT, produced by the phenelzine pretreatment, would be unveiled by lithium which also augments the efficacy of 5-HT neurons, probably by increasing the release of 5-HT from terminals (Treiser et al., 1981). Although these two clinical trials have been carried out in a small number of patients, their clear and consistent results constitute strong evidence in support of the notion that MAOIs might exert their therapeutic effect via the 5-HT system.

Other Antidepressant Treatments. The following treatments have also been shown to be efficacious in major depression: 5-hydroxytryptophan (van Praag, 1981), β_2 agonists (Lecrubier et al., 1980; Lerer et al., 1981), trazodone (Cassano et al., 1974; Feighner, 1980), and one night's sleep deprivation (Roy-Byrne et al., 1984). Although these treatments have not yet been thoroughly studied by electrophysiological means in animals, there exists some data suggesting that they might also exert their therapeutic effect via the 5-HT system. Chronic administration of 5-HTP, the immediate precursor of 5-HT, may result in an increase of 5-HT availability which would produce modifications in 5-HT neurotransmission similar to those induced by 5-HT reuptake blockade. The increased brain turnover of 5-HT measured after chronic administration of β_2 agonists most likely results from an increased plasma level of free tryptophan (Nimgaonkar et al., 1982). As a result, the availability of 5-HT is likely to be augmented by these adrenergic drugs, and this might enhance the efficacy of 5-HT neurons. In fact, β_2 agonists have been shown to potentiate a 5-HT behavioral syndrome in rats (Ortman et al., 1981). As is the case with TCA drugs and mianserin, the 5-MeODMT-induced head-twitch response is increased by repeated trazodone administration (Friedman et al., 1983). This suggests that trazodone sensitizes S_1 postsynaptic receptors. It remains to be determined whether this drug exerts the same effect on forebrain S_3 receptors. Given the potent inhibitory effect of trazodone on 5-HT raphe neurons (Scuvee-Moreau and Dresse, 1983), this drug could also exert its therapeutic effect via a 5-HT autoreceptor desensitization, as do 5-HT reuptake blockers and MAOIs. Finally, the responsiveness to 5-HT of rat hippocampal neurons is enhanced immediately after 24-hour sleep deprivation (Brunel and de Montigny, unpublished observations).

In summary, the results of the electrophysiological single-cell studies suggest that an increased 5-HT neurotransmission is produced by various types of antidepressant treatments. TCA drugs, ECT, mianserin and adinazolam may exert their therapeutic effect through sensitization of postsynaptic neurons to 5-HT. 5-HT reuptake blockers may relieve depression through a sustained blockade of the 5-HT membranal pump which results ultimately in an increased efficacy of the presynaptic element. Similarly, long-term MAOI administration, by decreasing 5-HT catabolism, may also enhance 5-HT neurotransmission.

Conclusion
==========

Intensification of 5-HT functions seems to be an effect common to all antidepressant treatments thus far investigated. However, several lines of evidence suggest that this modification may only be a link in a chain of events leading to an antidepressant response. For example, the presence of the NA system seems essential for the development of postsynaptic sensitization to 5-HT by ECT or TCA drugs as this enhanced responsiveness cannot be obtained in NA-denervated animals (Green and Deakin, 1979; Gravel and de Montigny, 1983). This suggests that monoamine systems are closely interdependent. Indeed, selective 5-HT depletion, by 5,7-dihydroxytryptamine or PCPA, has revealed functional links between 5-HT, NA and DA systems using either biochemical or electrophysiological approaches. In particular, the affinity of cortical adrenergic receptors is decreased and the responsiveness of these neurons to microiontophoretically-applied NA and DA is also diminished quite drastically (Ferron et al., 1982; Janowsky et al., 1982). A subsensitivity of the DA autoreceptor has been shown to result following administration of TCA drugs, ECT or phenelzine (for review, see Antelman et al., 1982). Interestingly, this decreased electrophysiological responsiveness depends primarily on passage of time following treatment initiation. However, the clinical significance of this neurobiological modification still awaits clinical verification. Further studies on the interactions between monoamine systems may reveal other neurobiological modifications that are essential to obtain an antidepressant response. Fortunately, this task has already been eased with the introduction of antidepressant drugs that are specific for certain neuronal processes, as opposed to TCA drugs.

In summary, extensive studies on the β adrenergic system have disclosed a deamplification of the NA signal by various classes of antidepressant treatments. However, several factors make it unlikely that this neurobiological modification is the sole basis for the therapeutic effect of antidepressant treatments. As for the modification of 5-HT neurotransmission, the notion that its augmentation might mediate its effect, as yet, is fully congruent with available clinical data. The 5-HT system has intimate relationships with other monoamine and non-monoamine systems. Hence, a better understanding of the neurobiological basis of the therapeutic effect of antidepressant treatments might be provided in the near future by disclosing the effect of an enhanced 5-HT neurotransmission on other chemospecific neuronal systems.

References

Aghajanian, G. K. (1978) Feedback regulation of central monoaminergic neurons: evidence from single cell recording studies. In: Essays in Neurochemistry and Neuropharmacology, vol. 3 (Youdim, M. B. H., Lovenberg, W., Sharman, D. F., and Lagnado, J. R., eds), John Wiley and Sons, New York, pp. 1-33.

Aghajanian, G. K. (1981) The modulatory role of serotonin of multiple receptors in brain. In: Serotonin Neurotransmission and Behavior (Jacobs, B. L. and Gelperin, A., eds), MIT Press, Cambridge, Mass., pp. 156-185.

Aghajanian, G. K., Graham, A. W., and Sheard, M. H. (1972) Serotonin-containing neurons in brain: depression of firing by monoamine oxidase inhibitors. Science 169, 1100-1102.

Anderson, J. L. (1983) Serotonin receptor changes after chronic antidepressant treatments: ligand binding, electrophysiological, and behavioral studies. Life Sci. 32, 1791-1801.

Antelman, S. M., Chiodo, L. A., and De Giovanni, L. A. (1982) Antidepressants and dopamine autoreceptors: implications for both a novel means of treating depression and understanding bipolar illness. In: Typical and Atypical Antidepressants (Costa, E. and Racagni, G., eds), Raven Press, New York, pp. 121-132.

Asberg, M., Traskman, L., and Thoren, P. (1976) 5-HIAA in the cerebrospinal fluid--a biochemical suicide predictor? Arch. Gen. Psychiatry 33, 1193-1197.

Baudry, M., Martres, M. P., and Schwartz, J. C. (1976) Modulation in the sensitivity of noradrenergic receptors in the CNS studied by the responsiveness of the cyclic AMP system. Brain Res. 116, 111-124.

Baumann, P. and Maitre, L. (1977) Blockade of presynaptic α-receptors and of amine uptake in the rat brain by the antidepressant mianserin. Naunyn-Schmiedeberg's Arch. Pharmacol. 300, 31-37.

Blackshear, M. A. and Sanders-Bush, E. (1982) Serotonin receptor sensitivity after acute and chronic treatment with mianserin. J. Pharmacol. Exp. Therap. 314, 303-308.

Blaschko, H. (1974) The natural history of amine oxidases. Rev. Physiol. Biochem. Pharmacol. 70, 83-148.

Blier, P. and de Montigny, C. (1980) Effect of chronic antidepressant treatment on the serotoninergic autoreceptor: a microiontophoretic study in the rat. Naunyn-Schmiedeberg's Arch. Pharmacol. 314, 123-128.

Blier, P. and de Montigny, C. (1983) Electrophysiological investigations on the effect of repeated zimelidine administration on serotonergic neurotransmission in the rat. J. Neurosci. 3, 1270-1275.

Blier, P. and de Montigny, C. (1983) Enhancement of serotoninergic neurotransmission by short-term lithium treatment: electrophysiological studies in the rat. Soc. Neurosci. Abstr. 9, 428.

Blier, P. and de Montigny, C. (1984) The effect of repeated administration of monoamine oxidase inhibitor on the firing activity of serotoninergic and noradrenergic neurons. Proc. Collegium Internationale Neuro-Psychopharmacologicum (in press).

Blier, P., de Montigny, C., and Tardif, D. (1984) Effects of two antidepressant drugs, mianserin and indalpine, on the serotoninergic system: single-cell studies in the rat. Psychopharmacology (in press).

Bloch, R. G., Dooneief, A. S., Buchberg, A. S., and Spellman, S. (1954) The clinical effect of isoniazid and iproniazid in the treatment of pulmonary tuberculosis. Ann. Int. Med. 40, 881-900.

Campbell, I. C., Murphy, D. L., Gallager, D. W., and Tallman, J.-F. (1979) Neurotransmitter-related adaptation in the central nervous system following chronic monoamine oxidase inhibition. In: Monoamine Oxidase: Structure, Function, and Altered Functions (Singer, T. P., Van Korff, R. W., and Murphy, D. L., eds), Academic Press, Inc., New York, pp. 517-530.

Campbell, I. C., Robinson, D. S., Lovenberg, W., and Murphy, D. L. (1979) The effects of chronic regimens of clorgyline and pargyline in the rat brain. J. Neurochem. 32, 49-55.

Cassano, G. B., Castrogiovanni, P., and Conti, L. (1974) Clinical evaluation of trazodone in the treatment of depression. In: Modern Problems in Pharmacopsychiatry, vol. 9 (Bonanz, T. A. and Silvestrini, B., eds), pp. 199-204.

Cedarbaum, J. M. and Aghajanian, G. K. (1977) Catecholamine receptors on locus coeruleus neurons: pharmacological characterization. Eur. J. Pharmacol. 44, 375-385.

Chazot, G., Renaud, B., Henry, J. F., and Schott, B. (1978) Open clinical trials in 40 depressed patients showed a strong and rapid antidepressant effect associated with pronounced inhibition of 5-HT uptake. Proc. World Congress Biological Psychiatry **2**, 143.

Classen, V. (1983) Review of the animal pharmacology and pharmacokinetics of fluvoxamine. Brit. J. Pharmacol. **15**, 349S-355S.

Clements-Jewery, S. (1978) The development of cortical β-adrenoceptor subsensitivity in the rat by chronic treatment with trazodone, doxepin and mianserin. Neuropharmacology **17**, 779-781.

Cohen, R. M., Ebstein, R. P., Daly, J. W., and Murphy, D. L. (1982) Chronic effects of a monoamine oxidase-inhibiting antidepressant: decreases in functional α-adrenergic autoreceptors precede the decrease in norepinephrine-stimulated cyclic adenosine 3':5'-monophosphate systems in rat brain. J. Neurosci. **2**, 1588-1595.

Coppen, A. (1967) The biochemistry of affective disorders. Brit. J. Psychiatry **113**, 1237-1264.

Coppen, A., Ramo Rao, V. A., Swade, C., and Wood, K. (1979) Zimelidine: a therapeutic and pharmacokinetic study in depression. Psychopharmacology **63**, 199-202.

Costain, D. W., Green, A. R., and Grahame-Smith, D. G. (1979) Enhanced 5-hydroxytryptamine-mediated behavioural responses in rats following repeated electroconvulsive shock: relevance to the mechanism of the antidepressive effect of electroconvulsive therapy. Psychopharmacology **61**, 167-170.

Cournoyer, G., de Montigny, C., Ouellette, J., Leblanc, G., Langlois, R., and Elie, R. (1984) Lithium addition in tricyclic-resistant unipolar depression: a placebo-controlled study. Proc. Collegium Internationale Neuro-Psychopharmacologicum (in press).

Cowen, P. J., Fraser, S., Grahame-Smith, D. G., Green, A. R., and Stanford, C. (1983) The effect of chronic antidepressant administration on β-adrenoceptor function of the rat pineal. Brit. J. Psychiatry **78**, 89-96.

Crane, G. E. (1957) Iproniazid (Marsilid) phosphate, a therapeutic agent for mental disorders and debilitating disease. Psychiatric Research Reports **8**, 142-152.

Crews, F. T., Paul, S. M., and Goodwin, F. K. (1981) Acceleration of β-receptor desensitization in combined administration of antidepressants and phenoxybenzamine. Nature (Lond.) **290**, 787-789.

Dahl, L. E., Lundin, L., LeFevre Honore, P., and Dencker, S. J. (1982) Antidepressant effect of femoxetine and desipramine and relationship to the concentration of amine metabolites in cerebrospinal fluid. Acta psychiatr. scand. 66, 9-17.

de Montigny, C. (1984) Electroconvulsive shock treatments enhance responsiveness of forebrain neurons to serotonin. J. Pharmacol. Exp. Therap. 228, 230-234.

de Montigny, C. and Aghajanian, G. K. (1978) Tricyclic antidepressants: long term treatment increases responsivity of rat forebrain neurons to serotonin. Science 202, 1301-1306.

de Montigny, C., Blier, P., Caille, G., and Kouassi, E. (1981a) Pre- and postsynaptic effect of zimelidine and norzimelidine on the serotonergic system: single cell study in the rat. Acta psychiatr. scand. 63, (Suppl. 290), 79-90.

de Montigny, C., Cournoyer, G., Morissette, R., Langlois, R., and Caille, G. (1983) Further studies on the antidepressant effect of lithium addition in patients not responding to a tricyclic antidepressant drug. Arch. Gen. Psychiatry 40, 1327-1334.

de Montigny, C., Grunberg, F., Mayer, A., and Deschesne, J. P. (1981b) Lithium induces rapid relief of depression in tricyclic antidepressant drug non-responders. Brit. J. Psychiatry 138, 252-256.

de Montigny, C. and Turmel, A. (1984) Early sensitization of forebrain neurons to serotonin by an antidepressant triazolobenzodiazepine, adinazolam: a single cell recording microiontophoretic study in the rat. Proc. Collegium Internationale Neuro-Psychopharmacologicum (in press).

Descarries, L., Watkins, K. C., Garcia, S., and Beaudet, A. (1982) The serotonin neurons in nucleus raphe dorsalis of adult rat: a light and electron microscope radioautographic study. J. Compar. Neurol. 207, 239-254.

Feighner, J. P. (1980) Trazodone, a triazolopyridine derivative, in primary depressive disorders. J. Clin. Psychiatry 41, 250-255.

Ferron, A., Descarries, L., and Reader, T. A. (1982) Altered neuronal responsiveness to biogenic amines in rat cerebral cortex after serotonin denervation or depletion. Brain Res. 231, 93-108.

Frazer, A., Pandey, G., and Mendels, J. (1974) The effect of tri-iodothyronine in combination with imipramine on ^{3}H-cyclic AMP production in slices of rat cerebral cortex. Neuropharmacology 13, 1131-1140.

Friedman, E., Cooper, T. B., and Dallob, A. (1983) Effects of chronic antidepressant treatment on serotonin receptor activity in mice. Eur. J. Pharmacol. 89, 69-76.

Fuxe, K., Ogren, S. O., Agnati, L. F., Benfenati, F., Fredholm, B., Andersson, K., Zini, I., and Eneroth, P. (1983) Chronic antidepressant treatment and central 5-HT synapses. Neuropharmacology 22, 389-400.

Gallager, D. W. and Bunney, W. E. Jr. (1979) Failure of chronic lithium treatment to block tricyclic antidepressant-induced 5-HT supersensitivity. Naunyn-Schmiedeberg's Arch. Pharmacol. 307, 129-133.

Gandolfi, O., Barbaccia, M. L., Chuang, D. M., and Costa, E. (1983) Daily bupropion injections for 3 weeks attenuates the norepinephrine stimulation of adenylate cyclase and the number of β-adrenergic recognition sites in rat frontal cortex. Neuropharmacology 22, 927-929.

Gastpar, M. and Gastpar, G. (1982) Preliminary studies with citalopram (LU10-171), a specific 5-HT reuptake inhibitor, as antidepressant. Prog. Neuro-Psychopharmacol. & Biol. Psychiatry 6, 319-325.

Gershon, S. A., Georgotas, R., Newton, R., and Bush, D. (1982) Clinical evaluation of two new antidepressants. Adv. Biochem. Psychopharmacol. 32, 57-68.

Gillespie, D. D., Manier, D. H., Steranka, L. R., and Sulser, F. (1983) Tryptophan hydroxylase inhibition by p-chlorophenylalanine (PCPA): effect on DMI-induced changes of the norepinephrine (NE) receptor coupled adenylate cyclase in rat cortex. Soc. Neurosci. Abstr. 9, 714.

Gillespie, D. D., Manier, D. H., and Sulser, F. (1979) Rapid subsensitivity of the norepinephrine receptor-coupled adenylate cyclase system in brain linked to down-regulation of β-adrenergic receptor. Commun. Psychopharmacol. 3, 191-194.

Glowinski, J. and Axelrod, J. (1964) Inhibition of uptake of tritiated noradrenaline in the intact rat brain by imipramine and structurally related compounds. Nature (Lond.) 204, 1318-1319.

Goodwin, F. K. and Post, R. M. (1975) Studies of amine metabolites in affective illness and in schizophrenia. A comparative analysis. In: Biology of the Major Psychoses (Friedman, D. X., ed.), Raven Press, New York, pp. 299-332.

Grahame-Smith, D. G. and Green, A. R. (1974) The role of brain 5-hydroxytryptamine in the hyperactivity produced in rats by lithium and monoamine oxidase inhibition. Brit. J. Pharmacol. 52, 19-26.

Gravel, P. and de Montigny, C. (1983) Noradrenergic deprivation prevents tricyclic antidepressant-induced sensitization of rat forebrain neurons to serotonin. Soc. Neurosci. Abstr. 9, 429.

Green, A. R. and Deakin, J. F. W. (1980) Brain noradrenaline depletion prevents ECS-induced enhancement of serotonin- and dopamine-mediated behaviour. Nature (Lond.) 285, 232-233.

Greengard, P. (1976) Possible role for cyclic nucleotides and phosphorylated membrane proteins in postsynaptic actions of neurotransmitters. Nature (Lond.) 260, 101-108.

Guelfi, J. D., Dreyfus, J. F., Boyer, P., and Pichot, P. (1981) A double blind controlled multicenter trial comparing indalpine with imipramine. Proc. World Congress of Biological Psychiatry 3, F1023.

Guelfi, J. D., Dreyfus, J. F., Pichot, P., and (1983) A double-blind controlled clinical trial comparing fluovoxamine with imipramine. Brit. J. Clin. Pharmacol. 15, 4115-4175.

Haigler, H. J. and Aghajanian, G. K. (1974) Lysergic acid diethylamide and serotonin: comparison of effects on serotonergic neurons and neurons receiving a serotonergic input. J. Pharmacol. Exp. Therap. 188, 688-699.

Haigler, H. J. and Aghajanian, G. K. (1975) Peripheral serotonin antagonists: failure to antagonize serotonin in brain areas receiving a prominent serotonergic input. J. Neural Transm. 35, 257-273.

Hall, H., Sallermak, M., and Ross, S. B. (1980) Clenbuterol, a central β-adrenoceptor agonist. Acta Pharmacol. Toxicol. 47, 159-160.

Heninger, G. R., Charney, D. S., and Sternberg, D. E. (1983) Lithium carbonate augmentation of antidepressant treatments. Arch. Gen. Psychiatry 40, 1335-1342.

Heninger, G. R. and Charney, D. S. (1983) Impaired serotonergic function in depressed patients: augmentation by antidepressant treatment and lith-

ium. Soc. Neurosci. Abstr. 9, 1053.
Herd, J. A. (1969) A new antidepressant M & B 9302. A pilot study and a double-blind controlled trial. Clinical Trials 6, 219-225.
Heydorn, W. E., Brunswick, D. J., and Frazer, A. (1982) Effect of treatment of rats with antidepressants on melatonin concentrations in the pineal gland and serum. J. Pharmacol. Exp. Therap. 222, 534-543.
Hyttel, J. (1982) Citalopram-pharmacological profile of a specific serotonin uptake inhibitor with antidepressant activity. Prog. Neuro-Psychopharmacol. & Biol. Psychiatry 6, 277-295.
Hyttel, J., Overo, F., and Arnt, J. (1983) Citalopram-biochemical effects in rats after long-term administration. Proc. International Catecholamine Symposium (in press).
Jacobs, B. L. and Klemfuss, M. (1975) Brain stem and spinal cord mediation of a serotonergic behavioral syndrome. Brain Res. 100, 450-457.
Janowsky, A., Okada, F., Manier, D. H., Applegate, G. D., Sulser, F., and Steranka, L. R. (1982) Role of serotonergic input in the regulation of the β-adrenergic receptor-coupled adenylate cyclase system. Science 218, 900-901.
Johnson, R. W., Reisine, T., Spotnitz, S., Wiech, N., Ursillo, R., and Yamamura, H. I. (1980) Effects of desipramine and yohimbine on α- and β-adrenoreceptor sensitivity. Eur. J. Pharmacol. 67, 123-127.
Jones, B. E. and Moore, R. Y. (1975) Ascending projections of the locus coeruleus in the rat. II. Autoradiographic study. Brain Res. 127, 23-53.
Jones, R. S. G. (1980) Long-term administration of atropine, imipramine, and viloxazine alters responsiveness of rat cortical neurons to acetylcholine. Can. J. Physiol. Pharmacol. 58, 531-535.
Joyce, P. R., Hewland, H. R., and Jones, A. V. (1983) Rapid response to lithium in treatment-resistant depression. Brit. J. Psychiatry 142, 204-214.
Kanof, P. D. and Greengard, P. (1978) Brain histamine receptors as targets for antidepressant drugs. Nature (Lond.) 272, 329-333.
Kay, D. W. K., Fahy, T., and Garside, R. F. (1970) A seven-month double-blind trial of amitriptyline and diazepam in ECT-treated depressed patients. Brit. J. Psychiatry 117, 667-671.

Kellar, K. J., Cascio, C. S., Butler, J. A., and Kurtze, R. N. (1981) Differential effects of electroconvulsive shock and antidepressant drugs on serotonin-2 receptors in rat brain. Eur. J. Pharmacol. 69, 515-518.

Kline, N. S. (1978) Clinical experience with iproniazid (Marsilid). J. Clin. Exp. Psychopathol. 19, (Suppl. 1), 72-78.

Kuhn, R. (1958) The treatment of depressive states with G22355 (imipramine hydrochloride). Am. J. Psychiatry 115, 459-464.

Langer, S. Z. (1977) Presynaptic receptors and their role in the regulation of transmitter release. Brit. J. Pharmacol. 60, 481-497.

Lecrubier, Y., Puech, A. J., Jouvent, R., Simon, P., and Widlocher, D. (1980) A beta-adrenergic stimulant (Salbutamol) versus clomipramine in depression--a controlled study. Brit. J. Psychiatry 136, 354-358.

Le Fur, G., Kabouche, M., and Uzan, A. (1978) On the regional and specific serotonin uptake inhibition by LM 5008. Life Sci. 23, 1959-1966.

Lerer, B., Ebstein, R. P., and Belmakon, R. M. (1981) Subsensitivity of human β-adrenergic adenylate cyclase after salbutamol treatment of depression. Psychopharmacology 75, 169-172.

Lindegaard Pedersen, O., Kragh-Sovensen, P., Bjerre, M., Fredricson Overo, K., and Gram, L. F. (1982) Citalopram, a selective serotonin reuptake inhibitor: clinical antidepressive and long-term effect--a phase II study. Psychopharmacology 77, 199-204.

Lipper, S., Murphy, D. L., Slater, S., and Buchsbaum, M. S. (1979) Comparative behavioral effects of clorgyline and pargyline in man: a preliminary evaluation. Psychopharmacology 62, 123-128.

Lucki, I. and Frazer, A. (1982) Prevention of the serotonin syndrome in rats by repeated administration of monoamine oxidase inhibitors but not tricyclic antidepressants. Psychopharmacology 77, 205-211.

Maj, J., Gorka, Z., Melzacka, M., Rawlow, A., and Pilc, A. (1983) Chronic treatment with imipramine: further functional evidence for the enhanced responsiveness of noradrenergic system. Naunyn-Schmiedeberg's Arch. Pharmacol. 322, 256-260.

Mann, J. J., Fox Aarrons, S., Frances, A., Bernstein, W., Douglas, C., and Sickles, M. (1982) Symptoms of atypical depression as a predictor of response to L-deprenyl. Psychopharmacol. Bull.

19, 333-335.
Meltzer, H. Y., Wiita, B., Tricou, B. J., Simonovic, M., Fang, V., and Manov, G. (1982) Effect of serotonin precursors and serotonin agonists on plasma hormone levels. In: Serotonin in Biological Psychiatry (Ho, B. T., Schoolar, J. C., and Usdin, E., eds), Raven Press, New York, pp. 117-139.
Mendlewicz, J. and Youdim, M. B. H. (1983) L-Deprenil, a selective monoamine oxidase type B inhibitor, in the treatment of depression: a double-blind evaluation. Brit. J. Psychiatry 142, 508-511.
Mendis, N., Pare, C. M. B., Sandler, M., Glover, V., and Stern, G. M. (1981) Is the failure of (-)deprenyl, a selective monoamine oxidase B inhibitor, to alleviate depression related to freedom from the cheese effect? Psychopharmacology 73, 87-90.
Mengel, H. and Lund, I. (1982) Kinetics and effects of femoxetine and norfemoxetine in man. Proc. Collegium Internationale Neuro-Psychopharmacologicum 13, 78.
Menkes, D. B., Aghajanian, G. K., and McCall, R. B. (1980) Chronic antidepressant treatment enhances α-adrenergic and serotonergic responses in the facial nucleus. Life Sci. 27, 45-55.
Menkes, D. B. and Aghajanian, G. K. (1981) Alpha-1-adrenoceptor-mediated responses in the lateral geniculate nucleus are enhanced by chronic antidepressant treatment. Eur. J. Pharmacol. 74, 27-35.
Menkes, D. B., Kehne, J. M., Gallager, D. W., Aghajanian, G. K., and Davis, M. (1983) Functional supersensitivity of CNS α-adrenoceptors following chronic antidepressant treatment. Life Sci. 33, 181-188.
Mishra, R., Gillespie, D. D., Youdim, M., and Sulser, F. (1982) Effect of selective inhibition of MAO A or MAO B on the norepinephrine (NE) receptor-coupled adenylate cyclase system in rat cortex. Fed. Proc. 41, 1066.
Mishra, R., Janowsky, A., and Sulser, F. (1979) Subsensitivity of NE receptor-coupled adenylate cyclase system in brain. Effects of nisoxetine or fluoxetine. Eur. J. Pharmacol. 60, 379-382.
Mishra, R., Janowsky, A., and Sulser, F. (1980) Action of mianserin and zimelidine on the norepinephrine receptor-coupled adenylate cyclase system in brain: subsensitivity without reduction in β-adrenergic receptor binding. Neuropharma-

cology 19, 983-987.
Mogilnicka, E., Arbilla, S., Depoortere, H., and Langer, S. Z. (1980) Rapid-eye-movement sleep deprivation decreases the density of ^{3}H-dihydroalprenolol and ^{3}H-imipramine binding sites in the rat cerebral cortex. Eur. J. Pharmacol. 65, 289-292.
Mogilnicka, E. and Klimek, V. (1979) Mianserin, danitracen and amitriptyline withdrawal increases the behavioural responses of rats to L-5-HTP. J. Pharmac. Pharmacol. 31, 704-705.
Moore, K. E., Carr, L. A., and Dominic, J. A. (1970) Functional significance of amphetamine-induced release of brain catecholamines. In: Amphetamine and Related Compounds (Costa, E. and Garaltini, S., eds), Raven Press, New York, pp. 371-384.
Murphy, D. L., Lipper, S., Pickar, D., Jimerson, D., Cohen, R. M., Garrick, N. A., Alterman, I. S., and Campbell, I. C. (1981) Selective inhibition of monoamine oxidase type A: clinical antidepressant effects and metabolic changes in man. In: Monoamine Oxidase Inhibitors: The State of the Art (Youdim, M. B. H. and Paykel, E. S., eds), John Wiley & Sons, New York, pp. 189-205.
Nagy, A. and Johansson, R. (1977) The demethylation of imipramine and clomipramine as apparent from their plasma kinetics. Psychopharmacology 54, 125-131.
Nelson, J. C. and Byck, R. (1982) Rapid response to lithium in phenelzine non-responders. Brit. J. Psychiatry 141, 85-86.
Nimgaonkar, V. L., Green, A. R., Cowen, P. J., Heal, D. J., Grahame-Smith, D. G., and Deakin, J. F. W. (1983) Studies on the mechanisms by which clenbuterol, a β-adrenoceptor agonist, enhances 5-HT mediated behaviour and increases metabolism of 5-HT in the brain of the rat. Neuropharmacology 22, 739-749.
Ofsti, E. (1982) Citalopram--a specific 5-HT-reuptake inhibitor as an antidepressant drug: a phase II multicentre trial. Prog. Neuro-Psychopharmacol. & Biol. Psychiatry 6, 327-335.
Olpe, H. R. and Schellenberg, A. (1980) Reduced sensitivity of neurons to noradrenaline after chronic treatment with antidepressant drugs. Eur. J. Pharmacol. 63, 7-13.
Olpe, H. R. and Schellenberg, A. (1981) The sensitivity of cortical neurons to serotonin: effect of chronic treatment with antidepressants, serotonin-uptake inhibitors and monoamine-oxidase blocking drugs. J. Neural Transm. 51, 233-244.

Olpe, H. R., Schellenberg, A., and Steinmann, M. W. (1981) Differential actions of mianserin and iprindole on the sensitivity of cortical neurons to noradrenaline: effect of chronic treatment. Eur. J. Pharmacol. 72, 381-385.

Ortmann, R., Martin, S., Radeke, E., and Delini-Sutla, A. (1981) Interaction of β-adrenoceptor agonists with the serotonergic system in rat brain: a behavioral study using the L-5-HTP syndrome. Naunyn-Schmiedeberg's Arch. Pharmacol. 36, 225-230.

Petrie, W. M., Maffucci, R. J., and Woosley, R. L. (1982) Propranolol and depression. Am. J. Psychiatry 139, 92-94.

Pyke, R. E., Cohn, J. B., Feighner, J. P., and Smith, W. T. (1983) Open-label studies of adinazolam in severe depression. Psychopharmacol. Bull. 19, 96-98.

Price, L. H., Conwell, Y., and Nelson, J. C. (1983) Lithium augmentation of combined neuroleptic-tricyclic treatment in delusional depression. Am. J. Psychiatry 3, 318-322.

Raft, D., Davidson, J., Wasik, J., and Mattox, A. (1981) Relationship between response to phenelzine and MAO inhibition in a clinical trial of phenelzine, amitriptyline and placebo. Neuropsychobiology 7, 122-126.

Reebye, P. N., Yiptong, C., Samsoon, J., Schulsinger, F., and Fabricius, J. (1982) A controlled double-blind study of femoxetine and amitriptyline in patients with endogenous depression. Pharmacopsychiatry 15, 164-169.

Reisine, T. D., U'Prichard, D. C., Wiech, N. L., Ursillo, R. C., and Yamamura, H. I. (1980) Effects of combined administration of amphetamine and iprindole on brain adrenergic receptors. Brain Res. 188, 587-592.

Riederer, P., Reynolds, G. P., and Youdim, M. B. H. (1981) Selectivity of MAO inhibitors in human brain and their clinical consequences. In: Monoamine Oxidase Inhibitors: The State of the Art (Youdim, M. B. H. and Paykel, E. S., eds), John Wiley & Sons, New York, pp. 87-102.

Robinson, D. S., Nies, A., Ravaris, C. L., Ives, J. O., and Bartlett, D. (1978) Clinical psychopharmacology of phenelzine: MAO activity and clinical response. In: Psychopharmacology: A Generation of Progress (Lipton, M. A., DiMascio, A., and Killam, K. F., eds), Raven Press, New York, 961-973.

Ross, S. B., Hall, H., Renyi, A. L., and Westerlund, D. (1981) Effects of zimelidine on serotoninergic and noradrenergic neurons after repeated administration in the rat. Psychopharmacology 72, 219-225.

Ross, S. B. and Renyi, A. L. (1975a) Tricyclic antidepressant agents. I. Comparison of the inhibition of the uptake of ^{3}H-noradrenaline and ^{14}C-5-hydroxytryptamine in slices and crude synaptosome preparations of midbrain-hypothalamus regions of the rat brain. Acta Pharmacol. Toxicol. 36, 382-394.

Ross, S. B. and Renyi, A. L. (1975b) Tricyclic antidepressant agents. II. Effect of oral administration of the uptake of ^{3}H-noradrenaline and ^{14}C-5-hydroxytryptamine in slices of the midbrain-hypothalamus region of the rat. Acta Pharmacol. Toxicol. 36, 395-408.

Ross, S. B. and Renyi, A. L. (1977) Inhibition of the neuronal uptake of 5-hydroxytryptamine and noradrenaline in rat brain by (Z)- and (E)-3-(4-bromophenyl)-N,N-dimethyl-3-(3-pyridyl) allylamines and their secondary analogues. Neuropharmacology 16, 57-63.

Roy-Byrne, P. P., Uhde, T. W., and Post, R. M. (1984) Antidepressant effects of one night's sleep deprivation: clinical and theoretical implications. In: Neurobiology of Mood Disorders (Post, R. M. and Ballenger, J. C., eds), Williams and Wilkins, Baltimore, pp. 817-835.

Saavedra, J. M. and Axelrod, J. (1976) Octopamine as a putative neurotransmitter. In: Advances in Biochemical Psychopharmacology, vol. 15 (Costa, E., Giacobini, E., and Paolotti, R., eds), Raven Press, New York, pp. 95-110.

Saletu, B., Schjerve, M., Grunberger, J., Schanda, H., and Arnold, O. H. (1977) Fluvoxamine--a new serotonin re-uptake inhibitor: first clinical and psychometric experiences in depressed patients. J. Neural Transm. 41, 17-36.

Sangdee, C. and Franz, D. N. (1978) Lithium-induced enhancement of 5-HT transmission at a central synapse. Commun. Psychopharmacol. 2, 191-198.

Savage, D. D., Frazer, A., and Mendels, J. (1979) Differential effects of monoamine oxidase inhibitors and serotonin reuptake inhibitors on ^{3}H-serotonin receptor binding in rat brain. Eur. J. Pharmacol. 58, 87-88.

Schildkraut, J. J. (1965) The catecholamine hypothesis of affective disorders: a review of supporting evidence. Am. J. Psychiatry 122, 509-522.

Schultz, J. (1976) Psychoactive drug effects on a system which generates cyclic AMP in brain. Nature (Lond.) 261, 417-418.

Schultz, J. E., Siggins, G. R., and Schocker, F. W. (1981) Effects of prolonged treatment with lithium and tricyclic antidepressants on discharge frequency, norepinephrine responses and beta receptor binding in rat cerebellum: electrophysiological and biochemical comparison. J. Pharmacol. Exp. Therap. 216, 28-38.

Scuvee-Moreau, J. (1981) Contribution experimentale à l'étude du mode d'action des substances antidepressives. D.Sc. thesis, Université de Liege.

Scuvee-Moreau, J. and Dresse, A. R. (1979) Effect of various antidepressant drugs on the spontaneous firing rate of locus coeruleus and dorsal raphe neurons of the rat. Eur. J. Pharmacol. 57, 219-225.

Scuvee-Moreau, J. J. and Dresse, A. (1983) Effect of trazodone on the firing rate of central monoaminergic neurons. Comparison with various antidepressants. Arch. Int. Pharmacodyn. 260, 299-301.

Scuvee-Moreau, J. J. and Svensson, T. H. (1982) Sensitivity in vivo of central α_2- and opiate receptors after chronic treatment with various antidepressants. J. Neural Transm. 54, 51-63.

Seager, C. P. and Bird, R. L. (1962) Imipramine with electrical treatment in depression. A controlled trial. J. Ment. Sci. 108, 704-707.

Segal, S. and Bloom, F. E. (1974) The action of norepinephrine in the rat hippocampus. I. Iontophoretic studies. Brain Res. 72, 79-97.

Selikoff, I. J., Robityck, E. H., and Ornstein, G. G. (1952) Toxicity of hydrazine derivatives of isonicotinic acid in chemotherapy of human tuberculosis. Quarterly Bulletin of Seaview Hospital 13, 17-26.

Sellinger-Barnette, M. M., Mendels, J., and Frazer, A. (1980) The effect of psychoactive drugs on beta-adrenergic receptor binding sites in rat brain. Neuropharmacology 19, 447-454.

Sheard, M. H., Zolovick, A., and Aghajanian, G. K. (1972) Raphe neurons: effect of tricyclic antidepressant drugs. Brain Res. 43, 690-694.

Shopsin, B., Friedman, E., and Gershon, S. (1976) Para-chlorophenylalanine reversal of tranylcypromine effects in depressed patients. Arch. Gen. Psychiatry 33, 811-819.

Shopsin, B., Gershon, S., Goldstein, F., Friedman, F., and Wilk, S. (1975) Use of synthesis inhibitors in defining a role for biogenic amines during imipramine treatment in depressed patients. Commun. Psychopharmacol. 1, 239-249.

Shopsin, B., Lefebvre, C., and Maulet, C. (1983) Indalpine (LM-5008): an open study in depressed outpatients. Curr. Ther. Res. 34, 239-252.

Sulser, F. (1983) Deamplification of noradrenergic signal transfer by antidepressants: a unified catecholamine-serotonin hypothesis of affective disorders. Psychopharmacol. Bull. 19, 300-304.

Sulser, F. and Janowsky, A. (1982) Receptors, receptor sensitivity, and receptor regulation in the CNS. In: Serotonin in Biological Psychiatry (Ho, B. T., Schoolar, J. C., and Usdin, E., eds), Raven Press, New York, pp. 141-153.

Svensson, T. H. and Usdin, T. (1978) Feedback inhibition of brain noradrenaline neurons by tricyclic antidepressants: α-receptor mediation. Science 202, 1089-1091.

Svensson, T. H., Dahlof, C., Engberg, G., and Hallberg, M. (1981) Central pre- and postsynaptic monoamine receptors in antidepressant therapy. Acta psychiatr. scand. 63 (Suppl. 290), 67-78.

Timmermans, P. B. and van Zwieten, P. A. (1982) α_2-Adrenoceptors: classification, localization, mechanisms and targets for drugs. J. Med. Chem. 25, 1389-1401.

Treiser, S. L., Cascio, C. S., O'Donohue, T. L., and Kellar, K. (1981) Lithium increases serotonin release and decreases serotonin receptors in the hippocampus. Science 213, 1529-1531.

Tsukamoto, T., Asakura, M., and Hasegawa, K. (1982) Long-term antidepressant treatment increases α_2-adrenergic receptor binding in rat cerebral cortex and hippocampus. Advances in the Biosciences 40, 147-151.

Turmel, A. and de Montigny, C. (1984) Sensitization of rat forebrain neurons to serotonin by adinazolam, an antidepressant triazolobenzodiazepine. Eur. J. Pharmacol. (in press).

van Praag, H. M. (1981) Management of depression with serotonin precursors. Biol. Psychiatry 16, 291-310.

Vetulani, J. and Pilc, A. (1982) Post-decapitation convulsions in the rat measured with an animex mobility meter: relation to central α_1-adrenoceptors. Eur. J. Pharmacol. 85, 269-275.

Vetulani, J., Stawarz, R. J., Dingell, J. V., and Sulser, F. (1976) A possible common mechanism of action of antidepressant treatments. Naunyn-Schmiedeberg's Arch. Pharmacol. **293,** 109-114.

Vetulani, J. and Sulser, F. (1975) Action of various antidepressant treatments reduce reactivity of noradrenergic cyclic AMP-generating system in limbic forebrain. Nature (Lond.) **257,** 495-496.

Vogel, G. W., Vogel, F., McAbee, R. S., and Thurmond, A. J. (1980) Improvement of depression by REM sleep deprivation: new findings and a theory. Arch. Gen. Psychiatry **37,** 247-253.

Waal, H. J. (1967) Propanolol-induced depression. Brit. Med. J. **2,** 50.

Wang, R. Y. and Aghajanian, G. K. (1980) Enhanced sensitivity of amygdaloid neurons to serotonin and norepineprhine after chronic antidepressant treatment. Commun. Psychopharmacol. **4,** 83-90.

Welch, J. J., Kim, K. H., and Liebman, J. (1981) Trazodone enhances locus coeruleus firing rates: evidence for relative lack of adrenoreceptor involvement. Soc. Neurosci. Abstr. **7,** 645.

Wheatley, D. (1970) Comparative trial of a new monoamine oxidase inhibitor in depression. Brit. J. Psychiatry **117,** 573-574.

Wolfe, B. B., Morden, T. K., and Sporn, J. R. (1978) Presynaptic modulation of beta-adrenergic receptors in rat cerebral cortex after treatment with antidepressants. J. Pharmacol. Exp. Therap. **207,** 446-457.

Youdim, M. B. H. and Finberg, J. P. M. (1983) Implications of MAO-A and MAO-B inhibition for antidepressant therapy. Modern Problems in Pharmacopsychiatry **19,** 63-74.

Young, W. S. and Kuhar, M. J. (1980) Noradrenergic α_1 and α_2 receptors: light microscopic autoradiographic localization. Proc. Nat. Acad. Sci. USA **77,** 1696-1700.

Zanko, M. T. and Biegon, A. (1983) Increased β-adrenergic receptor binding in human frontal cortex. Soc. Neurosci. Abstr. **13,** 719.

Zsilla, G., Barbaccia, M. L., Gandolfi, O., Knoll, F., and Costa, E. (1983) (L)-Deprenyl, a selective MAO 'B' inhibitor, increases ^{3}H-imipramine binding and decreases β-adrenergic receptor function. Eur. J. Pharmacol. **89,** 111-117.

12.

METABOLISM OF DRUGS USED IN AFFECTIVE DISORDERS

M. V. Rudorfer and W. Z. Potter

Given the serendipitous nature of the discovery of most of the drugs used in the treatment of affective disorders, it is not surprising that our understanding of how and why they work has lagged behind their clinical use. Thus in the 1950s an exaggerated view of the toxicity of these agents developed since, for instance, imipramine, was sometimes used in 600 mg intramuscular doses, iproniazid was combined unknowingly with tyramine-rich foods, and lithium was marketed casually as a salt substitute. After this, recommended doses were set rather low. Even at the present time, the sole therapeutic intervention required with some depressed patients referred to clinical psychopharmacologists consists of increasing (or decreasing) an inappropriate dose of the medication they are already taking. All of these examples have resulted from inadequate knowledge of how certain drugs are handled by the body.

With the development of specific and sensitive chemical assays, and in some cases bioassays, which permitted precise measurement of most antidepressant and antimanic compounds, metabolism of these agents became subject to study both in animals and humans. Pathways of drug biotransformation and understanding of the factors that can alter them are still under investigation.

In this chapter we will describe the current state of knowledge in this field, integrating basic and clinical investigations with the bridge of pharmacokinetics. Our underlying theme will be clinical application, as we explore how knowledge of metabolism of mood-altering drugs, including an appreciation of their kinetics, interactions, and active metabolites, can enhance their use in patients with affective illness.

Metabolism of Drugs Used in Affective Disorders

Biological Framework of Antidepressant Metabolism
==

As lipophilic exogenous compounds, antidepressants are subject to multiple biotransformation steps, yielding polar metabolites which are excreted renally. The major site of this drug metabolism is the liver, where tricyclic antidepressants (TCAs) undergo mainly demethylation and hydroxylation, followed by glucuronide coupling (Gram, 1974). Mixed-function oxidases in hepatic microsomes catalyze most of the oxidative reactions involved, centering in a hemoprotein (cytochrome P450) requiring NADPH and molecular oxygen (Gillette, 1971), with subsequent glucuronidation mediated by liver transferase enzymes. In addition to the intrinsic clearance represented by hepatic oxidation, the physiologic context of drug presentation to the liver, including factors such as hepatic blood flow and binding of drug to blood proteins and to tissues, influences the rate of antidepressant metabolism (Wilkinson and Shand, 1975).

In a series of experiments on TCA metabolism in various liver preparations of the rat, von Bahr (1972) demonstrated very high affinity of tricyclics and their metabolites for oxidized P450. This non-specific intracellular binding is associated with nearly complete hepatic uptake of both free and bound imipramine (IMI) (Stegmann and Bickel, 1977) or nortriptyline (NT) (von Bahr et al., 1973) in perfused rat liver. Studies in animal and human liver microsomes have demonstrated product inhibition of hydroxylation (von Bahr and Bertilsson, 1971; Mellstrom and von Bahr, 1981). TCA metabolism by specific pathways in these preparations agrees with in vivo clearance (Cl) results (Mellstrom et al., 1983a), with hydroxylation rate independent of glucuronide conjugation (von Bahr and Bertilsson, 1971). Evidence that IMI may be metabolised during intestinal absorption (Nagy, 1977), not seen during portal catheterisation (Dencker et al., 1976), was recently confirmed by direct incubation of labelled drug with small intestine microsomes from guinea pig (Christ et al., 1983), though metabolites appeared in proportions different from those from liver microsome transformation. Although TCA metabolism has also been observed in other organs, such as lung, in some species, it is hepatic metabolism that is felt to be of clinical relevance in man (Gram, 1974).

Metabolism of Drugs Used in Affective Disorders

First-Pass Metabolism

In TCA use in humans the above drug factors of high lipid solubility and extremely high affinity for hepatic microsomal cytochrome P450 result in significant 'first-pass' metabolism as drug flows through the liver via the portal vein to the hepatic vein prior to entering the systemic circulation. This is much greater following oral or (in animals) intraperitoneal administration compared with intravenous (IV) infusion or intramuscular (IM) injection (Nagy and Johansson, 1975). Consequently, bioavailability is maximal with intravenous administration, as calculated from the ratio of the area under the plasma concentration versus time curves (AUCs) following oral and IV presentation of the same dose, respectively, assuming complete absorption of the former (Crammer et al., 1969). Oral TCA dosing yields higher concentrations of demethylated (Nagy and Johansson, 1975) and hydroxylated metabolites (Alvan et al., 1977) than does parenteral administration, demonstrating that active drug metabolism, possibly saturable (Beaubien and Pakuts, 1979; Burch and Hullin, 1981; Erlandsen and Gram, 1982), and not just nonspecific TCA uptake and binding in the liver is responsible for the first-pass effect.

First-pass metabolism of several TCAs has been quantitated in man. Utilising the method of relative AUCs for oral and parenteral administration, Alexanderson et al. (1973) found a 30-44% extent of first-pass metabolism of NT. Other similar studies with this drug yielded comparable results of 41-54% in two investigations (Gram and Fredricson Overo, 1975; Niazi, 1976) and 26-59% in another (Alvan et al., 1977). A wider range of values has been seen with IMI, from 23-71% (Nagy and Johansson, 1975; Gram and Christiansen, 1975). In the absence of intravenous kinetic data, metabolism of other TCAs after oral dosing has been used to evaluate bioavailability (=1 - first-pass metabolism), assuming typical hepatic blood flow (Q) of 1500 ml/min, as equal to $Q/(Q + dose/AUC)$. By this technique, the estimated first-pass metabolism of protriptyline (PRO) was relatively small, with a range of 10-25% (Ziegler et al., 1978b). The most extensive first-pass metabolism has been reported for doxepin (DOX), averaging 70% (Virtanen et al., 1980; Faulkner et al., 1983) with a range of 55-87% (Ziegler et al., 1978c), consistent with the common clinical observation that chronic DOX use produces lower steady-state plasma concentrations than the same dose of other tricyclics. Thirty to 69% of an oral dose of amitriptyline (AT) is extracted during the first pass through the liver (Burch and Hullin, 1981).

Metabolic Routes of TCAs

Hepatic metabolism of antidepressants is so complete that very little of an administered dose is excreted unchanged. Gram (1974) has summarised findings in urine after IMI administration to humans as consisting of 1-4% IMI + DMI, 15-35% other nonconjugated metabolites, 40-60% glucuronide metabolites, and 20-30% nonextractable polar metabolites (Christiansen et al., 1967; Crammer et al., 1968). Use of a single oral dose of [^{14}C]-IMI (Crammer et al., 1969) yielded 15 identifiable metabolites in urine, resulting from various combinations of demethylation (to desipramine [DMI] and, to a lesser extent, didesmethylimipramine), dealkylation of the entire side-chain to iminodibenzyl (IDB), hydroxylation in the central ring system at the 2- (or 10-) position with subsequent conjugation, and N-oxidation in the side chain (Figure 12.1). Quantitatively, the most important IMI metabolites were 2-OH-DMI (free plus conjugated, 40%), 2-OH-IMI (25%), and 2-OH-IDB (15%). Methodological limitations may have interfered with identification of trace metabolites (Gram, 1977). Conjugated plus unconjugated OH-NT accounted for 55% of an oral dose of AT (Vandel et al., 1982). Similarly, the 10-hydroxy metabolite in urine represented 49% (Alexanderson and Borga, 1973) or 43% (Mellstrom et al., 1981) of an oral dose of NT, and 2-OH-DMI, an average of 38% of DMI 100 mg orally (Potter et al., 1982). The significance of the biologically active hydroxy metabolites will be considered below.

In considering the pattern of antidepressant metabolic routes, it should be noted that both TCAs and their metabolites undergo enterohepatic circulation (Dencker et al., 1976; Beaubien and Pakuts, 1979; Erlandsen and Gram, 1982). The failure to account for drug excretion via bile and feces may have contributed to the common recovery of only 60-70% of administered TCAs (Alexanderson and Borga, 1973; Vandel et al., 1982; Rudorfer et al., 1984b).

Distribution of TCAs to human brain has been quantitated in cases of fatal overdose. Bickel et al. (1967) reported high levels of DMI with no trace of 2-OH-DMI in the brain of a child who died 6-1/2 hr after ingestion of 2500 mg of DMI. However, multiple hydroxy metabolites as well as parent drug

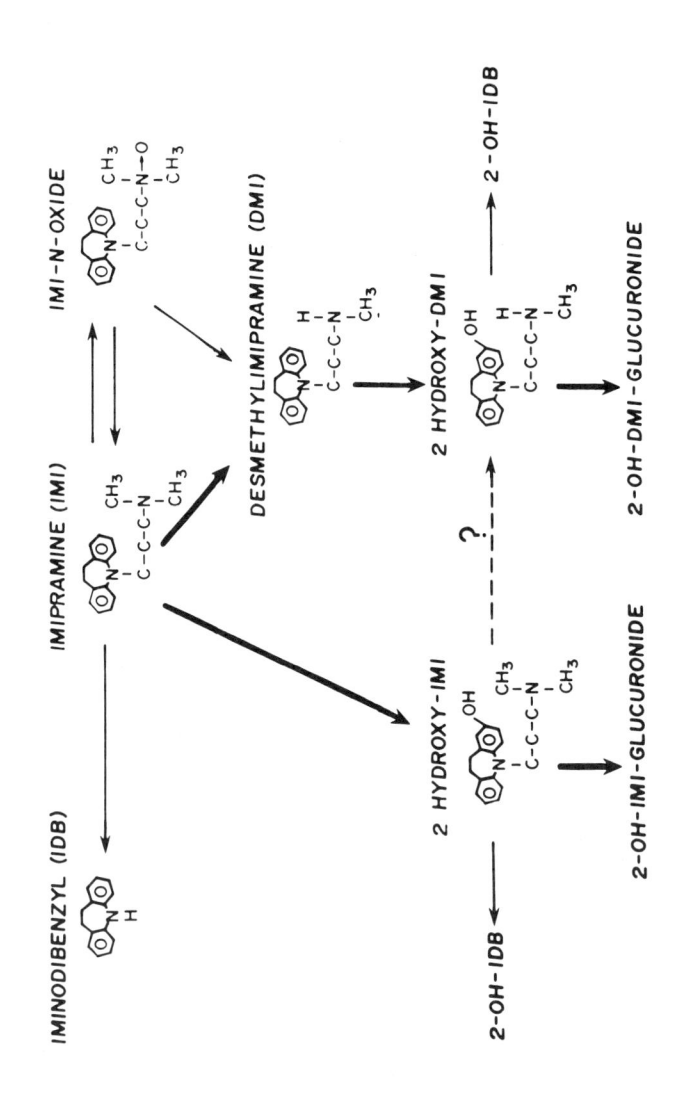

Metabolism of Drugs Used in Affective Disorders

Figure 12.1: Pathways of imipramine metabolism in man

were identified in the brain of an adult whose death occurred following an IMI overdose of unknown amount (Christiansen and Gram, 1973). More recently, uneven brain distribution, with mean concentrations of drugs and demethylated metabolites up to several times those in plasma, has been observed in rats given IMI and clomipramine (CMI) (Nagy, 1977; Friedman and Cooper, 1983). During actual clinical treatment of patients with IMI, concentrations of IMI plus DMI in the cerebrospinal fluid (CSF) equalled 12% of those in plasma, with a close correlation between drug levels in the two fluids (Muscettola et al., 1978), the latter in contrast to an earlier report (Sathananthan et al., 1976). A greater than 0.9 correlation has also been noted between plasma and CSF levels for drug and for 2-OH metabolite during DMI treatment (Potter et al., 1982).

Demethylation

Other aspects of TCA demethylation have attracted interest. In large series of patients the ratio between parent tertiary amine and demethylated secondary amine plasma concentration was about 1 for IMI (Gram et al., 1977; Muscettola et al., 1978), >1 for AT (Montgomery et al., 1979) and, in a small group, <0.5 for CMI (Linnoila et al., 1982) with wide inter-subject variability. IMI to DMI concentration in the CSF, however, was 0.8, lower than that in plasma (Muscettola et al., 1978). The inverse of this ratio, referred to as the 'demethylation rate', was correlated with clinical improvement in one group of AT-treated patients (Jungkunz and Kuss, 1978) but not another (Coppen and Rama Rao, 1979). It should be noted, however, that such a ratio is determined not just by the rate of demethylation of the parent drug, but also by the clearance of the demethylated metabolite, which is primarily dependent on hydroxylation (Potter et al., 1984).

More detailed studies of AT demethylation (Rollins et al., 1980) quantitated the fraction of a single oral dose converted to NT as the ratio of NT plasma AUCs under two conditions: after AT administration and again after direct administration of NT, yielding a wide range of 25-89% in 6 volunteers. In that study AT demethylation was significantly correlated with oral Cl of AT. Failure to measure any NT after intramuscular injection of AT (ibid.) was subsequently found to be a methodological error of the HPLC assay used (Mellstrom et al., 1982); with mass fragmentography NT AUC was equivalent with the two routes of AT administration, in contrast to the lack of desmethylCMI in 4 of 5 volunteers given IM CMI (Nagy and Johansson, 1977). The latter authors found a higher parent drug/demethylated metabolite ratio with IM versus oral use of either chronic CMI or chronic or acute (Nagy and Johansson, 1975) IMI: no other type of intervention or interaction is able to reduce the level of demethylated TCA metabolites (see below).

There is no correlation between plasma concentration of parent drug and demethylated metabolite for IMI (DeVane et al., 1981) or CMI (Linnoila et al., 1982) despite significant correlations between parent TCA and hydroxy metabolites, consistent with more variability in demethylation than in hydroxylation. Bock et al. (1982) found a modest but significant (r = 0.53) correlation between the sum of AT + NT concentrations and the total of all unconjugated hydroxy metabolites in AT-treated patients. That different factors in the hepatic P450 system are involved in these two metabolic pathways is supported by the lack of correlation between plasma Cl of AT by demethylation and the purported hydroxylation marker of urinary ratio of parent drug to hydroxy metabolite after single dose debrisoquine (Mellstrom et al., 1983b); the use of debrisoquine in pharmacogenetic studies will be discussed below.

Recent *in vitro* studies have demonstrated demethylation of hydroxy metabolites of TCAs, including conversion of 10-OH-AT to 10-OH-NT (B. Mellstrom and L. Bertilsson, personal communication) and 2-OH-IMI to 2-OH-DMI (T. Monks and J. R. Gillette, personal communication). Thus ultimate plasma levels of active drug forms depend on multiple pathways of formation and Cl. On the other hand, didesmethylated metabolites of TCAs are not considered clinically important (Potter and Linnoila, 1984) as only small amounts are recovered in urine following administration of IMI (Crammer et al., 1969) or NT (Alexanderson and Borga, 1973).

Methylation of TCAs has been reported to occur under certain circumstances but has not been confirmed in systematic series. *In vitro* studies have described methylation of several secondary amine tricyclics (NT, DMI, and PRO) by N-methyltransferase present in rabbit lung (Dingell and Sanders, 1966; Narasimhachari and Lin, 1976). In the only such clinical report (Narasimhachari et al., 1982), 15% of a group of patients treated with therapeutic doses of DMI had measurable amounts of the tertiary amine compound IMI in their blood, presumably resulting from direct methylation of the DMI. A case report of a fatal NT overdose (2 grams) described plasma drug concentrations approximately 12 hr after ingestion as 51 ng/ml of AT and 886 ng/ml of NT (Rudorfer and Robins, 1981); no AT was assayed in plasma from two patients with less serious NT overdoses.

Of course, overdose and therapeutic situations are not necessarily comparable, and at very high drug concentrations usual (first order kinetics) metabolic pathways may be saturated (Gram et al., 1983). This has been speculated to occur in the case of demethylation, such that the ratio of IMI to DMI in the brain after IMI overdose was disproportionately high (Christiansen and Gram, 1973). In plasma parent TCA to demethylated metabolite concentration ratios are double therapeutic values (>2) in more than 60% of IMI or AT overdoses (Bailey et al., 1978; Rudorfer and Robins, 1982) and progressively decline with time, as tertiary amine levels fall and secondary amine concentrations remain the same (Spiker et al., 1975) or rise (Gram et al., 1983). Gram and associates (1983) identified IMI-N-oxide in the plasma of patients early after IMI overdose but not in any patients taking therapeutic doses; they also found hydroxylation to be saturable even in the latter group. However, elimination half-life ($t_{1/2}$) is usually within normal limits for parent tricyclic and demethylated and hydroxylated metabolites after overdose (Gram et al., 1983) or chronic megadosing (Brown et al., 1978), though prolonged TCA plasma concentrations following overdose have been reported (Spiker et al., 1975; Spiker and Biggs, 1976).

Interindividual Variability in Antidepressant Kinetics

With the development of reliable assays for antidepressant compounds in body fluids in the 1960s, the clinical observation that 'therapeutic doses' of TCAs differed greatly among depressed patients was identified as resulting from wide variability in steady-state plasma concentrations to a given dose (Hammer and Sjoqvist, 1967). Intrinsic hepatic Cl differences among individuals, primarily of genetic origin but susceptible to environmental influences, were subsequently found to underlie this phenomenon (Alexanderson and Sjoqvist, 1971).

Metabolism of Drugs Used in Affective Disorders

Much of the basic pharmacokinetics of TCAs has been worked out in single dose studies with patients and healthy volunteers. In at least half of subjects, a two-compartment open model (Gibaldi and Perrier, 1982) best fit the disposition data, with other individuals' data more consistent with a single central compartment (Alexanderson, 1972; Fredricson Overo et al., 1975; DeVane et al., 1981; Findlay et al., 1981; Antal et al., 1982). Plasma protein binding is typically 90% for tricyclics, with free fraction of 6% for NT (Broga et al., 1969), 11% for IMI (Muscettola et al., 1978; Kristensen, 1983), and 14% for DMI (Muscettola et al., 1978). Plasma free fraction of TCAs is approximately equal to CSF drug concentration (Muscettola et al., 1978) and shows less than 100% interindividual variability (Kristensen, 1983); this is small in comparison to other kinetic parameters such as Cl, suggesting that plasma protein binding is not the prime locus of interindividual TCA kinetic variability. Although greater accuracy of results is obtained by accounting for free drug fraction in calculating 'intrinsic Cl' (see Potter et al., 1981a for discussion) most of the literature considers total Cl, as represented in single dose studies, as the ratio of dose (assuming complete absorption) to plasma concentration versus time AUC. Cl rates and $t_{1/2}$ of NT (Alexanderson, 1972) or DMI (Potter et al., 1980) do not differ in single versus multiple dose paradigms within a given individual (see Tables 12.1 and 12.3), consistent with the long-term stability of steady-state TCA plasma concentrations in patients maintained on a constant dose (Potter et al., 1980; Kragh-Sorensen and Larsen, 1980), suggesting lack of autoregulation of TCAs of their own metabolism. Slow Cl of NT in most of the patients in one study (Braithwaite et al., 1978) was felt to differ from kinetics in normals, but most investigators have found similar tricyclic or tetracyclic pharmacokinetics in depressives and healthy volunteers (Gruter and Poldinger, 1982; Faulkner et al., 1983; Maguire et al., 1982; Hrdina et al., 1983).

With the exception of protriptyline (PRO), which is cleared several times more slowly than the others, with an elimination $t_{1/2}$ averaging greater than 3 days (Moody et al., 1977; Ziegler et al., 1978b), TCA $t_{1/2}$s are generally on the order of a day (Table 12.1), with up to 5-fold interindividual variability (Amsterdam et al., 1980), permitting the common clinical practice of single daily (bedtime) dosing. Chronopharmacological studies indicated

Metabolism of Drugs Used in Affective Disorders

lack of a circadian effect on single dose kinetics of NT or AT in volunteers (Nakano and Hollister, 1978, 1983) other than a faster rate of AT absorption, with resulting increase in side effects, after morning rather than evening administration; completeness of absorption and other kinetic parameters--and presumably drug efficacy in the therapeutic situation--did not differ between the two time conditions. Similarly, patient studies comparing NT (Ziegler et al., 1977), DMI (Zielger et al., 1978a), or maprotiline (Gruter and Poldinger, 1982) given thrice daily versus once at night found no differences in steady-state plasma concentrations (Css) for any drug. The 'second generation' antidepressant nomifensine, with a $t_{1/2}$ of only 2 to 4 hr (Brogden et al., 1979) (Table 12.2), on the other hand, must be given at least 3 times a day.

Plasma elimination reflects metabolism to the 10-hydroxy metabolite in the case of NT (Alexanderson, 1973), with liver blood flow apparently the limiting factor in rapid hydroxylators. In a typical study, Reisby et al. (1977), utilizing a fixed daily dose (225 mg) of IMI in a large group of depressed patients, found steady-state concentrations of IMI between 6 and 300 ng/ml, with DMI levels ranging from 15 to 700 ng/ml. In contrast, amoxapine may exhibit less interindividual variability in kinetics, with only 6 to 7-fold differences in Css among volunteers (M. Bishop, personal communication). In our lab, 300 Chinese and Caucasian volunteers demonstrated a more than 10-fold range of total DMI Cl (18-221 L/hr) following a single 100 mg oral dose (Rudorfer et al., 1984b) (Table 12.3). In that study, specific hydroxylation Cl of DMI to 2-OH-DMI, calculated as (total amount of hydroxy metabolite excreted in urine)/(plasma DMI AUC) after a single dose varied 11-fold, from 6.7 to 77.1 L/hr. A similar, over 10-fold range, of NT hydroxylation was shown by Mellstrom et al. (1981) when poor and efficient hydroxylators were compared; stereospecificity of the hydroxylation reaction was seen, with E- but not Z-10-hydroxylation closely ($r = 0.96$) correlated with total plasma Cl of NT. Further aspects of TCA hydroxy metabolites will be considered below. Looking at a tissue compartment, Linnoila et al. (1978) found a strong positive correlation between plasma levels of each of several TCAs and their respective concentrations in red blood cells, with the latter in turn showing up to a 6-fold interindividual variability at a given plasma concentration. Such striking interindividual varia-

Table 12.1: Elimination half-lives of tricyclic antidepressants after a single dose

TCA	$t_{1/2}$ (hr) Mean	Range	Reference
Imipramine (IMI)	7.6	4.0 - 17.6	Nagy and Johansson, 1975
	8.6	6.0 - 11.2	Gram et al., 1976
	11.7	8.0 - 14.0	Gram and Christiansen, 1975
	12	7 - 22	Brunswick et al., 1979
	28.4	18.5 - 34.0	Potter et al., 1980
Desipramine (DMI)	17.1	12.5 - 24.7	Alexanderson, 1972b*
	20	12 - 30	Potter et al., 1980
	18.2	10.3 - 31.8	Rudorfer et al., 1984b**
Amitriptyline (AT)	17.1	15.5 - 19.5	Jorgensen and Hansen, 1976
	24.1	20.3 - 30.8	Rollins et al., 1980***
	36.1	31.0 - 46.6	Ziegler et al., 1978a
Nortriptyline (NT)	15	6 - 28	Nakano and Hollister, 1978
	26.8	18.2 - 35.0	Alexanderson, 1972b*
	28.2	22.0 - 39.4	Rollins et al., 1980***
	33.3	17.8 - 57.8	Gram et al., 1976
	46.4	21.5 - 88.1	Braithwaite et al., 1978

*Same subjects; **Caucasian subjects; ***same subjects

Table 12.1 (cont'd)

TCA	$t_{1/2}$ (hr) Mean	Range	Reference
Doxepin (DOX)	16.8 17.7 17.9	8.2 – 24.5 12.6 – 26.1 10.9 – 47.3	Ziegler et al., 1978d Faulkner et al., 1983 Virtanen et al., 1980
Protriptyline (PRO)	74.3 78.4	53.6 – 91.7 54.6 – 124.0	Ziegler et al., 1978c Moody et al., 1977
Clomipramine (CMI)	24.7	20.1 – 39.6	Nagy and Johansson, 1977
Dothiepin	25	17 – 42	Maguire et al., 1983

Table 12.2: Elimination half-lives of "second-generation" antidepressants after a single dose

Drug	Mean $t_{1/2}$ (hr)	Range	Reference
Maprotiline	43	27 – 58	Riess et al., 1975
Amoxapine	8		Greenblatt et al., 1978
Nomifensine	1.7 3.9	1.6 – 1.8 3.4 – 4.9	Heptner et al., 1977 Vereczkey et al., 1975
Trazodone	6.3 13.9		Yamato et al., 1976 Jauch et al., 1976
Mianserin	21.6	10.7 – 40.8	Hrdina et al., 1983
Bupropion	11.9	10.7 – 13.8	Findlay et al., 1981
Zimelidine	5.1	4.3 – 6.0	Brown et al., 1980

Metabolism of Drugs Used in Affective Disorders

bility in disposition kinetics has particular clinical importance for those drugs such as NT with a well-defined plasma concentration 'therapeutic window' (Asberg et al., 1971a; Ziegler et al., 1976a); the significance of therapeutic plasma level monitoring will be discussed in Chapter 14.

Genetic Factors

It is now well established that there is a genetic basis for the interindividual variability in hepatic metabolism and consequently steady-state plasma concentrations (Css) of TCAs, although the exact mode of transmission is unclear. In what remains the landmark work in this area, 39 healthy middle-aged twin pairs in separate Swedish households were administered low doses of NT for 8 days (Alexanderson et al., 1969). Among those not taking other medication, there was virtually no intrapair difference in Css for the monozygotic twins while 4 of the 11 such dizygotic twinships showed significant intrapair differences. As recalculated by Potter et al. (1981a) intrinsic Cl varied as much as 3.35 L/min within dizygotic twinships but not more than 1.08 L/min between monozygotic twins. Further investigations involving relatives of these twins suggested polygenic control of NT metabolism (Asberg et al., 1971b) but given that most of the fraternal twinships showed little intrapair Css differences, only a small number of genes appeared responsible. Concomitant use of other drugs eliminated the high concordance in NT Css within identical twin pairs, indicating the role of environmental as well as genetic factors (Alexanderson and Sjoqvist, 1971) as will be discussed later in this chapter. Css, in turn, is a composite parameter; using NT as a pharmacogenetic probe in some of these twin pairs, Alexanderson (1973) found separate genetic control of plasma $t_{1/2}$ and apparent volume of distribution (V), suggesting each of these factors contributes independently to Css. The most prominent genetically based difference was in the plasma elimination rate constant, representing metabolism of NT to 10-OH-NT.

Within individuals, degree of variability in metabolism of two or more TCAs may indicate regulation by common genetic and environmental factors (Alexanderson and Sjoqvist, 1971) or intrinsic differences between drugs (Gram, 1977). For example, metabolism of the secondary amines NT and DMI are closely related, chronic doses of each yielding highly correlated Css (Hammer et al., 1969; Alexanderson, 1972b). Plasma Cl of DMI is twice as rapid as that of NT after both single and multiple doses (Alexanderson, 1972b) but the two drugs' Cl values are highly correlated (r = 0.90) secondary to their similar $t_{1/2}$s despite marked differences in V. In contrast, Cl of NT is weakly correlated with that of IMI, the latter drug showing faster Cl, with smaller values for $t_{1/2}$ and V (Gram et al., 1976); single-dose kinetics of PRO also failed to correlate with those of DOX in healthy volunteers (Ziegler et al., 1978b) (Tables 12.1 and 12.3). These data are consistent with the in vitro work of von Bahr (1972), who found tertiary amine TCAs to have higher affinity to hepatic microsomal enzymes than did secondary amines. Looking at two tertiary amines, AT and CMI, in a crossover study, Mellstrom et al. (1979) found a 0.87 correlation between steady-state levels of the parent drugs and a 0.77 correlation for the respective desmethyl metabolites. The tetracyclic compound maprotiline, which is metabolised similarly to conventional TCAs (see below) correlated with IMI in terms of single dose kinetic parameters (Hrdina et al., 1980).

The metabolic pathway of hepatic acetylation, responsible for monoamine oxidase inhibitor (MAOI) disposition (Whitford, 1978) is also under polymorphic genetic control, the gene for slow acetylation being autosomally recessive. Population differences in rapid acetylation phenotype range from 95% in Eskimo to 32% among Swedes (Rawlins, 1974). Despite early suggestions that acetylation status might predict MAOI responsiveness, controlled studies do not support this idea (Rose, 1982) and indeed rapid acetylation of MAOIs might produce more toxic intermediate metabolites.

Pharmacogenetic Probes

Further understanding of the genetics of TCA breakdown has come from intraindividual comparison of tricyclic kinetics with that of marker drugs which undergo metabolism of known inheritance patterns. Clearance of antipyrine, under polymorphic genetic control, occurs via several pathways, and shows modest correlation with IMI, but not NT Cl (Gram et al., 1976; Bertilsson et al., 1980), possibly because demethylation is more important for the former TCA. With regard to psychotropic medications, antipyrine Cl is most closely correlated with that of benzodiazepines, including the triazolobenzodia-

Table 12.3: Plasma clearance of tricyclic antidepressants after an oral dose

TCA	Clearance (L/hr) Mean	Range	Reference
Imipramine (IMI)	79.0	39.5 - 172.4	Potter et al., 1980
	138.6	85.8 - 227.4	Gram et al., 1976*
	151.2	54.6 - 212.4	Gram and Christiansen, 1975
	184.8	64.8 - 300.0	Nagy and Johansson, 1975
Desipramine (DMI)	123.0	54.2 - 221.0	Rudorfer et al., 1984b##
	130.2#	70.0 - 202.3#	Alexanderson, 1972b
	130.2#	81.2 - 156.1#	DeVane et al., 1981
Amitriptyline (AT)	96.0	48.6 - 140.4	Rollins et al., 1980***
	148.2	58.2 - 204.6	Ziegler et al., 1978a
Nortriptyline (NT)	30.0	15.0 - 44.4	Rollins et al., 1980***
	53.9#	29.4 - 100.1#	Alexanderson, 1972b**
	62.4	38.4 - 85.2	Gram et al., 1976*
	172.2	55.8 - 254.4	Nakano and Hollister, 1978
Doxepin (DOX)	60.9#	49.0 - 80.5#	Faulkner et al., 1983
	65.1#	54.6 - 75.6#	Virtanen et al., 1980
	266.7#	107.8 - 557.2#	Ziegler et al., 1978c

#Corrected for 70 kg body wt; ##Caucasian subjects; *same subjects; **same subjects; ***same subjects

Table 12.3 (cont'd)

TCA	Clearance (L/hr) Mean	Range	Reference
Protriptyline (PRO)	11.9#	7.7 - 19.6#	Ziegler et al., 1978b
	14.9#	7.5 - 22.8#	Moody et al., 1977
Clomipramine (CMI)	64.2	35.4 - 119.4	Nagy and Johansson, 1977
Dothiepin	144.9#	44.8 - 353.5#	Maguire et al., 1983

#Corrected for 70 kg body wt

zepine compound alprazolam (Greenblatt et al., 1983a), with putative antidepressant properties. Drugs metabolised primarily by hydroxylation demonstrate the closest relationship to tricyclic disposition. Single dose $t_{1/2}$ of oxyphenylbutazone (Hammer et al., 1969) paralleled steady-state plasma concentrations of NT or DMI. Similarly, phenylbutazone has been used as a marker of TCA Cl; Perel et al. (1976) observed a positive correlation (magnitude unreported) between phenylbutazone $t_{1/2}$ and later Css of IMI + DMI in the same depressed individuals.

More recently much attention has focused on the anti-hypertensive compound debrisoquine (Kalow, 1982). Deficient hydroxylation of debrisoquine (D), commonly defined as a high ratio of D to 4-hydroxy D in an 8 hr urine sample after a single dose, is inherited as a single autosomal recessive trait (Mahgoub et al., 1977) and varies widely across populations, including 9% of British Caucasians (Price Evans et al., 1980) and >30% of Orientals (Inaba et al., 1981). This is relevant to the observation that TCA level outliers appear to belong to a different population from the rest (Hammer and Sjoqvist, 1967), such as the 5% of a mixed group of patients treated with DMI who exhibited unusually low hydroxy metabolite concentrations (Potter et al., 1982a). An association between D and TCA metabolism has been suggested by studies showing significant correlations between D-hydroxylation and E-hydroxylation Cl of NT (Mellstrom et al., 1981) and between D-hydroxylation and DMI Css (Bertilsson and Aberg-Wistedt, 1983). The latter 0.92 correlation was heavily dependent on the presence of 2 of 10 subjects with very high urinary D to 4-OHD ratios. However, we were recently unable to document a relationship between D-hydroxylation and total or hydroxylation Cl of single dose DMI in Caucasian or Chinese volunteers (Rudorfer et al., submitted), none of whom were slow D-hydroxylators in spite of interethnic differences in DMI Cl (Rudorfer et al., 1984b), suggesting that pathways other than hydroxylation were of major imnportance in DMI metabolism. One such candidate, that of demethylation, has also been shown to lack correlation with D-hydroxylation in the case of AT (Mellstrom et al., 1983b). Tricyclic metabolism in individuals already shown to exhibit a wide range of D metabolic ratios has not been reported and may shed further light on the relationship between the body's handling of the two types of drugs.

Metabolism of Drugs Used in Affective Disorders

Clinical Application

A potentially therapeutically useful application of these pharmacokinetic studies is the ability to relate single and chronic dosing kinetic parameters and thereby predict the dosing regimen required to achieve a desired steady-state plasma concentration based on data from single dose administration in the same individual. In the wake of the pioneering work of Alexanderson (1972a,b), who found correlations near unity between Cl after a single dose and Css on chronic administration for both NT and DMI, numerous investigators have extended and in some cases streamlined for clinical use the inverse relationship between these parameters: Css = AUC x maintenance dose/dosing interval x loading dose (Potter et al., 1980). Nagy and Johansson (1975) also used the single dose AUC to predict steady-state levels of IMI.

Employment of a single concentration measurement at a fixed time point after loading dose administration is a simpler procedure for patient dosing but dependent on the degree to which such a level reflects actual AUC (i.e. intrinsic Cl). In fact, Potter et al. (1980) found that while 24 hr concentration was somewhat less precise than complete AUC for predicting IMI or DMI Css in depressed patients, the observed variability was clinically acceptable for targeting the chronic plasma level within the therapeutic range. Thus, empirically derived high (r > 0.9) correlations have been demonstrated between Css and single time point levels at times between 24 (Cooper and Simpson, 1978) and 48 hr (Braithwaite et al., 1978) after a loading dose of NT. These associations do not diminish with advanced age (Dawling et al., 1980). Two blood samples drawn within 36 hr of single dose NT enabled patients to be dosed so as to achieve therapeutic steady-state levels (Browne et al., 1983). The linear relationship between 24 hr DMI concentrations and Css has been confirmed in inpatients (Brunswick et al., 1979) and, to a lesser degree, in outpatients (Rudorfer and Young, 1980). Elderly depressives' DMI Css (Antal et al., 1982), however, correlated with single dose Cl but not a 20 hr time point concentration. In the case of AT, the predictability of Css (AT + NT) based on single dose Cl (Garland et al., 1978) remained clinically useful (r = 0.85) when only the 24 hr loading dose plasma concentration was obtained (Brunswick et al., 1980), and the correlation coefficient increased to 0.92

(Madakasira et al., 1982) using the 36 hr blood sample. Similarly, 24 hr blood levels of dothiepin and its S-oxide metabolite after a single dose correlated with their respective concentrations during the fourth week of treatment (Maguire et al., 1983). PRO, the TCA with the longest $t_{1/2}$, showed comparable correlations between day 3 and steady-state plasma levels (Moody et al., 1977).

Individuals who are slow metabolisers of antidepressants may be at increased risk of toxic plasma concentrations after overdose (Rudorfer and Robins, 1982). Confirmation of this awaits prospective studies.

Other Biological Characteristics of Individuals

Age. Given the immaturity of the hepatic enzyme and renal systems at birth and the somewhat analogous decline in many bodily functions in advanced age, it is reasonable to postulate alterations in antidepressant metabolism with changes in stage of life. Conclusions are limited by the relative paucity of data, many studies neither accounting nor controlling for subjects' age, as well as the difficulty in factoring out other confounding variables (Potter et al., 1981a).

A comparison between young and elderly male volunteers' handling of single dose AT (Schulz et al., 1983) illustrated several of the issues involved. Cl was slightly (10%) but not significantly lower in the older subjects, attributed to the expected decrease in liver weight and hepatic blood flow. Mean $t_{1/2}$, however, was considerably (34%) elevated in the elderly, based not only on the reduction in Cl, but on an observed increase in V in these individuals; each of these factors can independently affect $t_{1/2}$, which = 0.693 V/Cl. Changes in V may relate to alterations in body composition with age or to variation in plasma protein binding; the latter was no different in the older subjects studied by Schulz et al. (1983). Concomitant somatic disease and dietary habits may affect the concentration of plasma proteins in the elderly. For instance, increases in alpha$_1$ acid glycoprotein with inflammation or malignancy results in decreased free fraction and increased total Css of antidepressants. However, as noted above, Cl and the unbound pharmacologically active drug concentration, and therefore drug effect, will not change. Cl was slower and $t_{1/2}$ prolonged after single dose NT in a group of elderly depressed inpatients (Dawling et al., 1980) but the presence of significant medical illness and concomitant polypharmacy compared to the young healthy volunteer control group limited interpretation.

Psychiatrically healthy individuals, most of them relatives of patients known to achieve unusually high plasma NT steady-state concentrations, showed no age effect on NT kinetics (Asberg et al., 1971b). Other studies in naturalistic patient settings have yielded mixed results. No significant effect of age on steady-state concentrations has emerged from most studies of AT and NT (Ziegler and Biggs, 1977; Linnoila et al., 1981), though Kragh-Sorensen and Larsen (1980) found higher NT levels over age 70. In a relatively young group of patients (Rudorfer and Robins, 1982) age was unrelated to plasma TCA concentrations after AT overdose. One frequently cited study (Nies et al., 1977) yielded an almost 3-fold increase in Css of IMI and DMI and longer $t_{1/2}$s of DMI in older patients, findings which were not replicated in a more recent study (Potter et al., 1980). Gram et al. (1977) also found generally higher IMI levels with advancing age, with a complex gender interaction, to be discussed below. In two fixed-dose CMI studies older patients also exhibited higher drug concentrations. This relationship was nonlinear in Traskman and associates' (1979) patients, with a steep rise of CMI levels in the upper age group; the desmethyl metabolite did not change in older subjects. In a similar investigation (John et al., 1980), endogenously depressed patients older than 65 yr developed higher Css of CMI and desmethylCMI than those less than 40 yr old; there was even an age differential among the elderly, those above 75 yr with higher drug levels than patients between 65 and 75 yr.

Five elderly depressed women, compared with results of younger adults in other studies, showed reduced Cl and longer $t_{1/2}$ of single dose IMI but 'normal' values of these parameters for the tetracyclic compound maprotiline (Hrdina et al., 1980). Metabolism of the new 'second generation' antidepressants is in most respects similar to that of the standard tricyclic compounds (see below). In terms of the age effect under discussion, mianserin has generally produced similar Css across age groups (Brogden et al., 1978) whereas in the case of zimelidine (Heel et al., 1982) prolonged $t_{1/2}$s and increased Css have been reported for both parent drug and demethylated metabolite in older versus younger patients. Longer $t_{1/2}$ and reduced Cls were seen in elderly men after a single dose of alprazolam (Greenblatt et al., 1983a).

A provocative report from Odense, Denmark (Bjerre et al., 1981), described dose-dependent kinetics of therapeutic doses of IMI in elderly depressed patients, whereby elevations of DMI plasma levels were disproportionately greater than the linear rises in parent drug concentrations with increases in IMI dose; NT, on the other hand, showed first-order kinetics at all dosages. These authors hypothesised saturability of IMI and DMI hydroxylation but not demethylation pathways to account for their findings (Gram et al., 1983). At least for DMI levels up to 150 ng/ml, our group (Potter et al., 1982a) has not found dose dependence of DMI hydroxylation.

The above alterations in pharmacokinetics in the aged have generally been ascribed to reductions in the rate of hepatic biotransformation of drugs. Only relatively recently has the role of renal function in antidepressant metabolism been fully appreciated. It has long been recognised that lithium (Li) does not undergo metabolism but is nearly completely excreted through the kidneys. Thus the normal decline in glomerular filtration rate (GFR) with age causes up to a 60% decrease in Li renal Cl, with lengthening of $t_{1/2}$ up to 36 hr in the elderly versus 24 hr in middle-aged adults (Prien, 1981).

While unchanged TCAs are not subject to renal excretion, their metabolites are. With the demonstration of biological activity of tricyclic hydroxy metabolites (Potter and Calil, 1981) came realisation of the clinical significance of changes in the elimination rate of these substances. It was originally shown by Alexanderson and Borga (1973) that the renal Cl of hydroxy-NT was over 100 ml/min. A similarly high urinary Cl has been shown for unconjugated hydroxy-DMI (Kitanaka et al., 1982), with a decrease in elderly depressed patients ($r = -0.73$ between age and 2-OH-DMI renal Cl) accompanied by an increase in the plasma OH-DMI/DMI ratio. This is interpreted to mean that the rate of DMI hydroxylation was not altered, since DMI plasma concentrations were the same in the elderly as in younger populations (Cutler et al., 1981). Even without truly elderly subjects (Rudorfer et al., 1984b) our Chinese and Caucasian volunteers demonstrated after single dose DMI a significant reduction in renal Cl of OH-DMI with increasing age (Potter et al., 1983). A weaker but still significant association has been noted between age and plasma OH-NT/NT ratio in patients treated with NT or AT (Sjoqvist, 1981; Pottash et al., 1983) despite unchanged levels of the unmetabolised drug. One group of IMI-treated patients which included 21% slow hydroxylators (Gram et al., 1983) did not show this higher hydroxy metabolite ratio in the elderly. In 45 DMI-treated patients with a nearly 4-fold age range (Bock et al., 1983) there was as well only a weak trend toward higher relative levels of hydroxy metabolite with increasing age. Therapeutic or toxic actions mediated by TCA hydroxy metabolites thus may be exaggerated in geriatric patients unless allowances are made in dosing.

Turning briefly to the category of monoamine oxidase inhibitors (MAOIs) in geriatric populations, Robinson (1981) retrospectively reviewed his group's experience with phenelzine in double-blind studies. He found a tendency for higher phenelzine plasma concentrations in older patients, with no effect of age on drug acetylator subtype, and postulated a slower rate of phenelzine Cl in the elderly.

Although specific data are even sparser than in the elderly, drug metabolism at the other extreme of the life cycle--infancy and childhood--is also frequently different from that in adults, in fact often resembling that in the aged. In the early months of life GFR is low, with the same implications for drug elimination as discussed above; by childhood, however, renal and hepatic functioning are at least equivalent (relative to body surface area) to adult values (Rane and Wilson, 1976). Von Bahr (1972) described 2-hydroxylation of DMI by fetal human livers, speculating potential teratological effect (hepatic centrolobular necrosis) of possible toxic intermediate epoxides. In vivo demonstration of TCA metabolism by a neonate was reported in a unique investigation of a young woman who took an overdose of NT one day prior to delivery (Sjoqvist et al., 1972). The child's plasma NT concentration at birth was 20% that of the mother, possibly related to decreased protein binding, while subsequent drug elimination revealed a $t_{1/2}$ in the newborn of 56 hr, 3 times that of the mother, although the contribution of immaturity of drug metabolising enzymes versus genetic factors could not be discerned; the Cl, albeit slow, of the NT, with documentation of 10-OH-NT in the infant's plasma and urine over several days, confirmed that NT metabolism was occurring in the neonate.

Tricyclic metabolism in children has been

reviewed by Rapoport and Potter (1981). Although on a mg/kg basis Css of DMI or, with IMI treatment, of IMI + DMI were similar in children and adults, apparent Cl of IMI by demethylation was more rapid in children, yielding a mean IMI/DMI ratio of 0.54, half that in adults. Ratios of OH-DMI to DMI, however, were similar in the two age groups. The lower extent of TCA protein binding that has been suggested to occur in children was thought not be clinically meaningful, as it would not affect free drug Css, as discussed above.

Sex. Most studies which have specifically compared male to female concentrations of NT (Alexanderson et al., 1969; Asberg et al., 1971b; Dawling et al., 1980), AT and/or NT (Ziegler and Biggs, 1977)--including after overdose (Rudorfer and Robins, 1982)--IMI (Glassman et al., 1977; Gram et al., 1983), or DMI (Bock et al., 1983) have not found a significant difference. The sole exception consisted of higher IMI Css in older males, compared with younger females (Gram et al., 1977). In our crosscultural DMI study mentioned above (Potter et al., 1983) the relationship between OH-DMI renal Cl and age, which was unaffected by race, did show a sex effect, with a significant correlation ($r = -0.69$) only for women (who exhibited a slightly wider age range), not men ($r = -0.30$).

Again the newer drugs are similar to the standard TCAs, other than a tendency for peak mianserin concentrations after a single dose to be slightly higher in males than females (Brogden et al., 1978). The atypical tricyclic dothiepin (Maguire et al., 1983) showed slower elimination $t_{1/2}$s of parent compound and northiaden, but not dothiepin S-oxide, in female patients and volunteers compared to males, suggesting sex-related differences in demethylation; however, age differences between the two groups (women older than men) confounded interpretation of this result. As already noted, the prolonged $t_{1/2}$ and reduced Cl in advanced age for alprazolam (Greenblatt et al., 1983a) was observed only in men.

Race. Most reports of antidepressant use do not account for the race of subjects under study. Ziegler and Biggs (1977) found 50% higher steady-state plasma NT concentrations in black patients than in whites (although this difference was small compared to the 7-fold overall variation in NT levels); in another group of patients treated with AT, a smaller racial difference was not significant.

Earlier studies had reported for blacks more rapid response to TCA and phenothiazine therapy (Overall et al., 1969), greater anxiety reduction in response to both antianxiety and antidepressant drugs (Henry et al., 1971), and more improvement on IMI at one week (Raskin and Crook, 1975). These older works presumably all reflected slower rates of TCA metabolism in black patients, but their interpretation is limited by their failure to assay TCA plasma concentrations and by diagnostic heterogeneity in treatment groups.

Following AT overdose blacks developed plasma total TCA levels adjusted for amount ingested twice that of whites (Rudorfer and Robins, 1982) with a nonsignificantly higher AT/NT concentration ratio, again pointing to a difference in rate of metabolism between the races.

Anecdotal reports (Yamamoto et al., 1979; Kleinman, 1981) have long described the need for lower routine doses of TCAs in Asian as opposed to Western countries, suggesting racially based pharmacokinetic differences. In the only English language report we are aware of documenting TCA plasma concentrations in Asian patients, Yamashita and Asano (1979) did not find elevated plasma levels in their uncontrolled sample and proposed that pharmacodynamic or psychosocial factors might explain the efficacy of low doses. However, healthy Asian volunteers had higher plasma drug concentrations for 24 hr after a single dose of CMI than their native British counterparts (Allen et al., 1977; Lewis et al., 1980).

Extending these investigations we traced the fate of a single oral dose of DMI over 5 days in healthy Chinese and Caucasian volunteers (Rudorfer et al., 1984b). Total DMI Cl was significantly slower in the Chinese (mean of 73.5 L/hr compared with 123 L/hr for the Caucasians), with a trimodal distribution including a minority of outliers in each group (29% Chinese, slow Cl; 25% Caucasians, rapid Cl). Surprisingly, there were no significant interethnic differences in specific hydroxylation Cl. The genetic implications of these findings have already been discussed.

Population differences in drug acetylation rate (Rawlins, 1974) would imply racial variability in MAOI metabolism (Whitford, 1978). Given an 85-95% rate of rapid acetylation in Asians versus < 50% in blacks and whites (ibid.) it has been speculated though not yet demonstrated that contrary to the situation with TCAs, dose requirements for MAOIs might actually be higher in Asians compared to other ethnic groups (Lin and Finder, 1984). However, a faster acetylator rate might cause increased levels of intermediate metabolites mediating toxicity, thus making the rapid metaboliser group more susceptible to adverse effects.

Interactions Affecting Antidepressant Metabolism

Activity of antidepressants can be greatly altered by the effects of concomitant drug or substance use. Pharmacodynamic intensification of adverse reactions is common, ranging from additive sedation or anticholinergic effects when tricyclics are combined with hypnotics or some analgesics to hypertensive crises from consumption of tyramine-rich foods by patients taking MAO inhibitors. Theoretically, any exogenous factor changing absorption or excretion characteristics of antidepressants can influence the amount of drug available systemically. In fact, the most clinically significant interactions are those which, by induction or inhibition of metabolising enzymes, determine the rate or extent of antidepressant breakdown and, consequently, steady-state concentrations.

Smoking

Tobacco smoke contains both inducers and retardants of drug oxidising enzymes. The net effect, that of stimulation of drug metabolism, probably occurs in organs, e.g. lung, other than liver (Vahakangas et al., 1983).
 There is contradictory evidence of a significant impact of smoking on TCA metabolism. Alexanderson et al. (1969) found no correlation between extent of smoking and steady-state NT plasma concentration. Two other studies also found no difference in AT and/or NT levels between smokers and nonsmokers (Ziegler and Biggs, 1977; Norman et al., 1977), although the latter report has been questioned on the methodological grounds of unusually great intraindividual variability in plasma NT concentrations. More recently, Bock et al. (1983) found no relationship between smoking habits and steady-state DMI or 2-OH-DMI plasma levels.
 On the other hand, there have been careful investigations demonstrating in smokers significantly lower Css of IMI and DMI (Perel et al., 1976), CMI (John et al., 1980) and of AT and/or NT (Lin-

noila et al., 1981). The reasons for this discrepancy in the literature are unclear. Careful prospective documentation of tobacco use by subjects in antidepressant studies should help clarify this issue and judge its practical importance.

Alcohol and Dietary Factors

Chronic heavy drinking, defined as daily consumption of alcoholic beverages containing at least 200 gm of absolute ethanol, can induce the metabolism of drugs handled by the hepatic cytochrome P450 enzyme system (Iber, 1977). In contrast, more moderate drinking by depressed patients did not affect steady-state AT and NT (Linnoila et al., 1981) or DMI or 2-OH-DMI (Bock et al., 1983) plasma concentrations. However, 11 depressed alcoholic men had an intrinsic Cl of IMI 2.5-fold higher than that of controls matched for smoking status (Ciraulo et al., 1982), resulting in lower Css not only of IMI but of 2-OH-IMI, DMI, and 2-OH-DMI as well in the alcohol-dependent group.

<u>Acute</u> alcohol loading can impair TCA Cl. Pretreatment with ethanol caused an increase in total TCA concentration (in brain and blood, respectively) of approximately 200% (mainly in parent drug) following single dose AT administration both in rat (Preskorn and Hughes, 1983) and in man (Dorian et al., 1982), apparently by decreasing AT hepatic first-pass extraction; the former authors speculated that consumption of alcohol by a patient prior to blood sampling may render a TCA plasma level measurement unreliable.

More difficult to control are dietary factors. Individuals from Western countries are probably exposed to more chemical enzyme inducers in their food than are people in the Third World. Vegetarians in London, most of them Asians, had longer $t_{1/2}$s of antipyrine (Fraser et al., 1976) than did native Britons. A challenge of charcoal-broiled beef for one week reduced the single dose AUC of phenacetin (Conney et al., 1976), presumably via hepatic enzyme induction by polycyclic hydrocarbons. However, this issue has not been specifically explored for antidepressant metabolism. Crossethnic studies, involving TCA administration to Asian (Allen et al., 1977; Lewis et al., 1980) or Chinese volunteers (Rudorfer et al., 1984b), took note of probable dietary differences between these subjects and their Caucasian controls, but were unable to factor out other confounding variables, most obviously racial/genetic considerations.

Metabolism of Drugs Used in Affective Disorders

Other Drug Interactions

Depressed patients often are prescribed multiple medications, with resulting potential for alteration of antidepressant kinetics. Among the most potent nonspecific inducers of hepatic microsomal metabolism are the barbiturates, capable of accelerating the breakdown of numerous other compounds (Gillette, 1971). Specific demonstrations with antidepressants include lower Css of NT in patients receiving concomitant barbiturates versus those on NT only (Alexanderson et al., 1969). Burrows and Davies (1971) similarly documented a dramatic fall in NT plasma level in a subject with the addition of amylobarbitone. Early in the literature on TCA concentrations (Hammer et al., 1966) a patient was described whose DMI Css was reduced by half on exposure to phenobarbitone. Controlled series have replicated the overall lower TCA concentrations in patients also taking barbiturates when compared to matched groups untreated with hypnotics; antidepressants studied have included IMI (Ballinger et al., 1974), PRO (Moody et al., 1977), and CMI (Traskman et al., 1979). Interestingly, and fortunately, the benzodiazepines do not share this effect on TCA metabolism. None of a variety of benzodiazepines altered Css of AT or NT (Silverman and Braithwaite, 1973), IMI (Ballinger et al., 1974; Gram et al., 1974), or PRO (Moody et al., 1977). Thus, in addition to therapeutic and toxicologic considerations, there is a sound kinetic basis for using a benzodiazepine rather than a barbiturate for antianxiety or sedative purposes when combined pharmacotherapy with a tricyclic compound is required.

As reviewed by Potter et al. (1981a) chlorpromazine may induce its own metabolism. This has not been described for the TCAs; the stability of long-term Css of these drugs has been noted above. Carbamazepine, an anticonvulsant agent with demonstrated efficacy in affective disorders (Ballenger and Post, 1980) is metabolised principally to its epoxide by the hepatic oxidase system; it is also a potent inducer of these enzymes, such that after 2 weeks of treatment autoinduction occurs, leading to a fall in mean $t_{1/2}$ from 30 to 18 hr with concomitant decline of previously steady-state plasma concentrations (Eichelbaum et al., 1975). Although the 'second generation' antidepressant bupropion is a weak to moderate inducer of hepatic drug metabolising enzymes in rats and mice (Schroeder, 1983), there is no evidence for this occurring at clinically relevant levels in humans.

Competition for the same degradative enzymes enables certain other psychotropic drugs, most notably antipsychotics and, to a lesser extent, stimulants, to block the metabolism of antidepressants and thereby lower the Cl of the latter compounds. Imipramine-treated rats showed elevation of tissue concentrations of both IMI and even more so of DMI when perphenazine (PPZ) was added (Gram, 1977); the higher affinity of IMI to microsomal cytochrome P450 (von Bahr, 1972) may render this compound less susceptible than DMI to displacement by neuroleptics. This effect in humans, which appeared to be dose-dependent, has been generalised to include a number of TCAs and a variety of phenothiazine and nonphenothiazine antipsychotics (Gram, 1977).

Doses and sequencing of drugs play a role in the TCA-neuroleptic interaction. Danish investigators (Gram and Fredericson Overo, 1972; Gram, 1974; Gram et al., 1974) reported that repeated oral doses of chlorpromazine or PPZ (in doses as high as 24-28 mg/day) had an inhibitory effect on the metabolism of single oral doses of IMI and NT. On the other hand, adding PPZ 12 mg/day to an established regimen of NT (Kragh-Sorensen et al., 1977) resulted in a slight increase in plasma NT concentrations in only two of six patients, with barely demonstrable reduction in Cl of NT to 10-OH-NT in one of them. Interestingly, in a similar paradigm with elderly patients at steady-state on IMI or NT (Bjerre et al., 1981) all five patients subsequently treated with concomitant PPZ (in daily doses as low as 8 mg) did show marked increase in tricyclic plasma levels (as expected, affecting DMI more so than IMI concentrations in IMI-treated individuals).

Large-scale reviews (Vandel et al., 1979; Linnoila et al., 1982a) of patients treated with AT or NT combined with a phenothiazine confirmed significantly elevated TCA levels compared to a control group on TCAs alone. Five such patients (Bock et al., 1982) had a lower proportion of 10-OH metabolites and a higher mean NT/AT ratio (Vandel et al., 1979) but no difference in AT and/or NT plasma concentrations versus control AT-only patients. A similar effect of antipsychotics on tricyclic hydroxylation was documented for DMI (Bock et al., 1983); combined treatment with PPZ, haloperidol, or thiothixene was associated with higher DMI plasma concentrations and reduced proportion of 2-OH metabolite. Relatively high IMI and DMI levels with low plasma concentrations of their hydroxy metabolites were assayed during combined IMI and fluphenazine decanoate treatment in a small uncontrolled study (Siris et al., 1982). Thioridizine also raised plasma DMI levels (Hirschowitz et al., 1983).

Although competitive inhibition of hepatic metabolism appeared responsible for this neuroleptic-antidepressant interaction, other actions of neuroleptics, including reduction in hepatic blood flow (Gram, 1977) or competition for nonmetabolising hepatic binding sites (Beaubien and Pakuts, 1980) may contribute to this effect. Decreased hepatic blood flow due to reduced cardiac output and competition for microsomal oxidising enzymes appeared to account for the elevation of maprotiline Css induced by addition of the beta-blocker propranolol in a recent report (Tollefson and Lesar, 1984); similar interactions would be expected with the older tricyclics as well. The resulting increase in TCA concentrations could have clinical significance if the new value is associated with toxicity or takes the patient out of (or into) the therapeutic range.

In vitro and patient studies of the central stimulant methylphenidate (Wharton et al., 1971) revealed a pattern (decreased TCA hydroxylation and less effect on demethylation, with resultant rise in plasma IMI and DMI levels) strikingly similar to that seen with neuroleptics; these authors were unable to replicate their findings with dextroamphetamine. However, the positive therapeutic value seen with the addition of methylphenidate to tricyclics (ibid.) has been attributed by other investigators (Drimmer et al., 1983) to a pharmacodynamic effect, without alteration of TCA concentrations.

A final example of an apparently identical pharmacokinetic interaction has involved the histamine H_2-receptor antagonist cimetidine, which over the past several years has gained widespread use in the treatment and prophylaxis of peptic ulcer disease and a variety of other gastric disorders. This medication can interfere with the metabolism of a wide variety of drugs handled by the hepatic P450 enzyme system, thereby reducing their Cl, elevating their Css and enhancing their therapeutic and/or toxic activity. With specific reference to the antidepressants under consideration in this chapter, cimetidine slowing of metabolism has been demonstrated for carbamazepine and multiple benzodiazepines (Somogyi et al., 1982) including alprazolam, which had a one-third prolongation of elimination $t_{1/2}$ (Abernethy et al., 1983). Case reports have described similar effects when cimetidine was combined with TCAs; one patient experienced a 40% decline in Cl of IMI with rise in tricyclic levels and toxicity (Miller and Macklin, 1983). Cimetidine has recently been shown to impair both demethylation of tertiary amine TCAs and hydroxylation of secondary amine tricyclics (Miller and Macklin, 1984).

While oral contraceptive (OC) steroids theoretically can inhibit hepatic microsomal oxidising enzymes as well (O'Malley et al., 1972), clinical data have been contradictory. First-pass metabolism of IMI was strikingly lower in a woman taking an OC than in three other volunteers (Gram and Christiansen, 1975) and elevated plasma CMI Css has been reported in patients taking OCs concurrently (Luscombe and Jones, 1977). Subsequently, John et al. (1980), upon failing to find any effect of OC use on plasma Css of CMI in depressed women, speculated that dose-dependence of this putative interaction could explain this disparity of results; the earlier studies used OCs containing high estrogen doses of at least 50 µg while in recent years common clinical practice (including their study) dictated a reduction of estrogen content to 30 µg or less.

Several kinetic interactions involving antidepressants and anticonvulsants have been reported though not yet fully explored. Seizure disorder patients maintained on combination anticonvulsant regimens exhibited lower single dose plasma levels of mianserin or nomifensine than did a control group (Nawishy et al., 1981), presumably by hepatic enzyme induction. Conversely, IMI can elevate plasma phenytoin concentrations (Perucca and Richens, 1977). Carbamazepine, now used for affective as well as seizure disorders, engaged in a 'double-drug interaction' with the antituberculous drug isoniazid (INH) (Wright et al., 1982), the latter drug causing elevated carbamazepine blood levels and toxicity (Valsalan and Cooper, 1982) with the presence of carbamazepine apparently rendering patients more vulnerable to INH-induced liver toxicity; presumably INH inhibits hepatic microsomal enzymes that metabolise carbamazepine, while the induction of liver enzymes characteristic of carbamazepine (Levy et al., 1983) could be responsible for a more rapid than usual buildup of a putative hepatotoxic intermediate metabolite of INH. Increase in carbamazepine levels has been reported to result from concomitant MAOI antidepressant therapy as well (Post and Uhde, 1984), consistent with *in vitro* data showing inhibition of hepatic oxidative microsomal enzymes by the MAOI tranylcypromine (Belanger and Atitse-

Metabolism of Drugs Used in Affective Disorders

Gbeassor, 1982). It is of note that presumed interactions of carbamazepine and Li have been of a pharmacodynamic nature, i.e. antidiuretic properties of carbamazepine counteracting the opposite effects of Li, and possible combined neurotoxicity, but no pharmacokinetic changes have resulted from the combination therapy (Ghose, 1980).

Activity of the anticoagulant warfarin can be altered by changes in its hepatic metabolism secondary to concomitant antidepressant use. Competitive inhibition of warfarin breakdown with resulting increase in prothrombin time has been produced both by standard TCAs such as AT (Loomis and Racz, 1980) and second generation drugs, e.g. mianserin (Warwick and Mindham, 1983). On the other hand, Massey (1983) found the presumed hepatic enzyme-inducing effect of carbamazepine to shorten the $t_{1/2}$ of warfarin and reduce clinical activity of the latter.

As noted above, the dependence of Li Cl on renal excretion means that concomitant drug treatment with agents that affect the kidney can produce interactions with Li. Such drugs include sodium-depleting diuretics, which lead to increased Li reabsorption and higher Li blood levels (Salzman, 1982) and a variety of nonsteroidal anti-inflammatory agents which, apparently by inhibiting prostaglandin-dependent renal mechanisms, decrease Li Cl with resultant elevation in Li plasma concentrations (Ragheb et al., 1980). Another potential alteration of antidepressant kinetics not specifically affecting metabolism per se consists of displacement of TCAs from their binding sites on alpha$_1$ acid glycoprotein; in an in vitro preparation (Muller et al., 1983) a variety of other psychotropic drugs ranging from benzodiazepines and phenothiazines to anticholinergics and carbamazepine displayed this activity, causing increase in free IMI fractions.

Organic Pathology and Disease

During the course of transit to their site of action in the central nervous system, antidepressant drugs are susceptible to alterations in their metabolism and disposition when illness changes the usual physiologic homeostasis. Such alterations can affect any pharmacokinetic parameter, as follows:

Absorption. Changes in gut pH or motility can influence absorption of the weakly basic TCAs. Increased exposure to gastric acidity, including delayed gastric emptying, may destroy drug and thereby reduce its bioavailability, whereas rapid movement of gastric contents can increase the amount of TCAs presented to the small intestine for absorption (Siris and Rifkin, 1981). Some intestinal disorders may directly limit absorption, though inflammatory bowel disease may be associated with increased vascularity or membrane damage causing increased amounts of drug to enter the blood. Nonetheless, since overall absorption of TCAs is so high, these variations are only likely to produce fluctuations in absolute peak levels and not average steady-state. Only minor consequences, most likely related to transient side effects, should result.

Distribution. As TCAs are generally at least 90% bound to proteins, particularly alpha$_1$ acid glycoprotein, lipoproteins, and albumin, changes in amount of protein or extent of binding may affect total TCA plasma concentrations. Plasma proteins are often reduced by hepatic or renal disease, poor dietary intake and aging, as discussed above, and are elevated in various other illness states. In particular, postoperative states, inflammatory disease (Kragh-Sorensen and Larsen, 1980), especially rheumatoid arthritis and Crohn's disease, and cancer (Schulz and Luttrell, 1982) are associated with increased plasma protein binding and consequently higher total TCA concentrations. However, as already noted, in these altered states of binding the free fraction of drug changes inversely to the change' in proteins, with reciprocal alteration of Css; thus the free, pharmacologically active concentration of drug generally remains constant (Potter et al., 1981a), rendering clinical effect unchanged but interpretation of (total) TCA blood levels tenuous. Acidosis from any cause may reduce binding affinity, thereby leading to higher concentrations of unbound drug; the opposite is true of alkalosis.

Hepatic Metabolism. Parenchymal damage or disease of the liver might seem a likely cause of altered kinetics of tricyclics, which are cleared primarily by hepatic mechanisms including a substantial first-pass effect. In fact, reduced drug metabolism does not necessarily occur even in severe liver impairment, the cytochrome P450 enzyme system generally functioning in diseased as well as healthy hepatic tissue. The limited studies in this area have focused on the benzodiazepines, presumably because of their widespread use in alcoholic patients. Thus long-acting benzodiazepines such as diazepam showed diminished Cl with alcoholic cirrhosis of the liver but no change was seen in shorter-acting drugs such as oxazepam (Wilkinson and Schenker, 1976; Sellers et al., 1977); alprazolam has not yet been reported on in this regard. Even in Gilbert Syndrome, a congenital defect in hepatic conjugating capacity, disposition of the short-acting benzodiazepines lorazepam and oxazepam, which are metabolised primarily by glucuronidation to inactive compounds, was not significantly different from that in normal populations (Shader et al., 1981).

TCA metabolism has not been systematically studied in liver disease. Indeed Ciraulo et al. (1982) specifically excluded individuals with impaired liver function in investigating IMI disposition in alcoholics. The decreased Cl and first-pass metabolism of the analgesics pentazocine and pethidine in cirrhotic patients (Neal et al., 1979) were hypothesised, but not shown, to extend to antidepressants. A single case report of disproportionately high AT and NT Css in a man with biopsy-proven alcoholic cirrhosis (Giller et al., 1979) could only speculate at a causal relationship between the two phenomena and has not been replicated.

Blood flow changes may directly or indirectly alter hepatic drug metabolism; Cl of highly extracted drugs is particularly sensitive to changes in hepatic blood flow (Williams, 1983). In portal hypertension enteric venous blood may circumvent the liver on the first pass, resulting in a greater than usual percentage of the administered dose reaching the systemic circulation. On the other hand, congestive heart failure has been speculated (Glassman et al., 1983) to induce alterations in hepatic blood flow with consequent reduction in demethylation of TCAs; such cardiac patients, when treated with IMI, yielded higher plasma concentrations of IMI and DMI than healthy controls (ibid.). The net effect of these pathophysiological sequelae of hepatic disease on drug metabolism is thus variable; Wood and associates (1978) found a nonsignificant fall in Cl of propranolol in patients with cirrhosis, but with elevation of V, $t_{1/2}$ was tripled compared to controls. Although first-pass effects, at least, could be reduced by parenteral drug administration, this is not usual practice with TCAs; slow careful titration of dose with plasma level monitoring remains the best clinical approach to TCA treatment of patients with liver disease. These effects on hepatic drug metabolism probably apply as well to MAOIs and second generation antidepressants (Hollister,

1983).

Renal excretion. Subject to renal elimination without biotransformation, lithium kinetics are susceptible to even minor changes in excretory function. The interaction between renal disease and Li retention is well established, with elevated Li serum concentrations in patients with diminished renal Cl (Amdisen, 1977), while the possibility of Li-induced kidney pathology remains under investigation (Jenner, 1979).

In contrast, throughout most of their history TCAs have been thought to depend little on renal elimination as a mode of termination of their activity as it was believed these drugs were nearly completely metabolised to inactive byproducts prior to reaching the kidney (e.g. Siris and Rifkin, 1981). However, with the recognition of biological activity of unconjugated hydroxy TCA metabolites (Potter and Calil, 1981) came realisation of the functional importance of renal Cl of these compounds (Potter et al., 1983); indeed renal Cl of these metabolites, measured as high as 500 ml/min, greatly exceeds GFR, suggesting active secretion (Potter et al., 1984). The clinical significance of reduced GFR and the resulting buildup of plasma concentrations of pharmacologically active TCA hydroxy metabolites has been reviewed above in the context of the elderly; parallel changes follow from impairment of excretory function secondary to kidney disease or drugs. For instance, the elimination $t_{1/2}$ of the second generation antidepressant nomifensine was prolonged in marked renal failure (Brogden et al., 1979).

Renal Cl of the hydroxy metabolite of the beta receptor antagonist metoprolol appeared reduced in elderly healthy volunteers (Lundborg et al., 1982) and correlated directly with GFR in four patients with impaired renal function (Hoffmann et al., 1980). In an initial study of 20 patients with chronic renal failure who were administered a single dose of NT, Dawling et al. (1981) found no changes in parent drug Cl or $t_{1/2}$ in patients compared to controls; these investigators speculated that hydroxy metabolites of NT might accumulate during renal insufficiency and proceeded to subsequently demonstrate this phenomenon, with elevated plasma concentrations of 10-OH-NT, in some of these same patients (Braithwaite and Dawling, 1981).

Clinically, antidepressant pharmacotherapy can thus be utilised in renal disease patients with conservative dosing (Hollister, 1983). The clinician must bear in mind the myriad possible pharmacodynamic influences on mood in these patients; steroids used for immunosuppression in kidney transplant cases or alphamethyldopa treatment of hypertension may contribute to the substantial incidence of secondary depression in individuals with end stage renal disease and may respond to changes in medical regimen short of specific antidepressant medication (ibid.). Moreover, the pharmacokinetic implications of polypharmacy have already been noted, including possible steroid-associated increase in TCA metabolism via induction of hepatic enzymes.

Active Metabolites of Antidepressants

Metabolism of antidepressant drugs yields a number of structurally related polar and nonpolar compounds, with only 1 to 3 percent of an administered TCA dose being excreted unchanged (Crammer et al., 1969). Considerable evidence, reviewed by Potter and Calil (1981), argues against a biologically active role for several IMI metabolites, including IDB and 2-OH-IDB (Figure 12.1). The status of the N-oxide metabolite is less clear. Antidepressant efficacy of AT-N-oxide was observed in an outpatient study (Rapp, 1978) flawed by the lack of placebo control of plasma level monitoring and by use of concomitant benzodiazepines in some subjects. Avoiding concurrent administration of other drugs, but otherwise subject to the same limitations as the preceding study, Borromei (1982) also found AT-N-oxide a very effective antidepressant in a heterogeneous group of depressives; the claimed superiority of this drug over AT must be viewed with caution, given the low doses of the latter compound taken by control patients. Nagy and Hansen (1978) documented in vivo formation of IMI and DMI from IMI-N-oxide in healthy volunteers and depressed patients treated with the latter, also with a positive therapeutic response. On the other hand, demethylated metabolites of tertiary amine TCAs (including NT and DMI, which are marketed separately from their parent drugs) and hydroxylated metabolites of all tricyclics demonstrate in vitro monoamine reuptake blockade (Bertilsson et al., 1979; Potter et al., 1979) though only the former group has been directly administered to patients.

By definition, active metabolites must be sufficiently lipid soluble at physiologic pH to cross the blood-brain barrier and enter the central nervous system. The metabolites are themselves subject to further biotransformation or conjugation; the latter process, to nonlipid-soluble substances, renders the metabolites inactive and susceptible to renal and potentially biliary excretion (Potter et al., 1984), with possible enterohepatic circulation, as discussed above for the parent drug.

Pharmacodynamic studies indicate that the demethylated, secondary amine TCAs are relatively specific for blockade of noradrenaline (NA) reuptake in vitro while their parent, tertiary amine counterparts act more on the serotonin (5-hydroxytryptamine; 5-HT) system initially (Ross and Renyi, 1975). This is expressed in vivo by relatively selective reduction of NA or serotonin turnover, using monoamine metabolites 3-methoxy-4-hydroxyphenylethylene glycol (MHPG; MOPEG) and 5-hydroxyindole-3-acetic acid (5-HIAA) as markers, by secondary or tertiary amines, respectively (Bertilsson et al., 1974). Administration of a tertiary amine TCA results in significant plasma concentrations of the demethylated metabolite as well, as discussed above; under such circumstances plasma levels of the parent drug correlate with decline in 5-HIAA whereas secondary amine concentrations relate to MHPG reduction (Muscettola et al., 1978; Traskman et al., 1979). Possible clinical implications of these biochemical differences have been reviewed by Goodwin et al. (1978). Hydroxy metabolites, in turn, are approximately equipotent reuptake blockers compared to the compounds from which they are derived in most in vitro systems (reviewed by Potter and Calil, 1981; Potter et al., 1984). Their action on other systems may differ from the parent drugs'; for example, 10-OH-AT and -NT are less anticholinergic than the corresponding nonhydroxylated TCAs (Hyttel et al., 1980).

The pharmacokinetics of demethylation have already been discussed in terms of the balance of metabolite formation and Cl (Potter et al., 1984). Very recently the kinetics of hydroxy metabolites have undergone scrutiny, as illustrated for example by the intensity of study of debrisoquine hydroxylation as a marker pathway. During treatment with AT, the three major active forms are AT, NT, and 10-OH-NT, with the latter two showing a 10-fold variation in concentration and the parent AT a 15-fold variability (Bock et al., 1982). This greater variability of the tertiary amine is consistent with its Cl being dependent on both demethylation and hydroxylation, which are independent of each other. Elimination of hydroxy metabolites has been described as the sum of two types of processes: conjugation or other metabolism (e.g. didemethylation) of the hydroxy form and direct renal Cl of the unconjugated hydroxy metabolite. Alteration of the latter pathway will be described below. Interindividual variability of metabolism of hydroxy metabolites has not been shown to be large and, given the overwhelming preponderance of the conjugation pathway, probably of minimal clinical importance with regard to the other processes (Potter et al., 1984).

Once formed, OH-metabolites of TCAs exhibit Css ranging from half (OH-DMI, Potter et al., 1982; OH-desmethylCMI, Linnoila et al., 1982b) or less (OH-CMI, Linnoila et al., 1982b) to greater than (OH-NT, Kragh-Sorensen et al., 1977; Bertilsson et al., 1979) that of the corresponding prehydroxylated compounds. Thus, at steady-state 2-OH-DMI concentrations are approximately 50% of those of DMI, whereas 10-OH-NT levels are 140% corresponding values for NT. 2-OH-DMI Css have been described as correlating positively with levels of DMI in some individuals (Potter and Calil, 1981) and negatively but nonsignificantly in others (Kitanaka et al., 1982). DMI concentrations have shown negative correlation with the concentration ratio of OH-DMI/DMI (Nelson et al., 1983); patients with very low hydroxy metabolite concentrations identified by Gram et al. (1983) demonstrated relatively high DMI levels felt to be consistent with poor hydroxylating ability of these individuals. Fraction of NT metabolised to the hydroxy compound has been reported as higher in rapid hydroxylators of the drug (Mellstrom et al., 1981); in the case of DMI the reverse was true (Rudorfer et al., 1984b), <u>slow</u> hydroxylators converting a larger fraction of an administered dose to the hydroxy metabolite than rapid hydroxylators. Significant (r = 0.63 and 0.75, respectively) associations between NT and OH-NT plasma levels were observed in two uncontrolled studies (Bertilsson et al., 1979; Ziegler et al., 1976b). It remains unclear what predictions of high NT concentrations imply in terms of concomitant OH-NT levels (Potter et al., 1984). While in our lab plasma concentrations of 2-OH-DMI + DMI correlate more closely with reduction in urinary MHPG during DMI treatment than do levels of parent drug alone, Nelson and associates (1983) found similar 2-OH-DMI concentrations in DMI responders and nonresponders, in contrast to the positive correlation they noted between DMI plasma levels and treatment response.

Metabolism of Drugs Used in Affective Disorders

As we have discussed elsewhere (Potter et al., 1983), metabolite concentration varies directly in a nonlinear fashion with Cl of parent drug to the metabolite and inversely with renal Cl of metabolite. The effects of altered renal function on hydroxy metabolite excretion have already been noted. Hydroxy metabolites are subject to conjugation or to further metabolic breakdown, none of which steps are known to demonstrate much interindividual variability (Potter et al., 1984). Decline of plasma hydroxy metabolite concentrations after TCA withdrawal paralleled those of the parent drug for both NT (Alexanderson and Borga, 1973; Alvan et al., 1977) and DMI (DeVane et al., 1981; Rudorfer et al., 1984b) as well as following IMI overdose (Gram et al., 1983). Similarly, the elimination $t_{1/2}$s of the demethylated and S-oxide metabolites of dothiepin were comparable to that of the parent TCA given as a single dose (Maguire et al., 1983).

One frequently cited study (Jandhyala et al., 1977) found greater cardiotoxicity of OH-IMI compared to an equal IV dose of the parent TCA; plasma drug concentrations were not controlled, thereby making it impossible to assess the true relative toxicities. We are aware of proposed protocols seeking to investigate the therapeutic and toxic activity as well as kinetics of tricyclic hydroxy metabolites administered to humans and animals. An initial effort at such an investigation has in fact been reported for one of the second generation antidepressants, the tetracyclic compound maprotiline. Schmidlin et al. (1982) documented decreased salivary flow and increased heart rate and blood pressure without alteration in plasma NA concentration in healthy volunteers given acute doses of OH-maprotiline, with the (+)-enantiomer more active than the (-) analogue. No drug concentrations were monitored in that study.

Other data on active metabolites of the newer antidepressant drugs are sparse at present, with some major exceptions. In contrast to the differential neurotransmitter effects of tertiary versus secondary amine TCAs noted above, norzimelidine, the demethylated metabolite of the bicyclic drug zimelidine (ZIM), is an even more potent 5-HT reuptake inhibitor than the parent compound (reviewed by Heel et al., 1982). As norzimeline plasma concentrations at steady-state are severalfold those of ZIM (Rudorfer et al., 1984c), the latter can be considered a prodrug. Clinical research on ZIM was abruptly halted by reports of neurotoxicity

(Rudorfer et al., 1984a). Recent speculation of an active metabolite of bupropion present in vivo in concentrations many times greater than the parent drug awaits confirmation. A heavily prescribed antidepressant of the 1980s, amoxapine, is notable for its 7-OH metabolite with dopamine receptor blocking activity (Fulton et al., 1982), presumed responsible for described antipsychotic properties of the drug as well as neuroleptic-like toxicity, e.g. galactorrhea, withdrawal and tardive dyskinesias (reviewed by Rudorfer et al., 1984a); 8-OH-amoxapine, which accumulates to much higher levels than the parent drug during treatment (Greenblatt et al., 1978; Cooper and Kelly, 1979; Wong and Waugh, 1983), probably accounts for much of the antidepressant effect. The primary, N-desmethyl, metabolite of maprotiline appears in plasma in significant concentrations at steady-state (Wong and Waugh, 1983), although maprotiline metabolites have not been accounted for thus far in clinical studies. Only one of the three principal metabolites of nomifensine (the 4-hydroxyphenyl derivative) has consistently demonstrated in vitro and in vivo biological activity (Brogden et al., 1979).

Metabolism of trazodone has not been reported in depressed patients. Healthy volunteer studies indicated the predominant species in plasma to be unchanged trazodone (Jauch et al., 1976; Yamato et al., 1976). In urine, the major metabolites after trazodone administration include the 4-hydroxy derivative, representing 20% of the dose, a dihydrodiol compound (15%), and a carboxylic acid resulting from oxidative cleavage (3.5%) (Jauch et al., 1976).

The major hydroxylated metabolite of the triazolobenzodiazepine alprazolam may have pharmacologic activity; early studies suggesting affinity of this metabolite to IMI binding sites have not been replicated by others (H. Bowen, personal communication). Furthermore, given some investigators' observation that very rapid Cl of the metabolite prevents in vivo accumulation of significant plasma concentrations (Greenblatt et al., 1983b), the clinical role of 4-hydroxyalprazolam awaits clarification. Similarly, of 6 identified renally excreted metabolites of bupropion (Schroeder, 1983), only 2 have any biological activity and these display less than half the potency of the parent drug.

Recent reports on the anticycling antidepressant carbamazepine have focused on its major, 10,11-epoxide metabolite, which reached a steady-state CSF concentration correlating with and nearly half that

of the parent drug (Post et al., 1983); in depressed
patients CSF levels of the metabolite but not of
carbamazepine itself were correlated with degree of
clinical improvement. Administration of the epoxide
to healthy volunteers (Tomson et al., 1983) has
served to better elucidate the kinetics of the metabolite; in the absence of a formation input, the
epoxide demonstrates an elimination $t_{1/2}$ 25% of that
of carbamazepine and is inactivated by a simple
hydration step.

Finally, conventional MAOI antidepressants are
not known to have any therapeutically active metabolites (Potter et al., 1984); an investigational
MAOI does have a minor alcohol derivative displaying
potent reversible inhibition of MAO type B (Dostert
et al., 1983). Formation of amphetamine compounds
from certain MAOIs has been noted (see below). However, as discussed above in the context of drug
interactions, intermediate byproducts of MAO inhibitors may contribute to tissue toxicity (reviewed by
Potter et al., 1981a).

Metabolism of Nontricyclic Antidepressants

Lithium

The Li cation is not metabolised per se. Although
its accompanying anion may undergo metabolism, this
has no effect on drug action as the purpose of the
anion is to facilitate Li absorption. As noted previously, the parameter of Li kinetics subject to
clinically significant interindividual variability
and alteration is renal excretion.

Second Generation Drugs

The spate of new antidepressant compounds developed
in recent years offers putative biochemical or clinical specificity and claimed improvements in side
effect profiles compared to conventional TCAs (see
Rudorfer et al., 1984a for review). Nonetheless,
the metabolic pathways mediating disposition of the
newer drugs are essentially the same as those for
the standard agents, i.e. hepatic demethylation and
oxidation with renal excretion of conjugated, polar
metabolites. Thus there appears to be no pharmacokinetic explanation for the reported differences in
activity between the two generations of antidepressants. Two-hr plasma levels of nomifensine did not
correlate with comparable values for AT in the same

volunteers in a single dose crossover study (Chan et al., 1980) but actual Cl rates were not determined.
Some of the specific, unique features of several of the second generation antidepressants have been cited in the preceding sections on drug interactions and active metabolites. Otherwise the differences among these drugs and between them and the older compounds are more quantitative than qualitative; for example, the $t_{1/2}$ of the tetracyclic maprotiline is approximately 2 days (Gruter and Poldinger, 1982) (Table 12.2), about twice that of standard TCAs other than PRO (Table 12.1), while at the other extreme, nomifensine's $t_{1/2}$ is only 2 to 4 hr in patients with normal renal functioning (Brogden et al., 1979) (see Tables 12.2 and 12.4). It should be noted that, as in the case of the TCAs, active metabolites affect the kinetics as well as function of the second generation drugs, e.g. the two active metabolites 8-OH- and 7-OH-amoxapine display $t_{1/2}$s of 30 and 4 hr, respectively (Greenblatt et al., 1978), versus 8 hr for the parent drug; Potter et al. (1981b) noted withdrawal $t_{1/2}$ of 7.8 hr for ZIM but 30.6 hr for norzimelidine.

Monoamine Oxidase Inhibitors

With intensive clinical research in affective (including atypical depression) and phobic disorders over the past decade has come a renewed niche for MAO inhibitors in the psychopharmacologic armamentarium (Nies and Robinson, 1982). Even more recently, the distinction between two types of the enzyme has led to the development of specific MAOIs acting either on MAO type A (e.g. clorgyline) or type B (e.g. L-deprenyl) (Potter et al., 1982b; Rudorfer et al., 1984a).
As most MAOIs are 'hit and run' drugs (Baldessarini, 1979) with enzyme-inhibiting effects long outlasting the drug's physical presence in detectable plasma levels (the latter measurements only recently available) (Cooper et al., 1978), indirect biochemical indices of drug effect have been used to monitor MAOI activity. These include platelet MAO inhibition, a probable marker of MAO-B (Robinson et al., 1978) and urinary MHPG levels as a reflection of MAO-A (Linnoila et al., 1982c); increase of the former or reduction in the latter parameter is associated with marked inhibition of the respective subtype of the enzyme.
For these reasons, understanding of the metabolism of MAOIs is somewhat rudimentary. The member

Table 12.4: Plasma clearance of 'second generation' antidepressants after an oral dose

Drug	Clearance (L/hr) Mean	Range	Reference
Maprotiline	41.1	5.5 – 20.0	Alkalay et al., 1980
Amoxapine	250.0		Unpublished**
Nomifensine	78.9	63.1 – 89.7	Vereczkey et al., 1975
Trazodone	8.9		Unpublished**
Mianserin	36.4*	23.1 – 56.7*	Hrdina et al., 1983
	68.6*	32.9 – 122.5*	Maguire et al., 1982
Bupropion	148.7*	136.9 – 155.8*	Findlay et al., 1981
Zimelidine	120.0	86.4 – 177.6	Brown et al., 1980

*Corrected for 70 kg body weight; **Lederle Laboratories, data on file; ***Mead Johnson & Co., Product Monograph, 1982

of this class most thoroughly investigated is the hydrazine derivative phenelzine. Much of the information on its handling is based on inferences from its chemical similarity to drugs such as INH and the sulfonamides which are subject to hepatic acetylation under polymorphic genetic control (Rawlins, 1974). Extrapolating from INH actions in tuberculosis patients, speculations that rapid acetylators of phenelzine experience greater side effects and clinical response than slow metabolisers has received considerable study with mixed, generally negative results (Rose, 1982). Indeed, Nies and Robinson (1982) did not find higher plasma concentrations of phenelzine in slow acetylators; these investigators questioned the importance of acetylation in MAOI metabolism. Moreover, some serious side effects of MAOIs such as hepatotoxicity or development of a lupus-like syndrome may be more pronounced in rapid acetylators and mediated by the development of free radicals or other toxic intermediate metabolites from the acetylhydrazine moiety via hepatic microsomal mixed function oxidases (ibid.).

Another important metabolic pathway of MAOIs consists of the formation of phenylethylamine metabolites by monoamine oxidase itself, first described by Clineschmidt and Horita (1969). In a study that identified 3 deaminated MAOI metabolites (with the acid derivative most prevalent in rat brain) Benedetti and Dow (1983) found a specific type B MAOI to be metabolised by the A form of the enzyme. Substitution of deuterium atoms for the 4 hydrogens in the phenelzine molecule that are removed by MAO created stronger bonds less susceptible to degradation by this enzyme and thus potentiated biochemical and behavioural effects of the antidepressant in a rat model (Dourish et al., 1983). Actual interferences by MAOIs of their own metabolism in the clinical situation has been hypothesised but not proven (Raft et al., 1981).

Another pathway of MAOI metabolism of potential clinical importance is the formation of methamphetamine and amphetamine from the specific MAO-B inhibitor L-deprenyl (Karoum et al., 1983), documented both in Parkinsonian patients and in rats; these active metabolites were believed to mediate the decreased urinary excretion of NA metabolites in these patients. Amphetamine, reported present in the plasma after tranylcypromine overdose but not routine therapeutic doses (Reynolds et al., 1980) may be responsible for the occasional instance of apparent addiction to that nonspecific MAOI.

In conclusion, metabolism of antidepressant drugs has been shown to vary widely between and within individuals, subject to both genetic and environmental factors. While the clinical significance of some aspects of drug metabolism, such as the prediction of steady-state concentrations, is clear, the role of other parameters, e.g. active metabolites and *in vivo* methylation, continues to evolve. The recently available 'second generation' compounds are more similar to than different from the standard drugs in terms of their disposition. As the remaining questions about antidepressant metabolism are answered, clinical use of current medications and the development of new agents are both likely to benefit.

References

Abernethy, D. R., Greenblatt, D. J., Divoll, M., Moschitto, L. J., Harmatz, J. S., and Shader, R. I. (1983) Interaction of cimetidine with the triazolobenzodiazepines alprazolam and triazolam. Psychopharmacology **80**, 275-278.

Alexanderson, B. (1972a) Pharmacokinetics of nortriptyline in man after single and multiple oral doses: the predictability of steady-state plasma concentrations from single-dose plasma-level data. Eur. J. Clin. Pharmacol. **4**, 82-91.

Alexanderson, B. (1972b) Pharmacokinetics of desmethylimipramine and nortriptyline in man after single and multiple oral doses--a cross-over study. Eur. J. Clin. Pharmacol. **5**, 1-10.

Alexanderson, B. (1973) Prediction of steady-state plasma levels of nortriptyline from single oral dose kinetics: a study in twins. Eur. J. Clin. Pharmacol. **6**, 44-53.

Alexanderson, B. and Borga, O. (1973) Urinary excretion of nortriptyline and five of its metabolites in man after single and multiple oral doses. Eur. J. Clin. Pharmacol. **5**, 174-180.

Alexanderson, B., Borga, O., and Alvan, G. (1973) The availability of orally administered nortriptyline. Eur. J. Clin. Pharmacol. **5**, 181-185.

Alexanderson, B., Price Evans, D. A., and Sjoqvist, F. (1969) Steady-state plasma levels of nortriptyline in twins: influence of genetic factors and drug therapy. Brit. Med. J. **4**, 764-768.

Alexanderson, B. and Sjoqvist, F. (1971) Individual differences in the pharmacokinetics of monomethylated tricyclic antidepressants: role of genetic and environmental factors and clinical importance. Ann. N.Y. Acad. Sci. **179**, 739-751.

Alkalay, D., Wagner, W. E. Jr., Carlsen, S., Khemani, L., Volk, J., Bartlett, M. F., and LeSher, A. (1980) Bioavailability and kinetics of maprotiline. Clin. Pharmacol. Ther. **27**, 679-703.

Allen, J. J., Rack, P. H., and Vaddadi, K. S. (1977) Differences in effects of clomipramine on English and Asian volunteers. Preliminary report on a pilot study. Postgrad. Med. J. **53** (Suppl. 4), 79-86.

Alvan, G., Borga, O., Lind, M., Palmer, L., and Siwers, B. (1977) First pass hydroxylation of nortriptyline: concentrations of parent drug and major metabolites in plasma. Eur. J. Clin. Pharmacol. **11**, 219-224.

Amdisen, A. (1977) Serum level monitoring and clinical pharmacokinetics of lithium. Clin. Pharmacokinet. 2, 73-92.

Amsterdam, J., Brunswick, D., and Mendels, J. (1980) The clinical application of tricyclic antidepressant pharmacokinetics and plasma levels. Am. J. Psychiatry 137, 653-662.

Antal, E. J., Lawson, I. R., Alderson, L. M., Chapron, D. J., and Kramer, P. A. (1982) Estimating steady state desipramine levels in noninstitutionalized elderly patients using single dose disposition parameters. J. Clin. Psychopharmacol. 2, 193-198.

Asberg, M., Cronholm, B., Sjoqvist, F., and Tuck, R. (1971a) Relationship between plasma level of nortriptyline and therapeutic effect. Brit. Med. J. 3, 331-334.

Asberg, M., Price Evans, D. A., and Sjoqvist, F. (1971b) Genetic control of nortriptyline kinetics in man. A study of relatives of propositi with high plasma concentrations. J. Med. Genetics 8, 129-135.

Bailey, D. N., Van Dyke, C., Langou, R. A., and Jatlow, P. I. (1978) Tricyclic antidepressants: plasma levels and clinical findings in overdose. Am. J. Psychiatry 135, 1325-1328.

Baldessarini, R. J. (1979) Status of psychotropic drug blood level assays and other biochemical measurements in clinical practice. Am. J. Psychiatry 136, 1177-1180.

Ballenger, J. C. and Post, R. M. (1980) Carbamazepine in manic-depressive illness: a new treatment. Am. J. Psychiatry 137, 782-790.

Ballinger, B. R., Presly, A., Reid, A. H., and Stevenson, I. H. (1974) The effects of hypnotics on imipramine treatment. Psychopharmacologia (Berl.) 39, 267-274.

Beaubien, A. R. and Pakuts, A. P. (1979) Influence of dose on first-pass kinetics of ^{14}C-imipramine in the isolated perfused rat liver. Drug Metab. Disp. 7, 34-39.

Beaubien, A. R. and Pakuts, A. P. (1980) Effect of thioridizine on the first-pass kinetics of [^{14}C]imipramine in perfused rat liver: interaction at hepatic binding sites. Xenobiotica 10, 235-242.

Belanger, P.-M. and Atitse-Gbeassor, A. (1982) Inhibitory effect of tranylcypromine in hepatic drug metabolism in the rat. Biochem. Pharmacol. 31, 2679-2683.

Bertilsson, L. and Aberg-Wistedt, A. (1983) The debrisoquine hydroxylation test predicts steady-state plasma levels of desipramine. Brit. J. Clin. Pharmacol. 15, 388-390.

Bertilsson, L., Asberg, M., and Thoren, P. (1974) Differential effect of chlorimipramine and nortriptyline on cerebrospinal fluid metabolites of serotonin and noradrenaline in depression. Eur. J. Clin. Pharmacol. 7, 365-368.

Bertilsson, L., Eichelbaum, M., Mellstrom, B., Sawe, J., Schulz, H.-U., and Sjoqvist, F. (1980) Nortriptyline and antipyrine clearance in relation to debrisoquine hydroxylation in man. Life Sci. 27, 1673-1677.

Bertilsson, L., Mellstrom, B., and Sjoqvist, F. (1979) Pronounced inhibition of noradrenaline uptake by 10-hydroxy-metabolites of nortriptyline. Life Sci. 25, 1285-1292.

Bickel, M. H., Brochon, R., Friolet, B., Hermann, B., and Stofer, A. R. (1967) Clinical and biochemical results of a fatal case of desipramine intoxication. Psychopharmacologia (Berl.) 10, 431-436.

Bjerre, M., Gram, L. F., Kragh-Sorensen, P., Kristensen, C. B., Pedersen, O. L., Moller, M., and Thayssen, P. (1981) Dose-dependent kinetics of imipramine in elderly patients. Psychopharmacology 75, 354-357.

Bock, J. L., Giller, E., Gray, S., and Jatlow, P. (1982) Steady-state plasma concentrations of cis- and trans-10-OH amitriptyline metabolites. Clin. Pharmacol. Ther. 31, 609-616.

Bock, J. L., Nelson, J. C., Gray, S., and Jatlow, P. I. (1983) Desipramine hydroxylation: variability and effect of antipsychotic drugs. Clin. Pharmacol. Ther. 33, 322-328.

Borga, O., Azarnoff, D. L., Plym-Forshell, G., and Sjoqvist, F. (1969) Plasma protein binding of tricyclic antidepressants in man. Biochem. Pharmacol. 18, 2135-2143.

Borromei, A. (1982) A new antidepressant agent: amitriptyline-N-oxide. Adv. Biochem. Psychopharmacol. 32, 43-47.

Braithwaite, R. A. and Dawling, S. (1981) The pharmacokinetics and metabolism of tricyclic antidepressant drugs in patients with chronic renal failure. In: Clinical Pharmacology in Psychiatry: Neuroleptic and Antidepressant Research (Usdin, E., Dahl, S. G., Gram, L. F., and Lingjaerde, O., eds), Macmillan, London, pp. 285-295.

Braithwaite, R. A., Montgomery, S., and Dawling, S. (1978) Nortriptyline in depressed patients with high plasma levels. II. Clin. Pharmacol. Ther. 23, 303-308.

Brogden, R. N., Heel, R. C., Speight, T. M., and Avery, G. S. (1978) Mianserin: a review of its pharmacological properties and therapeutic efficacy in depressive illness. Drugs 16, 273-301.

Brogden, R. N., Heel, R. C., Speight, T. M., and Avery, G. S. (1979) Nomifensine: a review of its pharmacological properties and therapeutic efficacy in depressive illness. Drugs 18, 1-24.

Brown, D., Scott, D. H. T., Scott, D. B., Meyer, M., Westerlund, D., and Lundstrom, J. (1980) Pharmacokinetics of zimelidine: systemic availability of zimelidine and norzimelidine in human volunteers. Eur. J. Clin. Pharmacol. 17, 111-116.

Brown, G. M., Stancer, H. C., Moldofsky, H., Harman, J., Murphy, J. T., and Gupta, R. N. (1978) Withdrawal from long-term high-dose desipramine therapy. Clinical and biological changes. Arch. Gen. Psychiatry 35, 1261-1264.

Browne, J. L., Perry, P. J., Alexander, B., Sherman, A. D., Tsuang, M. T., Dunner, F. J., and Pfohl, B. M. (1983) Pharmacokinetic protocol for predicting plasma nortriptyline levels. J. Clin. Psychopharmacol. 3, 351-356.

Brunswick, D. J., Amsterdam, J. D., Mendels, J., and Stern, S. L. (1979) Prediction of steady-state imipramine and desmethylimipramine plasma concentrations from single-dose data. Clin. Pharmacol. Ther. 25, 605-610.

Brunswick, D. J., Amsterdam, J. D., Schless, A., Rothbart, M., Sandler, K., and Mendels, J. (1980) Prediction of steady-state plasma levels of amitriptyline and nortriptyline from a single dose 24 hr. level in depressed patients. J. Clin. Psychiatry 41, 337-340.

Burch, J. E. and Hullin, R. P. (1981) Amitriptyline pharmacokinetics. A crossover study with single doses of amitriptyline and nortriptyline. Psychopharmacology 74, 35-42.

Burrows, G. D. and Davies, B. (1971) Antidepressants and barbiturates. Brit. Med. J. 4, 113.

Chan, M.-Y., Ehsanullah, R., Wadsworth, J., and McEwen, J. (1980) A comparison of the pharmacodynamic profiles of nomifensine and amitriptyline in normal subjects. Brit. J. Clin. Pharmacol. 9, 247-253.

Christ, W., Hecker, W., Junge, H., and Stille, G. (1983) Phase I metabolism of imipramine by microsomes of small intestine in comparison with metabolism by liver microsomes. Naunyn-Schmiedeberg's Arch. Pharmacol. 323, 176-182.

Christiansen, J. and Gram, L. F. (1973) Imipramine and its metabolites in human brain. J. Pharm. Pharmacol. 25, 604-608.

Christiansen, J., Gram, L. F., Kofod, B., and Rafaelsen, O. J. (1967) Imipramine metabolism in man. A study of urinary metabolites after administration of radioactive imipramine. Psychopharmacologia (Berl.) 11, 255-264.

Ciraulo, D. A., Alderson, L. M., Chapron, D. J., Jaffe, J. H., Subbarao, B., and Kramer, P. A. (1982) Imipramine disposition in alcoholics. J. Clin. Psychopharmacol. 2, 2-7.

Clineschmidt, B. V. and Horita, A. (1969) The monoamine oxidase catalyzed degradation of phenelzine-1-^{14}C, an irreversible inhibitor of monoamine oxidase--I. Studies in vitro. Biochem. Pharmacol. 18, 1011-1020.

Conney, A. H., Pantuck, E. J., Hsiao, K. C., Garland, W. A., Anderson, K. E., Alvares, A. P., and Kappas, A. (1976) Enhanced phenacetin metabolism in humans fed charcoal broiled beef. Clin. Pharmacol. Ther. 20, 633-642.

Cooper, T. B. and Kelly, R. G. (1979) GLC analysis of loxapine, amoxapine, and their metabolites in serum and urine. J. Pharm. Sci. 68, 216-219.

Cooper, T. B., Robinson, D. S., and Nies, A. (1978) Phenelzine measurement in human plasma: a sensitive GLC-ECD procedure. Commun. Psychopharmacol. 2, 505-512.

Cooper, T. B. and Simpson, G. M. (1978) Prediction of individual dosage of nortriptyline. Am. J. Psychiatry 135, 333-335.

Coppen, A. and Rama Rao, V. A. (1979) Amitriptyline and its demethylation-rate. Lancet i, 49.

Crammer, J. L., Scott, B., and Rolfe, B. (1969) Metabolism of ^{14}C-imipramine: II. Urinary metabolites in man. Psychopharmacologia (Berl.) 15, 207-225.

Crammer, J. L., Scott, B., Woods, H., and Rolfe, B. (1968) Metabolism of ^{14}C-imipramine: I. Excretion in the rat and in man. Psychopharmacologia (Berl.) 12, 263-277.

Cutler, N. R., Zavadil, A. P. III, Eisdorfer, C., Ross, R. J., and Potter, W. Z. (1981) Concentrations of desipramine in elderly women. Am. J. Psychiatry 138, 1235-1237.

Dawling, S., Crome, P., and Braithwaite, R. (1980) Pharmacokinetics of single oral doses of nortriptyline in depressed elderly hospital patients and young healthy volunteers. Clin. Pharmacokin. 5, 394-401.

Dawling, S., Lynn, K., Rosser, R., and Braithwaite, R. (1981) The pharmacokinetics of nortriptyline in patients with chronic renal failure. Brit. J. Clin. Pharmacol. 12, 39-45.

Dencker, H., Dencker, S. J., Green, A., and Nagy, A. (1976) Intestinal absorption, demethylation, and enterohepatic circulation of imipramine. Clin. Pharmacol. Ther. 19, 584-586.

DeVane, C. L., Savett, M., and Jusko, W. J. (1981) Desipramine and 2-hydroxydesipramine pharmacokinetics in normal volunteers. Eur. J. Clin. Pharmacol. 19, 61-64.

Dingell, J. V. and Sanders, E. (1966) Methylation of desmethylimipramine by rabbit lung in vitro. Biochem. Pharmacol. 15, 599-605.

Dorian, P., Sellers, E. M., Warsh, J. J., Reed, K. L., Hamilton, C., and Fan, T. (1982) Decreased hepatic first-pass extraction of oral drugs: mechanism of ethanol-amitriptyline interaction. Clin. Pharmacol. Ther. 31, 219.

Dostert, P., Strolin Benedetti, M., and Guffroy, C. (1983) Different stereo-selective inhibition of monoamine oxdiase-B by the R- and S-enantiomers of MD 780236. J. Pharm. Pharmacol. 35, 161-165.

Dourish, C. T., Dewar, K. M., Dyck, L. E., and Boulton, A. A. (1983) Potentiation of the behavioural effects of the antidepressant phenelzine by deuterium substitution. Psychopharmacology 81, 122-125.

Drimmer, E. J., Gitlin, M. J., and Gwirtsman, H. E. (1983) Desipramine and methylphenidate combination treatment for depression: case report. Am. J. Psychiatry 140, 241-242.

Eichelbaum, M., Erbom, K., Bertilsson, L., Ringberger, V., and Rane, A. (1975) Plasma kinetics of carbamazepine and its epoxide metabolite in man during single and multiple dosing. Eur. J. Clin. Pharmacol. 8, 337-341.

Erlandsen, E. J. and Gram, L. F. (1982) Imipramine kinetics in the single pass rat liver perfusion model. Acta Pharmacol. Toxicol. 50, 137-147.

Faulkner, R. D., Pitts, W. M., Lee, C. S., Lewis, W. A., and Fann, W. E. (1983) Multiple-dose doxepin kinetics in depressed patients. Clin. Pharmacol. Ther. 34, 509-515.

Findlay, J. W. A., Van Wyck Fleet, J., Smith, P. G., Butz, R. F., Hinton, M. L., Blum, M. R., and Schroeder, D. H. (1981) Pharmacokinetics of bupropion, a novel antidepressant agent, following oral administration to healthy subjects. Eur. J. Clin. Pharmacol. 21, 127-135.

Fraser, H. S., Bulpitt, C. J., Khan, C., Mould, G., Mucklow, J. C., and Dollery, C. T. (1976) Factors affecting antipyrine metabolism in West African villagers. Clin. Pharmacol. Ther. 20, 369-376.

Fredricson Overo, K., Gram, L. F., and Hansen, V. (1975) Kinetics of nortriptyline in man according to a two compartment model. Eur. J. Clin. Pharmacol. 8, 343-347.

Friedman, E. and Cooper, T. B. (1983) Pharmacokinetics of chlorimipramine and its demethylated metabolite in blood and brain regions of rats treated acutely and chronically with chlorimipramine. J. Pharmacol. Exp. Ther. 225, 387-390.

Fulton, A., Norman, T., and Burrows, G. D. (1982) Ligand binding and platelet uptake studies of loxapine, amoxapine and their 8-hydroxylated derivatives. J. Affec. Disorders 4, 113-119.

Garland, W. A. and Min, B. H. (1978) The kinetics of amitriptyline following single oral dose administration to man. Res. Commun. Chem. Pathol. Pharmacol. 22, 475-484.

Ghose, K. (1980) Interaction between lithium and carbamazepine. Brit. Med. J. 280, 1122.

Gibaldi, M. and Perrier, D. (1982) Pharmacokinetics, 2nd edn, Marcel Dekker, New York, pp. 45-111.

Giller, E. L. Jr., Bialos, D. S., Docherty, J. P., Jatlow, P., and Harkness, L. (1979) Chronic amitriptyline toxicity. Am. J. Psychiatry 136, 458-459.

Gillette, J. R. (1971) Factors affecting drug metabolism. Ann. N.Y. Acad. Sci. 179, 43-66.

Glassman, A. H., Johnson, L. L., Giardina, E.-G. V., Walsh, B. T., Roose, S. P., Cooper, T. B., and Bigger, J. T. Jr. (1983) The use of imipramine in depressed patients with congestive heart failure. J. Am. Med. Assoc. 250, 1997-2001.

Glassman, A. H., Perel, J. M., Shostak, M., Kantor, S. J., and Fleiss, J. L. (1977) Clinical implications of imipramine plasma levels for depressive illness. Arch. Gen. Psychiatry 34, 197-204.

Goodwin, F. K., Cowdry, R. W., and Webster, M. H. (1978) Predictions of drug response in the affective disorders: toward an integrated approach. In: Psychopharmacology--A Generation of Progress (Lipton, M., DiMascio, A., and Killam, K., eds),

Raven Press, New York, pp. 1277-1288.

Gram, L. F. (1974) Metabolism of tricyclic antidepressants. Dan. Med. Bull. 21, 218-231.

Gram, L. F. (1977) Factors influencing the metabolism of tricyclic antidepressants. Dan. Med. Bull. 24, 81-89.

Gram, L. F., Andreasen, P. B., Fredricson Overo, K., and Christiansen, J. (1976) Comparison of single dose kinetics of imipramine, nortriptyline and antipyrine in man. Psychopharmacology 50, 21-27.

Gram, L. F., Bjerre, M., Kragh-Sorensen, P., Kvinesdal, B., Molin, J., Pedersen, O. L., and Reisby, N. (1983) Imipramine metabolites in blood of patients during therapy and after overdose. Clin. Pharmacol. Ther. 33, 335-342.

Gram, L. F. and Christiansen, J. (1975) First-pass metabolism of imipramine in man. Clin. Pharmacol. Ther. 17, 555-563.

Gram, L. F. and Fredricson Overo, K. (1972) Drug interaction: inhibitory effect of neuroleptics on metabolism of tricyclic antidepressants in man. Brit. Med. J. 1, 463-465.

Gram, L. F. and Fredricson Overo, K. (1975) First-pass metabolism of nortriptyline in man. Clin. Pharmacol. Ther. 18, 305-314.

Gram, L. F., Fredricson Overo, K., and Kirk, L. (1974) Influence of neuroleptics and benzodiazepines on metabolism of tricyclic antidepressants in man. Am. J. Psychiatry 131, 863-866.

Gram, L. F., Sondergaard, I., Christiansen, J., Petersen, G. O., Bech, P., Reisby, N., Ibsen, I., Ortmann, J., Nagy, A., Dencker, S. J., Jacobsen, O., and Krautwald, O. (1977) Steady-state kinetics of imipramine in patients. Psychopharmacology 54, 255-261.

Greenblatt, D. J., Divoll, M., Abernethy, D. R., Moschitto, L. J., Smith, R. B., and Shader, R. I. (1983a) Alprazolam kinetics in the elderly. Arch. Gen. Psychiatry 40, 287-290.

Greenblatt, D. J., Divoll, M., Abernethy, D. R., and Shader, R. I. (1983b) Clinical pharmacokinetics of alprazolam, a triazolo benzodiazepine. In: The Affective Disorders (Davis, J. M. and Maas, J. W., eds), American Psychiatric Press, Washington, D.C., pp. 367-378.

Greenblatt, E. N., Hardy, R. A. Jr., and Kelly, R. G. (1978) Amoxapine. Pharmacol. Biochem. Prop. Drug Sub. 2, 1-19.

Gruter, W. and Poldinger, W. (1982) Maprotiline. Mod. Prob. Pharmacopsychiatry 18, 17-48.

Hammer, W., Idestrom, C.-M., and Sjoqvist, F. (1966) Chemical control of antidepressant drug therapy. In: *Proceedings First International Symposium on Antidepressant Drugs* (Garattini, S. and Dukes, M. N. G., eds), Exerpta Medica International Congress Series, Milan, No. 122, pp. 301-310.

Hammer, W., Martens, S., and Sjoqvist, F. (1969) A comparative study of the metabolism of desmethylimipramine, nortriptyline, and oxyphenylbutazone in man. *Clin. Pharmacol. Ther.* **10**, 44-49.

Hammer, W. and Sjoqvist, F. (1967) Plasma levels of monomethylated tricyclic antidepressants during treatment with imipramine-like compounds. *Life Sci.* **6**, 1895-1903.

Heel, R. C., Morley, P. A., Brogden, R. N., Carmine, A. A., Speight, T. M., and Avery, G. S. (1982) Zimelidine: a review of its pharmacological properties and therapeutic efficacy in depressive illness. *Drugs* **24**, 169-206.

Henry, B. W., Overall, J. E., and Markette, J. (1971) Comparison of major drug therapies for alleviation of anxiety and depression. *Dis. Nerv. Syst.* **32**, 655-667.

Hirschowitz, J., Bennett, J. A., Zemlan, F. P., and Garver, D. L. (1983) Thioridazine effect on desipramine plasma levels. *J. Clin. Psychopharmacol.* **3**, 376-379.

Hoffmann, K.-J., Regardh, C.-G., Aurell, M., Ervik, M., and Jordo, L. (1980) The effect of impaired renal function on the plasma concentration and urinary excretion of metoprolol metabolites. *Clin. Pharmacokin.* **5**, 181-191.

Hollister, L. E. (1983) Treating depressed patients with medical problems. In: *The Affective Disorders* (Davis, J. M. and Maas, J. W., eds), American Psychiatric Press, Washington, D.C., pp. 393-408.

Hrdina, P. D., Lapierre, Y. D., McIntosh, B., and Oyewumi, L. K. (1983) Mianserin kinetics in depressed patients. *Clin. Pharmacol. Ther.* **33**, 757-762.

Hrdina, P. D., Rovei, V., Henry, J. F., Hervy, M. P., Gomeni, R., Forette, F., and Morselli, P. L. (1980) Comparison of single-dose pharmacokinetics of imipramine and maprotiline in the elderly. *Psychopharmacology* **70**, 29-34.

Hyttel, J., Christiansen, A. V., and Fjalland, B. (1980) Neuropharmacological properties of amitriptyline, nortriptyline and their metabolites. *Acta Pharmacol. Toxicol.* **47**, 53-57.

Iber, F. L. (1977) Drug metabolism in heavy consumers of ethyl alcohol. Clin. Pharmacol. Ther. 22, 735-742.

Inaba, T., Otton, S. V., and Kalow, W. (1981) Debrisoquine hydroxylation capacity: problems of assessment in two populations. Clin. Pharmacol. Ther. 33, 394-399.

Jandhyala, B. S., Steenberg, M. L., Perel, J. M., Manian, A. A., and Buckley, J. P. (1977) Effects of several tricyclic antidepressants on the hemodynamics and myocardial contractibility of the anesthetized dogs. Eur. J. Pharmacol. 42, 403-410.

Jauch, Von R., Kopitar, Z., Prox, A., and Zimmer, A. (1976) Pharmakokinetik und stoffwechsel von trazodone beim menschen. Arzneim.-Forsch. 26, 2084-2089.

Jenner, F. A. (1979) Lithium and the question of kidney damage. Arch. Gen. Psychiatry 36, 888-890.

John, V. A., Luscombe, D. K., and Kemp, H. (1980) Effects of age, cigarette smoking and the oral contraceptive on the pharmacokinetics of clomipramine and its desmethyl metabolite during chronic dosing. J. Int. Med. Res. 8 (Suppl. 3), 88-95.

Jorgensen, A. and Hansen, V. (1976) Pharmacokinetics of amitriptyline infused intravenously in man. Eur. J. Clin. Pharmacol. 10, 337-341.

Jungkunz, G. and Kuss, H. J. (1978) Amitriptyline and its demethylation-rate. Lancet ii, 1263-1264.

Kalow, W. (1982) The metabolism of xenobiotics in different populations. Can. J. Physiol. Pharmacol. 60, 1-12.

Karoum, F., Chuang, L.-W., Eisler, T., Calne, D. B., Liebowitz, M. R., Quitkin, F. M., Klein, D. F., and Wyatt, R. J. (1982) Metabolism of (-) deprenyl to amphetamine and methamphetamine may be responsible for deprenyl's therapeutic benefit: a biochemical assessment. Neurology 32, 503-509.

Kitanaka, I., Ross, R. J., Cutler, N. R., Zavadil, A. P. III, and Potter, W. Z. (1982) Altered hydroxydesipramine concentrations in elderly depressed patients. Clin. Pharmacol. Ther. 31, 51-55.

Kleinman, A. (1981) Culture and patient care: psychiatry among the Chinese. Drug Ther. 11, 134-140.

Kragh-Sorensen, P., Borga, O., Garle, M., Hansen, L. B., Hansen, C. E., Hvidberg, E. F., Larsen, N.-E., and Sjoqvist, F. (1977) Effect of simultaneous treatment with low doses of perphenazine on plasma and urine concentrations of nortriptyline and 10-hydroxynortriptyline. Eur. J. Clin. Pharmacol. 11, 479-483.

Kragh-Sorensen, P. and Larsen, N.-E. (1980) Factors influencing nortriptyline steady-state kinetics: plasma and saliva levels. Clin. Pharmacol. Ther. 28, 796-803.

Kristensen, C. B. (1983) Imipramine serum protein binding in healthy subjects. Clin. Pharmacol. Ther. 34, 689-694.

Levy, R. H., Lane, E. A., Guyot, M., Brachet-Liermain, A., Cenraud, B., and Loiseau, P. (1983) Analysis of parent drug-metabolite relationship in the presence of an inducer: application to the carbamazepine-clobazam interaction in normal man. Drug Metab. Dispos. 9, 286-292.

Lewis, P., Vaddadi, K. S., Rack, P. H., and Allen, J. J. (1980) Ethnic differences in drug response. Postgrad. Med. J. 56 (Suppl. 1), 46-49.

Lin, K.-M. and Finder, E. (1984) Different doses of neuroleptics for genetically different groups. Am. J. Psychiatry 141, 158.

Linnoila, M., Dorrity, F. Jr., and Jobson, K. (1978) Plasma and erythrocyte levels of tricyclic antidepressants in depressed patients. Am. J. Psychiatry 135, 557-561.

Linnoila, M., George, L., and Guthrie, S. (1982a) Interaction between antidepressants and perphenazine in psychiatric inpatients. Am. J. Psychiatry 139, 1329-1331.

Linnoila, M., George, L., Guthrie, S., and Leventhal, B. (1981) Effect of alcohol consumption and cigarette smoking on antidepressant levels of depressed patients. Am. J. Psychiatry 138, 841-842.

Linnoila, M., Insel, T., Kilts, C., Potter, W. Z., and Murphy, D. L. (1982b) Plasma steady-state concentrations of hydroxylated metabolites of clomipramine. Clin. Pharmacol. Ther. 32, 208-211.

Linnoila, M., Karoum, F., and Potter, W. Z. (1982c) Effect of low-dose clorgyline on 24-hour urinary monoamine excretion in patients with rapidly cycling bipolar affective disorder. Arch. Gen. Psychiatry 39, 513-516.

Loomis, C. W. and Racz, W. J. (1980) Drug interactions of amitriptyline and nortriptyline with warfarin in the rat. Res. Commun. Chem. Pathol. Pharmacol. 30, 41-58.

Lundborg, P., Regardh, C. G., and Landahl, S. (1982) The pharmacokinetics of metoprolol in healthy elderly individuals. Clin. Pharmacol. Ther. 31, 246.

Luscombe, D. K. and Jones, R. B. (1977) Effects of concomitantly administered drugs on plasma levels of clomipramine and desmethylclomipramine in depressive patients receiving clomipramine therapy. Postgrad. Med. J. 53 (Suppl. 4), 77-78.

Madakasira, S., Preskorn, S. H., Weller, R., and Pardo, M. (1982) Single dose prediction of steady state plasma levels of amitriptyline. J. Clin. Psychopharmacol. 2, 136-139.

Maguire, K. P., Norman, T. R., Burrows, G. D., and Scoggins, B. A. (1982) A pharmacokinetic study of mianserin. Eur. J. Clin. Pharmacol. 21, 517-520.

Maguire, K. P., Norman, T. R., McIntyre, I., and Burrows, G. D. (1983) Clinical pharmacokinetics of dothiepin. Single-dose kinetics in patients and prediction of steady-state concentrations. Clin. Pharmacokin. 8, 179-185.

Mahgoub, A., Idle, J. R., Dring, L. G., Lancaster, R., and Smith, R. L. (1977) Polymorphic hydroxylation of debrisoquine in man. Lancet ii, 584-586.

Massey, E. W. (1983) Effect of carbamazepine on coumadin metabolism. Ann. Neurol. 13, 691-692.

Mellstrom, B., Alvan, G., Bertilsson, L., Potter, W. Z., Sawe, J., and Sjoqvist, F. (1982) Nortriptyline formation after single oral and intramuscular doses of amitriptyline. Clin. Pharmacol. Ther. 32, 664-667.

Mellstrom, B., Bertilsson, L., Birgersson, C., Goransson, M., and von Bahr, C. (1983a) E- and Z-10-hydroxylation of nortriptyline by human liver microsomes--methods and characterization. Drug Metab. Dispos. 11, 115-119.

Mellstrom, B., Bertilsson, L., Lou, Y.-C., Sawe, J., and Sjoqvist, F. (1983b) Amitriptyline metabolism: relationship to polymorphic debrisoquine hydroxylation. Clin. Pharmacol. Ther. 34, 516-520.

Mellstrom, B., Bertilsson, L., Sawe, J., Schulz, H.-U., and Sjoqvist, F. (1981) E- and Z-10-hydroxylation of nortriptyline: relationship to polymorphic debrisoquine hydroxylation. Clin. Pharmacol. Ther. 30, 189-193.

Mellstrom, B., Bertilsson, L., Traskman, L., Rollins, D., Asberg, M., and Sjoqvist, F. (1979) Intraindividual similarity in the metabolism of amitriptyline and chlorimipramine in 41 depressed patients. Pharmacology 19, 282-287.

Mellstrom, B. and von Bahr, C. (1981) Demethylation and hydroxylation of amitriptyline, nortriptyline, and 10-hydroxyamitriptyline in human liver microsomes. Drug Metab. Dispos. 9, 565-568.

Miller, D. D. and Macklin, M. (1983) Cimetidine-imipramine interaction: a case report. Am. J. Psychiatry 140, 351-352.

Miller, D. D. and Macklin, M. (1984) Cimetidine-imipramine interaction: case report and comments. Am. J. Psychiatry 141, 153.

Montgomery, S. A., McAuley, R., Sani, S. J., Montgomery, D. B., Dawling, S., and Braithwaite, R. A. (1979) Amitriptyline plasma concentrations and clinical response. Brit. Med. J. 1, 230-231.

Moody, J. P., Whyte, S. F., MacDonald, A. J., and Naylor, G. J. (1977) Pharmacokinetic aspects of protriptyline plasma levels. Eur. J. Clin. Pharmacol. 11, 51-56.

Muller, W. E., Stillbauer, A. E., and El-Gamal, S. (1983) Psychotropic drug competition for ^{3}H-imipramine binding further indicates the presence of only one high-affinity drug binding site on human alpha-1-acid glycoprotein. J. Pharm. Pharmacol. 35, 684-686.

Muscettola, G., Goodwin, F. K., Potter, W. Z., Claeys, M. M., and Markey, S. P. (1978) Imipramine and desipramine in plasma and spinal fluid. Relationship to clinical response and serotonin metabolism. Arch. Gen. Psychiatry 35, 621-625.

Nagy, A. (1977) Blood and brain concentrations of imipramine, clomipramine and their monomethylated metabolites after oral and intramuscular administration in rats. J. Pharm. Pharmacol. 29, 104-107.

Nagy, A. and Hansen, T. (1978) The kinetics of imipramine-N-oxide in man. Acta pharmacol. toxicol. 42, 58-67.

Nagy, A. and Johansson, R. (1975) Plasma levels of imipramine and desipramine in man after different routes of administration. Naunyn-Schmiedeberg's Arch. Pharmacol. 290, 145-160.

Nagy, A. and Johansson, R. (1977) The demethylation of imipramine and clomipramine as apparent from their plasma kinetics. Psychopharmacology 54, 125-131.

Nakano, S. and Hollister, L. E. (1978) No circadian effect on nortriptyline kinetics in man. Clin. Pharmacol. Ther. 23, 199-203.

Nakano, S. and Hollister, L. E. (1983) Chronopharmacology of amitriptyline. Clin. Pharmacol. Ther. 33, 453-459.

Narasimhachari, N. and Lin, R.-L. (1976) Structure-activity relationships among desmethyl derivatives of neuroleptics and antidepressants for substrate specificity to indolethylamine N-methyltransferase from rabbit lung. Psychopharmacol. Commun. 2, 27-38.

Narasimhachari, N., Saady, J. J., Joseph, A., Ettigi, P., and Friedel, R. O. (1982) Evidence for in vivo methylation of the secondary amino antidepressant desipramine to imipramine in humans. J. Clin. Psychopharmacol. 2, 413-416.

Nawishy, S., Hathway, N., and Turner, P. (1981) Interactions of anticonvulsant drugs with mianserin and nomifensine. Lancet ii, 871-872.

Neal, A., Meffin, P., Gregory, P., and Blaschke, T. (1979) Enhanced bioavailability and decreased clearance of analgesics in patients with cirrhosis. Gastroenterology 77, 96-102.

Nelson, J. C., Bock, J. L., and Jatlow, P. I. (1983) Clinical implications of 2-hydroxydesipramine plasma concentrations. Clin. Pharmacol. Ther. 33, 183-189.

Niazi, S. (1976) Comparison of observed and predicted first-pass metabolism of nortriptyline in humans. J. Pharm. Sci. 65, 1535-1536.

Nies, A. and Robinson, D. S. (1982) Monoamine oxidase inhibitors. In: Handbook of Affective Disorders (Paykel, E. S., ed.), Guilford Press, New York, pp. 246-261.

Nies, A., Robinson, D. S., Friedman, M. J., Green, R., Cooper, T. B., Ravaris, C. L., and Ives, J. O. (1977) Relationship between age and tricyclic antidepressant plasma levels. Am. J. Psychiatry 134, 790-793.

Norman, T. R., Burrows, G. D., Maguire, K. P., Rubinstein, G., Scoggins, B. A., and Davies, B. (1977) Cigarette smoking and plasma nortriptyline levels. Clin. Pharmacol. Ther. 21, 453-456.

O'Malley, K., Stevenson, I. H., and Crooks, J. (1972) Impairment of human drug metabolism by oral contraceptive steroids. Clin. Pharmacol. Ther. 13, 552-557.

Overall, J. E., Hollister, L. E., Kimbell, I. Jr., and Shelton, J. (1969) Extrinsic factors influencing responses to psychotherapeutic drugs.

Arch. Gen. Psychiatry **21**, 89-94.

Perel, J. M., Shostak, M., Gann, E., Kantor, S. J., and Glassman, A. H. (1976) Pharmacodynamics of imipramine and clinical outcome in depressed patients. In: Pharmacokinetics of Psychoactive Drugs (Gottschalk, L. A. and Merlis, S., eds), Spectrum Press, New York, pp. 229-241.

Perucca, E. and Richens, A. (1977) Interactions between phenytoin and imipramine. Brit. J. Clin. Pharmacol. **4**, 485-486.

Post, R. M. and Uhde, T. W. (1984) Carbamazepine as a treatment for refractory depressive illness and rapidly cycling manic-depressive illness. In: Special Treatments for Resistant Depression (Zohar, J. and Belmaker, R. H., eds), Spectrum Press, New York (in press).

Post, R. M., Uhde, T. W., Ballenger, J. C., Chatterji, D. C., Greene, R. F., and Bunney, W. E. Jr. (1983) Carbamazepine and its -10, 11-epoxide metabolite in plasma and CSF. Arch. Gen. Psychiatry **40**, 673-676.

Pottash, A. L. C., Martin, D. M., Extein, I., Mas, F., Jarvis, A. H., Zirk, R. G., and Gold, M. S. (1983) The prediction of therapeutic nortriptyline dosage regimes and related plasma concentrations of hydroxylated metabolites in geriatric depressives. Soc. Neurosci. Abstr. **9**, 428.

Potter, W. Z., Bertilsson, L., and Sjoqvist, F. (1981) Clinical pharmacokinetics of psychotropic drugs: fundamental and practical aspects. In: The Handbook of Biological Psychiatry: Part VI, Practical Applications of Psychotropic Drugs and Other Biological Treatments (van Praag, H. M., Rafaelson, O., Lader, M., and Sachar, A., eds), Marcel Dekker, New York, pp. 71-134.

Potter, W. Z. and Calil, H. M. (1981) Metabolites of tricyclic antidepressants: biological activity and clinical implications. In: Clinical Pharmacology in Psychiatry (Usdin, E., ed.), Elsevier, New York, pp. 311-324.

Potter, W. Z., Calil, H. M., Extein, I., Gold, P. W., Wehr, T. A., and Goodwin, F. K. (1981) Specific norepinephrine and serotonin uptake inhibitors in man: a crossover study with pharmacokinetic, biochemical, neuroendocrine and behavioral parameters. Acta psychiatr. scand. **63** (Suppl. 290), 152-165.

Potter, W. Z., Calil, H. M., Manian, A. A., Zavadil, A. P. III, and Goodwin, F. K. (1979) Hydroxylated metabolites of tricyclic antidepressants: preclinical assessment of activity. Biol. Psychia-

try **14**, 601-613.
Potter, W. Z., Calil, H. M., Sutfin, T. A., Zavadil, A. P. III, Jusko, W. J., Rapoport, J., and Goodwin, F. K. (1982a) Active metabolites of imipramine and desipramine in man. Clin. Pharmacol. Ther. **31**, 393-401.
Potter, W. Z., Lane, E. A., and Rudorfer, M. V. (1983) Hydroxy metabolite concentrations: role of renal clearance. In: Clinical Pharmacology in Psychiatry: Bridging the Experimental-Therapeutic Gap (Gram, L. F., Usdin, E., Dahl, S. G., Kragh-Sorensen, P., Sjoqvist, F., and Morselli, P. L., eds), Macmillan Press, London, pp. 203-216.
Potter, W. Z. and Linnoila, M. (1984) Tricyclic antidepressant concentrations: clinical and research implications. In: Neurobiology of Mood Disorders (Post, R. M. and Ballenger, J. C., eds), Williams and Wilkins, Baltimore, pp. 698-709.
Potter, W. Z., Murphy, D. L., Wehr, T. A., Linnoila, M., and Goodwin, F. K. (1982b) Clorgyline: a new treatment for patients with refractory rapid-cycling disorder. Arch. Gen. Psychiatry **39**, 505-510.
Potter, W. Z., Rudorfer, M. V., and Lane, E. A. (1984) Active metabolites of antidepressants: pharmacodynamics and relevant pharmacokinetics. In: Frontiers in Biochemical and Pharmacological Research in Depression (Usdin, E., Bertilsson, L., and Sjoqvist, F., eds), Raven Press, New York, pp. 373-390.
Potter, W. Z., Zavadil, A. P. III, Kopin, I. J., and Goodwin, F. K. (1980) Single-dose kinetics predict steady-state concentrations of imipramine and desipramine. Arch. Gen. Psychiatry **37**, 314-320.
Preskorn, S. H. and Hughes, C. W. (1983) Ethanol effects on brain concentrations of amitriptyline and the relationship to psychomotor function. Psychopharmacology **80**, 217-220.
Price Evans, D. A., Mahgoub, A., Sloan, T. P., Idle, J. R., and Smith, R. L. (1980) A family and population study of the genetic polymorphism of debrisoquine oxidation in a white British population. J. Med. Genetics **17**, 102-105.
Prien, R. F. (1981) Age-related changes in lithium pharmacokinetics. In: Age and the Pharmacology of Psychoactive Drugs (Raskin, A., Robinson, D. S., and Levine, J., eds), Elsevier, New York, pp. 163-169.

Raft, B., Davidson, J., Wasik, J., and Mattox, A. (1981) Relationship between response to phenelzine and MAO inhibition in a clinical trial of phenelzine, amitriptyline, and placebo. Neuropsychobiology **7**, 122-126.

Ragheb, M., Ban, T. A., Buchanan, D., and Frolich, J. C. (1980) Interaction of indomethacin and ibuprofen with lithium in manic patients under a steady-state lithium level. J. Clin. Psychiatry **41**, 397-398.

Rane, A. and Wilson, J. T. (1976) Clinical pharmacokinetics in infants and children. Clin. Pharmacokin. **1**, 2-24.

Rapoport, J. L. and Potter, W. Z. (1981) Tricyclic antidepressants and children. In: Age and the Pharmacology of Psychoactive Drugs (Raskin, A., Robinson, D. S., and Levine, J., eds), Elsevier, New York, pp. 105-123.

Rapp, W. (1978) Comparative trial of amitriptyline-N-oxide and amitriptyline in the treatment of out-patients with depressive syndromes. Acta psychiatr. scand. **58**, 245-255.

Raskin, A. and Crook, T. H. (1975) Antidepressants in black and white inpatients: differential response to a controlled trial of chlorpromazine and imipramine. Arch. Gen. Psychiatry **32**, 643-649.

Rawlins, M. D. (1974) Variability in response to drugs. Brit. Med. J. **4**, 91-94.

Reisby, N., Gram, L. F., Bech, P., Nagy, A., Petersen, G. O., Ortmann, J., Ibsen, I., Dencker, S. J., Jacobsen, O., Krautwald, O., Sondergaard, I., and Christiansen, J. (1977) Imipramine: clinical effects and pharmacokinetic variability. Psychopharmacology **54**, 263-272.

Reynolds, G. P., Rausch, W.-D., and Riederer, P. (1980) Effects of tranylcypromine stereoisomers on monoamine oxidation in man. Brit. J. Clin. Pharmacol. **9**, 521-523.

Riess, W., Dubey, L., Funfgeld, E. W., Imhof, P., Hurzeler, H., Matussek, N., Rajagopalan, T. G., Raschdorf, F., and Schmid, K. (1975) The pharmacokinetic properties of maprotiline (Ludiomil®) in man. J. Int. Med. Res. **3** (Suppl. 2), 16-41.

Robinson, D. S. (1981) Monoamine oxidase inhibitors and the elderly. In: Age and the Pharmacology of Psychoactive Drugs (Raskin, A., Robinson, D. S., and Levine, J., eds), Elsevier, New York, pp. 157-162.

Robinson, D. S., Nies, A., Ravaris, C. L., Ives, J. O., and Bartlett, D. (1978) Clinical pharmacology of phenelzine. Arch. Gen. Psychiatry 35, 629-635.

Rollins, D. E., Alvan, G., Bertilsson, L., Gillette, J. R., Mellstrom, B., Sjoqvist, F., and Traskman, L. (1980) Interindividual differences in amitriptyline demethylation. Clin. Pharmacol. Ther. 28, 121-129.

Rose, S. (1982) The relationship of acetylation phenotype to treatment with MAOIs: a review. J. Clin. Psychopharmacol. 2, 161-164.

Ross, S. B. and Renyi, A. L. (1975) Tricyclic antidepressant agents. I. Comparison of the inhibition of the uptake of ^{3}H-noradrenaline and ^{14}C-5-hydroxytryptamine in slices and crude synaptosome preparations of the midbrain-hypothalamus region of the rat brain. Acta Pharmacol. Toxicol. 36, 382-392.

Rudorfer, M. V., Golden, R. N., and Potter, W. Z. (1984a) Second generation antidepressants. In: 'Clinical Psychopharmacology' (Lake, C. R., ed.), Psychiatr. Clin. North Am. (in press).

Rudorfer, M. V., Lane, E. A., Chang, W.-H., Zhang, M., and Potter, W. Z. (1984b) Desipramine pharmacokinetics in Chinese and Caucasian volunteers. Brit. J. Clin. Pharmacol. 17 (in press).

Rudorfer, M. V., Lane, E. A., and Potter, W. Z. Interethnic dissociation between debrisoquine and desipramine hydroxylation (submitted).

Rudorfer, M. V. and Robins, E. (1981) Fatal nortriptyline overdose, plasma levels, and in vivo methylation of tricyclic antidepressants. Am. J. Psychiatry 138, 982-983.

Rudorfer, M. V. and Robins, E. (1982) Amitriptyline overdose: clinical effects on tricyclic antidepressant plasma levels. J. Clin. Psychiatry 43, 457-460.

Rudorfer, M. V., Scheinin, M., Karoum, F., Ross, R. J., Potter, W. Z., and Linnoila, M. (1984c) Reduction of norepinephrine turnover by serotonergic drug in man. Biol. Psychiatry 19, 179-193.

Rudorfer, M. V. and Young, R. C. (1980) Plasma desipramine levels after single dosage and at steady state in outpatients. Commun. Psychopharmacol. 4, 185-188.

Salzman, C. (1982) Primer on geriatric psychopharmacology. Am. J. Psychiatry 139, 67-74.

Sathananthan, G. L., Gershon, S., Almeida, M., Spector, N., and Spector, S. (1976) Correlation between plasma and cerebrospinal levels of imipramine. Arch. Gen. Psychiatry 33, 1109-1110.

Schmidlin, O., Gundert-Remy, U., Maurer, W., and Weber, E. (1982) Differences of sympathomimetic and anticholinergic action of OH-maprotiline and its R(-)-enantiomer. Brit. J. Clin. Pharmacol. 14, 799-804.

Schroeder, D. H. (1983) Metabolism and kinetics of bupropion. J. Clin. Psychiatry 44 (Sec. 2), 79-81.

Schulz, P. and Luttrell, S. (1982) Increased plasma protein binding of imipramine in cancer patients. J. Clin. Psychopharmacol. 2, 417-420.

Schulz, P., Turner-Tamiyasu, K., Smith, G., Giacomini, K. M., and Blaschke, T. F. (1983) Amitriptyline disposition in young and elderly normal men. Clin. Pharmacol. Ther. 33, 360-366.

Sellers, E. M., MacLeod, S. M., Greenblatt, D. J., and Giles, H. G. (1977) Influence of disulfiram and disease on benzodiazepine disposition. Clin. Pharmacol. Ther. 21, 117.

Shader, R. I., Divoll, M., and Greenblatt, D. J. (1981) Kinetics of oxazepam and lorazepam in two subjects with Gilbert syndrome. J. Clin. Psychopharmacol. 1, 400-402.

Silverman, G. and Braithwaite, R. A. (1973) Benzodiazepines and tricyclic antidepressant plasma levels. Brit. Med. J. 3, 18-20.

Siris, S. G., Cooper, T. B., Rifkin, A. E., Brenner, R., and Lieberman, J. A. (1982) Plasma imipramine concentrations in patients receiving concomitant fluphenazine decanoate. Am. J. Psychiatry 139, 104-106.

Siris, S. G. and Rifkin, A. (1981) The problem of psychopharmacotherapy in the medically ill. In: 'The Medically Ill Patient' (Strain, J. J., ed.), Psychiatr. Clin. North Am. 4, 379-390.

Sjoqvist, F. (1981) General issues related to age and the pharmacology of psychoactive drugs. In: Age and the Pharmacology of Psychoactive Drugs (Raskin, A., Robinson, D. S., and Levine, J., eds), Elsevier, New York, pp. 195-204.

Sjoqvist, F., Gosta Bergfors, P., Borga, O., Lind, M., and Ygge, H. (1972) Plasma disappearance of nortriptyline in a newborn infant following placental transfer from an intoxicated mother: evidence of drug metabolism. J. Pediatr. 80, 496-500.

Somogyi, A. and Gugler, R. (1982) Drug interactions with cimetidine. Clin. Pharmacokin. 7, 23-41.

Spiker, D. G. and Biggs, J. T. (1976) Tricyclic antidepressants: prolonged plasma levels after overdose. J. Am. Med. Assoc. 236, 1711-1712.

Spiker, D. G., Weiss, A. N., Chang, S. S., Ruwitch, J. F. Jr., and Biggs, J. T. (1975) Tricyclic antidepressant overdose: clinical presentation and plasma levels. Clin. Pharmacol. Ther. 18, 539-546.

Stegmann, R. and Bickel, M. H. (1977) Dominant role for tissue binding in the first-pass extraction of imipramine by the perfused rat liver. Xenobiotica 7, 737-746.

Strolin Benedetti, M. and Dow, J. (1983) A monoamine oxidase-B inhibitor, MD 780236, metabolized essentially by the A form of the enzyme in the rat. J. Pharm. Pharmacol. 35, 238-245.

Tollefson, G. and Lesar, T. (1984) Effect of propranolol on maprotiline clearance. Am. J. Psychiatry 141, 148-149.

Tomson, T., Tybring, G., and Bertilsson, L. (1983) Single-dose kinetics and metabolism of carbamazepine-10,11-epoxide. Clin. Pharmacol. Ther. 33, 58-65.

Traskman, L., Asberg, M., Bertilsson, L., Cronholm, B., Mellstrom, B., Neckers, L. M., Sjoqvist, F., Thoren, P., and Tybring, G. (1979) Plasma levels of chlorimipramine and its demethyl metabolite during treatment of depression. Clin. Pharmacol. Ther. 26, 600-610.

Vahakangas, K., Pelkonen, O., and Sotaniemi, E. (1983) Cigarette smoking and drug metabolism. Clin. Pharmacol. Ther. 33, 375-380.

Valsalan, V. C. and Cooper, G. L. (1982) Carbamazepine intoxication caused by interaction with isoniazid. Brit. Med. J. 285, 261-262.

Vandel, B., Sandoz, M., Vandel, S., Allers, G., and Volmat, R. (1982) Biotransformation of amitriptyline in depressive patients: urinary excretion of seven metabolites. Eur. J. Clin. Pharmacol. 22, 239-245.

Vandel, B., Vandel, S., Allers, G., Bechtel, P., and Volmat, R. (1979) Interaction between amitriptyline and phenothiazine in man: effect on plasma concentration of amitriptyline and its metabolite nortriptyline and the correlation with clinical response. Psychopharmacology 65, 187-190.

Vereczkey, L., Bianchetti, G., Garattini, S., and Morselli, P. L. (1975) Pharmacokinetics of nomifensine in man. Psychopharmacologia (Berl.) 45,

225-227.
Virtanen, R., Scheinin, M., and Iisalo, E. (1980) Single dose pharmacokinetics of doxepin in healthy volunteers. Acta pharmacol. toxicol. 47, 371-376.
von Bahr, C. (1972) Metabolism of tricyclic antidepressant drugs: pharmacokinetic and molecular aspects. Thesis, Karolinska Institute, Stockholm.
von Bahr, C. and Bertilsson, L. (1971) Hydroxylation and subsequent glucuronide conjugation of desmethylimipramine in rat liver microsomes. Xenobiotica 1, 205-212.
von Bahr, C., Borga, O., Fellenius, E., and Rowland, M. (1973) Kinetics of nortriptyline (NT) in rats in vivo and in the isolated perfused liver: demonstration of a 'first pass disappearance' of NT in the liver. Pharmacology 9, 177-186.
Warwick, H. M. C. and Mindham, R. H. S. (1983) Concomitant administration of mianserin and warfarin. Brit. J. Psychiatry 143, 308.
Wharton, R. N., Perel, J. M., Dayton, P. G., and Malitz, S. (1971) A potential clinical use for methylphenidate with tricyclic antidepressants. Am. J. Psychiatry 127, 1619-1625.
Whitford, G. M. (1978) Acetylator phenotype in relation to monoamine oxidase inhibitor antidepressant drug therapy. Int. Pharmacopsychiatry 13, 126-132.
Wilkinson, G. R. and Schenker, S. (1976) Effects of liver disease on drug disposition in man. Biochem. Pharmacol. 25, 2675-2681.
Wilkinson, G. R. and Shand, D. G. (1975) A physiological approach to hepatic drug clearance. Clin. Pharmacol. Ther. 18, 377-390.
Williams, R. L. (1983) Drug administration in hepatic disease. N. Engl. J. Med. 309, 1616-1622.
Wong, S. H. Y. and Waugh, S. W. (1983) Determination of the antidepressants maprotiline and amoxapine, and their metabolites, in plasma by liquid chromatography. Clin. Chem. 29, 314-318.
Wood, A. J. J., Kornhauser, D. M., Wilkinson, G. R., Shand, D. G., and Branch, R. A. (1978) The influence of cirrhosis on steady-state blood concentrations of unbound propranolol after oral administration. Clin. Pharmacokin. 3, 478-487.
Wright, J. M., Stokes, E. F., and Sweeney, V. P. (1982) Isoniazid-induced carbamazepine toxicity and vice versa: a double-drug interaction. N. Engl. J. Med. 307, 1325-1327.

Yamamoto, J., Fung, D., Lo, S., and Reece, S. (1979) Psychopharmacology for Asian Americans and Pacific Islanders. Psychopharmacol. Bull. 15, 29-31.

Yamashita, I. and Asano, Y. (1979) Tricyclic antidepressants: therapeutic plasma level. Psychopharmacol. Bull. 15, 40-41.

Yamato, C., Takahashi, T., and Fujita, T. (1976) Studies on metabolism of trazodone. III. Species differences. Xenobiotica 6, 295-306.

Ziegler, V. E. and Biggs, J. T. (1977) Tricyclic plasma levels: effect of age, race, sex, and smoking. J. Am. Med. Assoc. 238, 2167-2169.

Ziegler, V. E., Biggs, J. T., Ardekani, A. B., and Rosen, S. H. (1978a) Contribution to the pharmacokinetics of amitriptyline. J. Clin. Pharmacol. 18, 462-467.

Ziegler, V. E., Biggs, J. T., Rosen, S. H., Meyer, D. A., and Preskorn, S. H. (1978b) Imipramine and desipramine plasma levels: relationship to dosage schedule and sampling time. J. Clin. Psychiatry 39, 660-663.

Ziegler, V. E., Biggs, J. T., Wylie, L. T., Coryell, W. H., Hanifl, K. M., Hawf, D. J., and Rosen, S. H. (1978c) Protriptyline kinetics. Clin. Pharmacol. Ther. 23, 580-584.

Ziegler, V. E., Biggs, J. T., Wylie, L. T., Rosen, S. H., Hawf, D. J., and Coryell, W. H. (1978d) Doxepin kinetics. Clin. Pharmacol. Ther. 23, 573-579.

Ziegler, V. E., Clayton, P. J., Taylor, J. R., Co, B. T., and Biggs, J. T. (1976a) Nortriptyline plasma levels and therapeutic response. Clin. Pharmacol. Ther. 20, 458-463.

Ziegler, V. E., Fuller, T. A., and Biggs, J. T. (1976b) Nortriptyline and 10-hydroxy-nortriptyline plasma concentrations. J. Pharm. Pharmacol. 28, 849-850.

Ziegler, V. E., Knesevich, J. W., Wylie, L. T., and Biggs, J. T. (1977) Sampling time, dosage schedule, and nortriptyline plasma levels. Arch. Gen. Psychiatry 34, 613-615.

13.

TECHNIQUES FOR ANALYSIS OF DRUGS USED IN THE TREATMENT OF AFFECTIVE DISORDERS

D. F. LeGatt and G. R. Jones

Introduction
============

The clinical importance of monitoring antidepressant levels has become generally accepted. Wide interpatient variability in blood levels and clinical response after particular doses, and correlations between levels and clinical response, are the two primary reasons which justify therapeutic monitoring of antidepressants. Consequently, accurate and precise analytical methods are required to accomplish this. This chapter is not intended to be a comprehensive review of the literature, but rather a review of the types of procedures available for quantitation of antidepressants, concentrating on methods published within the last half-decade. Physicians and clinical chemists who are considering antidepressant monitoring should find this review particularly useful. Further investigation should be directed towards the appropriate specific articles. Structures of some of the more common antidepressants are displayed in Table 13.1.

Gas Chromatography

A considerable number of papers has been published on the analysis of antidepressants by gas chromatography (GC). The vast majority of these deal with tricyclic or tetracyclic antidepressants and differ mostly in the methods of extraction rather than radical differences in chromatography.

Glassware. Many gas chromatographic methods are not reproducible in the µg/L range because of drug loss as a consequence of adsorption to glassware. The greatest amount of adsorption is likely to occur at

Techniques for Drug Analysis

Table 13.1: Structures of selected antidepressants

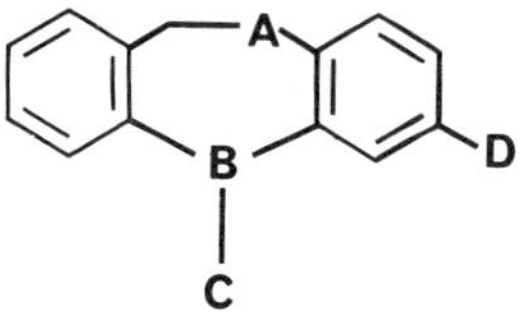

	A	B	C	D
Amitriptyline	CH_2	C	$=CHCH_2CH_2N(CH_3)_2$	H
Nortriptyline	CH_2	C	$=CHCH_2CH_2NHCH_3$	H
Imipramine	CH_2	N	$-CH_2CH_2CH_2N(CH_3)_2$	H
Desipramine	CH_2	N	$-CH_2CH_2CH_2NHCH_3$	H
Clomipramine	CH_2	N	$-CH_2CH_2CH_2N(CH_3)_2$	Cl
Trimipramine	CH_2	N	$-CH_2CHCH_3CH_2N(CH_3)_2$	H
Doxepin	O	C	$=CHCH_2CH_2N(CH_3)_2$	H

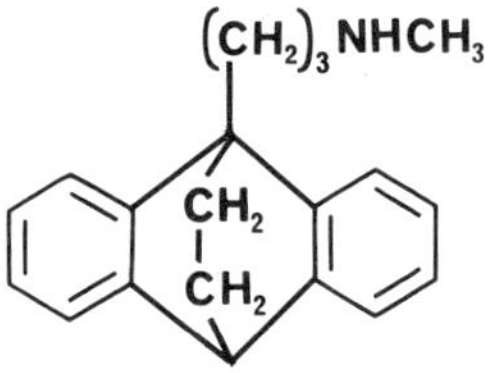

Maprotiline

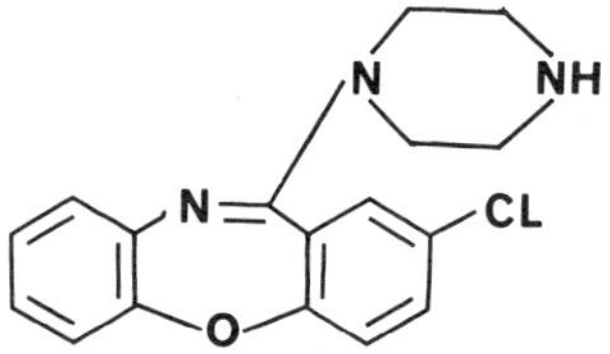

Amoxapine

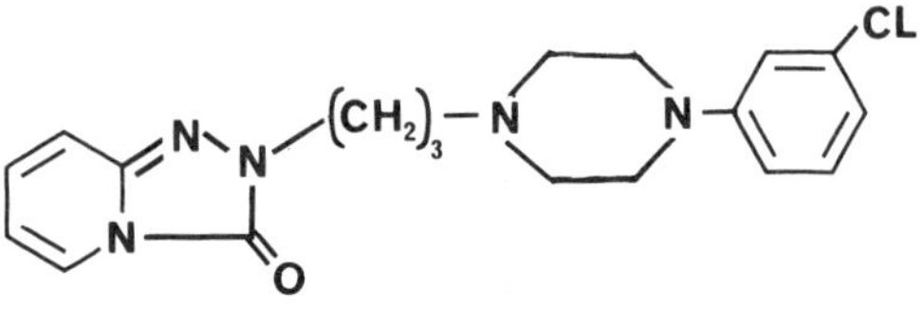

Trazodone

the stage where the final solvent extract is separated from the polar aqueous portion and is evaporated to dryness. Some authors have overcome the problem of adsorption by the addition of 0.04% triethanolamine in chloroform to the final extract (Norman et al., 1977; Norman et al., 1979). However, the majority of papers use either acid washing or silation of glassware. Hydrochloric acid (1N or similar) has been used by some laboratories and chromic acid has been used by others, followed by a deionized water rinse, or ammonium hydroxide and water. Others have used a variety of silating reagents (DMCS, TMCS, DCDMS, BTSA) in a solvent such as toluene, or in the vapour phase (Chinn et al., 1980). Many methods use both acid washing and silation.

An alternative to conventional silation is siliconization using a commercial solution such as Surfasil® (Pierce Chemical Co.) or Serva® Siliconizing Solution. Clean glassware is rinsed with the siliconizing solution, briefly drained, and baked at 100°C for 60 minutes in an oven, in order to bond an alkylsiloxane film to the surface.

Extraction. The extraction step varies in the tricyclic antidepressant papers published. However, most fall into two categories: those which use single extractions and those which involve a back-extraction.

Many of the published methods using single extraction can give results which are as reproducible, sensitive and accurate as those involving back-extraction or "clean-up" steps. However, it is the opinion of these authors that for a routine clinical assay, the extra time spent on a back-extraction is well advised. Even if a nitrogen selective detector is used, contamination from collection procedures (e.g. blood tubes, syringes) or co-administered drugs and/or their metabolites may interfere with the analyte or internal standard. Most single extraction procedures use non-polar solvents, such as heptane or hexane, in an effort to minimize the amount of extraneous co-extracted material. However, use of a non-polar solvent can lead to problems of adsorption in the final evaporation stage, unless rigorous precautions are taken to counter this.

Columns or cartridges packed with C_{18}-bonded silica phase or with diatomaceous earth have been used successfully for HPLC analyses; however, such methods tend to extract too much extraneous material to be useful in most gas chromatography assays.

pH. Many methods use sodium hydroxide to basify plasma to pH 12 or greater, although others use either a borate or a carbonate/bicarbonate buffer to adjust the pH between 9 and 11, normally pH 10. It is likely that a lower pH such as 10 is less destructive to protein and other endogenous material and so minimizes the formation of interfering substances. In fact, Hebb and others (1982) found that a pH between 8 and 9 gave better recoveries of imipramine than the more alkaline pH of 11-12 (1-chlorobutane/ether 3:1 solvent). A comprehensive evaluation of the effect of pH and organic solvent on extraction efficiencies has been published by Weder and Bickel (1968). There seems to be no clear advantage of using hydrochloric acid over sulfuric acid, or vice versa; both appear to be equally effective and are generally used at a concentration of 0.1 N.

Most authors use the same basifying agent in the final stage as they use for the initial extraction, whether that is sodium hydroxide or a buffer of lower pH. If buffers are used, however, some find it convenient to nearly neutralize the acidic back extract with sodium hydroxide and then add a fixed volume of buffer to finally adjust the pH, without having to use a pH meter.

Solvents. The final organic extraction is generally accomplished with the same solvent composition used for the first extraction. The majority, though by no means all, of the papers reviewed used hexane or heptane plus isoamyl alcohol. This combination of a hydrocarbon with an alcohol gives good recoveries of the tertiary and secondary tricyclic antidepressants but is sufficiently apolar to minimize extraction of potential interfering endogenous materials, as compared to a stronger solvent such as ethyl acetate. The concentration of isoamyl alcohol used has varied from 1%-5%, although concentrations greater than 2% do not enhance recoveries, but increase the amount of interference (Hebb et al., 1982). Isoamyl alcohol also helps to minimize emulsion formation.

Some authors have used a small volume of solvent in order to avoid a final evaporation step (which can lead to losses of analyte). For example, butyl acetate (100 µL) has been used as the final extraction solvent by Dawling and Braithwaite (1978). However, in our hands such short-cuts have proved less satisfactory than more commonly used methods.

In another variation, other investigators (Midha et al., 1980; Charette and McGilveray, 1981) made an initial extract of pH 9 with cyclohexane, and back-extracted into 50 μL 2% 1N HCl in methanol which was then evaporated to dryness prior to derivatization and GC analysis. This procedure is, however, closer to a single extraction than a back-extraction method.

Detection. The vast majority of gas chromatography procedures use nitrogen phosphorus (NP) detectors (also called alkali-flame ionization detectors or thermionic specific detectors). This detector is more sensitive than the flame ionization detector (FID) and, since it responds almost exclusively to compounds containing nitrogen or phosphorus, is considerably more selective. While some methods have been published based on FID detectors (Norman et al., 1977; Burch et al., 1979; Cooper et al., 1979; Karkkainen and Seppala, 1980), they lack the sensitivity and/or specificity for routine clinical application, and generally require quite large volumes of plasma or serum. An extensive account of the use of a NP detector for psychotropic drug monitoring has been published by Cooper (1981).

Electron capture (EC) detectors have been applied successfully to the analysis of secondary amine antidepressants (e.g. desipramine, nortriptyline, maprotiline) following derivatization with a halogenated acylating reagent (e.g. trifluoroacetic anhydride, pentafluoropropionic anhydride, heptafluorobutyric anhydride). Some tertiary antidepressants may also be chromatographed with an EC detector if they already contain an electrophoric group (e.g. zimelidine [Larsen and Marinelli, 1978], fluoxetine [Nash et al., 1982], loxapine [Cooper and Kelly, 1979]).

Columns. The vast majority of antidepressant papers use 5% phenylmethylsilicone gums (OV-17, SP-2250) on a variety of supports as the column packings. The percentage of liquid phase ranges from 1% to as high as 10%, although most methods use 3%. Similarly, the solid support used tends to be a matter of individual choice rather than scientific necessity, although Chromosorb W® is commonly used with OV-17 and Supelcoport® commonly used with SP-2250.

A well prepared, carefully packed 3% OV-17 on 80/100 mesh Chromosorb W® generally gives good results (relatively sharp peaks and baseline separation of the tertiary amine antidepressants from the desmethyl metabolites). Supelco® market a SP-2250 packing material specifically prepared and tested for tricyclic antidepressants, which they show to chromatograph one nanogram of amitriptyline and nortriptyline with very little peak tailing. However, any column is difficult to keep in good condition and give consistently symmetrical peaks, unless great care is taken with the material which is injected onto it. For this reason, methods which extract only strong bases, and which eliminate acidic and neutral substances (i.e. methods which include a back-extraction) are likely to result in longer column life and less interference from other drugs, metabolites, and plasticizers. Such methods, while they take longer to perform than those which only involve a single extraction, are usually much more reliable and trouble-free in routine clinical monitoring. Single extraction methods can be made to work and are quicker, but are less reliable than back-extraction methods.

Columns other than 5% phenylmethylsilicone (e.g. OV-17) have been used by some workers. Kristinsson (1981) used 3% OV-225 for a number of tricyclic antidepressants and claimed significantly less adsorption than with 3% OV-17, although in the reproduced chromatograms the secondary amines particularly show significant peak tailing. One of the major advantages of OV-225 is the separation of the secondary amines (e.g. nortriptyline, maprotiline) from the corresponding desmethyl metabolites (e.g. desmethylnortriptyline and desmethylmaprotiline). However, the measurement of these primary amines has not yet been demonstrated to be clinically useful. Separation of the cis- and trans-isomers of doxepin was also possible using OV-225.

At least two other centres have used Carbowax/KOH columns. Karkkainen and Seppala (1980) used 1.4% Carbowax 20M plus 1.4% KOH for the assay of maprotiline in serum. They also demonstrated the separation and good peak shape of a number of other tricyclic antidepressants, without derivatization of the secondary amine, suggesting cyproheptadine as an internal standard. Chinn and others (1980) used a 2% Carbowax 20M plus 0.5% KOH phase for the near baseline separation of amitriptyline, nortriptyline, imipramine and desipramine, as part of a GC/MS assay using deuterated internal standards. This stationary phase has the disadvantage that it has to be used at or very close to its maximum operating temperature in order to elute the tricyclic antidepres-

sants. However, the excellent peak shape attainable with these columns for both the secondary and tertiary amines makes it worthy of further consideration.
Capillary columns have also been used for the quantitation of antidepressants. Bailey and Barron (1980) used a 20 m, 0.3 mm i.d. open tubular Pyrex column coated with OV-225 for the analysis of tranylcypromine. Rosseel and others (1978) obtained separation of cis- and trans-doxepin and the N-trifluoroacetyl derivatives of the corresponding desmethyl metabolites. They used a 20 m, 0.5 mm i.d. glass capillary column coated with OV-17. A direct on-column injection technique was used with a 0.2 µL injection volume. Rovei and others (1980) used an open tubular glass column coated with SE-30 for the analysis of several tricyclic antidepressants in a comparison with a 3% SP-2250 packed column. Good separations and, after derivatization with heptafluorobutric anhydride (HFBA), good peak shapes were obtained with both systems, although a generally high C.V. was obtained in several replicate analyses of spiked samples with the SE-30 (capillary) system, compared with the SP-2250 (packed) system.
More recently, Van Brunt (1983) has used a DB-5 (similar to SE-54) fused silica capillary column (J & W Inc.) for the quantitation of amitriptyline, nortriptyline, imipramine, desipramine, and protriptyline. An excellent review is given of the problems and considerations in setting up an assay for tricyclic antidepressants and a viable method presented. The chromatography time was 10-12 minutes and injections were made in the split mode (1:150) using an NP detector. Extracts were run underivatized. However, the use of a DB-5 column appears to present little advantage over conventional packed columns, in terms of the resolution of parent drug and metabolites, or in the speed of chromatography. Furthermore, the lowest calibration point shown for all the tricyclic antidepressants was 100 µg/L. In many of the patient values presented, the individual tertiary and secondary amine plasma levels are less than 100 µg/L, although they are within the normally accepted therapeutic range. Good calibration is necessary at levels less than 100 µg/L where adsorption and other factors start to affect accuracy and precision most. The comprehensive list of retention times for other drugs is presented, which can be used to assess potential interference.
While peak shapes are invariably better with a good fused silica column than with a packed column, capillary systems (injection liner and column) are

at least as susceptible as packed columns to contamination from co-extracted endogenous substances (lipids, etc.) and other substances (e.g. accidentally injected buffers, acids). Injection liners may be cleaned, although the affected part of the column (e.g. front 5-10 cm) may have to be removed. Thus, capillary columns should not be used as a short-cut for omitting a clean-up or back-extraction stage in the extract preparation.

Derivatization. Whether to derivatize or not to derivatize? That is the question posed in most papers on tricyclic antidepressant analyses published to date. Derivatization is recommended by many authors for two reasons: firstly, to improve the peak shape of the secondary amine (e.g. nortriptyline, desipramine, protriptyline) and secondly, to improve the sensitivity of the NP detector to secondary amines. (Without derivatization, sensitivity is approximately half that for the corresponding tertiary amines, even allowing for peak shape and area.) Conversely, others regard derivatization as unnecessary if good chromatography is employed.

It is our opinion derivatization of the secondary (and if applicable, primary) amines is desirable for routine assays. A good GC column will give acceptable peak shapes for most underivatized secondary amines. However, in routine work, it is extremely difficult to maintain columns in their original condition, even if the glass wool and first one or two inches of packing is replaced on a regular basis. A review of most of the papers where secondary amines are chromatographed underivatized shows them to be tailing significantly, and sometimes considerably more than the corresponding tertiary amines. If a GC peak tails, the analyte is being adsorbed to the column packing or some other part of the GC system. Proportionally more will be adsorbed at lower concentrations than higher concentrations and therefore measurements will be less reproducible and the calibration will probably deviate from linearity.

Derivatization normally takes the form of acylation. Acetyl derivatives have been used for maprotiline (Gupta et al., 1977; Sioufi and Richard, 1980; Charette and McGilveray, 1981). However, acetyl derivatives tend to be significantly less volatile than the underivatized form. Excess acetic anhydride and liberated acetic acid are also more difficult to remove than the corresponding fluoroacyl anhydrides more commonly used.

Trifluoroacetyl (TFA) derivatives are most commonly used (Bailey and Jatlow, 1976a,b; Connor et al., 1977; Rosseel et al., 1978; Cooper and Kelly, 1979; Dhar and Kutt, 1979); however, pentafluoropropionyl (PFP) (Nash et al., 1982) and heptafluorobutyryl (HFB) (Bailey and Barron, 1980; Rovei et al., 1980) derivatives have also been used successfully. The choice of reagent may depend on separations of specific antidepressants required or other considerations such as cost or availability of reagents rather than effectiveness of derivatization. Conditions of derivatization reported in the literature vary. Some methods use the acylating reagent neat, whereas in others, the reagent is diluted 25% to 50% or greater with solvents such as ethyl acetate and heptane. Reaction conditions vary from ambient temperature for 5 min to 60-80°C for 20 min. However, most secondary amines are fully derivatized within 5 min at 60° C.

However, derivatization is not without its problems. Great care has to be taken to ensure that all traces of acylating reagent (anhydride) or liberated acid are 'blown off' from the extract prior to reconstitution and GC analysis. This is easily accomplished, although one has to be careful not to 'over-evaporate' the extract and so cause loss or oxidation of the residual drugs. Fortunately trifluoroacetic acid (and the anhydride) have a very pungent odor and residual traces are easily detected. Failure to remove all of the anhydride or acid results in 'acidification' of the GC column and subsequently peak tailing of the antidepressants.

Caution should be exercised in derivatization of desipramine and other imipramine-related secondary amines (e.g. desmethyltrimipramine and desmethylclomipramine). If conditions are too severe, additional peaks appear in the chromatogram due to degradation of imipramine and the N-acyl desipramine. This phenomenon has been previously reported (Claeys et al., 1976), although it does not seem to be widely recognized in the antidepressant analytical literature. A milder derivatizing reagent (trifluoroacetylimidazole, TFAI) has been proposed for desipramine and for imipramine analogues. This reagent, from our own experience, prevents formation of the degradation products of imipramine and desipramine.

Internal Standards. Use of an internal standard is essential to any GC assay and virtually all HPLC assays. It is added to measured aliquots of the original biological sample plus calibration standards and, if properly chosen, compensates for differences in binding of the analyte to one sample matrix compared to another, differences in transfer volumes of solvent, differences in GC injection volume and differences in the loss of analyte from sample to sample due to adsorption to glassware and the GC column. It also serves as a gross check of correct buffer pH at the different extraction stages and, if applicable, a check of proper derivatization.

Ideally, an internal standard should be virtually identical in physical properties, chemical properties, and structure to the analyte. This is nearly possible with ^{13}C analogues and to a slightly lesser extent with ^{2}H (deuterium) analogues. However, stable isotope analogues usually have virtually identical retention times and are therefore only suitable as internal standards in GC/mass spectrometry analyses. Usually chemical analogues are chosen, differing in substituents (e.g. fluoro, chloro, methyl) but not in functional groups. Normally it is convenient to choose an analogous drug, or at least another drug or chemical with identical functional groups and a close retention time.

Several of the papers reviewed used internal standards that were close analogues, for example, 7-methylmianserin for mianserin (Vink and Van Hal, 1980); methylbutriptyline for butriptyline (Gonzalez and Kraml, 1980), and others. Although most of the other papers reviewed showed acceptable or good calibration plots, many fell short of using a good internal standard. Some, for example, used the same internal standard for both the tertiary and secondary amine analyte. Whilst the internal standard chosen was usually a structurally related antidepressant, tertiary and secondary amines can differ significantly in their degree of extractability by a given solvent and degree of binding to active sides on glassware and GC columns. In one case, the internal standard chosen was a benzodiazepine (oxazepam) which, in the first place, is virtually neutral and secondly, is thermally unstable by gas chromatography (Szyszko and Wejman, 1981). It is not uncommon for internal standards to be added in the initial extraction solvent (Connor et al., 1977). Whilst it may be agreed that an equilibrium will eventually be formed, one of the purposes of an internal standard is to 'check' the extraction process and compensate for small variations in extraction efficiency. If an internal standard is added

Techniques for Drug Analysis

in the extraction solvent, it cannot adequately do this. Ideally, an internal standard should be added to the biological sample in a small volume of water, or if it is not soluble, in a water miscible solvent (e.g. methanol). Furthermore, the internal standard should be allowed to equilibrate in the sample for 5-10 minutes before the buffering agent is added. 'Internal standards' added at the end of the procedure, prior to final evaporation of the sample, are more correctly termed 'external standards'. Such standards are not acceptable in a quantitative GC assay unless they are added in addition to a proper internal standard, in order to check the relative recoveries of the analyte in the assay procedure.

Occasionally, though, chemically similar substances other than antidepressants have been successfully used as internal standards. For example, methadone (a tertiary amine) has been used as an internal standard for the measurement of amitriptyline and other tertiary tricyclic amines. Methadone has the advantage of eluting prior to all commonly used tricyclic antidepressants and tetracyclic antidepressants. The authors of this chapter used this internal standard in their laboratories for the tertiary amine parent drugs, using secondary amine tricyclic antidepressants as internal standards of the secondary amine metabolites.

Typical GC traces obtained in our laboratories are shown in Figure 13.1. These traces represent extracts obtained from sera containing 250 µg/L each of the following antidepressants and internal standard: methadone (I), imipramine (II), clomipramine (III), desipramine-TFA (IV), maprotiline-TFA (V), desmethylclomipramine-TFA (VI), amitriptyline (VII), cis- and trans-doxepin (VIII), nortriptyline-TFA (IX), trans-desmethyldoxepin-TFA (X). Conditions: GP 3% SP-2250 on 80/100 Supelcoport, 4 ft column; oven temp. 225° held for 4.5 min, rate 30°/min to 260° and held for 2 min (NP detector).

Other Methods. While most of the GC methods for analyses of the antidepressants are variations of one of the original papers by Hucker and Stauffer (1974), some differ markedly in their approach. Karlsson (1981) proposed a two-phase derivatization of amitriptyline by extraction from an aqueous solution containing sodium iodide into methylene chloride containing dichlorophenylchloroformate to form a stable chloroformate ester with good chromatographic properties and excellent EC detection response. Although the method is interesting and may have

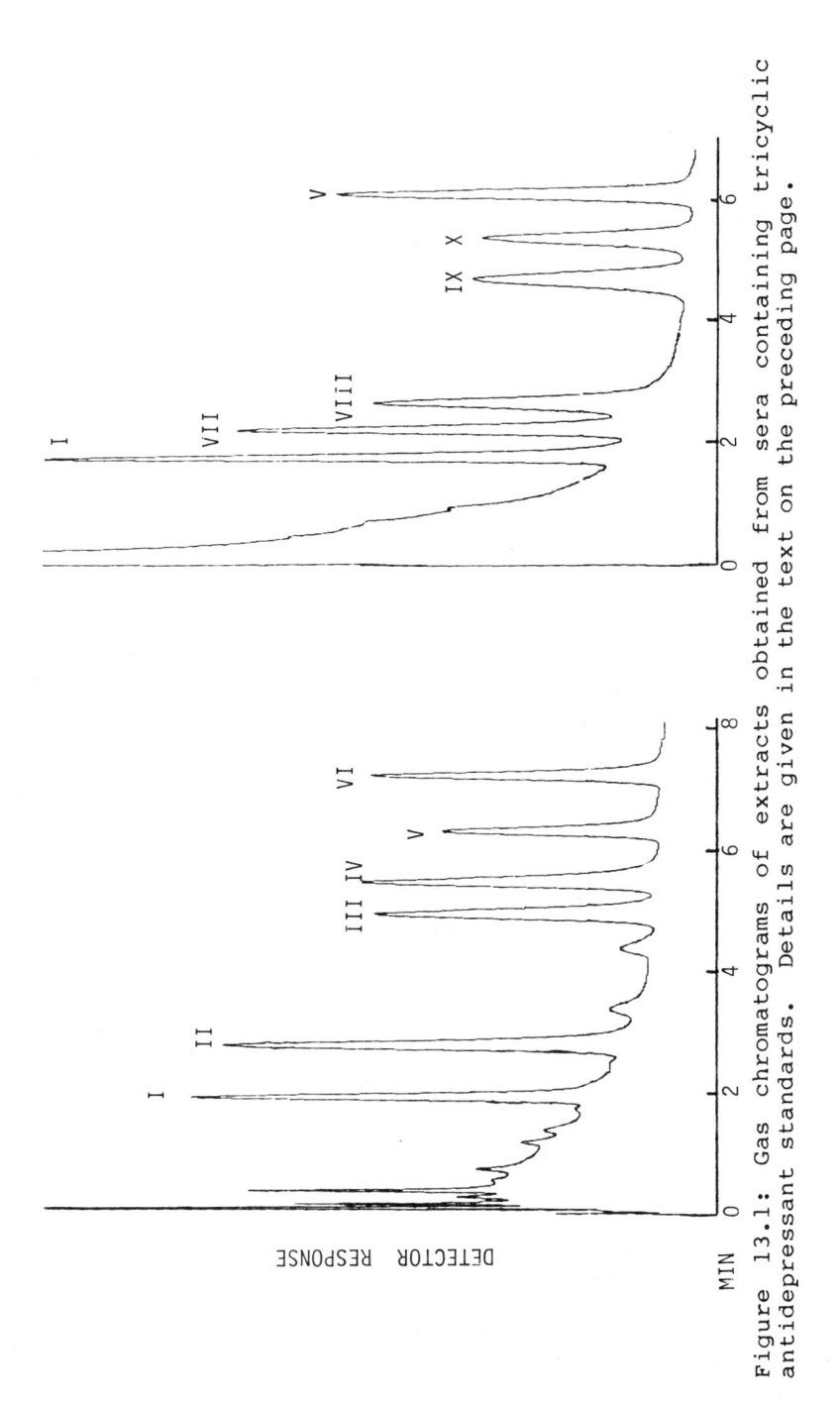

Figure 13.1: Gas chromatograms of extracts obtained from sera containing tricyclic antidepressant standards. Details are given in the text on the preceding page.

future application, it has yet to be proven useful for routine clinical applications.

Another sensitive but unusual method for the determination of amitriptyline in plasma has been published by Hartvig and co-workers (1976). Amitriptyline is separated from the biological matrix, nortriptyline, and other metabolites by column chromatography and then oxidized to anthraquinone with ceric sulphate. Chloroamitriptyline was also added as an internal standard. The anthraquinone (together with 2-chloroanthraquinone from the internal standard) was separated and measured on an OV-17 column connected to an EC detector. The method is undoubtedly sensitive, but is not suitable for routine clinical monitoring since the secondary amine, nortriptyline, is not measured. Furthermore, methods which involve gross degradation of an analyte to a much simpler derivative are rightly viewed with some scepticism by most clinical chemists.

Phenelzine

The monoamine oxidase inhibitor phenelzine is undoubtedly one of the most challenging antidepressants to analyze. Only in 1976 was the first analysis of phenelzine in biological fluids reported (Caddy et al., 1976), and only then for relatively high concentrations in urine. Since phenelzine is very unstable in alkaline solution, it was first converted to the acetonide by reaction with acetone, using phendimetrazine as the internal standard. However, the reaction was only about 20% efficient.

Later, Caddy and Stead (1977) reported an even more indirect gas chromatography method of determining phenelzine in urine, by iodate oxidation of phenelzine to 2-phenylethanol. However, this method was still not sensitive enough to measure phenelzine in plasma, except in cases of massive overdose.

Cooper and others (1978) first published a GC assay for the reliable measurement of phenelzine in plasma suitable for pharmacokinetic studies after a single 30 mg dose. Phenelzine was extracted into benzene:ethyl acetate (4:1) from plasma after adjustment to pH 6.8 with a phosphate buffer. The free phenelzine was then back extracted into 0.05M sulphuric acid, buffered to pH 6.8 and re-extracted into benzene containing triethylamine and the internal standard 1-phenyl(propyl)hydrazine. The extract was subsequently concentrated and the phenelzine and internal standard derivatized with heptafluorobutyric anhydride (HFBA). Analysis was performed on an

OV-17 column connected to an EC detector. The assay is quite lengthy, but probably owes some of its success to the use of a closely related analogue as the internal standard, although it is not clear why this is not added at the beginning of the assay rather than after the acidic back-extraction. The authors stress the importance of not subjecting phenelzine to a pH greater than 7.

Jindal et al. (1980a) reported a GC/MS assay for phenelzine capable of measuring blood plasma levels down to 2 µg/L with 10% precision. Deuterated phenelzine (d_7) was synthesized from phenylacetic acid-d_7 and used as the internal standard. Phosphate buffer (pH 6.7) was added to plasma and the internal standard, followed by pentafluorobenzaldehyde. This solution was mixed for 15 min to allow formation of the corresponding hydrazones. The hydrazones were then extracted into benzene, concentrated, and partially purified on a small Sephadex LH-20 column. The fraction containing the hydrazones was then concentrated and analyzed by GC/MS in the selected ion monitoring mode. Overall recovery of phenelzine from spiked plasma was 65%, with excellent sensitivity and reproducibility.

Mass Spectrometry

Mass spectrometry (MS) is probably one of the most selective and sensitive methods of quantitating antidepressants in biological fluids. It is normally used in combination with gas chromatography (GC), and most of the considerations that apply to GC methods apply to GC/MS methods. In fact, the mass spectrometer is merely being used as a very selective detector.

The technique of using mass spectrometry for quantitative work is called selected ion monitoring (SIM) or mass fragmentography. One or two fragment ions unique at any given retention time to the analyte (or internal standard) are monitored to the exclusion of all others whilst that particular compound is eluting from the chromatograph. Thus two compounds having the same retention time but differing mass spectra may be measured simultaneously. Thus analytes may be accurately measured in the presence of other co-eluting substances.

About half the procedures reviewed used extraction methods involving an acid back-extraction. The remainder used single organic extractions from alkaline solution into an organic solvent, or similar procedures with modifications. Whilst it is true that the use of mass spectrometry may enable methods to by-pass clean-up steps and still usually get 'clean chromatograms', problems may still be encountered. For example, co-extracted endogenous material can rapidly build up at the head of the GC column, causing adsorption and/or breakdown of the analytes and subsequently cause peak tailing. Also, compounds with long retention times can elute from previous injections causing an undesirable background or interference due to broad peaks. Most fatty acids or fatty acid esters and cholesterol have extremely complex spectra and give ions at most m/z values.

However, some single extraction procedures have included steps which are likely to make the method more selective. Chinn and others (1980) have used a solvent system (toluene:heptane:isoamyl alcohol; 70:20:10) which minimizes the extraction of endogenous compounds, in combination with a polar stationary phase (0.5% KOH plus 2.5% Carbowax 20M) which retains many unwanted co-extractants. The addition of KOH to the stationary phase enables the secondary amines to be chromatographed with minimal peak tailing.

Most methods use GC columns packed with OV-17 on Chromosorb® or a similar material. Virtually every paper used fluoroacyl derivatives of the secondary tricyclic amines. This has the advantage, mentioned previously, of improving the GC peak shape, but also can make the method more selective. Underivatized, many of the secondary tricyclic amines give EI mass spectra which have an abundant m/z 44 ion and few, if any, ions of abundances are greater than 5% and are often less than 1%. Unfortunately, the ion m/z 44 is common to the mass spectra of a great many compounds. However, fluoroacyl derivatives usually give mass spectral ions of relatively large mass and high abundance. For example, underivatized, the only major ion in the EI mass spectra of both nortriptyline and desmethyldoxepin is m/z 44. However, the trifluoroacetyl derivatives of nortriptyline and desmethyldoxepin give major ions at m/z 232 and m/z 234 respectively. Generally, the higher the mass ion monitored, the less likely it is interference will result from other compounds.

There seems to be no particular advantage of using quadrapole mass spectrometers compared with magnetic sector instruments or vice versa. Older magnetic sector mass spectrometers tend to be slower in switching from mass to mass than quadrapole instruments; however, modern magnetic sector mass spectrometers are very fast. Two thirds of the papers reviewed used electron impact (EI) ionization with a third using chemical ionization (CI). Again, this distribution probably reflects the number of instruments with or without CI capability. In fact, most authorities regard CI as being preferable to EI for SIM work because (a) less fragmentation occurs (the signal tending to be localized in a small number of ions), and (b) abundant ions tend to occur at much higher m/z values, where there is less background.

Most of the chemical ionization methods used methane, although two papers used isobutane. Isobutane is generally preferred for CI because it tends to give just quasi-molecular ions with no additional reactant ions as does methane (e.g. $M + C_2H_5$, $M + C_3H_5$). However, purified isobutane is quite expensive and many mass spectroscopists find methane quite acceptable. In fact, Claeys and others (1976) found methane gave greater <u>absolute</u> abundances for MH^+ ions than did isobutane. One method even used methanol as the reactant gas (Lapin and Karobath, 1980) --introduced from a side arm of the direct inlet probe. However, these authors do not indicate that there is any analytical advantage in using methanol over methane or isobutane.

One of the major advantages of GC/mass spectrometry as a quantitative technique, apart from the high degree of selectivity obtainable, is that stable isotope analogues can be used as internal standards. Deuterated analogs of at least amitriptyline, nortriptyline, imipramine, and desimipramine are available commercially as stock items. However, many authors synthesized their own internal standards. Methods of synthesis range from a relatively simple acid-catalyzed exchange in D_2O (deuterium oxide) (Claeys et al., 1976; de Ridder et al., 1977; Lapin and Karobath, 1980) to more complex synthetic procedures (Alfredsson et al., 1977; Garland et al., 1979; Crampton et al., 1980; Jindal et al., 1980b, 1982).

For example, Lapin and Karobath (1980) heated clomipramine and desmethylclomipramine in a 1:1 mixture of DCl and D_2O at 80°C in a sealed tube for four days. Most of the ethylene bridge protons in each compound were replaced with deuterium, giving a high yield of d_4 substitution with virtually no d_0 species.

As a more complex example, Jindal and others (1980b) synthesized [N-CD$_3$]-substituted maprotiline. Desmethyl maprotiline was reacted with ethylchlorocarbonate to form the corresponding carbonate, which was then reduced with lithium aluminium deuteride in tetrahydrofuran to form the desired [N-CD$_3$]maprotiline.

The importance of choosing a suitable internal standard has been examined by Claeys and others (1977). These authors reviewed the factors which can affect the reproducibility of a GC/MS assay and how the efficiency of an internal standard can be evaluated.

The majority of GC/MS methods reviewed deal with the measurement of amitriptyline or imipramine and their metabolites (Frigerio et al., 1972; Biggs et al., 1976; Alvan et al., 1977; Garland, 1977; Ziegler et al., 1977; Heck et al., 1978; Alkalay et al., 1979; Garland et al., 1979; Chinn et al., 1980; Breutzmann and Bowers, 1981; Narasimhachari, 1981; Narasimhachari et al., 1981; Potter et al., 1982). Others deal with doxepin (Biggs et al., 1976; Narasimhachari, 1981; Davis et al., 1983), maprotiline (Alkalay et al., 1979a; Jindal et al., 1980), clomipramine (Alfredsson et al., 1977; Alkalay et al., 1979b; Gaskell, 1980; Lapin and Karobath, 1980; Bertilsson, 1981), mianserin (de Ridder et al., 1977; Vink and Van Hal, 1980a; Jindal et al., 1982), dothiepin (Crampton et al., 1980; Maguire et al., 1981), protriptyline (Biggs et al., 1976; Narasimhachari, 1981) and lofepramine (Matsubayashi et al., 1977). Some of these papers also cover the analyses of the hydroxylated metabolites in plasma, including in some instances, the syntheses of deuterated internal standard analogs (Garland et al., 1979; Narasimhachari et al., 1981).

As discussed for the GC assays, most of the GC/MS assays are similar in principle but differ in detail. However, Narasimhachari (1981) has used C$_{18}$-Sep-Pak® cartridges (Waters Associates). Although many workers avoid the use of extraction cartridges for GC assays because they tend to extract too much extraneous material, Narasimhachari found that with GC/MS, the extracts appeared as clean as using a conventional liquid/liquid extraction system. In addition, his method was quicker and simpler. Absolute recoveries of the drugs were also greater.

A novel approach was used by Heck and others (1978) in devising an assay using HPLC and field ionization mass spectrometry (FI-MS). The drug imipramine and the corresponding deuterated internal standard were extracted using a conventional liquid/

liquid procedure with extensive clean-up steps (including two separate acid back-extractions). The final extract was applied to an HPLC column, the 'imipramine peak' collected and this aliquot concentrated and applied to a field ionization (FI) direct insertion probe. The probe was then inserted into the mass spectrometer and FI spectra recorded. The ratio between the deuterated and non-deuterated imipramine was determined. Clearly, this method is hardly routine in most laboratories, but the authors claimed subnanogram sensitivity--about ten-fold better than most GC/MS assays.

High Performance Liquid Chromatography

Scoggins and co-workers (1980) predicted high performance liquid chromatography (HPLC) would gain in popularity as a technique for quantitation of tricyclic antidepressants. HPLC is now one of the most widely employed techniques for quantitation of tricyclic and non-tricyclic antidepressants alike. In addition to high precision and accuracy, and the ability to resolve and quantitate structurally-related compounds and associated active metabolites, HPLC for most applications does not require derivatization of the sample extract--a necessity in many gas chromatographic assays.

Sample Preparation. Specimens, whether serum, plasma or whole blood, require pretreatment prior to HPLC analysis. The two major reasons are firstly, to eliminate endogenous compounds which may contaminate the chromatographic column and interfere with the analysis, and secondly, to concentrate the drug, permitting more sensitive analysis. Pretreatment generally involves basification of the biological specimen to pH 10-12 and extraction with an organic solvent. The non-aqueous phase is either evaporated to dryness, followed by reconstitution with a small volume of mobile phase or water-miscible solvent, or mixed with a small volume of an acidic solution such as 0.1N HCl. The reconstituted extract is then subjected to HPLC analysis. Back-extraction techniques have also been incorporated into many of the procedures (Brodie et al., 1977; Kraak and Bijster, 1977; Mellstrom and Tybring, 1977; Mellstrom and Braithwaite, 1978; Godbillon and Gauron, 1981; Kabra et al., 1981; Suckow and Cooper, 1981; Haefelfinger, 1982; Suckow and Cooper, 1982; Suckow et al., 1982), eliminating endogenous constituents which may potentially interfere with chromatographic analysis.

Techniques for Drug Analysis

For determination of hydroxylated antidepressant metabolites in plasma, hydrolysis of the glucuronide conjugates with β-glucuronidase (Bock et al., 1982) or acid (Kraak and Bijster, 1977) is required.

Recoveries of antidepressants and metabolites in procedures utilizing manual extraction procedures ranged from 53-95%.

Disposable extraction columns (Clin. Elut.®, Analytichem International) packed with an inert matrix of large surface area have been used for the quantitation of antidepressants and associated metabolites in serum or plasma (Thoma et al., 1979; Tasset and Hassan, 1982). The procedure is based upon the principle of liquid/liquid extraction. After addition of sodium carbonate buffer, serum or plasma is applied to the top of the column. Adsorbed analytes are subsequently eluted by application of organic solvent. Back-extraction with a small volume of methanolic HCl solvent is done prior to chromatography. Recoveries are acceptable to good (69-89%). Bond-Elut® C_{18} extraction columns (Analytichem International) have also been applied to the extraction of tricyclic and tetracyclic antidepressants from serum (Bierle and Hubbard, 1983a, b). Compared to manual extraction procedures, use of extraction columns eliminates mixing, centrifuging and transferring of extracts. Thus, technical time and losses due to adsorption are reduced.

An automated technique for extraction of antidepressants from serum using the Prep I®Automated Sample Processor (Dupont Co.) has been described (Koteel et al., 1982). The Prep I® is a reversible centrifuge which allows solvents to pass through disposable resin cartridges, packed with Type W styrene divinylbenzene copolymer, into two separate collection cups. A clockwise rotation of the rotor allows for loading of the sample onto the column. The first cup collects liquid, unadsorbed solutes, and wash solution dispensed on the column to flush remaining interfering substances. Rotation is reversed and the eluting solvent is applied to the column. Solvent containing the analytes is collected in the second cup and automatically dried under air or nitrogen. Recoveries are 72-97%. Reduction in dedicated technologist time compared to manual extraction is the most significant advantage of this technique.

A sophisticated example of automation for quantitation of tricyclic antidepressants is the Technicon 'FAST-LC' system (Technicon Instruments

Corp.) (Bannister et al., 1981). This system gives on-line extraction of serum or plasma, followed by HPLC analysis of the extract, all under direction of a microprocessor. The only manual manipulation required is pipetting the serum sample into the sample tray. Adsorption of the antidepressants onto components of the system is minimized with the use of fluorelastomer Acidflex® pump tubes and maintenance of sample pH < 2. Recovery of the tertiary and and secondary amine drugs approximates 95% and 76% respectively. Although the major advantage of this system is the elimination of all manual pretreatment steps, the system cost may be a deterrent for most clinical laboratories.

Chromatography. Liquid chromatographic resolution of antidepressants utilizes normal phase (adsorption), reversed-phase, reversed-phase/ion pair, ion pair or phase-bonded conditions.

For normal phase liquid chromatographic analysis, columns are packed with silica gel. The majority of these methods utilize a 5 µm (Watson and Stewart, 1977; Westenberg et al., 1977a,b; Emanuelsson and Moore, 1978; Vandermark et al., 1978; Sutfin and Jusko, 1979; Whall and Dokladalova, 1979; Streator et al., 1980; Godbillon and Gauron, 1981; Edelbroek et al., 1982; Haefelfinger, 1982; Smith et al., 1982) as opposed to a 10 µm packing (Moyes and Moyes, 1979; Dixon and Martin, 1981; Sonsalla et al., 1982a,b). Two methods discuss separation on columns of both pore sizes (Bierle and Hubbard, 1983a,b). Procedures using columns with 10 µm silica (column length = 25-30 cm) have achieved separation of amitriptyline, clomipramine, trimipramine, protriptyline, imipramine, doxepin, and associated demethylated metabolites. Resolution of the hydroxylated metabolites of amitriptyline and nortriptyline from the parent compounds has been reported (Dixon and Martin, 1981). Sensitivities reported for 10 µm columns range from 5-20 µg/L in the original specimen (1-2 mL). This is sufficient for therapeutic drug monitoring purposes. However, columns containing 5 µm particle size silica have replaced the former as columns of choice for adsorption chromatography of antidepressants. These columns are generally shorter (10 cm), offer increased sensitivity (as low as 0.1 µg/L [Haefelfinger, 1982]), and provide greater resolving power. Beirle and Hubbard (1983a,b), who compared the efficiency of 5 and 10 µm silica columns, concluded that the 5 µm column gives sharper peaks and increased resolution. A typical chromatogram is shown in Figure 13.2. Severe tailing of maprotiline found with a 10 μm column was corrected with a 5 μm column. However, even the 5 μm column was not successful in separating amoxapine from the active metabolite, 8-hydroxyamoxapine (Bierle and Hubbard, 1983b).

Mobile phases for adsorption chromatography generally are organic mixtures, the most common combination being methanol/acetonitrile, ammonia also being added to increase the pH as a means of suppressing ionization. Vandermark and co-workers (1978) have found a concentration of ammonium hydroxide of 7 mL/L in an acetonitrile mobile phase results in satisfactory separation of amitriptyline and imipramine (and mono-demethylated metabolites), and also eliminates interference of plasma matrix components. Addition of 10% isopropranol to acetonitrile permitted reduction of the ammonia concentration to 2 mL/L, resulting in increased column lifetime to greater than two hundred analyses. Beirle and Hubbard (1983a) used an acetonitrile/ethanol/tert-butylamine mobile phase to achieve the co-elution of seven tricyclic antidepressants. Although pH of the mobile phase was 10.0-10.4, no major deterioration in chromatographic performance was noted after nine hundred injections on the 5 μm silica column. The absence of an aqueous component (e.g. ammonia solution) in the mobile phase was the contributory factor to the long column life. Of the thirteen alkylamines tested, tert-butylamine gave the best resolution. Ethanol compared to methanol and isopropanol had the greatest resolving strength.

Ambient temperature, for the most part, is applied to adsorption chromatography of antidepressants. However, maintenance of column temperatures between 27°-65°C has been described (Emanuelsson and Moore, 1978; Vandermark et al., 1978; Whall and Dokladalova, 1979). The decreased chromatographic time resulting from the increased temperature is usually offset by a decrease in column life.

Adsorption chromatography is capable of separating geometric isomers of antidepressants. The cis- and trans-isomers of doxepin (Whall and Dokladalova, 1979; Bierle and Hubbard, 1983a) and desmethyldoxepin (Bierle and Hubbard, 1983a) have been resolved. However, the clinical significance of the ratios of the cis- and trans-isomer for doxepin and the major active metabolite has not been established (Bierle and Hubbard, 1983a).

Adsorption chromatography offers advantages over reversed-phase chromatography. Reversed-phase

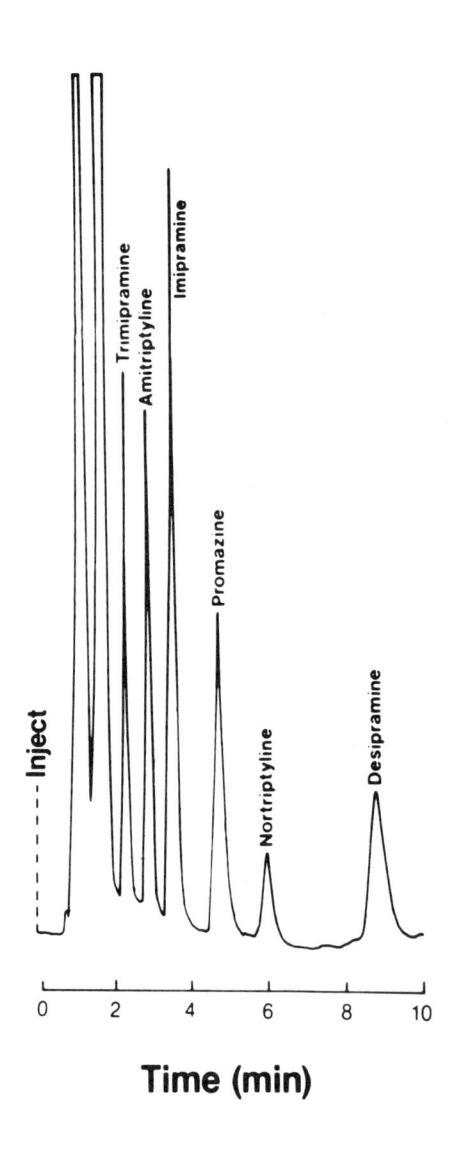

Figure 13.2: High-performance liquid chromatogram of a serum control on a 5 µm Supelco silica column (4.6 x 250 mm). Source: F. A. Bierle and R. W. Hubbard, Ther. Drug Monit., 5 (1983), Figure 7A, p. 285.

chromatography is less selective with regard to subtle differences in the tricyclic ring system. Westenberg and co-workers (1977a) were unable to resolve clomipramine from desipramine on a reversed-phase system, but achieved success using adsorption chromatography. The lifetime of a normal phase column generally is longer than that of a reversed-phase column. Thirdly, silica gel columns can function well at pH > 10, whereas reversed-phase systems deteriorate rapidly at pH > 7.5. Finally, reversed-phase columns are generally more expensive than adsorption phase columns.

A modified form of adsorption chromatography, bonded-phase liquid chromatography, has been used for antidepressant quantitation (Thoma et al., 1979; Ketchum et al., 1983). Bonded phase columns--polar cyanopropyl groups chemically bonded to silica through Si-C linkages--offer a medium polarity stationary phase, excellent for separation of moderately polar and non-polar compounds. These columns are versatile, permitting operation in either an adsorption or reversed-phase mode, and in addition, offer excellent stability. Equilibration time is reduced and the shifting of retention times may be minimized when compared to silica adsorption columns. The lifetime of a CN-bonded column may vary from one month of infrequent use (Ketchum et al., 1983) to ten months of daily use (Thoma et al., 1979). This variability may be related to column maintenance. Of the six antidepressants (amitriptyline, nortriptyline, doxepin and their major demethylated metabolites) studied on a CN-bonded column (Thoma et al., 1979), only amitriptyline and nortriptyline were not resolved from doxepin and desmethyldoxepin in a 6 min run at 60°C. The inability to resolve the two antidepressants and their metabolites is not serious, as concomitant administration of two tricyclic antidepressants in clinical practice is a rare occurrence. Ketchum and co-workers (1983) used CN-bonded columns to analyze amoxapine, the active metabolite 8-hydroxyamoxapine, and the inactive metabolite 7-hydroxyamoxapine. Although the 7- and 8-hydroxy metabolites were not resolved completely from each other, both were separated from amoxapine. The mobile phase utilized for bonded adsorption columns is usually a mixture of acetonitrile/phosphate buffer (approximate pH = 7.0) and methanol. Sensitivities of the methods range from 10 to 25 µg/L.

Ion-pair liquid chromatography has been applied to the quantitation of zimelidine (Westerlund et al., 1979), clomipramine (Mellstrom and Tybring, 1977), amitriptyline (Mellstrom and Braithwaite, 1978) and various metabolites in plasma and whole blood. In this technique, an ionic compound or counter-ion of opposite charge to the solute comprises the stationary phase. A neutral ion pair is formed and subsequently partitioned between the stationary and mobile phase. Chromatographic systems comprise a support phase of polar silica micro particles (5-10 µm) with an acidic perchlorate solution or hydrochloric acid/tetrapropyl ammonium hydrogen sulphate stationary phase. Mobile phases are organic in nature. The stationary phase is usually precoated onto the silica support phase in slurry form. Ion-partition chromatography can also be accomplished without precoating by using a mobile phase under-saturated with an aqueous phase containing the counter-ion (Mellstrom and Braithwaite, 1978). As for other types of liquid chromatography, a 5 µm support phase results in sharper peaks and increased resolution when compared to a 10 µm support. Westerlund et al. (1979), using a 5 µm precoated column, achieved excellent resolution of zimelidine, norzimelidine, and the E-isomer of norzimelidine (internal standard) within 8 min. Sensitivity of the assay is 1 µg/L for both parent drug and metabolite when 1 mL of plasma or whole blood is extracted, and can be increased to 0.1 µg/L after extraction of 5 mL of specimen. Mellstrom and Tybring (1977), on a 10 µm precoated column, achieved separation of clomipramine, desmethylclomipramine and the didemethylated metabolite in a 7 min analysis. Accurate quantitation was possible to 10 µg/L and 18 µg/L for clomipramine and desmethylclomipramine respectively. Understandably, peak width is broader than in procedures utilizing 5 µm packing.

Reversed-phase liquid chromatography has been applied extensively to the quantitation of antidepressants in clinical situations (Biggs et al., 1977; Brodie et al., 1977a,b; Kraak and Bijster, 1977; Biggs et al., 1979; Hackett and Dusci, 1979; Reece et al., 1979; Westerlund and Erixson, 1979; Ankier et al., 1981; Breutzmann and Bowers, 1981; Gitlian and Mason, 1981; Kabra et al., 1981; Kuss and Feistenauer, 1981; Wallace et al., 1981; Bock et al., 1982; Jozefczak et al., 1982; Kimball and Lampert, 1982; Linnoila et al., 1982; Oyehang et al., 1982; Tasset and Hassan, 1982; Bierle and Hubbard, 1983b; Wong and Waugh, 1983). The stationary phase is hydrophobic, usually an alkyl- or arylsilane compound. A pre-column or guard column is frequently used for protecting the main column from particulate matter and impurities which may become irreversibly adsorbed. The guard column is composed of a similar packing material and must maintain the high efficiency capability of the separating system. Mobile phases are aqueous/organic mixtures using water-miscible organic solvents, such as acetonitrile and methanol. Separation is dependent on the hydrophobic character of the compound, with the more hydrophobic substances having greater retention. Mobile phase pH is very critical for reversed-phase chromatography, as a pH of < 7.0 is essential for maintaining column integrity. The composition of mobile phases used with reversed-phase columns varies widely, and resolution of the antidepressants concerned is critically dependent on this composition. Kabra and co-workers (1981) achieved simultaneous resolution of amitriptyline, nortriptyline, imipramine, desipramine, doxepin and nordoxepin using a mobile phase of acetonitrile/phosphate buffer (21:79) containing n-nonylamine (600 µL). Resolution of amitriptyline, nortriptyline, desmethylnortriptyline, cis-10-hydroxynortriptyline, trans-10-hydroxynortriptyline, and trans-10-hydroxyamitriptyline was done in 10 min on reversed-phase material (C-8 bonded) with a mobile phase of water/methanol/dichloromethane/propylamine (Kraak and Bijster, 1977). A methanol concentration of 60% was selected, as higher concentrations resulted in reduced column selectivity while a decreased concentration reduced sensitivity. Dichloromethane was added to the polar water/methanol mobile phase to improve selectivity. The effects of bases such as hexylamine, ethylamine, propylamine, and ammonia on capacity, selectivity and peak shape were investigated. Propylamine was found to be the best choice.

Reversed-phase chromatography has applications for quantitation of novel antidepressants. Zimelidine, a nontricyclic antidepressant, and the pharmacologically active metabolite norzimelidine have been determined in plasma (10 min analysis) using a Nucleosil® (Machery-Nagel) C_{18} (5 µm) column and acetonitrile/phosphate buffer (pH 2)/N,N-dimethyl-N-octylamine mobile phase (Westerlund and Erixson, 1979). Detection limits in plasma (1 mL) were approximately 1.5 and 0.7 µg/L for zimelidine and norzimelidine respectively. This sensitivity is improved over an adsorption (normal phase) method (25 µg/L) (Emanuelsson and Moore, 1978) and is comparable to sensitivity (1 µg/L) offered by an ion-partition assay (Westerlund et al., 1979). The simultaneous determination of indalpine and its major plasma metabolite was accomplished with a µBondapak® (Waters Associates) C_{18} (10 µm) column and a methanol/potassium phosphate/acetic acid mobile phase (Jozefczak, 1982). Chromatography time was a lengthy 20 min. Extraction of 2 mL of plasma gave a sensitivity of 2 µg/L for indalpine. A sensitive and selective method has been developed for the quantitation of the novel tricyclic antidepressant citalopram and its methylamino and amino metabolites in plasma (Oyehang et al., 1982). A 5 µm Spherisorb® (Phase Separations) ODS reversed-phase column and acetonitrile/phosphate buffer (pH 3) permitted the resolution of the three compounds in a 9 min analysis. Peak symmetry was excellent. The detection limits were 1-2 µg/L for citalopram and the methylamino metabolite, and 0.5-1 µg/L for the primary amino metabolite. Viloxazine, a psychotropic drug with antidepressant activity, has been resolved from five of its metabolites on a reversed-phase column of unspecified composition using a mobile phase composed of acetonitrile, triethylamine and phosphate buffer (pH 3.2) (Gitlian and Mason, 1981). The detection limit in plasma (0.5 ml) was 25 µg/L. A novel antidepressant, trazodone, a triazolo-pyridine derivative, has been quantitated in human plasma utilizing a reversed-phase column (Spherisorb® S5 ODS) (Phase Separations) and an acetonitrile/sulphuric acid mobile phase in an 8 min analysis (Ankier et al., 1981). Sensitivity of the assay is 20 µg/L. The metabolite of trazodone (2-[3-carboxypropyl]-1,2,4-triazolo[4,3-a]pyridin-3(2H)-one] does not interfere. Amoxapine, a tetracyclic antidepressant is metabolized to 7- and 8-hydroxyamoxapine, the latter metabolite recognized as being active. Consequently, any analytical procedure must be capable of resolving amoxapine from the two metabolites. Wong and Waugh (1983) have achieved complete resolution of amoxapine and the metabolites. However, two separate procedures of extraction and analysis are required for concomitant determination. In a single procedure, Kimball and Lampert (1982) achieved separation of amoxapine and the active metabolite 8-hydroxyamoxapine. Unfortunately, 7-hydroxyamoxapine co-eluted with the active metabolite, preventing the accurate quantitation of the former metabolite. Tasset and Hassen (1982) in a single procedure achieved the complete resolution of all three compounds. Using a µBondapak® (Waters Associates) C_{18} reversed-phase column and a mobile phase of acetonitrile/water/n-butylamine, an 8 min analysis achieved resolution. However, the limit of sensitivity of this latter amoxapine assay for both active components was determined at 50 µg/L (1 mL serum) compared to 2 µg/L (2 mL plasma) (Wong and Waugh, 1983) and 20 µg/L (1 mL plasma) (Kimball and Lampert, 1982).

As with normal adsorption chromatography, modified reversed-phase columns are used for quantitating antidepressants. With a µBondapak-CN® (Waters Associates) reversed-phase column, Koteel and co-workers (1982) analyzed nine antidepressants simultaneously, although doxepin was not completely resolved from amitriptyline, and retention time data was not provided for maprotiline. Incorporation of the -CN moiety reduces the polarity of the reversed-phase column and consequently offers different selectivity. The serum detection limits (1 mL sample volume) are 5 and 6 µg/L for the secondary and tertiary amines respectively. Hydroxylated metabolites were not investigated.

Reversed-phase liquid chromatography has been compared with the more sophisticated and expensive technique (GC/MS). Biggs and co-workers (1977) have developed an HPLC method for quantitation of amitriptyline and nortriptyline in plasma using a C_{18} Partisil® (Whatman Ltd.) column and an acetonitrile/potassium dihydrogen orthophosphate mobile phase. An EI SIM procedure was also developed for the two compounds. The limit of sensitivity of the HPLC assay was 5 µg/L of plasma compared with 0.1 µg/L for the GC/MS method. However, the concentrations obtained by HPLC analysis were not compared with those quantitated by the GC/MS method. Breutzman and Bowers (1981) have compared measurement of four antidepressants (desipramine, imipramine, nortriptyline and amitriptyline) by the two analytical methods. The HPLC method utilized a µBondapak® (Waters Associates) C_{18} column and an acetonitrile/phosphate buffer mobile phase. The gas chromatograph/mass spectrometer was a Finnigan model 3200 instrument with a 3% OV-17 on Chromosorb W (HP) column. Complete resolution of the four antidepressants was accomplished within 12 min. Calibration curve concentrations ranged from 25-250 µg/L. Statistical comparison of the two methods demonstrated excellent correlation for imipramine, amitriptyline and nortriptyline. Correlation coefficients for the three compounds were 0.98, 0.99 and 0.97 respectively. Slopes and "Y" intercepts ranged from 0.96-1.07 and -6.2-6.0 respectively.

Ion-pair reversed-phase HPLC is described for

the quantitation of antidepressants (Proelss et al., 1978; Suckow and Cooper, 1981, 1982; Suckow et al., 1982; Lagerstrom et al., 1983). This technique, however, is usually applied for completely ionized compounds. As with normal or adsorption phase ion-pair chromatography, an ion-pair is formed by the interaction of the solute with an ionic compound (counter-ion) of opposite charge, the latter added to the mobile phase. The neutral ion-pair is partitioned into the hydrophobic stationary phase, resulting in selective retention on the column. The rationale for using a counter-ion with a reversed-phase column is to eliminate ionization of the antidepressants while permitting elution at a pH < 7 to ensure reasonable column life. Heptanesulphonate, pentanesulphonate and phosphate are the counter-ions applied in this technique. A representative chromatogram is shown in Figure 13.3. Quantitation of six antidepressants (imipramine, amitriptyline, doxepin, trimipramine, clomipramine, mianserin) and various metabolites has been reported for this particular technique. However, the application of ion-pairing to reversed-phase chromatography of antidepressants has been challenged by two investigators. Bannister and co-workers (1981) evaluated reversed-phase analysis with and without ion-pairing. Although they found ion-pairing reduced column variability and improved band shape, one major problem was found: slow column equilibration after daily column regeneration. Breutzmann and Bowers (1981) compared the reversed-phase chromatographic separation of five antidepressants with and without ion-pairing. They found no improvement in selectivity using ion-pairing reagents.

Detection. Detection of antidepressants by HPLC is accomplished by ultraviolet, fluorescence or electrochemical detectors. The majority of methods employ either fixed or variable wavelength ultraviolet detectors. Wavelength selection ranges from the near (longer wavelength) to far (shorter wavelength) ultraviolet range (258-200 nm). The near ultraviolet is utilized to a greater extent with 254 nm, the most common wavelength selected. This wavelength has applications to the quantitation of tricyclic, tetracyclic, and novel antidepressants alike. Clomipramine and desmethylclomipramine have been quantitated using a wavelength setting of 250 nm, though a higher absorbance occurs at 220 nm (Westenberg et al., 1977b). The former wavelength is selected to eliminate the solvent impurity interferences which

Techniques for Drug Analysis

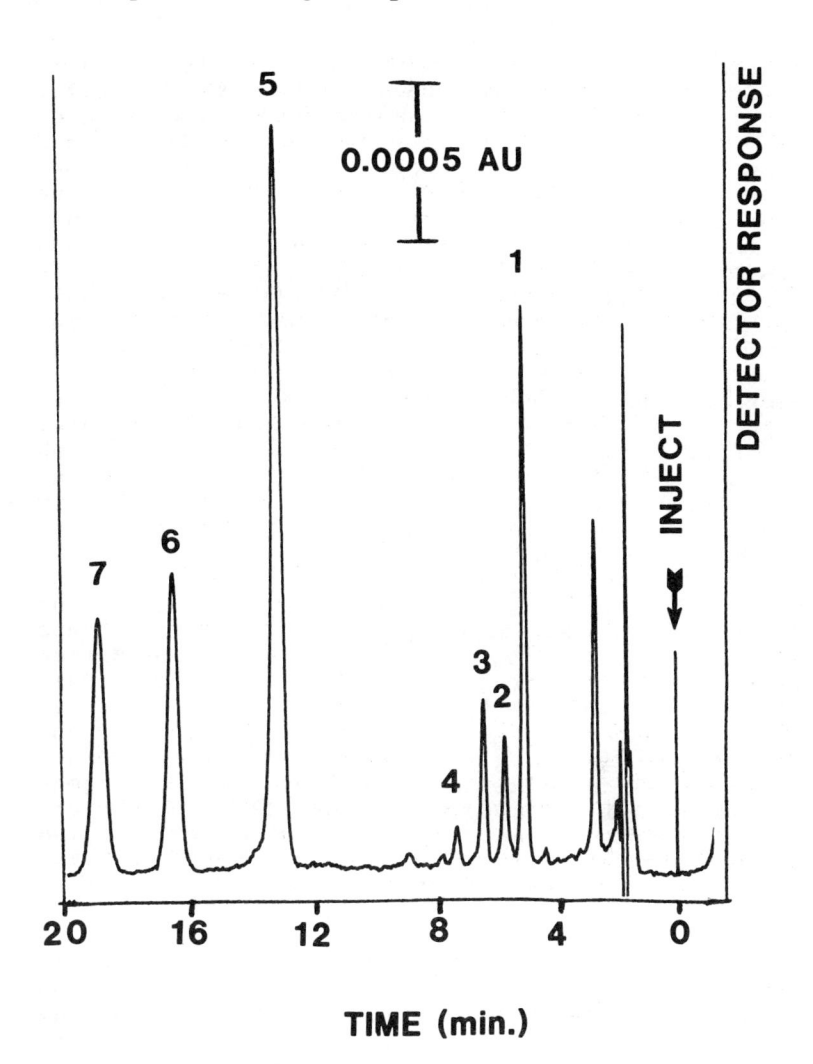

Figure 13.3: Sample chromatogram of a plasma sample (1 mL) from a patient receiving amitriptyline analyzed on a 5 μm reversed-phase (trimethylsilyl) column, using the counter-ion heptane sulfonate. Compounds resolved include (1) trans-10-OH-nortriptyline, (2) trans-10-OH-amitriptyline, (3) cis-10-OH-nortriptyline, (4) cis-10-OH-amitriptyline, (5) loxapine (internal standard), (6) nortriptyline, and (7) amitriptyline. (From: R. F. Suckow and T. B. Cooper [1982] J. Chromatogr., 230, Fig. 4, p. 398).

occur at 220 nm. An intermediate range of wavelengths (240-230 nm) has been utilized for the quantitation of tricyclic antidepressants and their metabolites, which is near the maximal absorbance for this antidepressant group. In liquid chromatography, the mobile phase must not contribute to absorbance at the selected wavelength. Ethyl acetate should be avoided, for this solvent has substantial absorbance in this intermediate ultraviolet range. The far ultraviolet region (220-200 nm) has been utilized for the specific determination of maprotiline (Kuss and Feistenauer, 1981; Bierle and Hubbard, 1983b; Wong and Waugh, 1983) and other antidepressants (Vandermark et al., 1978; Moyes and Moyes, 1979; Thoma et al., 1979; Bannister et al., 1981; Kabra et al., 1981; Wallace et al., 1981; Bock et al., 1982; Kimball and Lampert, 1982; Smith et al., 1982). Increased sensitivity is the advantage claimed for operating at wavelengths in the far- as opposed to the near-ultraviolet spectrum. However, sensitivities reported for detection in the far-ultraviolet region (2 µg/L) are claimed by researchers using the near-ultraviolet region. The use of far-ultraviolet wavelengths may enhance the detection of interfering drugs such as the benzodiazepines.

Fluorescence detection offers one major advantage over ultraviolet for the quantitation of antidepressants--an increase in sensitivity to a limit as low as 0.1 µg/L (Haefelfinger, 1982). However, the use of fluorescence to date is restricted to the quantitation of imipramine, imipramine analogs, viloxazine and citalopram--the latter two compounds being bicyclic antidepressants (Gitlian and Mason, 1981).

Electrochemical detectors have also been utilized for antidepressant quantitation (Suckow and Cooper, 1981; Linnoila et al., 1982; Suckow et al., 1982). Sensitivity of the assays are comparable to those using instruments with ultraviolet detectors. At present the use of electrochemical detectors is limited to the quantitation of imipramine, clomipramine, mianserin, and structurally related compounds (i.e. metabolites). Under the analytical conditions described (Suckow and Cooper, 1981), nortriptyline, 10-hydroxynortriptyline, protriptyline, amitriptyline and 10-hydroxyamitriptyline are either not detected or do not elicit a substantial response. In addition, benzodiazepines (flurazepam, chlordiazepoxide, diazepam) and related metabolites are electrochemically unresponsive under conditions described (Suckow et al., 1982), namely, a detector cell potential of +1.05 V versus a silver-silver chloride reference electrode. This is a distinct advantage over methods using ultraviolet detection, where the benzodiazepines are liable to cause interference.

High performance liquid chromatography has come of age in application to the quantitation of antidepressants in the clinical situation. The advent of automated HPLC systems with autosamplers and programmable injection sequences, high speed-low volume detectors, and high resolution columns has contributed to this development. The selectivity of HPLC is the major advantage of this method over some others discussed in this chapter. The ability to resolve hydroxylated, demethylated, and N-oxide metabolites, and also geometric isomers of metabolites from each other, is not rivalled by any other method discussed. However, HPLC methods for antidepressant quantitation may be open to interference from other co-administered drugs such as benzodiazepines and antipsychotic drugs. Therefore, the procurement of the complete medication profile of the patient is essential for detection of any possible interferences.

Thin Layer Chromatography (TLC)

Several TLC methods for the quantitation of tricyclic antidepressants have been developed over the last ten years. Most of the procedures reviewed consist of a solvent extraction at alkaline pH, separation of the tricyclic antidepressant from its major metabolites by one-dimensional TLC, chemical visualization, and quantitative measurement by densiometry.

Prior to the wide acceptance of the NP detector for GC, TLC methods provided a more sensitive and relatively selective alternative to methods previously developed using flame ionization detection.

Nagy and Treiber (1973) separated imipramine and desipramine on silica gel plates after extraction from plasma, followed by visualization with nitrous gases as intense yellow spots. The intensity of the spots was determined by densiometric measurement, using transmission and reflectance simultaneously. Standard curves were produced by means of spiked plasma. The sensitivity of the assay was reported as 5 µg/L using a 5 mL plasma sample, although increased sensitivity was claimed if larger samples were used.

Lang and others (1978) formed the highly fluorescent 1-diethylaminonapthalene-5-sulphonic acid derivative of tranylcypromine, prior to chromatographic separation on silica gel plates and fluorescent scanning of the plates. The method requires 5 mL of plasma, but is sufficiently sensitive to perform pharmacokinetic studies on single therapeutic doses (20 mg).

Amitriptyline and nortriptyline were measured by Haefelfinger (1978) after conversion to azo-dyes following separation by thin layer chromatography. The drugs were sequentially nitrated, reduced, and finally the products coupled with N-(1-napthyl)-ethylenediamine. The method is sensitive down to 0.5 µg/L based on a 1 mL sample, which is greater than the majority of GC methods, and is suitable for single dose pharmacokinetic studies.

The TLC method described by Kaul et al., (1978) differs from others in that amitriptyline extracted from blood is then quaternized with 9-bromomethylacridine. The amitriptyline quaternary product is separated from the 10-hydroxy and 10,11-dihydroxy metabolites of amitriptyline on silica gel plates. Fluorescent products are subsequently formed by photolysis with ultraviolet light *in situ*, individually eluted from the plate, and measured in 0.001N sulfuric acid by spectrofluorimetry. The assay is designed for amitriptyline concentrations from 20-200 µg/L, based on a 3 mL blood sample. However, this method has limited clinical applicability since the major active metabolite, nortriptyline, is not measured.

Zuleski and others (1977) used radioactive (^{14}C)-acetic anhydride for derivatization and subsequent measurement of nortriptyline. Their method was an improvement over other similar methods published, in that the ^{14}C-acetylnortriptyline was separated from other acetylated impurities prior to elution of the TLC spot and scintillation counting. Calibrators down to 3 µg/L were prepared, based on a 1 mL plasma sample, making it useful for single dose pharmacokinetic studies of nortriptyline (though not amitriptyline).

Fenimore and co-workers (1977) used high performance thin layer chromatography (HPTLC) to quantitate amitriptyline and nortriptyline, or imipramine and desipramine, with sensitivities down to 5 µg/L, based on 1 mL of serum. The drugs were chromatographed and measured underivatized by ultraviolet scanning *in situ* using a chromatographic spectrophotometer. Unlike most of the other TLC methods published, this method used an internal standard (loxapine) to help compensate for any losses of drug during extraction and chromatography. A 'carrier' (perphenazine) was also added to the sample to minimize losses during the extraction and chromatographic process.

However, most TLC methods are unsuitable for routine clinical measurement of antidepressants in blood or plasma, either because they are too time-consuming to perform, or because they require a very high degree of technical skill and equipment not normally required with more routine TLC work.

Radioimmunoassay

Radioimmunoassay (RIA) has been used for the quantitation of antidepressants in serum or plasma, and almost exclusively the published methods refer to tricyclic antidepressants and associated metabolites. Three major components comprise any RIA procedure: antibody, labelled antigen (radioligand), and unlabelled antigen in the patient specimen. Unlabelled antigen competes with the radioligand for binding to the antibody, consequently lowering the degree of bound radioligand. The free and bound label are physically separated prior to counting of the bound or free fraction. Concentration of the particular drug in the patient specimen is determined from a calibration curve.

Antiserum specificity is an important determinant of the routine application of any RIA procedure. If a high degree of cross-reactivity exists for compounds which are frequently co-administered with antidepressants, these interferences must first be removed to permit accurate quantitation. This is time-consuming. Antisera are prepared by injecting the antidepressant (or analog) bound to bovine serum albumin (BSA) into rabbits or sheep. Examples of such complexes are given in Table 13.2.

For tricyclic antidepressants, two major antigenic determinants have been identified: the tricyclic ring and the aliphatic side chain. Maguire and co-workers (1978) investigated both determinants. They used a nortriptyline/BSA conjugate (side chain coupling) for production of antiserum. The conjugate resembled a tertiary amine, which explains the stronger binding of antiserum to the tertiary drugs. Substitution on the tricyclic ring structure either drastically or moderately reduced binding, depending on the position of substitution. The 2-hydroxy metabolite of imipramine gave less than 5%

cross reactivity whereas clomipramine with a chlorine atom in the 3-position on the tricyclic nucleus gave 30-40% cross reactivity relative to nortriptyline.

Major tricyclic nucleus modifications such as a change to a six- from a seven-membered ring (e.g. maprotiline, chlorpromazine) have been shown to severely restrict binding. Additionally, bicyclic antidepressants such as zimelidine and nomifensine do not bind. For development of an RIA assay for clomipramine, Read and co-workers (1977, 1978) coupled BSA to the 10/11-hydroxy metabolites of the drug via the 10/11 bridge position on the tricyclic ring instead of the aliphatic side chain. The conjugate resulted in an antiserum which cross reacted equally between clomipramine and the 10/11-hydroxy metabolite, but did not react with desmethylclomipramine, the active metabolite, or any other metabolites by greater than 5%. The 10/11-hydroxy metabolite is a minor metabolite in plasma, and would not contribute greatly to the determined level of clomipramine. Although these assays are specific for clomipramine, their clinical usefulness is debatable as plasma levels of the active desmethylmetabolite were not considered.

All other tricyclic antidepressant RIA procedures referred to in this chapter solely involve coupling of BSA to the aliphatic side chain of a particular drug analog. This results in cross-reactivity between the parent and monodemethylated active metabolites. The cross-reactivity of hydroxylated metabolites in these latter procedures is generally minimal (i.e. < 5%). However, some of the didemethylated metabolites demonstrate appreciable cross-reactivity (> 20%) (Robinson et al., 1978; Brunswick et al., 1978), creating the potential for inflation of the true values of the parent and monodemethylated metabolite. In the procedures performing simultaneous quantitation of the parent tricyclic drug and the active demethylated metabolite, reactivities of the particular antiserum with the two compounds are generally not equivalent. The RIA methods of Midha et al. (1978) and Mould et al. (1978) for simultaneous amitriptyline/nortriptyline quantitation are exceptions. Some researchers have overcome this problem by performing selective extraction prior to the RIA analysis which separates the demethylated metabolite from the parent drug (Lucek and Dixon, 1977; Brunswick et al., 1978, 1979; Virtanen, 1980; Virtanen et al., 1980). For example, Lucek and Dixon (1977) quantitatively

Table 13.2: Drug – BSA complexes for preparation of antidepressant antisera

Compound	Antidepressants Analyzed
N-succinylnortriptyline – BSA	Amitriptyline, nortriptyline, doxepin, desmethyldoxepin, imipramine
N-4-aminobutylnortriptyline – BSA	Amitriptyline, nortriptyline
Nortriptyline – succinylated – BSA	Amitriptyline, nortriptyline
10/11-hydroxyclomipramine hemi-succinate – BSA	Clomipramine
N-(2-carboxyethyl)nortriptyline – BSA	Doxepin, desmethyldoxepin amitriptyline, nortriptyline
N-(8-nomifensine)succinamic acid – BSA	Nomifensine
N-(3-carboxypropionyl)nortriptyline – BSA	Amitriptyline, nortriptyline
N-(3-carboxyethyl)desipramine – BSA	Imipramine, desipramine

extracted amitriptyline from plasma at pH 5, with 96% of nortriptyline left in the aqueous phase. The remaining aqueous phase was buffered to pH 9 and extracted to remove the nortriptyline. The individual organic extracts containing the two drugs were back-extracted into aqueous media for RIA analysis. Individual standard curves were prepared for quantitative determination. Brunswick and co-workers (1979) co-extracted amitriptyline and nortriptyline prior to conversion of nortriptyline to its succinyl derivative. Succinylnortriptyline was subsequently extracted into dilute base, while the underivatized parent drug was extracted into dilute acid. Again, two separate RIAs were performed to obtain a combined antidepressant level. Kamel and associates (1979), by performing the assay at pH 9.0, equalized the cross-reactivities of amitriptyline and nortriptyline. This eliminated the requirement for time-consuming extraction procedures and individual RIA procedures for each drug. The remaining methods for simultaneous quantitation of parent and active demethylated metabolite do not compensate for unequal cross-reactivities and do not undertake isolation techniques. Additionally, only one calibration curve is used to quantitate both drug entities. Thus, extreme caution must be taken in interpreting the quantitative results from such assays, as the total tricyclic levels obtained are only approximations. These latter assays are not suitable for routine therapeutic drug monitoring of antidepressants.

One of the determinants of the limit of sensitivity of a RIA assay is the specific activity of the radioligand. The most widely used tracers are tritiated imipramine (^{3}H-imipramine) and amitriptyline (^{3}H-amitriptyline), with specific activities ranging from 3.2-23 Ci/mmole for the former and 2-28 Ci/mmole for the latter label. Limits of sensitivity have been shown to vary from 0.5-10 µg/L. It should be noted that the sensitivity limits are also defined by the inclusion of an extraction step to isolate or purify analytes before RIA analysis (i.e. extraction decreases sensitivity), and by the volume of patient specimen used for quantitation (50-500 µL). An assay for clomipramine in plasma utilized a radioligand with high specificity, namely, [10,11-^{3}H$_2$] clomipramine (specific activity = 39 Ci/mmole) (Read and Riad-Fahmy, 1978). The limit of sensitivity of this assay was determined at 0.175 µg/L from analysis of 50 µL of patient plasma. As this method did not have an extraction procedure, the individual quantitation of the active metabolite desmethylclomipramine is not possible. The tracer [^{3}H]-Succinylnortriptyline was applied to measuring nortriptyline levels to 2.3 µg/L from a 50 µL plasma sample (Brunswick et al., 1979). The specific activity of the crude product was 13.6 Ci/mmole. Tritiated nomifensine with a specific activity of approximately 5 Ci/mmole was used for quantitation of levels as low as 0.3 µg/L of the novel antidepressant in 100 µL plasma specimens (Heptner et al., 1977). For determination of total nomifensine, acidification was done to split the acid-labile conjugate prior to RIA analysis. This was accomplished using a separate plasma specimen. However, McIntyre and associates (1981), using the same radioligand, achieved a sensitivity limit of 1 µg/L. In order to eliminiate potential cross-reactivity of conjugated nomifensine in the assay for free nomifensine, an extraction procedure, using 1 mL of plasma, was undertaken to selectively remove conjugated nomifensine prior to quantitation. Fluorescein isothiocyanate or N-acetyl-L-histidine derivatives of nortriptyline have been radioiodinated to produce nortriptyline radioligands (Kamel et al., 1979). The iodinated histidine conjugate gave high immunoreactivity and was obtained in a higher yield. With the isothiocyanate derivative, however, a compromise is made between yield and product immunoreactivity. Compared to tritiated analogs, instrument counting times are reduced from 10 min to 20 sec. Sensitivity of these assays are 2.8 to 3.6 µg/L with analysis of 25-50 µl of patient specimen.

After reaction of the patient sample and antiserum with the radioligand, the free and bound radioligand must be physically separated to allow quantitation of the bound fraction. This is a procedural necessity for RIA, a heterogeneous immunoassay. Separation is accomplished by one of four methods. Dextran-coated charcoal is the most frequently used. After a predetermined incubation period, charcoal suspension is added to the mixture of radioligand, antiserum, and patient specimen. Any radioligand not bound to antiserum becomes adsorbed to the charcoal. After centrifugation, the supernatant containing the bound radioligand is transferred to a scintillation vial containing scintillation fluid for counting. This method is simple, rapid and is efficient in separating the bound and free fractions. An alternative to charcoal is a more complex procedure using saturated ammonium sulphate (pH 7.4), which precipitates the antibody-bound radioligand (Lucek and Dixon, 1977). After addition of the saturated solution and centrifugation, the supernatant is aspirated and discarded, and the precipitate resuspended in 50% saturated ammonium sulphate (pH 7.4). After centrifugation, the washed precipitate is dissolved in water, Aquasol® added, followed by scintillation counting. Kamel and co-workers (1979) have described two sophisticated methods for separating bound from free radioligand with the use of liquid-phase or magnetizable solid-phase second-antibody radioimmunoassays. For the liquid-phase procedure, antirabbit serum is added after the initial incubation of antinortriptyline serum with patient sample and radioligand. The anti-rabbit serum precipitates out the bound ligand. After centrifugation and aspiration of the supernatant containing the free ligand, counting is performed. The magnetizable solid-phase assay requires coupling of whole sheep anti-(rabbit immunoglobulin G) serum to cellulose/iron oxide particles. After incubation, this anti-rabbit magnetizable solid-phase is added to the assay mixture. After a specified time, the rack containing the tubes is placed on the flat surface of a multipolar ferrite magnet to sediment the solid-phase ligand bound complex. The supernatants are aspirated and the sedimented particles are counted. The solid-phase second-antibody procedure eliminates centrifugation but requires a magnet for operation.

Interferences from other compounds as a consequence of appreciable cross-reactivities with a particular antiserum are commonplace, and must be thoroughly investigated for each antidepressant radioimmunoassay. Such interferences are not always detrimental and may prove beneficial for quantitation of all clinically active forms of a particular drug. However, cross-reactivities of all such active substances are usually not equal and this must be taken into consideration for accurate quantitation. Cross-reactivity as it pertains to metabolites has been mentioned previously in a discussion on antiserum specificity. Other parent antidepressants and their metabolites may exhibit cross-reactivity in a particular antidepressant method. As stated in the discussion of HPLC, tricyclic antidepressants are rarely administered concurrently in clinical practice and therefore this cross-reactivity should not prove to be a problem. Antipsychotic drugs such as perphenazine, chlorpromazine, trifluoperazine and haloperidol do not exhibit appreciable cross-reactivity with the published RIA methods for tricyclic antidepressants. Nomifensine antisera (Heptner et al., 1977; McIntyre et al., 1981) have been found not to exhibit any cross-reactivity with the three known metabolites or with eight other psychotropic drugs.

With the exception of three methods (Robinson et al., 1977; Midha and Charette, 1980; Virtanen, 1980), validity of RIA procedures for antidepressants has been evaluated by comparison with other analytical techniques such as HPLC, GC, GC-MS, double radioisotope derivative assays, and other RIA methods. Some evaluations are incomplete. A comparison of one RIA procedure with a GC method only involved a graphic representation which was plotted incorrectly (Aherne et al., 1977). RIA data was plotted on the "X" axis and reference GC data on the "Y" axis. For method evaluation, the reference method data should be represented on the "X" axis. Although a statement was made inferring a significant correlation, a correlation coefficient value was not given. When comparisons are made, not only should correlation coefficients be given, but values for the slope and "Y" intercept of the best fit straight line should be quoted. Correlation coefficients alone may be misleading and may mask tendencies for over- or underestimation of results. Although six publications (Heptner et al., 1977; Braithwaite et al., 1978; Brunswick et al., 1978; Mould et al., 1978; Brunswick et al., 1979; Kamel et al., 1979) gave correlation coefficients ranging from 0.88 to 0.997, no additional comparison data was provided. However, some researchers insert tables of raw data from which one can calculate the slope and "Y" intercept. Seven investigative groups provide adequate comparison data with correlation coefficients, slopes, and "Y" intercepts ranging from 0.89 to 0.996, 0.87 to 1.07, and -7.08 to 2.6 µg/L respectively. In general, validation of RIA procedures providing the appropriate data was accomplished.

A commercial kit for quantitating tricyclic antidepressants in plasma has been marketed by Wein Laboratories. The antiserum raised in rabbits against a succinylnortriptyline-BSA complex cross-reacts with tertiary and secondary tricyclic antidepressants, including amitriptyline, nortriptyline, imipramine, desipramine, protriptyline, and doxepin. A standard curve is prepared using imipramine, and for all drugs a corrected concentration is determined by using specific cross-reactivity factors supplied with the kit. To optimize quantitation, standards and controls are available as accessory components. Maguire and associates (1980) evaluated kit performance for the quantitation of nortriptyline. The cross-reactivity factor for nortriptyline supplied with the kit (1.6) varied from 1.0 at 50 µg/L to 1.4 at 200 and 400 µg/L, but did not approach the quoted value of 1.6. Therefore, the potential for reporting erroneously high values is very real. Comparison of the kit with a GC/MS procedure (Biggs et al., 1976) gave a correlation coefficient of 0.90 and a slope of 1.06, but an unacceptably high "Y" intercept of 43.6 µg/L. The latter value is explained by the fact the Wein Laboratories kit measures nortriptyline, didesmethylnortriptyline, and the 2-hydroxy metabolite of nortriptyline, while the GC/MS procedure specifically monitors only nortriptyline. This lack of selectivity has probably been the primary reason RIA kits for tricyclic quantitation have not been extensively marketed.

Radioimmunoassay, although sensitive and with great potential for analysis of many specimens simultaneously, has not evolved into one of the primary methods for quantitation of antidepressants. A single test by GC or HPLC enables simultaneous and individual quantitation of antidepressants and their active and non-active metabolites. A simple radioimmunoassay cannot do this. Specific quantitation by RIA can only be accomplished after selective extraction. However, this is not a practical routine procedure.

Radioreceptor Assays

As stated by Smith and associates (1980), "radioreceptor (RR) blood level assays measure the amount of substance in the blood which binds to a specific type of receptor prepared from brain tissue membranes". The particular substance competes with a radiolabelled ligand of high specific activity for receptor binding.

Nortriptyline has been shown to bind to muscarinic cholinergic receptors and post-synaptic α-adrenergic receptors in brain, as assessed by displacement of [^{3}H]quinuclidinyl benzilate (^{3}H-QNB) and WB-4101 binding respectively (Smith et al., 1980). Consequently, Smith and co-workers (1980) assessed displacement of QNB or WB-4101 binding to rat cortex membrane preparations in patient samples containing nortriptyline, or in blank plasma to which varying concentrations of nortriptyline were added. Prior to incubation with labelled ligand and the membrane preparation, the particular plasma sample was extracted and an aliquot of this extract (100 µL) utilized in the radioreceptor assay. Details of the extraction were not given. Incubation of the three major components was carried out at 37°C (20 min) to permit the nortriptyline in the specimen extract to compete with the particular radioligand for binding to the membrane preparation. The incubation mixtures were filtered, with radioligand bound to membrane retained on the filters. The isolated filters were suspended overnight in scintillation fluid and the next day the radioactivity of the samples determined. The amount of radioactivity present on the filters is inversely proportional to the nortriptyline concentration in the original specimen. Calculations were made from log probit plots of the percentage inhibition of QNB or WB-4101 binding versus nortriptyline concentration. Validity of the method has been assessed by comparison with a previously described GC method (Chojnacki et al., 1981). Results were not promising. No relationship was found between the GC and RR assay values for nortriptyline regardless of whether the QNB or WB-4101 ligands were used. With the exception of three values, 11 steady-state plasma nortriptyline levels were grossly over-estimated by the RR method using WB-4101 as the radioligand. A similar result was found in assays with QNB as radioligand where all 16 steady-state values were overestimated by the RR assay. The most probable explanation for the discrepancies is a substantial lack of specificity of the RR assay. Desmethylnortriptyline and associated hydroxylated metabolites may also bind with the membrane preparations, resulting in inflated values. The patients may have been taking other drugs with the potential for binding to the cholinergic and α-adrenergic receptors. Interference of nortriptyline metabolites was not evaluated and no reference was made to concomitant medications.

An RR assay for tertiary amine tricyclic antidepressants has been developed by Paul and associates (1980). "High affinity" binding sites for ^{3}H-imipramine, distinct from adrenergic, cholinergic, serotoninergic, and histaminergic receptors were utilized in this assay. These binding sites in human brain are also located on human platelets and appear to be specific for tertiary amine tricyclic antidepressants. Preliminary studies revealed that the drug-free plasma used directly inhibited binding of ^{3}H-imipramine. Plasma samples were either processed by basification and organic solvent extraction or diluted 1:4 with assay buffer prior to assay. Crude platelet membrane preparations were incubated with radioligand and either plasma dilution or extract. Specific binding was defined as binding difference in the presence and absence of 5 µM desipramine. Filters were isolated after filtration and scintillation counting was performed. Calibration curves were plotted on log probit paper as inhibition of binding. Initial extraction of plasma samples prior to RR assay resulted in sensitivities for amitriptyline and imipramine of 2-5 µg/L when 0.5-2.0 mL of initial plasma specimen was used. However, the time-consuming extraction could be eliminated, as radioreceptor assays on diluted plasma samples gave comparable results to assays performed with plasma extracts (data not shown). Interference from secondary amine analogs in routine measurement is unlikely as the corresponding secondary amines exhibited potency up to seventeen-fold less than the parent compounds. Desmethylclomipramine is an exception, with almost equal potency to clomipramine. However, the hydroxy analogs may pose some interference as 2-hydroxyimipramine exhibited an inhibition of binding approximately one-half the potency of imipramine. Interference by psychotropic drugs at expected plasma concentrations was not found. Validity of the assay was established by comparison with a GC-MS and an HPLC procedure. No specific references for the two other techniques were given. The correlation coefficient was 0.95 for both comparisons. Although 'Y' intercepts are not quoted, the comparison with HPLC results demonstrated an underestimation of results by the RR assay. As combined imipramine and 2-hydroxyimipramine results were considered for the correlation determination, the reduced potency of the two hydroxy analogs to bind to receptors compared to the parent is the most likely cause of the depressed results.

A third RR assay for tricyclic antidepressants has used membrane-bound rat brain cholinergic receptors and ^{3}H-QNB radioligand (Innis and Snyder, 1981). A time-consuming extraction/back-extraction technique was utilized to eliminate non-specific effects experienced by direct use of as little as 100 µL of plasma. A large volume of plasma (5 mL) is required. Assay sensitivity was established at 2, 1, 3, 6, and 1 µg/L of original plasma or serum for nortriptyline, amitriptyline, imipramine, desipramine, and doxepin respectively. Assay validity

Techniques for Drug Analysis

was assessed by analyzing only seven plasma samples by the RR and a GC method (Jorgensen, 1975). The only comparison data provided was a correlation coefficient of 0.99. Due to the differences between the tertiary and secondary antidepressants in their potencies in inhibiting ^{3}H-QNB binding, differential extraction was required to separate the compounds prior to assay. Binding interference from the phenothiazine derivatives (especially thiorizadine) atropine, benztropine, and trihexyphenidyl eliminates the use of this assay for patients on concurrent therapy with tricyclic antidepressants and any of the previously mentioned compounds.

Radioreceptor assays, at present, offer limited usefulness for the routine clinical monitoring of tricyclic antidepressants in plasma or serum. Binding interference and an inability to offer simultaneous analysis of parent drugs and metabolites are the two major reasons other methodologies such as GC and HPLC remain the mainstay of antidepressant quantitation.

Enzyme Immunoassay

Therapeutic drug monitoring in the past five years has been revolutionized by the advent of enzyme immunoassay techniques. Rapid, sensitive, and accurate procedures are commercially available for the quantitation of, at present, eighteen drugs and their metabolites (Syva Inc.).

The operational principle of enzyme immunoassay is competitive protein binding. A drug labelled with an enzyme competes with drug in patient specimen for binding to antibodies raised against the drug or structurally-related compound. After a specified period of time, enzyme activity of the unbound drug-enzyme or bound drug-enzyme-antibody complexes are monitored. Enzyme activity correlates with concentration of drug in the patient specimen.

A non-commercial double-antibody immunoassay technique has been developed for nortriptyline (Al-Bassam et al., 1978a; Al-Bassam et al., 1978b). The nortriptyline antiserum was raised in sheep against a nortriptyline-BSA conjugate. α-D-galactosidase from Escherichia coli conjugated to desmethylnortriptyline served as drug-enzyme complex. By use of the cross-linking reagent dimethyladipimidate, 75% of the enzyme was conjugated to desmethylnortriptyline with 80% of the bound enzyme retaining activity after conjugation. Initially, nortriptyline standard or patient sample (100 µL) was mixed with diluent buffer followed by addition of drug-enzyme complex and antiserum. A 90 min incubation was carried out at 4°C. An antibody raised against the initial antiserum was added to separate free antigen (drug-enzyme) from antigen bound to the first antibody by precipitating out the latter. After an overnight equilibration the precipitate was isolated, substrate solution (O-nitrophenyl-α-D-galactopyranoside) was added and a 2 h incubation (20°C) begun. Any enzyme present as drug-enzyme-antibody complex in the precipitate enzymatically converted the substrate to an end product, the formation of which was monitored spectrophotometrically at 420 nm. Thus, if a large amount of nortriptyline is in the patient specimen, a small portion of the antibody will be bound to the drug-enzyme complex. Consequently, little absorbance will be monitored at 420 nm. The converse results if a minimal drug concentration is present. Calibration curves were plotted as the ratio of the fraction of enzyme-labelled nortriptyline bound at a given nortriptyline concentration to the fraction bound when no nortriptyline is present. Nortriptyline concentrations for the calibration ranged from 1 to 20 µg/L. Assay conditions would have to be modified to accommodate the quantitation of concentrations within the therapeutic range of 50-150 µg/L (Orsulak and Schildkraut, 1979; Risch et al., 1981). Cross-reactivity of other drugs was evaluated and the assay has been found not to be specific for nortriptyline. The cross-reactivities ranged from 153% for amitriptyline to < 3% for carbamazepine of the eight drugs evaluated. Imipramine, desmethylnortriptyline, protriptyline, and desipramine gave intermediate but substantial cross-reactivities. No cross-reaction was demonstrated for the major nortriptyline metabolites, the hydroxylated compounds. Activity of the enzyme-drug complex is quite stable as storage for 6 months at 4°C resulted in only a 10% decrease in activity. Validity of the enzyme immunoassay was evaluated by comparison with RIA and GC methods. Correlation coefficients and slopes were acceptable. However, the 'Y' intercepts indicated a tendency of the enzyme immunoassay to overestimate results.

A single antibody enzyme immunoassay, trademarked EMIT®, is commercially available for the qualitative determination of tricyclic antidepressants and their metabolites in serum or plasma (Syva, Inc., 1982). The patient specimen is mixed with two reagents: Reagent A contains antibodies made in sheep against a desipramine derivative, the co-enzyme nicotinamide adenine dinucleotide (NAD), and glucose-6-phosphate. Reagent B contains a desipramine derivative chemically coupled to bacterial glucose-6-phosphate dehydrogenase. Both reagents are stable for 12 weeks after reconstitution. Initial addition of reagent A to the sample results in binding of the antibody to drug recognized in the patient specimen. Once reagent B is added, any remaining antibody binding sites become coupled to the enzyme-labelled drug. Once bound, the enzyme is no longer active, unlike the previous double antibody method (Al-Bassam et al., 1978a; Al-Bassam et al., 1978b) in which the enzyme retained activity after antibody binding. Unbound enzyme remains active, capable of metabolizing glucose-6-phosphate, which in turn results in conversion of NAD to NADH. The final absorbance change to NADH is measured spectrophotometrically.

Utilization of the co-enzyme NAD eliminates interference from endogenous serum G6PDH which functions with nicotinamide adenine dinucleotide phosphate (NADP). This assay, unlike the other enzyme immunoassay, is homogeneous--physical separation of bound from unbound enzyme is not required for analysis. Total analysis time for the Emit® method is approximately 20 min as compared to the overnight analysis required for the double antibody enzyme immunoassay (Al-Bassam et al., 1978a; Al-Bassam et al., 1978b).

However, the Emit® method, as stated previously, is only qualitative and therefore not suitable for therapeutic drug monitoring. The Emit® Serum Tricyclic Antidepressants Calibrator and Control contain 0, 300, and 1,000 µg/L of nortriptyline for the negative control, calibrator, and positive control respectively. The antibody cross-reacts with virtually all tricyclic antidepressants and metabolites, including the hydroxylated derivatives. Amoxapine and the tetracyclic maprotiline are not detected. No clinically relevant interference has been demonstrated from stimulants, narcotics, hypnotics, and antipsychotics, with the exception of chlorpromazine in high therapeutic or toxic concentrations.

Enzyme immunoassays available at present are not suitable for routine therapeutic drug monitoring of antidepressants. With the development of more specific antibodies and an increase in sensitivity, enzyme immunoassay products such as Emit® could become widely used methods for quantitation of this group of drugs.

Techniques for Drug Analysis

Double Radioisotope Derivative Analysis

A number of isotope derivative dilution procedures for tricyclic antidepressants have been published since Hammer and Brodie (1967) described the analysis of desipramine and nortriptyline. Maguire and others (1976) modified the basic procedure to include an internal standard. Nortriptyline was extracted from alkalinized plasma samples using n-heptane and subsequently derivatized with [^{3}H]acetic anhydride. [^{14}C]Nortriptyline was added prior to the extraction as an internal standard. Nortriptyline was then separated from other co-extracted materials by thin layer chromatography, eluted from the plate, and counted for [^{3}H] and [^{14}C] content.

Using a similar method, Carnis and others (1976) devised a procedure for the measurement of clomipramine and desmethylclomipramine. Respective [^{14}C] analogues were used as internal standards. Desmethylclomipramine extracted from the sample was derivatized with [^{3}H]acetic anhydride and then separated from clomipramine and other acetylated material by TLC. The eluted [^{3}H]acetyldesmethylclomipramine was then counted for both ^{3}H and ^{14}C (internal standard). Then the clomipramine was eluted from the silica gel plate and reacted with trichloroethyl chloroformate. The resulting urethane was then saponified and decarboxylated to form desmethylclomipramine, which in turn was [^{3}H]acetylated, purified by TLC, eluted, and measured by scintillation counting. Although the sensitivity for the desmethyl metabolite was 2 µg/L, the sensitivity for the parent drug was only 15 µg/L.

Methods have been published for other antidepressants. However, whilst double isotope dilution assays are stated to be "sensitive, specific, precise, rapid and relatively inexpensive" (Scoggins et al., 1980), they are still regarded as unsuitable for routine clinical assays. The TLC manipulations are a drawback to some laboratories, but more importantly, the availability of ^{14}C analogues for most antidepressants is poor and the use of relatively potent ^{3}H-containing reagents should be discouraged if other methods are available (e.g. GC, HPLC).

Lithium

Lithium (Li) is well recognized as an effective treatment for acute mania and as a preventor of relapses in bipolar mood disorders. Monitoring of serum Li concentrations is an important adjunct to successful treatment with the drug and serves to prevent the development of toxic symptoms which may occur at concentrations near the therapeutic range.

Flame emission photometry and atomic absorption spectroscopy are the two mainstay methodologies available for determining Li in serum. Levy and Katz (1970) compared flame photometry and atomic absorption spectrophotometry for determination of Li in serum. These authors found no significant difference in the results reported by the two methods. Flame photometry was found to be more sensitive and easier to use but not as precise as atomic absorption spectrophotometry. Most flame photometers measuring sodium (Na) and potassium (K) with Li as internal standard can be easily converted to measuring Na and Li with K as internal standard. Measurement of serum Li by atomic absorption involves either manual dilution of the specimen prior to analysis (Pylus and Briers, 1970) or direct determination using flow-injection analysis (FIA) (Rocks et al., 1982). With flow injection, the sample is injected into a continuously flowing stream of deionized water and pumped to the nebulizer of the instrument. A transient signal response proportional to Li quantity in the sample is generated. FIA not only eliminates sample pretreatment, but permits use of a low sample volume (5 µL).

The Li erythrocyte/plasma ratio, which may be of greater diagnostic value for toxicity than serum concentrations, has been determined by direct measurement in erythrocytes by flame emission photometry (Eisenberg and Lentz, 1977) and by an indirect hematocrit measurement using atomic absorption spectrophotometry (Hisayasu et al., 1977). No method offers overwhelming superiority for ratio determination.

There is little to choose between flame emission and atomic absorption for lithium quantitation. However, the relative operational ease and inexpense of flame emission photometry may make this technique more accessible to a greater number of laboratories.

Conclusion

The most widely applied methods for quantitating antidepressants in a routine clinical setting at present are GC and HPLC. Specificity is the major advantage of these two methods. GC/MS, although a very routine and specific analytical tool in some laboratories for clinical monitoring, is unlikely to become a widely accepted method because of the expense and operational expertise involved. RIA is a sensitive method, but generally lacks the specificity of GC, HPLC, and GC/MS. Radioreceptor assays at present also lack specificity and thus have not been extensively applied to routine determinations. TLC and double radioisotope derivative assays are not suitable for clinical monitoring because of the general tediousness involved, but may be useful for pharmacokinetic/research studies. The method group which has the greatest potential for application to clinical antidepressant monitoring is immunoassay. Although only a qualitative enzyme immunoassay is available at present (Syva®), utilization of monoclonal antibodies and application of sophisticated techniques such as fluorescence polarization immunoassay (Abbott®) will result in development of sensitive, accurate, specific, and rapid methods for quantitation of antidepressants and respective active metabolites.

References

Aherne, G. W., Marks, V., Mould, G., and Stout, G. (1977) Radioimmunoassay for nortriptyline and amitriptyline. Lancet i, 1214.

Al-Bassam, M. N., O'Sullivan, M. J., Gnemmi, E., Bridges, J. W., and Marks, V. (1978a) Nortriptyline enzyme immunoassay. In: Enzyme Labelled Immunoassay of Hormones and Drugs (Pal, S. B., ed.), Walter de Gruyter, Berlin, pp. 375-386.

Al-Bassam, M. N., O'Sullivan, M. J., Gnemmi, E., Bridges, J. W., and Marks, V. (1978b) Double-antibody enzyme immunoassay for nortriptyline. Clin. Chem. 24, 1590-1594.

Alfredsson, G., Wiesel, F.-A., Fyro, B., and Sedvall, G. (1977) Mass fragmentographic analysis of clomipramine and its mono-demethylated metabolite in human plasma. Psychopharmacology 52, 25-30.

Alkalay, D., Carlsen, S., Khemani, L., and Bartlett, M. F. (1979a) Selected ion monitoring assay for the antidepressant maprotiline. Biomed. Mass Spec. 6, 435-438.

Alkalay, D., Volk, J., and Carlsen, S. (1979b) A sensitive method for the simultaneous determination in biological fluids of imipramine and desipramine or clomipramine and N-desmethylclomipramine by gas chromatography mass spectrometry. Biomed. Mass Spec. 6, 200-204.

Alvan, G., Borga, O., Lind, M., Palmer, L., and Siwers, B. (1977) First pass hydroxylation of nortriptyline: concentrations of parent drug and major metabolites in plasma. Eur. J. Clin. Pharmacol. 11, 219-224.

Ankier, S. I., Martin, B. K., Rogers, M. S., Carpenter, P. K., and Graham, C. (1981) Trazodone--a new assay procedure and some pharmacokinetic parameters. Brit. J. Clin. Pharmacol. 11, 505-509.

Antal, E., Mercik, S., and Kramer, P. A. (1980) Technical considerations in the gas chromatographic analysis of desipramine. J. Chromatogr. 183, 149-157.

Bailey, D. N. and Jatlow, P. I. (1976a) Gas-chromatographic analysis for therapeutic concentrations of amitriptyline and nortriptyline in plasma, with use of a nitrogen detector. Clin. Chem. 22, 771-781.

Bailey, D. N. and Jatlow, P. I. (1976b) Gas-chromatographic analysis for therapeutic concentrations of imipramine and desipramine in plasma, with use of a nitrogen detector. Clin. Chem. 22, 1697-1701.

Bailey, E. and Barron, E. J. (1980) Determination of tranylcypromine in human plasma and urine using high-resolution gas-liquid chromatography with nitrogen-sensitive detection. J. Chromatogr. **183,** 25-31.

Bannister, S. J., van der Wal, S., Dolan, J. W., and Snyder, L. R. (1981) Liquid chromatographic analysis for common tricyclic antidepressant drugs and their metabolites in serum or plasma with the Technicon Fast LC system. Clin. Chem. **27,** 849-855.

Bertilson, L. (1981) Quantitative mass fragmentography: a valuable tool in clinical psychopharmacology. In: Clinical Pharmacology in Psychiatry (Usdin, E., ed.), Elsevier, New York, pp. 35-42.

Bierle, F. A. and Hubbard R. W. (1983a) Liquid chromatographic separation of antidepressant drugs: I. Tricyclics. Ther. Drug Monit. **5,** 279-292.

Bierle, F. A. and Hubbard R. W. (1983b) Liquid chromatographic separation of antidepressant drugs: II. Amoxapine and maprotiline. Ther. Drug Monit. **5,** 293-301.

Biggs, J. T., Holland, W. H., Chang, S., Hipps, P. P., and Sherman, W. R. (1976) Electron beam ionization mass fragmentographic analysis of tricyclic antidepressants in human plasma. J. Pharm. Sci. **65,** 261-268.

Biggs, S. R., Brodie, R. R., Hawkins, D. R., and Midgley, I. (1977) The use of high pressure liquid chromatography and mass spectrometry for the analysis of amitriptyline and its metabolites in plasma. In: Clinical Toxicology (Leonard, B. J. and Duncan, W. A. M., eds), Excerpta Medica, vol. 18, pp. 174-176.

Biggs, S. R., Chasseaud, L. F., Hawkins, D. R., and Midgley, I. (1979) Determination of amitriptyline and its major basic metabolites in human urine by high-performance liquid chromatography. Drug. Metab. Dispos. **7,** 233-236.

Bock, J. L., Giller, E., Gray, S., and Jatlow, P. (1982) Steady-state plasma concentrations of cis- and trans-10-OH amitriptyline metabolites. Clin. Pharmacol. Ther. **31,** 609-616.

Braithwaite, R. A., Montgomery, S., and Robinson, J. D. (1978) A radioimmunoassay for amitriptyline and nortriptyline. Brit. J. Pharmacol. **63,** 370P-371P.

Breutzmann, D. A. and Bowers, L. D. (1981) Reversed-phase liquid chromatography and gas chromatography/mass fragmentography compared for determination of tricyclic antidepressant drugs. Clin.

Chem. **27**, 1907-1911.
Brodie, R. R., Chassaud, L. F., and Hawkins, D. R. (1977a) Separation and measurement of tricyclic antidepressant drugs in plasma by high performance liquid chromatography. J. Chromatogr. **143**, 535-539.
Brodie, R. R., Chassaud, L. F., Crampton, E. L., Hawkins, D. R., and Risdall, P. C. (1977b) High performance liquid chromatographic determination of dothiepin and northiaden in human plasma and serum. J. Int. Med. Res. **5**, 387-390.
Brunswick, D. J., Neidelman, B., and Mendels, J. (1978) Radioimmunoassay of imipramine and desmethylimipramine. Life Sci. **22**, 137-146.
Brunswick, D. J., Neidelman, B., and Mendels, J. (1979) Specific radioimmunoassay of amitriptyline and nortriptyline. Brit. J. Clin. Pharmacol. **7**, 343-348.
Burch, J. E., Raddats, M. A., and Thompson, S. G. (1979) Reliable routine method for the determination of plasma amitriptyline and nortriptyline by gas chromatography. J. Chromatogr. **162**, 351-366.
Caddy, B. and Stead, A. H. (1977) Indirect determination of phenelzine in urine. Analyst **102**, 42-49.
Caddy, B. and Stead, A. H. (1978) Three cases of poisoning involving the drug phenelzine. J. Forens. Sci. Soc. **18**, 207-208.
Caddy, B., Tilstone, W. J., and Johnstone, E. C. (1976) Phenelzine in urine: assay and relation to acetylator status. Brit. J. Clin. Pharmacol. **3**, 633-637.
Carnis, G., Godbillon, J., and Metayer, J. P. (1976) Determination of clomipramine and desmethylclomipramine in plasma or urine by the double-radioisotope derivative technique. Clin. Chem. **22**, 817-823.
Charette, C. and McGilveray, I. J. (1981) Gas-liquid chromatographic procedure with alkali flame ionization detection for the determination of maprotiline in plasma. J. Chromatogr. **224**, 128-132.
Chinn, D. M., Jennison, T. A., Crouch, D. J., Peat, M. A., and Thatcher, G. W. (1980) Quantitative analysis for tricyclic antidepressant drugs in plasma or serum by gas chromatography-chemical-ionization mass spectrometry. Clin. Chem. **26**, 1201-1204.
Chojnacki, M., Kralik, P., Allen, R. H., Ho, B. T., Schoolar, J. C., and Smith, R. C. (1981) Neuroleptic-induced decrease in platelet MAO activity in schizophrenic patients. Am. J. Psychiatry

138, 838-842.

Claeys, M., Markey, S. P., and Maenhaut, W. (1977) Variance analysis of error in selected ion monitoring assays using various internal standards. A practical study case. Biomed. Mass Spec. 4, 122-128.

Claeys, M., Muscettola, G., and Markey, S. P. (1976) Simultaneous measurement of imipramine and desipramine by selected ion recording with deuterated internal standards. Biomed. Mass Spec. 3, 110-116.

Connor, J. N., Johnson, G. F., and Solomon, H. M. (1977) Quantitation of amitriptyline and nortriptyline in human serum. J. Chromatogr. 143, 415-421.

Cooper, S., Albert, J.-M., Dugal, R., Bertrand, M., and Elie, R. (1979) Gas chromatographic determination of amitriptyline, nortriptyline and perphenazine in plasma of schizophrenic patients after administration of the combination of amitriptyline with perphenazine. Arzneim.-Forsch./Drug Res. 29, 158-161.

Cooper, T. B. (1981) Nitrogen phosphorous detector: experiences in psychotropic drug level monitoring. In: Clinical Pharmacology in Psychiatry (Usdin, E., ed.), Elsevier, New York, pp. 35-42.

Cooper, T. B., Allen, D., and Simpson, G. M. (1975) A sensitive GLC method for the determination of imipramine and desmethylimipramine using a nitrogen detector. Psychopharmacol. Commun. 1, 445-454.

Cooper, T. B. and Kelly, R. G. (1979) GLC analysis of loxapine, amoxapine, and their metabolites in serum and urine. J. Pharm. Sci. 68, 216-219.

Cooper, T. B., Robinson, D. S., and Nies, A. (1978) Phenelzine measurement in human plasma: a sensitive GLC-ECD procedure. Commun. Psychopharmacol. 2, 505-512.

Crampton, E. L., Glass, R. C., Marchant, B., and Rees, J. A. (1980) Chemical ionisation mass fragmentographic measurement of dothiepin plasma concentrations following a single oral dose in man. J. Chromatogr. 183, 141-148.

Davis, T. P., Veggeberg, S. K., Hameroff, S. R., and Watts, K. L. (1983) Sensitive and quantitative determination of plasma doxepin and desmethyldoxepin in chronic pain patients by gas chromatography and mass spectrometry. J. Chromatogr. 273, 436-441.

Dawling, S. and Braithwaite, R. A. (1978) Simplified method for monitoring tricyclic antidepressant

therapy using gas-liquid chromatography with nitrogen detection. J. Chromatogr. 146, 449-456.
de Ridder, J. J., Koppens, P. C. J. M., and van Hal, H. J. M. (1977) Mass fragmentographic assay of nanogram amounts of the antidepressant drug mianserin hydrochloride (Org GB 94) in human plasma. J. Chromatogr. 143, 289-297.
Dhar, A. K. and Kutt, H. (1979) An improved gas-liquid chromatographic procedure for the determination of amitriptyline and nortriptyline levels in plasma using nitrogen-sensitive detectors. Ther. Drug Monit. 1, 209-216.
Dixon, R. and Martin, D. (1981) Tricyclic antidepressants: a simplified approach for the routine clinical monitoring of parent drug and metabolites in plasma using HPLC. Res. Commun. Chem. Pathol. Pharmacol. 33, 537-545.
Edelbroek, P. M., de Haas, E. J. M., and de Wolff, F. A. (1982) Liquid chromatographic determination of amitriptyline and its metabolites in serum with adsorption onto glass minimized. Clin. Chem. 28, 2143-2148.
Eisenberg, R. and Lantz, R. (1977) Erythrocyte lithium analysis. Clin. Chem. 23, 900.
Emanuelsson, B. and Moore, R. G. (1978) Quantitation of zimelidine and norzimelidine in plasma using high-performance liquid chromatography. J. Chromatogr. 146, 113-119.
Fenimore, D. C., Meyer, C. J., Davis, C. M., Hsu, H., and Zlatkis, A. (1977) High-performance thin-layer chromatographic determination of psychopharmacologic agents in blood serum. J. Chromatogr. 142, 399-409.
Frigerio, A., Belvedere, G., de Nadai, F., Fanelli, R., Pantarotto, C., Riva, E., and Morselli, P. L. (1972) A method for the determination of imipramine in human plasma by gas-liquid chromatography-mass fragmentography. J. Chromatogr. 74, 201-208.
Garland, W. A. (1977) Quantitative determination of amitriptyline and its principal metabolite, nortriptyline, by GLC-chemical ionization mass spectrometry. J. Pharm. Sci. 66, 77-81.
Garland, W. A., Muccino, R. R., Min, B. H., Cupano, J., and Fann, W. E. (1979) A method for the determination of amitriptyline and its metabolites nortriptyline, 10-hydroxyamitriptyline, and 10-hydroxynortriptyline in human plasma using stable isotope dilution and gas chromatography-chemical ionization mass spectrometry (GC-CIMS). Clin. Pharmacol. Ther. 25, 844-856.

Gaskell, S. J. (1980) Gas chromatography/high-resolution mass spectrometry as a reference method for clomipramine determination. Postgrad. Med. J. 56, 90-93.

Gitlian, R. and Mason, W. D. (1981) High pressure liquid chromatographic determination of viloxazine in human plasma and urine. J. Pharm. Sci. 70, 220-221.

Godbillon, J. and Gauron, S. (1981) Determination of clomipramine or imipramine and their mono-demethylated metabolites in human blood or plasma by high-performance liquid chromatography. J. Chromatogr. 204, 303-311.

Gonzalez, R. and Kraml, M. (1980) Butriptyline: improved gas-liquid chromatographic method using a nitrogen-phosphorus detector for its determination in serum. Clin. Biochem. 13, 141-143.

Gupta, R. N., Molnar, G., and Gupta, M. L. (1977) Estimation of maprotiline in serum by gas-chromatography, with use of a nitrogen-specific detector. Clin. Chem. 23, 1849-1852.

Hackett, L. P. and Dusci, L. J. (1979) The use of high performance liquid chromatography in clinical toxicology. II. Tricyclic antidepressants. Clin. Toxicol. 15, 55-61.

Haefelfinger, P. (1978) Determination of amitriptyline and nortriptyline in human plasma by quantitative thin-layer chromatography. J. Chromatogr. 145, 445-451.

Haefelfinger, P. (1982) Sensitive assay for the tricyclic antidepressant Ro 11-2465 in biological fluids by high-performance liquid chromatography and fluorescence detection. J. Chromatogr. 233, 269-278.

Hammer, W. H. and Brodie, B. B. (1967) Application of isotope derivative technique to assay of secondary amines: estimation of desipramine by acetylation with ^{3}H-acetic anhydride. J. Pharmacol. Exp. Ther. 157, 503-508.

Hartvig, P., Strandberg, S., and Naslund, B. (1976) Determination of plasma amitriptyline by electron-capture gas chromatography after oxidation to anthraquinone. J. Chromatogr. 118, 65-74.

Hebb, J. H. Jr., Crooks, C. R., Caplan, Y. H., and Mergner, W. J. (1982) A method for the determination of therapeutic and toxic concentrations of tricyclic antidepressant drugs in post mortem fluids and tissues. J. Anal. Toxicol. 6, 206-208.

Heck, H. d'A., Flynn, N. W., Buttrill, S. E. Jr., Dyer, R. L., and Anbar, M. (1978) Determination of imipramine in plasma by high pressure liquid chromatography and field ionization mass spectrometry: increased sensitivity in comparison with gas chromatography mass spectrometry. Biomed. Mass Spec. 5, 250-257.

Heptner, W., Badian, M. J., Baudner, S., Christ, O. E., Fraser, H. M., Rupp, W., Weiner, K. E., and Wissmann, H. (1977) Determination of nomifensine by a sensitive radioimmunoassay. Br. J. Clin. Pharmacol. 4, 123S-127S.

Hisayasu, G. H., Cohen, J. L., and Nelson, R. W. (1977) Determination of plasma and lithium concentrations by atomic absorption spectrophotometry. Clin. Chem. 23, 41-45.

Hucker, H. B. and Stauffer, S. (1974) GLC method for quantitative determination of amitriptyline in human plasma. J. Pharm. Sci. 63, 296-297.

Innis, R. B. and Snyder, S. H. (1981) Radioreceptor assay: techniques and applications to psychopharmacology. In: Clinical Pharmacology in Psychiatry (Usdin, E., ed.), Elsevier, North Holland, pp. 103-120.

Jindal, S. P., Lutz, T., and Cooper, T. B. (1980a) Determination of phenelzine in human plasma with gas chromatography-mass spectrometry using an isotope-labeled internal standard. J. Chromatogr. 221, 301-308.

Jindal, S. P., Lutz, T., and Vestergaard, P. (1980b) GLC-mass spectrometric determination of maprotiline and its major metabolite using stable isotope-labeled analog as internal standard. J. Pharm. Sci. 69, 684-687.

Jindal, S. P., Lutz, T., and Vestergaard, P. (1982) Selected ion monitoring assay for the antidepressant mianserin in human plasma with stable isotope-labeled analog as internal standard. J. Anal. Toxicol. 6, 34-37.

Jorgensen, A. (1975) A gas chromatographic method for the determination of amitriptyline and nortriptyline in human sera. Acta pharmacol. toxicol. 36, 79-90.

Jozefczak, C., Ktorza, H., and Uzan, A. (1982) High performance liquid chromatographic determination of indalpine, a new non-tricyclic anitdepressant in human plasma. J. Chromatogr. 230, 87-95.

Kabra, P. M., Mar, N. A., and Marton, L. J. (1981) Simultaneous liquid chromatographic analysis of amitriptyline, nortriptyline, imipramine, desipramine, doxepin and nordoxepin. Clin. Chim.

Acta 111, 123-132.

Kamel, R. S., Landon, J., and Smith, D. S. (1979) Novel ^{125}I-labelled nortriptyline derivatives and their use in liquid-phase or magnetizable solid-phase second-antibody radioimmunoassays. Clin. Chem. 25, 1997-2002.

Karkkainen, S. and Seppala, E. (1980) Gas chromatographic analysis of therapeutic concentrations of maprotiline in serum, using flame-ionization detection. J. Chromatogr. 221, 319-326.

Karlsson, K.-E. (1981) Two-phase derivatization of amitriptyline and structurally related tertiary amines for gas chromatography with electron-capture detection. J. Chromatogr. 219, 373-378.

Kaul, P. N., Whitfield, L. R., and Clark, M. L. (1978) Quantitative determination of amitriptyline in blood. J. Pharm. Sci. 67, 60-62.

Ketchum, C., Robinson, C. A., and Scott, J. W. (1983) Analysis of amoxapine, 8-hydroxyamoxapine, and maprotiline by high pressure liquid chromatography. Ther. Drug Monit. 5, 309-312.

Kimball, D. F. and Lampert, A. A. (1982) Analysis of amoxapine and its metabolites in human plasma by high pressure liquid chromatography. S. D. J. Med. 35, 31-33.

Koteel, P., Mullins, R. E., and Gadsden, R. H. (1982) Sample preparation and liquid-chromatographic analysis for tricyclic antidepressants in serum. Clin. Chem. 28, 462-466.

Kraak, J. C. and Bijster, P. (1977) Determination of amitriptyline and some of its metabolites in blood by high-pressure liquid chromatography. J. Chromatogr. 143, 499-512.

Kristinsson, J. (1981) A gas chromatographic method for the determination of antidepressant drugs in human serum. Acta pharmacol. toxicol. 49, 390-398.

Kuss, H. J. and Feistenauer, E. (1981) Quantitative high-performance liquid chromatographic assay for the determination of maprotiline and oxaprotiline in human plasma. J. Chromatogr. 204, 349-353.

Lagerstrom, P., Marle, I., and Persson, B. (1983) Solvent extraction of tricyclic amines from blood plasma and liquid chromatographic determination. J. Chromatogr. 273, 151-160.

Lang, V. A., Geibler, H. E., and Mutschler, E. (1978) Fluorimetrische bestimmung von tranylcypromin in plasma als 1-dimethylamino-naphthalin-5-sulfonsaure-derivat durch direkte quantitative dunnschichtchromatographie. Arzneim.-Forsch./Drug Res. 28, 575-577.

Lapin, A. and Karobath, M. (1980) Determination of chlorimipramine and desmethylchlorimipramine in plasma using selected ion monitoring with chemical ionization. Biomed. Mass Spec. 7, 588-591.

Larsen, N.-E. and Marinelli, K. (1978) Determination of zimelidine and its demethylated metabolite in human plasma by gas chromatography. J. Chromatogr. 156, 335-339.

Levy, A. and Katz, E. M. (1970) Comparison of serum lithium concentrations by flame photometry and atomic absorption spectrophotometry. Clin. Chem. 16, 840-842.

Linnoila, M., Insel, T., Kilts, C., Potter, W. Z., and Murphy, D. L. (1982) Plasma steady-state concentrations of hydroxylated metabolites of clomipramine. Clin. Pharmacol. Ther. 32, 208-211.

Lucek, R. and Dixon, R. (1977) Specific radioimmunoassay for amitriptyline and nortriptyline in plasma. Res. Commun. Chem. Pathol. Pharmacol. 18, 125-136.

Lundgren, R., Olsson, A., and Forshell, G. P. (1977) Gas chromatographic determination of lofepramine and desmethylimipramine in plasma. Acta Pharm. Suec. 14, 81-94.

Maguire, K. P., Burrows, G. D., Coghlan, J. P., and Scoggins, B. A. (1976) Rapid radioisotopic procedure for determination of nortriptyline in plasma. Clin. Chem. 22, 761-764.

Maguire, K. P., Burrows, G. D., Norman, T. R., and Scoggins, B. A. (1980) Evaluation of a kit for measuring tricyclic antidepressants. Clin. Chem. 26, 529.

Maguire, K. P., Burrows, G. D., Norman, T. R., and Scoggins, B. A. (1978) A radioimmunoassay for nortriptyline (and other tricyclic antidepressants) in plasma. Clin. Chem. 24, 549-554.

Maguire, K. P., Norman, T. R., and Burrows, G. D. (1981) Simultaneous measurement of dothiepin and its major metabolites in plasma and whole blood by gas chromatography-mass fragmentography. J. Chromatogr. 222, 399-408.

Matsubayashi, K., Hakusui, H., and Sano, M. (1977) Mass fragmentographic determination of lofepramine and its metabolites in human plasma and urine using deuterated internal standards. J. Chromatogr. 143, 571-580.

McIntyre, I. M., Norman, T. R., Burrows, G. D., and Maguire, K. P. (1981) Determination of nomifensine plasma concentrations: a comparison of radioimmunoassay and gas chromatography. Brit. J. Clin. Pharmacol. 12, 691-694.

Mellstrom, B. and Braithwaite, R. (1978) Ion-pair chromatography of amitriptyline and metabolites in plasma. J. Chromatogr. 157, 379-385.

Mellstrom, B. and Tybring, G. (1977) Ion-pair liquid chromatography of steady-state plasma levels of clomipramine and desmethylclomipramine. J. Chromatogr. 143, 597-605.

Midha, K. K. and Charette, C. (1980) Radioimmunoassay for total doxepin and N-desmethyl doxepin in plasma. Commun. Psychopharmacol. 4, 11-15.

Midha, K. K., Charette, C., Cooper, J. K., and McGilveray, I. J. (1980) Comparison of a new GLC-AFID method with a GLC-MS selected ion monitoring technique and a radioimmunoassay for the determination of plasma concentrations of imipramine and desipramine. J. Anal. Toxicol. 4, 237-243.

Midha, K. K., Loo, J. C. K., Charette, C., Rave, M. L., Hubbard, J. W., and McGilveray, I. J. (1978) Monitoring of therapeutic concentrations of psychotropic drugs in plasma by radioimmunoassays. J. Anal. Toxicol. 2, 185-192.

Mould, G. P., Stout, G., Aherne, G. W., and Marks, V. (1978) Radioimmunoassay of amitriptyline and nortriptyline in body fluids. Ann. Clin. Biochem. 15, 221-252.

Moyes, R. B. and Moyes, I. C. A. (1979) Metabolism and pharmacokinetics of clomipramine--measurement of plasma antidepressant levels by high performance liquid chromatography. Postgrad. Med. J. 53, 117-123.

Nagy, A. and Treiber, L. (1973) Quantitative determination of imipramine and desipramine in human blood plasma by direct densitometry of thin-layer chromatograms. J. Pharm. Pharmacol. 25, 599-603.

Narasimhachari, N. (1981) Evaluation of C_{18} Sep-Pak cartridges for biological sample clean-up for tricyclic antidepressant assays. J. Chromatogr. 225, 189-195.

Narasimhachari, N., Saady, J., and Friedel, R. O. (1981) Quantitative mapping of metabolites of imipramine and desipramine in plasma samples by gas chromatographic-mass spectrometry. Biol. Psychiatry 16, 937-944.

Nash, J. F., Bopp, R. J., Carmichael, R. H., Farid, K. Z., and Lemberger, L. (1982) Determination of fluoxetine and norfluoxetine in plasma by gas chromatography with electron-capture detection. Clin. Chem. 28, 2100-2102.

Norman, T. R., Burrows, G. D., Davies, B. M., and Wurm, J. M. E. (1979) Determination of viloxazine in plasma by GLC. Brit. J. Clin. Pharmacol. 8,

169-171.
Norman, T. R., Maguire, K. P., and Burrows, G. D. (1977) Determination of therapeutic levels of butriptyline in plasma by gas-liquid chromatography. J. Chromatogr. 134, 524-528.
Orsulak, P. J. and Schildkraut, J. J. (1979) Guidelines for therapeutic monitoring of tricyclic antidepressant plasma levels. Ther. Drug Monit. 1, 199-208.
Oyehang, E., Ostensen, E. T., and Salvesen, B. (1982) Determination of the antidepressant agent citalopram and metabolites in plasma by liquid chromatography with fluorescence detection. J. Chromatogr. 227, 129-135.
Paul, S. M., Rehavi, M., Hulihan, B., Skolnick, P., and Goodwin, F. G. (1980) A rapid and sensitive radioreceptor assay for tertiary amine tricyclic antidepressants. Commun. Psychopharmacol. 4, 487-494.
Potter, W. Z., Calil, H. M., Sutfin, T. A., Zavadil, A. P., Jusko, W. J., Rapoport, J., and Goodwin, F. K. (1982) Active metabolites of imipramine and desipramine in man. Clin. Pharmacol. Ther. 31, 393-401.
Proelss, H. F., Lohmann, H. J., and Miles, D. G. (1978) High-performance liquid-chromatographic simultaneous determination of commonly used tricyclic antidepressants. Clin. Chem. 24, 1948-1953.
Pylus, J. and Briers, G. N. (1970) Measurement of serum lithium by atomic absorption spectroscopy. Clin. Chem. 16, 139-143.
Read, G. F. and Riad-Fahmy, D. (1978) Determination of a tricyclic antidepressant clomipramine (Anafranil) in plasma by a specific radioimmunoassay procedure. Clin. Chem. 24, 36-40.
Read, G. F., Riad-Fahmy, D., and Walker, R. F. (1977) A specific radioimmunoassay procedure for plasma clomipramine. Postgrad. Med. J. 53 (Suppl. 4), 110-116.
Reece, P. A., Zacest, R., and Barrow, C. G. (1979) Quantification of imipramine and desipramine in plasma by high-performance liquid chromatography and fluorescence detection. J. Chromatogr. 163, 310-314.
Risch, S. C., Kalin, N. H., Janowsky, D. S., and Huey, L. Y. (1981) Indications and guidelines for plasma tricyclic antidepressant concentration monitoring. J. Clin. Psychopharmacol. 1, 59-63.

Robinson, J. D., Aherne, G. W., and Risby, D. (1977) A radioimmunoassay for amitriptyline and related compounds in blood. In: Clinical Toxicology (Leonard, B. J. and Duncan, W. A. M., eds), Excerpta Medica, pp. 168-170.

Robinson, J. D., Risby, D., Riley, G., and Aherne, G. W. (1978) A radioimmunoassay for the determination of combined amitriptyline and nortriptyline concentrations in microlitre samples of plasma. J. Pharmacol. Exp. Ther. 205, 499-502.

Rocks, B. F., Sherwood, R. A., and Riley, C. (1982) Direct determination of therapeutic concentrations of lithium in serum by flow injection analysis with atomic absorption spectroscopic detection. Clin. Chem. 28, 440-443.

Rosseel, M. T., Bogaert, M. G., and Claeys, M. (1978) Quantitative GLC determination of cis- and trans-isomers of doxepin and desmethyldoxepin. J. Pharm. Sci. 67, 802-805.

Rovei, V., Sanjuan, M., and Hrdina, P. D. (1980) Analysis of tricyclic antidepressant drugs by gas chromatography using nitrogen-selective detection with packed and capillary columns. J. Chromatogr. 182, 349-357.

Scoggins, B. A., Maguire, K. P., Norman, T. R., and Burrows, G. D. (1980) Measurement of tricyclic antidepressants. Part 1. A review of methodology. Clin. Chem. 26, 5-17.

Sioufi, A. and Richard, A. (1980) Gas chromatographic determination of maprotiline and its N-desmethyl metabolite in human blood using nitrogen detection. J. Chromatogr. 221, 393-398.

Smith, G. A., Schulz, P., Giacomini, K. M., and Blaschke, T. F. (1982) High-pressure liquid chromatographic determination of amitriptyline and its major metabolites in human whole blood. J. Pharm. Sci. 71, 581-583.

Smith, R. C., Vroulis, G., Misra, C. H., Schoolar, J., John, C. D., Korivi, P., Leelavathi, D. E., and Arzu, D. (1980) Receptor techniques in the study of plasma levels of neuroleptics and antidepressant drugs. Commun. Psychopharmacol. 4, 451-465.

Sonsalla, P. K., Jennison, T. A., and Finkle, B. S. (1982a) Quantitative liquid chromatographic technique for the simultaneous assay of tricyclic antidepressant drugs in plasma and serum. Clin. Chem. 28, 457-461.

Sonsalla, P. K., Jennison, T. A., and Finkle, B. S. (1982b) Importance of evaporation conditions and two internal standards for quantitation of amitriptyline and nortriptyline. Clin. Chem. 28, 1401-1402.
Streator, J. J., Eichmeier, L. S., and Caplis, M. E. (1980) Determination of tricyclic antidepressants in serum by high pressure liquid chromatography on a silica column. J. Anal. Toxicol. 4, 58-62.
Suckow, R. F. and Cooper, T. B. (1981) Simultaneous determination of imipramine, desipramine, and their 2-hydroxy metabolites in plasma by ion-pair reversed-phase high-performance liquid chromatography with amperometric detection. J. Pharm. Sci. 70, 257-261.
Suckow, R. F. and Cooper, T. B. (1982) Simultaneous determination of amitriptyline, nortriptyline and their respective isomeric 10-hydroxy metabolites in plasma by liquid chromatography. J. Chromatogr. 230, 391-400.
Suckow, R. F., Cooper, T. B., Quitkin, F. M., and Stewart, J. W. (1982) Determination of mianserin and metabolites in plasma by liquid chromatography with electrochemical detection. J. Pharm. Sci. 71, 889-892.
Sutfin, T. A. and Jusko, W. J. (1979) High-performance liquid chromatographic assay for imipramine, desipramine and their 2-hydroxylated metabolites. J. Pharm. Sci. 68, 703-705.
Syva Inc. (1982) Serum tricyclic antidepressants assay--for use in the quantitative enzyme immunoassay of tricyclic antidepressants in human serum or plasma. Package insert.
Szyszko, E. and Wejman, W. (1981) Gas chromatographic determination of noxyptyline in substance, tablets and in biological material. J. Chromatogr. 219, 291-296.
Tasset, J. J. and Hassan, F. M. (1982) Liquid-chromatographic determination of amoxapine and 8-hydroxyamoxapine in human serum. Clin. Chem. 28, 2154-2157.
Thoma, J. J., Bondo, P. B., and Kozak, C. M. (1979) Tricyclic antidepressants in serum by a Clin. Elut® column extraction and high pressure liquid chromatographic analysis. Ther. Drug Monit. 1, 335-358.
Van Brunt, N. (1983) Application of new technology for the measurement of tricyclic antidepressants using capillary gas chromatography with a fused silica DB5 column and nitrogen phosphorus detec-

tion. Ther. Drug Monit. 5, 11-37.
Vandermark, F. L., Adams, R. F., and Schmidt, G. J. (1978) Liquid-chromatographic procedure for tricyclic drugs and their metabolites in plasma. Clin. Chem. 24, 87-91.
Vink, J. and Van Hal, H. J. M. (1980a) Comparative statistical study of assay methods using mass fragmentography and gas chromatography with nitrogen detection for determination of the tetracyclic antidepressant mianserin in human plasma. J. Chromatogr. 181, 115-119.
Vink, J. and Van Hal, H. J. M. (1980b) Simplified method for determination of the tetracyclic antidepressant mianserin in human plasma using gas chromatography with nitrogen detection. J. Chromatogr. 181, 25-31.
Virtanen, R. (1980) Radioimmunoassay for tricyclic antidepressants. Scand. J. Clin. Invest. 40, 191-197.
Virtanen, R., Salonen, J. S., Scheinin, M., Iisalo, E., and Mattila, V. (1980) Radioimmunoassay for doxepin and desmethyldoxepin. Acta pharmacol. toxicol. 47, 274-278.
Wallace, J. E., Shimek, E. L. Jr., and Harris, S. C. (1981) Determination of tricyclic antidepressants by high-performance liquid chromatography. J. Anal. Toxicol. 5, 20-23.
Watson, I. D. and Stewart, M. J. (1977) Quantitative determination of amitriptyline and nortriptyline in plasma by high-performance liquid chromatography. J. Chromatogr. 132, 155-159.
Weder, H. J. and Bickel, M. H. (1968) Separation and determination of imipramine and its metabolites from biological samples by gas-liquid chromatography. J. Chromatogr. 37, 181-189.
Westenberg, H. G. M., Drenth, B. F. H., De Zeeuw, R. A., De Cuyper, H., Van Praag, H. M., and Korf, J. (1977a) Determination of clomipramine and desmethylclomipramine in plasma by means of liquid chromatography. J. Chromatogr. 142, 725-733.
Westenberg, H. G. M., De Zeeuw, R. A., De Cuyper, H., Van Praag, H. M., and Korf, J. (1977b) Bioanalysis and pharmacokinetics of clomipramine and desmethylclomipramine in man by means of liquid chromatography. Postgrad. Med. J. 53, 124-130.
Westerlund, D. and Erixson, E. (1979) Reversed-phase chromatography of zimelidine and similar dibasic amines. I. Analysis in biological material. J. Chromatogr. 185, 593-603.
Westerlund, D., Nilsson, L., and Jaksch, Y. (1979) Straight-phase ion-pair chromatography of zimeli-

dine and similar divalent amines. J. Liq. Chromatogr. **2**, 373-405.
Whall, T. J. and Dokladalova, J. (1979) High performance liquid chromatographic determination of (Z)- and (E)- doxepin hydrochloride isomers. J. Pharm. Sci. **68**, 1454-1456.
Wong, S. H. Y. and Waugh, S. W. (1983) Determination of the antidepressants maprotiline and amoxapine and their metabolites in plasma by liquid chromatography. Clin. Chem. **29**, 314-318.
Ziegler, V. E., Knesevich, J. W., Wylie, L. T., and Biggs, J. T. (1977) Sampling time, dosage schedule, and nortriptyline plasma levels. Arch. Gen. Psychiatry **34**, 613-615.
Zuleski, F. R., Loh, A., and Di Carlo, F. J. (1977) Assay of human plasma for nortriptyline by radioacetylation and thin-layer chromatography. J. Chromatogr. **132**, 45-49.

14.

ANTIDEPRESSANT PLASMA CONCENTRATIONS AND CLINICAL EFFICACY

S. Montgomery

Introduction

The tricyclic antidepressants were introduced nearly a generation ago and have represented tremendous progress in the relief of suffering of depressed patients. Nevertheless they have well-recognised shortcomings both in terms of safety and acceptability. They are dangerous in overdose and approximately 3% of overdose cases in the U.K. have a fatal outcome. Even in therapeutic doses they are associated with significant cardiotoxicity. Their anticholinergic side effects make them unacceptable to many patients and may compromise compliance with tablet-taking. These disadvantages might be accepted as a regrettable necessity if the antidepressants were effective in a much higher proportion of patients than they in fact are.

Estimates vary as to the proportion of patients who will not respond to pharmacotherapy or whose response will be equivocal, but even the most optimistic reports suggest there will be at least 20% of patients who have a poor response. More reliable studies suggest that the rate of nonresponse lies between 40 and 50%, depending on the number of placebo responders included. In hospital practice it is the common experience that a third of patients have a good response to standard antidepressants, a third have a moderate response, leaving a third of patients with a poor response. There are several different approaches to refining treatment in order to select those patients for whom treatment is appropriate and to improve response ratios. In this chapter the approaches considered are the clinical and the pharmacological.

Briefly, the clinical approach has been to

observe and define the group of patients who apparently and most reliably respond to antidepressant drugs. The broad clinical features such as age, sex, previous psychiatric history, premorbid personality, etc., as well as the carefully observed presenting symptoms of the present episode, are all taken into consideration. Conversely, the group of patients who do not respond to antidepressants are examined in an attempt to find any common characteristics which may be markers of nonresponse. The characteristics which appear to be most reliably associated with better response are the more biological features associated with 'endogenous' depression such as diurnal variation of mood, early morning waking, and retardation. Drug related efficacy is less convincing in the 'non-endogenous' type of depression. It has indeed been difficult to demonstrate efficacy of an antidepressant compared with placebo except in those studies which were conducted on patients suffering from defined 'endogenous' depression.

The pharmacological approach has been to seek the determinants of therapeutic response, or indeed the lack of it, in the pharmacological actions of the drugs, and also in their pharmacokinetic and pharmacodynamic properties.

Clearly, little progress will be made in the investigation of depressive illness if any one approach is adopted without taking account of the information provided by other sources. This is certainly apparent in the extensive literature on the relationship between therapeutic efficacy and drug plasma concentrations of antidepressant drugs.

Interindividual Variability of Drug Plasma Concentrations

It has long been known that patients treated with the same dose of tricyclic antidepressants may achieve widely differing drug plasma concentrations, varying by as much as thirty-fold. This interindividual variability is a phenomenon common to many drugs, not just to antidepressants. The steady-state plasma concentrations of an antidepressant achieved by a patient appears to be a reproducible characteristic providing that external factors are held reasonably constant. The most important factor in determining the levels achieved has been shown to be the rate of clearance and much of the variability seen is genetically determined.

Clinical Significance of Plasma Concentrations

The issue for researchers in depressive illness is not whether there is significant interindividual variability of drug plasma concentrations but whether these varying levels are of clinical significance in determining response. The possibility of patients achieving unexpectedly high plasma concentrations of an antidepressant is of course an important consideration for treatment. Very high plasma concentrations of some antidepressants may be expected to be toxic. For example, a correlation has been shown between cardiotoxicity and plasma concentrations of amitriptyline and nortriptyline. This should encourage the clinician to keep the levels low. Tricyclic antidepressants as a group are dangerous in overdose and therefore must be regarded as toxic at very high plasma levels.

A possible relationship between drug plasma concentrations and therapeutic response is, however, more complex, and there is considerable disagreement in the literature as to what kind of relationship might exist. If a relationship can be demonstrated it might account for some of the anomalies of response seen in the treatment of depressed patients. Even when patients have been carefully selected as potential responders a third or more may have a poor response. If response is more closely related to plasma concentrations achieved than to dose given, it might explain some of the variability of response.

A relationship between plasma concentrations and therapeutic efficacy is of interest for several reasons. The relationship can provide objective confirmation of the therapeutic effect of the pharmacological action of the drug as distinct from a non-specific placebo effect. This is important because some 25% or more of patients with clearly defined depression may respond to random variables such as admission to hospital and the response may be erroneously ascribed to the concurrent pharmacotherapy. A plasma level response relationship should provide important information in determining appropriate dosages, and this is of practical concern when a new antidepressant is being introduced. Early in the development of a potential antidepressant there is little rational means of selecting an appropriate dose, and open dose ranging studies do not adequately answer the problem. A plasma concentration response relationship can provide information on which to base rational decisions as to recommended dosages. It may also be used to indicate where adjustments to therapy might improve the response of individual patients. A relationship may also provide some information on the mechanism of action of the drugs, although it must be remembered that measuring the plasma concentrations is not the same as measuring the activity of the drug at the physiologically significant site of action.

Methodological Issues

Plasma concentration/clinical response relationships have provided a fruitful area of investigation, but not all the findings have been in accord. However, some of the disagreement may be more apparent than real and may be due in large part to methodological differences between the studies. In particular, some of the earlier investigations have not always paid sufficient attention to appropriately stringent methodology, and this must be borne in mind in the interpretation of findings.

Studies are unlikely to demonstrate a relationship between plasma concentrations and response unless they take adequate care with the following factors:

1. Sample size
2. Diagnosis
3. Placebo responders and treatment-resistant depressives
4. Length of study
5. Dosage regime
6. Standardised measures of plasma concentrations
7. Compliance
8. Sensitivity of measures of response

Sample Size. To demonstrate a relationship the drug plasma concentrations achieved by patients should ideally be spread widely across the possible range. In any group studied there may by chance be insufficient numbers of patients developing a particular range of drug plasma concentrations to adequately test a plasma concentration response hypothesis. Large numbers of patients are needed to overcome this problem. It is of course possible that a comparatively small study may by chance have sufficient patients above and below a critical level to produce a significant result. It is also obviously true that testing for the more complex nonlinear relationships requires even larger numbers of patients. A report that no relationship has been demonstrated in a relatively small study probably means simply that insufficient numbers of patients were included to test the hypothesis adequately.

Diagnosis. In the absence of a simple, adequate or even promising biochemical or physiological marker for the presence of depressive illness, it is necessary for researchers in this field to keep close to validated clinical criteria. The word depression is commonly used to indicate anything from minor, transient irritability or the lowering of spirits in the face of setbacks to a profound and persistent melancholia preoccupied with delusions of guilt, ruin and utter despair. In the presence of such a heterogenous variety of states described by the same term, it is of crucial importance that studies of any aspect of depressive illness should use an adequate description of the patients under investigation.

Early attempts to define depression more closely were based entirely on presenting psychopathological features and took no account of the history or other conditions. The Medical Research Council criteria of 1965, requiring a persistent alteration of mood and only one other psychopathological feature, are altogether too thin and unreliable. The Present State Examination (Wing et al., 1974), although based on a standardised interview to assess the signs and symptoms present, fails to distinguish between primary depression and depression secondary to alcohol, drugs, etc.

The operational definitions of the criteria of the St Louis group, usually referred to as the Feighner criteria (Feighner et al., 1972), have been most widely adopted as research criteria for primary affective disorder. They continue to provide possibly the most reliable identification of patients suffering from primary depression in spite of more recent nosological offerings such as the DSM III. These criteria are softer than the Feighner criteria, and it may be possible for patients not suffering from depressive illness still to fulfil the depressive criteria. The Feighner criteria also correlate more closely with the clinician's diagnosis than the DSM III (Angst et al., 1981). This is good evidence of the loss of validity of the DSM III. A further categorisation of patients into the 'endogenous' and other forms of depression is also desirable since this division appears to have treatment implications. Response to antidepressants appears to be associated with the more biological features of 'endogenous' depressive illness. The therapeutic efficacy of antidepressants in patients suffering from other forms of depression, variously termed 'neurotic', 'reactive', or 'non-endogenous', is less convincing. Roth and the Newcastle group created weighted diagnostic scales to differentiate endogenous depression from reactive depression and depression from the anxiety states (Carney et al., 1965; Gurney et al., 1972). These diagnostic scales, used in conjunction with a set of criteria, e.g. those of Feighner et al. which separate primary from secondary depression, provide a sufficiently thorough categorisation of the depressed group studied to allow comparisons with other populations as well defined.

Failure to use careful diagnostic criteria may have the effect of increasing variance which will obscure interesting findings. It is now customary in studies of antidepressant efficacy to investigate patients who fulfil well-defined research diagnostic criteria for depressive illness, but this has not always been the case.

Placebo Responders and Treatment-Resistant Depressives. Even if a study has a large enough number of well-diagnosed depressed patients, a relationship between plasma concentrations and therapeutic response may be obscured by the inclusion of patients who are resistant to antidepressant therapy. An obvious requirement for this kind of study is that the patients be likely to respond to antidepressant therapy, but this is not necessarily easy to fulfil. Clinical differentiation can indicate patients more likely to respond, but even in a homogenous group there will be a significant proportion with a poor response. The inclusion of treatment-resistant depressives is likely to obscure any relationship and is to be avoided if at all possible. There is no secure way of excluding such patients, although careful history-taking can exlude some patients who are clearly nonresponders to pharmacotherapy.

The presence of placebo responders who respond to random variables can also have the effect of obscuring possible relationships. The inclusion of a placebo run in period can weed out some obvious placebo responders and reduce some of the effect of placebo response, although this still remains a possible source of variance.

Length of Study. One of the drawbacks to therapy with all the antidepressants currently available is the delay in the onset of antidepressant action. Some two to three weeks elapse before their antidepressant effect begins to be seen, and a significant difference between an antidepressant and placebo may not be established before the fourth week. It would be unrealistic, therefore, to expect to see a difference in response between different categories of plasma concentrations of an antidepressant in a short study, and negative results from short studies cannot be regarded as conclusive. There is good evidence that a longer trial period is needed before a relationship becomes apparent and that significant differences may not emerge until between the fourth and sixth week. For example, in our studies of amitriptyline a worsening of depression was observed between four and six weeks in patients developing high drug concentrations. The deleterious effects of high plasma concentrations of amitriptyline and nortriptyline would not have been so easily detected in a shorter study.

Dosage Regime. In order to establish that a relationship exists between plasma concentrations and response, a fixed dosage should be used. If it takes four weeks to establish efficacy of an antidepressant against placebo, then changing the dose during that period will add so many extra variables that it will generally be impossible to establish which dose or plasma level would be associated with the response or nonresponse observed. Plasma level results from nonblind dosage adjustments are contaminated further by allowing investigator bias to affect clinical assessment. The most common, but scientifically unsupported, clinical practice of raising the dose in patients who do not show improvement inevitably biasses the results.

Plasma Concentration Determination. We know so little about what it is that makes a particular drug effective that it is unlikely any assumptions about peak drug plasma levels or trough levels are clinically relevant. It is also unclear whether it is the peak level of the drug or its steady-state concentration over time that is of greater importance in mediating the antidepressant effect. It has been assumed because of the delay in antidepressant effect that the steady-state level is the significant factor, and this average level is used as the measure in plasma level response studies. The steady-state level appears to be constant over time although there may be some day-to-day variations.

Most studies take the average level from several weeks of treatment, which evens out minor fluctuations. If the time of sampling is not held constant this could have the effect of producing unaccountable variations in levels. Sampling time must be held constant for all patients on all occasions to avoid fluctuations related to absorption time or metabolism of the drug.

Compliance. Some minor intraindividual fluctuations in plasma concentrations can be accommodated by using the average steady-state concentration as a measure. However, noncompliance with treatment or erratic tablet-taking may lead to greatly fluctuating and spurious results. In a study of plasma concentration/clinical response relationships it is very important to check on compliance as a source of error. The inclusion of outpatients, who are known to have a poorer compliance with treatment, is likely to increase this source of variance, and tablet counts do not seem to overcome the problem.

Measures of Response. The differences to be observed in biological studies are likely to be small, and a relationship between plasma concentrations and response may be obscured by using a blunt measuring instrument. If the improvement in the depression is to be attributed to particular drug plasma concentrations, it is necessary to use the most sensitive and valid measures of the severity of depression. The severity of the depressive illness must be considered quite separately from the diagnosis, and different instruments must be used for measurement. Some of the standard instruments used for rating severity were constructed on a rather ad hoc basis from a collection of items that seemed suitable. Some are contaminated by the inclusion of diagnostic items. Quite often such items are not particularly sensitive to treatment changes and the usefulness of the scales is reduced. Observer-rating scales are more likely to measure differences than self-rating scales, which have a wide interindividual variability of reporting which reduces their sensitivity. They also cannot be used in poorly educated populations, and they often cannot be used in the severely ill patient.

The Montgomery and Asberg Depression Rating Scale (Montgomery and Asberg, 1979) was constructed for depressive illness using sensitivity and accuracy of change estimates as major criteria for inclusion of items. The ten items included were selected from a larger pool as the most sensitive to change in severity. The performance of the scale was tested against the Hamilton Rating Scale as part of its initial testing in treatment studies where both scales were used. The power of the Montgomery and Asberg scale to discriminate response categories was markedly better than the Hamilton Rating Scale. This scale has also been used in studies of plasma concentration/response relationships where its sensitivity has been demonstrated. For example, a relationship between mianserin plasma concentrations and response was shown using the Montgomery and Asberg scale at a higher level of significance than with the Hamilton Rating Scale. In the same study the self-rating scale used, the Beck, was unable to demonstrate this relationship. The Hamilton Rating Scale has until now been the scale most used, although it has disadvantages in loss of sensitivity. A further complication has arisen since several different versions have been produced by different investigators so that it is not always easy to interpret results. Some studies, particularly in the United States, have used versions with extra items, and this is unfortunately not always made clear in the reports.

Plasma Concentration Response Studies
==

Nortriptyline

A review of the plasma level/antidepressant response literature provides an excellent example of the influence of good and poor clinical methodology on the results. Nortriptyline, which is the most easily measured tricyclic, has been the subject of a number of plasma concentration response studies. Six of the studies reported a relationship between plasma nortriptyline concentrations and response, and only three did not demonstrate a relationship. The failure to find a relationship in these studies may, however, be affected by certain weaknesses of methodology.

For example, the study of Lyle and coworkers (Lyle et al., 1974), which did not demonstrate a relationship, did not give a definition of depression and reported no diagnostic criteria. The studies of the Burrows group specifically excluded severe depression and also did not give diagnostic criteria (Burrows et al., 1972, 1974). Three of the studies which did demonstrate a relationship used the Newcastle criteria to define endogenous depression, which probably led to the inclusion of a more homogenous population. There is evidence that plasma concentration response relationships will be best demonstrated in endogenous depression.

There appears to be a consensus that in treating endogenous depression with nortriptyline the best clinical response is associated with steady-state plasma concentrations between approximately 50-175 or 200 µg/l and that a poorer response is seen in patients with concentrations outside this range. The results indicate a self-inhibiting effect of high levels of nortriptyline. In the study of Montgomery et al. (1978) there was no further response after two weeks in the group who developed high concentrations, whereas the group with concentrations within the range 80-200 µg/l continued to improve. Since improvement due either to random variables or to spontaneous remission would have been expected, the result is interesting. Kragh-Sorensen demonstrated the significant clinical advantage of adjusting the dosage of patients to bring their plasma nortriptyline concentrations from above to within the optimum range between the fourth and sixth week of treatment (Kragh-Sorensen et al., 1976).

Amitriptyline

The association of high concentrations of nortriptyline with a poorer response was of particular interest because it is the major active metabolite of amitriptyline, still one of the most commonly used antidepressants. There have been a large number of studies with amitriptyline and results have not all been in agreement, whether the measure is of amitriptyline or nortriptyline alone or amitriptyline plus the metabolite combined.

The majority of studies have demonstrated a significant relationship between therapeutic response and plasma concentrations of amitriptyline plus nortriptyline (Montgomery, 1980). All but one of these have reported either a curvilinear relationship or had findings consistent with the curvilinear hypothesis that optimum antidepressant effect is associated with intermediate plasma concentrations of amitriptyline plus its active metabolite nortriptyline of between approximately 80 and 200 µg/l.

The positive correlation between levels and response reported in some studies does not in itself refute the curvilinear hypothesis. In studies where there were very few patients achieving plasma concentrations in the upper range, a positive correlation might simply be reflecting one side of a curvilinear relationship.

A careful analysis of some of the negative studies indicates that some of the findings may be consistent with the hypothesis that a relationship exists. For example, in the study of Liisberg's group, which was conducted on a rather small number of patients, two of the three patients with high drug concentrations were nonresponders, and this is consistent with the hypothesis that best response is associated with intermediate concentrations (Liisberg et al., 1978). Likewise, in the WHO study high concentrations of nortriptyline were associated with significantly poorer response as measured by percentage change of the Hamilton Rating Scale. The likelihood of detecting a relationship in this study was probably reduced by the inherent weakness of all multicentre studies. They tend to suffer from increased variance introduced by different patient populations and differing rater habits. The centres in the WHO study were in different parts of Europe, and some differences in presenting psychopathology and in rater attitudes would be expected which would increase variance. No quantification of this source of variance is possible in this study as no intercentre rater reliabilities are reported. The WHO study is also open to criticism because of the very low overall response rate achieved. It has been suggested that the response rate of only 35% reported in this study indicates rather poor selection of patients likely to respond to pharmacotherapy. Another large study which did not report a relationship also had a very low response rate, and as far as one can tell this was a group of relatively difficult outpatients suffering from atypical depression who were unlikely to respond to tricyclic antidepressants (Robinson et al., 1979).

A curvilinear relationship between plasma concentrations and response, with best response associated with intermediate levels of amitriptyline plus nortriptyline, has been reported by three separate groups, reviewed by Montgomery (1980), and by a fourth group in 1982 (Breyer-Pfaff et al., 1982). It seems that at least in endogenous depression high concentrations should be avoided.

Drug Plasma Concentrations

Imipramine

The findings from investigations of imipramine show much less agreement than has been reached concerning the association of high levels of nortriptyline and poor response. The discussion has also been complicated by disagreement as to whether the most important factor might be the level of the parent compound, the metabolite desimipramine, or the ratio between them.

An association between higher levels and better response has been reported by three research studies of adequate size (Glassman et al., 1977; Gram et al., 1976; Reisby et al., 1977). Later studies have not, however, confirmed these findings. It seems, therefore, that the association is still open to question.

Methodological flaws make the interpretation of some of the studies on imipramine difficult. Flexible dosages have been used, which confuses the relationship between level and response. In the study of Glassman and Perel, the retrospective exclusion of severely depressed psychotic patients would have the unavoidable effect of biassing the sample. The study of Gram et al. reported that responders fell into the higher concentration category, but there was much overlap and the authors point out that one poor responder with high concentrations responded when the dose was reduced.

More recent studies have not demonstrated an association between high levels and better response. In 1982 a study which used a standard dose reported that previously published plasma concentration categories failed to discriminate responders and nonresponders on all of the measures used except one (Simpson et al., 1982). In another study of 25 patients by our group, there was also no relationship found between good response and high levels (Montgomery et al., 1983).

It seems unlikely that the effect of high concentrations of imipramine on response will be fully explored since there are other reasons for avoiding very high plasma concentrations. There is, for example, the possibility of associated increased subjective side effects and cardiotoxicity, etc. It is not easy to establish a relationship between plasma concentrations of a drug and subjectively experienced side effects because of the variability in patients' tolerance and reporting of unwanted effects. However, a relationship with at least some side effects is likely to exist. It has been shown, for example in depressed patients, that high concentrations of desimipramine are associated with a greater suppression of salivation than are low levels. It has also been shown that cardiotoxicity of some tricyclic antidepressants is related to plasma concentrations in therapeutic doses and in overdose.

Clomipramine

The interpretation of a possible clinical response/plasma concentration relationship is difficult in the presence of active metabolites and particularly so with a drug like clomipramine, whose active metabolite, desmethylclomipramine, has a pharmacological effect different from the parent compound. In arriving at the steady-state plasma concentration, the rate of demethylation cannot be ignored since there is likely to be a time difference between achieving steady state of the parent compound and the metabolite. The study of Montgomery and coworkers in 1980, which investigated the possible relation between levels and response, reported that in a six-week study steady-state plasma concentrations of desmethylclomipramine had still not been reached by some patients. In that study there was no significant relationship between plasma concentrations and response, although there was a trend for high desmethylclomipramine concentrations to be associated with a poorer response (Montgomery et al., 1980). A curvilinear relationship exists between plasma level and response in patients with obsessional neurosis, but this is a difficult finding to interpret in view of the kind of patient studied.

Maprotiline

Maprotiline, although frequently described as a tetracyclic, is a tricyclic antidepressant with a minor structural change. In the early studies there was a hint that high levels could be associated with nonresponse, although the number of patients with high levels was very small. Later systematic studies from several groups have not confirmed the presence of an association between high levels and poor response. Maprotiline is, however, very close in structure to the tricyclics and has some of their disadvantages, particularly risk in overdose. It is therefore prudent to avoid high doses which might lead to unacceptably high plasma concentrations.

Lofepramine

Lofepramine is a tricyclic antidepressant which has recently been introduced into the U.K. Its desmethyl metabolite is desipramine, and studies of the possible relationship between plasma concentration and therapeutic efficacy would therefore be of interest in view of the discordant findings with imipramine. No systematic studies are currently available. The drug has not yet been sufficiently widely used in the U.K. to gain definitive experience of its safety, particularly in overdose, but since it is a tricyclic antidepressant caution is recommended with respect to high plasma concentrations.

Newer Antidepressants

The newer generation of antidepressants has been developed to try to overcome some of the shortcomings and disadvantages of the traditional tricyclic antidepressants. The attempt has been made to increase their safety and reduce their unacceptable side effects, and in many instances they represent an advance. They do not appear to have the narrow therapeutic window seen with the tricyclics. Excessively high concentrations following standard doses do not appear to occur as frequently, and the relevance of plasma monitoring seems less at issue than with the more dangerous tricyclics.

The possibility of a relationship between high concentrations and poor response is of less practical clinical interest but remains of research interest since there is evidence that a relationship exists between response and plasma concentrations with at least some of the newer compounds.

A curvilinear relationship was reported with mianserin by Montgomery et al. in 1978, with best response associated with intermediate levels. Patients with both endogenous and non-endogenous depression as defined by the Newcastle Scales were included in this study, and it appears that the plasma level/response relationship was seen only in the endogenous depression group. In two smaller studies a linear relationship between level of mianserin and response was demonstrated, and these results may be consistent with a curvilinear hypothesis. Coppen's group in 1978 in a study of 17 patients did not find a relationship (reviewed by Montgomery, 1980). The studies on mianserin completed later reveal that there are rather few patients developing high levels. The conclusions from our early study were tentative and based on only six patients developing high levels. From later studies it does not appear that high levels of mianserin are associated with poor response.

The other newer antidepressant where a relationship has been demonstrated is zimelidine, which has subsequently been withdrawn. The finding of a relationship remains of interest, however, since a number of similar 5-HT uptake inhibitors are being introduced. Three of the early studies reported a poor response associated with high plasma concentrations (Montgomery et al., 1981; Walinder et al., 1981; Wood et al., 1982). The study of Montgomery et al. showed as well a relationship between plasma concentrations of norzimelidine and certain gastrointestinal side effects. This type of side effect turned out in other studies to be a common occurrence and was a cause of noncompliance with medication. In retrospect it appears that the recommendation from the early plasma level based research studies to reduce drastically the dose used was correct. It will be interesting to see with the range of new 5-HT uptake inhibitors whether the same sort of phenomena will be observed.

Other second generation antidepressants introduced after the traditional tricyclics include nomifensine and trazodone. A relationship between levels and therapeutic response has not been demonstrated with either of these drugs. Nomifensine is of course very rapidly metabolised and eliminated, and therefore the concept of steady-state plasma concentrations may not be appropriate.

Plasma level monitoring of the newer antidepressants remains a research technique which can shed light on the mechanism of action or on the appropriate dosage in a more reliable way than dose ranging studies. The plasma level investigations of zimelidine gave an early indication of the clinical disadvantage of high plasma levels and of the increased side effects associated with these high levels. They also indicated that very high levels of uptake inhibition offer no extra clinical advantage and may even offer some disadvantage.

Conclusion
==========

The disadvantages of the older antidepressants were primarily related to their toxicity and in some cases to their narrow therapeutic range. The newer

Drug Plasma Concentrations

antidepressants have been selectively tested before they enter the clinic to ensure fewer side effects and less toxicity. It is therefore not surprising that the practical relevance of plasma level monitoring in the clinic is less important with the newer antidepressants. The common clinical practice in Europe, rather than monitoring old toxic antidepressants, is now to use relatively less dangerous drugs with a wider safety margin and a wider range of effective plasma levels.

References

Angst, J., Grigo, H., and Lanz, M. (1981) Classification of depression. Acta psychiat. scand. **63** (Suppl. 290), 23-28.

Breyer-Pfaff, U., Gaertner, H. J., and Giedke, H. (1982) Plasma levels, psychophysiological variables and clinical response to amitriptyline. Psychiatry Res. **6**, 223-234.

Burrows, G. D., Davies, B., and Scoggins, B. A. (1972) Plasma concentrations of nortriptyline and clinical response in depressive illness. Lancet **ii**, 619-623.

Burrows, G. D., Scoggins, B. A., Turecek, L. T., and Davies, B. (1974) Plasma nortriptyline and clinical response. Clin. Pharmacol. Ther. **16**, 639-644.

Carney, M. W. P., Roth, M., and Garside, R. F. (1965) The diagnosis of depressive syndromes and the prediction of ECT response. Brit. J. Psychiatry **3**, 659-674.

DSM III (1979) Diagnostic and Statistical Manual, American Psychiatric Association.

Feighner, J. P., Robins, E., Guze, S. B., Woodruff, R. A., Winokur, G., and Munoz, R. (1972) Diagnostic criteria for use in psychiatric research. Arch. Gen. Psychiatry **26**, 57.

Glassman, S. H., Perel, J. M., Shostak, M., Kantor, S. J., and Fleiss, J. L. (1977) Clinical implication of imipramine plasma levels for depressive illness. Arch. Gen. Psychiatry **34**, 197-204.

Gram, L. F., Reisby, N., Ibsen, I., Nagy, A., Dencker, S. J., Bech, P., Petersen, G. O., and Christiansen, J. C. (1976) Plasma levels of antidepressant effect of imipramine. Clin. Pharmacol. Ther. **19**, 318-324.

Gurney, C., Roth, M., Garside, R. F., Kerr, T. A., and Schapira, K. (1972) Studies in the classification of affective disorder. Brit. J. Psychiatry **121**, 162-166.

Kragh-Sorensen, P., Eggert-Hansen, C., Baastrup, P. C., and Hvidberg, E. F. (1976) Self inhibiting action of nortriptyline's antidepressant effect at high plasma levels. Psychopharmacologia (Berl.) **45**, 305-316.

Liisberg, P., Mose, H., Amdisen, A., Jorgensen, A., and Hopfner-Petersen, H. E. (1978) A clinical trial comparing sustained release amitriptyline and conventional amitriptyline tablets in endogenously depressed patients with simultaneous determination of serum levels of amitriptyline and nortriptyline. Acta psychiat. scand. 57, 426-435.

Lyle, W. H., Brooks, P. W., Early, D. F., Leggett, W. P., Silverman, G., Braithwaite, R. A., Cuthill, J. M., Goulding, R., Pearson, I. B., Smith, R. P., and Strang, G. E. (1974) Plasma concentration of nortriptyline as a guide to therapy. Postgrad. Med. J. 50, 282-287.

Medical Research Council Criteria (1965) Clinical trial of the treatment of depressive illness. Brit. Med. J. 1, 881-886.

Montgomery, S. A. (1980) Measurement of serum drug levels in the assessment of antidepressants. Brit. J. Clin. Pharmacol. 10, 411-416.

Montgomery, S. A. and Asberg, M. (1979) A new depression scale designed to be sensitive to change. Brit. J. Psychiatry 134, 382-389.

Montgomery, S. A., Braithwaite, R., Dawling, S., and McAuley, R. (1978) High plasma nortriptyline levels in the treatment of depression. Clin. Pharmacol. Ther. 32, 309-314.

Montgomery, S. A., McAuley, R., and Montgomery, D. B. (1978) Relationship between mianserin plasma levels and antidepressant effect in a double-blind trial comparing a single night-time and divided daily dose regimens. Brit. J. Clin. Pharmacol. 5, 71S-76S.

Montgomery, S. A., McAuley, R., Montgomery, D. B., Dawling, S., and Braithwaite, R. A. (1980) Plasma concentration of clomipramine and desmethyl clomipramine and clinical response in depressed patients. Postgrad. Med. J. 56 (Suppl. 1), 130-133.

Montgomery, S. A., McAuley, R., Rani, J., Roy, D., and Montgomery, D. B. (1981) A double blind comparison of zimelidine and amitriptyline in endogenous depression. Acta psychiat. scand. 63 (Suppl. 290), 314-327.

Montgomery, S. A., Roy, D., Wynne-Willson, S., Robinson, C., and Montgomery, D. B. (1983) Plasma levels and clinical response with imipramine in a study comparing efficacy with mianserin and nomifensine. Brit. J. Clin. Pharmacol. 15, 205S-211S.

Reisby, N., Gram, L. F., Bech, P., Nagy, A., Petersen, G. O., Ottman, J., Obsen, I., Dencker, S. J., Jacobsen, O., Krautwald, O., Sondergaard, I., and Christiansen, I. (1977) Imipramine. Clinical effects and pharmacokinetic variability. Psychopharmacology **54**, 263-272.

Simpson, G. M., White, K. I., Boyd, J. L., Cooper, T. B., Halaris, G., Wilson, I. C., Raman, E. J., and Ruther, E. (1982) Relationship between plasma antidepressant levels and clinical outcome for inpatients receiving imipramine. Am. J. Psychiatry **139**, 358-360.

Robinson, D. S., Cooper, T. B., Ravaris, C., Ives, J. O., Nies, A., Bartlett, D., and Lambourn, K. R. (1979) Plasma tricyclic drug levels in amitriptyline treated depressed patients. Psychopharmacology **63**, 223-231.

Walinder, J., Carlsson, A., and Persson, R. (1981) 5-HT Reuptake inhibitors plus tryptophan in endogenous depression. Acta psychiat. scand. **63** (Suppl. 290), 179-190.

Wing, J. K., Cooper, J. E., and Sartorius, N. (1974) The Measurement and Classification of Psychiatric Symptoms: An Instruction Manual for the PSE and Catego Program. Cambridge University Press.

Wood, K. M., Swade, C. C., and Coppen, A. J. (1982) Zimelidine: a pharmacokinetic and pharmacodynamic study in depressive illness. Brit. J. Clin. Practice, Suppl. 19, 42-47.

15.

CHILDHOOD DEPRESSION

D. R. Offord and R. T. Joffe

Introduction

Symptoms of unhappiness or sadness have been reported as occurring in children for over a century (Kashani et al., 1981). However, the concept of depression as a syndrome where the dysphoric mood occurs regularly with a number of other symptoms indicating affective, motivational, and cognitive changes as well as vegetative and psychomotor disturbances has not been accepted so readily (Cantwell and Carlson, 1980; Costello, 1980; Lefkowitz, 1980; Lefkowitz and Burton, 1978). The most frequent views up until the last decade were that either depressive disorder did not occur in childhood or that if it did occur, the clinical picture did not resemble that of adult depressive disorder (Cantwell and Carlson, 1980). More recently, there has been increasing acceptance that the syndrome of childhood depression exists and that the clinical picture is similar to that of adult depressive disorder (Cantwell and Carlson, 1980).

This chapter reviews critically the literature on the syndrome of childhood or prepubertal depression. When the term 'childhood depression' is used in the chapter, it refers to a syndrome rather than to individual symptoms. No distinction is made between syndrome and disorder. That is, the term 'disorder' is not considered to indicate evidence of the validity of a syndrome (Cantwell and Carlson, 1980). The following topics are covered: diagnosis and classification, instrumentation, associated disorders, epidemiology, etiologic factors, natural history, and treatment approaches.

Childhood Depression

Diagnosis and Classification

Diagnostic Criteria

Many authors have outlined their criteria for the diagnosis of childhood depression. The items used in operationalizing the criteria of these various investigators have been listed and summarized (Kovacs and Beck, 1977; Cytryn et al., 1980). The most commonly used criteria for depression, derived from the study of children, appear to be those developed by Weinberg and his associates (Weinberg et al., 1973) and modified by Petti (Petti, 1978), Cytryn and McKnew (Cytryn and McKnew, 1972), and Kovacs and Beck (Kovacs and Beck, 1977). The Weinberg criteria arose from those proposed for adults by Feighner and his associates (Feighner et al., 1972). Cytryn and McKnew developed their criteria from the intensive study of children referred to the inpatient unit of the Children's Hospital of the District of Columbia. The items used by Kovacs and Beck are a modification of the adult Beck Depression Inventory (BDI) (Beck, 1972) and are termed the Childhood Depression Inventory (CDI) (Beck and Kovacs, 1977).

Table 15.1 lists the DSM III criteria (American Psychiatric Association, 1980) for major depressive disorder and shows the extent to which the items used by Weinberg, Cytryn and McKnew, and Beck and Kovacs to fulfill their criteria also are appropriate to the DSM III criteria. It is clear that the three sets of diagnostic criteria are similar. It is evident also that the items employed in these three sets of criteria overlap considerably with each other and with the items associated with the DSM III criteria for major depressive disorder (American Psychiatric Association, 1980; Cytryn et al., 1980). Because of the similarity between the DSM III criteria for depressive disorder and those employed to arrive at a diagnosis of childhood depression, there has been a recognition that the child and adult criteria for affective disorder are closely similar (Cytryn et al., 1980). Indeed, there has been an increasing acceptance of DSM III as a reasonable classification system for depression in children (Cytryn et al., 1980). However, the extent to which the DSM III criteria for affective disorder identify a valid syndrome in childhood is not known. The one essential criterion for the establishment of the validity (accuracy) of this diag-

Table 15.1: A comparison of items of three diagnostic criteria for childhood depression with DSM III criteria for major depressive disorder

DSM III Criteria	Weinberg Criteria	Cytryn & McKnew	CDI
A Mood			
Dysphoric	+	+	
Sad	+	+	+
Hopeless	+	+	+
Irritable	+		+
B (1) Poor appetite	+	+	+
(2) Sleep disturbance	+	+	+
(3) (a) Psychomotor Retardation	+	+	+
(b) Psychomotor Agitation	+	+	+
(4) Loss of interest or pleasure	+	+	+
(5) Loss of energy	+		+
(6) Feelings of guilt	+		+
(7) Diminished concentration	+	+	+
(8) Suicidal thoughts	+	+	+

nostic category is that it must be shown to differ on some variable or variables other than the symptoms which define it (Rutter, 1978). These variables could include ones associated with etiology, course, response to treatment, or some other aspect of the disorder. It will be seen in this chapter that the needed data in these areas are almost nonexistent. Thus it is reasonable for investigators at this time to employ various diagnostic criteria for depression with the same groups of children in an effort to determine both the extent of congruity among the diagnostic systems and to provide the background against which the diagnostic validity of these various criteria can be tested. As mentioned previously, there is increasing acceptance that the DSM III criteria for adult depression are appropriate for children, and certainly these criteria should be one of the sets employed in any study aiming to establish the validity of the diagnosis of childhood depression.

Classification

Table 15.2 presents various classification systems for childhood depression. It can be seen that the organizational principles underlying the systems vary and include developmental stage, symptomatology, treatment needs, etiology, severity, and empirical analysis of data. Masked depression is a subtype in several of the classifications. This concept implies that the child's depression is covered up or masked by other symptoms and thus the child rarely experiences the depressive feelings directly. The child is thought to be depressed because of the depressive themes in fantasies, dreams, and through responses to projective tests (Kovacs and Beck, 1977). The variety of symptoms implicated in the concept of masked depression includes almost the full gamut of childhood psychopathology (Kovacs and Beck, 1977). There is increasing evidence in the majority of cases of masked depression that the depressive symptomatology can be elicited if it is asked about in a systematic way, and thus the mask, if present, is thin and should be viewed primarily as representing presenting complaints (Carlson and Cantwell, 1980).

Glaser's classification (Glaser, 1967, 1968) centers on the concept of masked depression and sees the symptomatology of the 'mask' as different depending on the developmental level of the child. In the infant and young child the depression can

Table 15.2: Classification of childhood depression

Author	Organizational Principles	Subtypes
Glaser, 1967, 1968	Developmental stage	1. Masked presenting as developmental retardation in infants and preschoolers 2. Masked presenting as behaviour problems, psychoneurosis or psychophysiologic reactions
Frommer, 1968	Symptomatology; treatment needs	1. Enuretic or encopretic 2. Uncomplicated 3. Phobic or anxiety states
Malmquist, 1971	Developmental stage; symptomatology; etiology	1. Organic disease 2. Deprivation syndrome 3. Difficulties in individuation 4. Latency age 5. Adolescent
Cytryn and McKnew, 1972	Etiology; severity	1. Masked 2. Acute 3. Chronic
McConville et al., 1973	Empirical analysis of data	1. Affectual 2. Negative self-esteem 3. Guilt

Table 15.2 (cont'd)

Author	Organizational Principles	Subtypes
Lucas, 1977	Developmental stage symptomatology; etiology	1. Deprivation syndrome 2. Organic disease 3. Reactive 4. Masked 5. Endogenous unipolar 6. Endogenous bipolar
Chambers et al., 1982	History	1. Endogenous 2. Nonendogenous

present as developmental retardation; in the adolescent it can present itself in a variety of ways, including behaviour problems, psychoneuroses, or psychophysiologic reactions. Frommer (1968) grouped into three categories 264 youngsters ages 3 to 16 whom she felt were depressed: (1) enuretic or encopretic depressives where the most common symptoms were moodiness, weepiness, and immaturity and the disorder was longstanding; (2) uncomplicated depression characterized by irritability, weepiness, and a tendency to temper outbursts; and (3) depressive phobic anxiety state where the children suffered from weepiness, tension, and irritability but where they were less moody and more apathetic than in the other two groups.

Malmquist's classification (Malmquist, 1971) is based on developmental stage, symptomatology, and etiology, and he defines five subtypes as outlined in Table 15.2. Cytryn and McKnew (1972) used both the parameters of etiology and severity in arriving at their classification of childhood depression. The first category, masked depressive reaction of childhood, is characterized by a chronic history of acting out aggressive behaviour in families with severe psychopathology. The depression becomes manifest through fantasies and projective tests and through verbal productions in the interview situation. It appears that if inquiries were made about depression, the mask disappeared. The second subtype was termed acute depressive reaction of childhood. Here the child's depressive symptomatology was directly experienced and expressed in patients with good premorbid history and was secondary to traumatic events such as the loss of a parenting figure. The third and last category, chronic depressive reaction of childhood, was characterized by the presence of chronic depressed mood and suicidal ideation in families where one parent was depressed and the child had experienced multiple separations.

McConville and his associates (1973) proposed their subtypes based on data gathered by staff in an inpatient unit. Information was collected on 75 children ages 6 to 13 where depression was seen as a target symptom. The items recorded on these children clustered into three subtypes. The affectual depression group expressed sadness, helplessness, and hopelessness; the negative self-esteem depression group included children who had fixed ideas of negative self-esteem including worthlessness and being unloved; and the guilt depression group felt

537

that they were wicked and should be dead or killed. The first group was most common in children 6 to 8 years old; the second was more frequent after age 8 through to age 11; and the third was rare and occurred usually after the age of 11.

Lucas (1977) attempted to integrate elements of several classification systems and proposed six subcategories. It can be seen from Table 15.2 that he included categories, such as reactive, endogenous unipolar and bipolar, which have usually been associated with adult depressive disorder.

Lastly, Chambers et al. (1982) classified 58 prepubertal children into endogenous and nonendogenous subtypes of depression based on Research Diagnostic Criteria (Spitzer et al., 1981). All types of hallucinations were more common in the endogenous than in the nonendogenous group. For instance, 14 of 29 children in the endogenous subtype reported auditory hallucinations, while this occurred in 7 of 29 in the nonendogenous group. All of the children were seen in a child psychiatric clinic specializing in depression and thus the role of selection factors was probably particularly important in this sample.

It is evident that the classification of childhood depression is in its infancy. This is not surprising since the diagnostic validity of the general entity has not been firmly established. None of the subtypes of childhood depression arising from these classificatory systems has been shown to have adequate validity (Rutter, 1978). Two steps will be needed to accomplish this task. First, the validity of the general syndrome will have to be established; and second, a particular subtype within the general syndrome will have to be shown to differ reliably from the rest of the children within the syndrome in ways other than its presenting symptoms. These can include etiology, course or response to treatment. The end result is that currently any sub-categorization of childhood depression should be viewed as preliminary and in need of further investigation.

Instrumentation
================

Table 15.3 provides a list of instruments which have been used in the study of childhood depression (Orvashel et al., 1980; Kazdin, 1981). The majority have been employed to assess the severity of depression rather than its presence or absence, but of course various cut-off points can and have been used to indicate the presence or absence of depression

Table 15.3: Instruments used to assess childhood depression*

---

1. Self-Reports

    - Children's Depression Inventory (CDI)
    - Short Children's Depression Inventory (SCDI)
    - Children's Depression Scale (CDS)

2. Interviews

    - Interview Schedule for Children (ISC)
    - Bellevue Index of Depression (BID)
    - Children's Depression Rating Scale (CDRS)
    - Children's Affective Rating Scale (CARS)
    - Diagnostic Interview for Children and Adolescents (DICA)
    - NIMH Interview
    - Kiddie-SADS (K-SADS)

3. Projective Techniques

4. Peer Ratings

    - Peer Nomination Inventory for Depression (PNID)

---

*Based primarily on Kazdin, 1981

(Kazdin, 1981).
   The first category listed in Table 15.3 is self-report measures. The most widely used is the Children's Depression Inventory (CDI) (Kovacs and Beck, 1977) which is an adaptation of the adult Beck Depression Inventory (BDI) (Beck, 1972). The instrument consists of 27 items with each item having a three-point response scale. Based on administration to clinical and normative samples, ages 7 to 17, cut-off scores have been obtained for the presence or absence of depression and for degrees of severity of depression (Carlson and Cantwell, 1980). Preliminary data are available on internal consistency and construct validity (Kovacs et al., 1977; Carlson and Cantwell, 1980; Kazdin, 1981). The Short Children's Depression Inventory (SCDI) (Carlson and Cantwell, 1979, 1980) is a modification of the short form of the BDI and is administered to children ages 7 to 17. It contains 13 items with

each item scored on a four-point scale. The only psychometric property reported is beginning data on construct validity where children who scored > 8 were more likely to be clinically diagnosed as primary affective disorder using DSM III criteria (Kazdin, 1981). The last self-report scale is the Children's Depression Scale (Lang and Tisher, 1978) designed for children 9 to 16. This scale consists of 66 items of which 48 focus on depressive symptoms and 18 on positive experiences. Each item is rated on a five-point scale and versions of the instrument suitable for parents and siblings in addition to children are available. Internal consistency has been reported to be high, and there is evidence that scores on the CDS can distinguish depressed children from both other clinical samples of children and normal children.

The second category of instruments in Table 15.3 is interviews. Here the respondent, usually the child, answers questions and the rater, most often a clinician, is able to employ follow-up clarification queries. This of course is not possible with checklist data.

The Interview Schedule for Children (ISC) focuses on children 8 to 13 (Kovacs and Beck, 1977). Data are gathered from the child about depression and associated characteristics such as aggression and hyperactivity. Beginning data on construct validity indicate a 'moderate' correlation beetween ratings of depression based on the interview and scores on CDI (Kazdin, 1981).

The Bellevue Index of Depression (BID) (Pettie, 1978) collects data through interviews with the child, parent or other. The forty items in the scoring system are based on the earlier Weinberg criteria for childhood depression (Ling et al., 1970; Weinberg et al., 1973) and were developed for children ages 6 to 12. Each problem is rated on both severity and duration, and both parameters are used in judging whether or not an item is present. Agreement between independent raters using the diagnostic scale is over 80% (Pettie, 1978).

The Children's Depression Rating Scale (CDRS) (Poznanski et al., 1979) follows a similar format to the Hamilton Rating Scale for adults. The scale was developed in a children's inpatient setting and the 15 items were scored after interviews with the child and others such as the parents and nursing staff. High correlations in the range of 0.90 were obtained between the total item scores and the global ratings of depression by two psychiatrists. A recent revision of the scale, the CDRS-R (Poznanski et al., 1984), has a total of 17 items and a revised scoring system. Again, the correlation of the CDRS-R with a global rating of depression was high ($r = 0.87$), as was the interrater reliability ($r = 0.86$) and the test-retest reliability over a four-week period ($r = 0.81$).

The Children's Affective Rating Scale (CARS) (McKnew and Cytryn, 1979; McKnew et al., 1979) consists of three subscales which address depressive mood and behaviour, verbal experience, and fantasy. Each subscale is scored from 0 to 10 after interviewing the child. Beginning data on construct validity indicate that the scores on the CARS correlate positively with the diagnosis of depression using the Weinberg criteria. Interobserver agreement among judges scoring the interview has ranged between $r = 0.79$ to 0.95.

The Diagnostic Interview for Children and Adolescents (DICA) (Herjanic and Campbell, 1977) is a structured interview administered to the child and to the parents. It covers a wide range of diagnostic categories, including depression, and is tied closely to DSM III (American Psychiatric Association, 1980). Thus the diagnostic orientation is a categorical one and psychiatric symptomatology is assessed during the child's lifetime. Each interview takes between one and one and a half hours, and the instrument is suitable for children ages 9 to 17. Some pretesting has occurred, particularly with regard to the reliability and correspondence of diagnoses according to source of information, that is, parent and child (Reich et al., 1982). The interrater reliability for individual symptoms was high with two raters agreeing 85% of the time. In addition, the interview was able to distinguish samples of psychiatrically disturbed and non-disturbed children (Herjanic and Campbell, 1977).

The NIMH interview is a modification of the DICA and is now called the DISC. Extensive pilot work on the test-retest reliability and construct validity and the performance of lay compared to clinical interviewers has recently been completed (Costello, 1984).

The last of the interviews to be mentioned is the Kiddie-SADS. It is modelled after the Schedule for Affective Disorder and Schizophrenia (SADS) for adults developed by Spitzer and Endicott (1978). Like the DICA, it is a structured psychiatric interview with a categorical orientation and is designed primarily as a diagnostic instrument for children between the ages of 6 to 17. It is administered directly to children or to parents about their children. The interview lasts between forty-five minutes to one hour and a half and requires a trained interviewer. The first version (K-SADS-P) (Puig-Antich et al., 1978) focused on the current psychiatric state of children and adolescents, while a later version (K-SADS-E) (Puig-Antich et al., 1978), for use in epidemiological surveys, is designed to identify both past and current episodes of psychopathology. Both versions gather data on ten disorders included in DSM III, but the interview is particularly detailed in covering depression and its subtypes. Preliminary testing of the SADS-P found excellent interrater reliability for the major diagnostic syndromes and it ranged from 0.65 to 0.96 for individual symptoms (Orvashel et al., 1980). Sensitivity to change on repeated measures before and after imipramine treatment has been demonstrated (Orvashel et al., 1980). In addition, there is evidence that the K-SADS-E does diagnose as depressed children who a year earlier (on average) had been diagnosed as depressed according to the K-SADS-P. The testing to date of the psychometric properties of these two instruments has been based on small samples, usually under 20 children.

Projective techniques have been used to gauge the extent of underlying depressive fantasy in cases where overt manifestations of depression are not evident (Kazdin, 1981). Several investigators (Cytryn and McKnew, 1972, 1974; Polvan and Cebiroglu, 1972; Rapoport, 1976) have used various projective tests in this way, but only one (Rapoport, 1976) reported psychometric properties of the procedure. Here, interrater reliability ratings were high ($r = 0.94$).

The last type of instrument used to assess childhood depression is that based on peer ratings. The Peer Nomination Inventory for Depression (PNID) (Lefkowitz and Tesing, 1980) requires that children rate their peers on questions aimed at characterizing depression in childhood. Each child ends up with a score on depression which is a sum of the ratings he or she has received across all questions. A good deal of work on the psychometric properties of this instrument has been completed (Lefkowitz and Tesing, 1980). This includes measures of internal consistency (item-total correlations varied between 0.34 and 0.71), test-retest ($r = 0.79$), and interrater agreement (alpha = 0.75). Some of the validation data, however, are not encouraging. For example, the correlation between the peer ratings of the PNID and the self-report ratings on CDI were weak (r = 0.23). It did predict, nevertheless, other facets of the child's adjustment such as performance at school, self-concept, teacher ratings of work skills, and social behaviour.

In summary, the development of instruments for the identification and measurement of childhood depression is in its preliminary stages. It is clear that a distinction must be made between instruments that are to be used in large scale community surveys and those that are to be employed to measure degrees of severity or changes among patients already diagnosed as depressed. In the former, the goal is to identify efficiently and accurately children with a valid syndrome of childhood depression. A more limited goal for such an instrument might be to identify children, some of whom on a second-stage procedure, will be diagnosed as depressed. In this case, the specificity of the screening instrument must be high; that is, there cannot be many false negatives while false positives can be tolerated more easily. On the other hand, an instrument to be employed with cases already diagnosed will have to be especially sensitive to detecting clinically important changes in severity such as would be expected during treatment studies.

Regardless of the type of instrument, the issue of the sources of data to be tapped must be considered. There is evidence, for instance, that parents and teachers identify almost completely separate groups of children who are eventually seen as being disturbed by clinicians (Gould et al., 1981). Certainly more than one source should be employed. Parents, teachers, and the children themselves and, in a clinical setting, the appropriate staff are all potential respondents. Work needs to be done to determine which combination of sources at which ages of children and for what kinds of instruments provide data which allow a valid diagnosis of childhood depression to be made.

Studies on the psychometric properties of the existing instruments are scarce and of uneven quality. The samples used in such studies are usually small and the selection factors are not well understood. The reliability data are usually presented in terms of percentage of agreement instead of a kappa statistic (Cohen, 1960) which takes into account agreement due to chance. Since there is no 'gold' standard, criterion validity is not possible and one is left with establishing construct validity for any instrument. This will involve showing that the instrument behaves in hypothesized ways with a variety of samples of children along many predicted dimensions.

At present, none of the self-report measures has sufficiently developed psychometric properties to justify its use in either epidemiologic or clinic work. The most promising interview is clearly the NIMH one on which extensive pilot work has recently been completed centering primarily on reliability and validity. Other issues with this instrument will include its ability to measure clinically important changes in depressed children and its cost if it is to be employed in large community surveys. The extent to which checklist data, which obviously can be more efficiently obtained, can substitute for interview data is a question of utmost importance in epidemiological work.

Associated Disorders
====================

Children who have received a diagnosis of childhood depression appear to have, in a significant proportion of cases, other psychiatric diagnoses. These have included hyperactivity, conduct disorder, anxiety states, and other forms of depression.

One study (Brumback and Warren, 1977), for instance, noted that of 223 children, representing three cohorts of consecutively referred children to an educational diagnostic center, 136 (61%) were diagnosed as depressed according to the Weinberg criteria. Of these 136, 86 (63%) were also diagnosed as hyperactive based on Stewart's criteria (Stewart, 1970). The sources of data on which these diagnoses were based were parent and teacher self-administered questionnaires and clinical assessment of the children. The depressed children who were also hyperactive were either chronically hyperactive or had episodes of hyperactivity which worsened or occurred only during periods of depression. In the latter cases, hyperactivity decreased with resolution of the depression. In two similar studies (Weinberg et al., 1973; Staton and Brumback, 1981) depressed children were also diagnosed as hyperactive in a sizeable proportion of cases, the percentages being 48 and 55 respectively.

A recent report (Puig-Antich, 1982) focused on the relationship between prepubertal depression and conduct disorder. Forty-three latency-aged boys were a consecutive sample accepted for treatment of major depression in the Child Depression Clinic at New York State Psychiatric Institute. Their diagnosis of major depression was based on the K-SADS and the K-SADS-P (Chambers et al., 1978; Puig-Antich et al., 1979; Hirsch et al., 1980). Sixteen (37%) of the 43 were also found to have a diagnosis of conduct disorder. Thirteen of these 16 responded to antidepressant medication and in 11 of the 13, the full antidepressant response was associated with no evidence of conduct disorder.

It is clear that not only does the full-blown diagnosis of childhood depression overlap considerably with both hyperactivity and conduct disorder, but that part of the depressive symptomatology, that is, individual symptoms, occur in certainly a third and perhaps in the majority of children with conduct disorder and hyperactivity (Carlson and Cantwell, 1980).

Anxiety disorders (separation anxiety, overanxious, avoidant or phobic disorder) according to DSM III criteria (American Psychiatric Association, 1980) also are found in a significant percentage of depressed children. For instance, it has been reported, in a study utilizing DSM III criteria (American Psychiatric Association, 1980) and gathering data from self-administered parent and child checklists and a semi-structured child psychiatric interview (ISC) (Kovacs and Beck, 1977), that 14 of 42 children with major depression disorder were also diagnosed as having anxiety disorder, and 10 of 28 with dysthymic disorder and 3 of 11 with adjustment disorder with depressed mood also received a diagnosis of anxiety disorder. This same article provides evidence of the overlap among the DSM III diagnoses of depression. For instance, 16 of 42 children with major depressive disorder also had dysthymic disorder and, conversely, 16 of 28 children with dysthymic disorder were also diagnosed as having major depressive disorder. This study makes it clear that children referred to a psychiatric out-patient clinic who received a diagnosis of some form of depression according to DSM III criteria (American Psychiatric Association, 1980) also tended strongly to receive other DSM III diagnoses. The percentages of children with adjustment disorder with depressed mood, major depressive disorder, and dysthymic disorder receiving other diagnoses were 45, 79, and 93 respectively.

One additional finding deserves mention (Hughes, 1984). It focuses on a report on 23 children who presented with the major complaint of recurrent abdominal pain for which no organic cause could be determined. These patients represented 15% of the consecutive referrals over a six-month period to a psychiatric consultation liaison service in a children's hospital. All of these 23 children met the DSM III diagnostic criteria for major depressive disorder.

The findings with regard to depression and overlapping psychiatric disorders are similar to those found with conduct disorder (Offord and Waters, 1983). It may be that once individual childhood psychiatric disorders are defined in a mutually exclusive manner, a child with any psychiatric diagnosis will have only one diagnosis in a minority of instances. In the case of childhood depression, it will be important to learn the frequency and type of associated disorders in an unselected comunity sample. The data thus far are based on various clinic samples where generalization even to other clinic samples is dangerous. Further, it is necessary to determine whether childhood depressive illnesses, with and without overlapping psychiatric disorders, are valid subtypes of prepubertal depressive disorder with unique characteristics in terms of etiology, family history, natural history, and especially response to treatment.

Epidemiology

Tables 15.4 and 15.5 list prevalence studies of childhood depression. The investigations tabulated in Table 15.4 took place in various clinical settings. These settings, the sources of data, the instrumentation and the diagnostic criteria were seldom comparable in different studies and thus it is not surprising that the prevalence rates for depression vary widely from a low of 7% in a pediatric inpatient population (Kashani et al., 1981) to a high of 59% in a children's psychiatric inpatient unit (Petti, 1978).

As Table 15.5 notes, there are only six surveys of childhood depression carried out on non-clinic populations. In three of them (Albert and Beck, 1975; Kashani and Simonds, 1979; Leon et al., 1981) the samples were small and the factors affecting sample selection were unknown. In one of these (Albert and Beck, 1975) adolescents were included and the only source of data was children's self-reports. In another (Leon et al., 1980) only

Table 15.4: Prevalence studies of childhood depression in clinic populations

AUTHORS	SETTING	AGE AND SEX OF SAMPLE	SOURCES OF DATA	DIAGNOSTIC CRITERIA	RESULTS
Bauersfeld, 1972	School psychiatric centre	Most between 8-13 years; no sex breakdown	Parents, children and teachers	Unspecified	307 (14%) of 2238 with depressed mood or other depressive conditions
Cebiroglu et al., 1972	University department of child psychiatry	3-16 years; no sex breakdown	Unspecified	Unspecified	85 (0.8%) of 10,661 with depression
Meierhofer, 1972	Residential nurseries	0-6 years; no sex breakdown	Unspecified	Unspecified	25% of more than 50 children with depressive states
Weinberg et al., 1973; Brumbach et al., 1977	Eduational diagnostic centre	6.5-12.7 years; 50 boys, 22 girls	Parents and children	Weinberg criteria	42 (58%) of 72 depressed
Pearce, 1978	Hospital department of child psychiatry	3-17 years; no sex breakdown	Unspecified	Symptom of morbid depression	126 (23%) of 547 depressed

Table 15.4 (cont'd)

AUTHORS	SETTING	AGE AND SEX OF SAMPLE	SOURCES OF DATA	DIAGNOSTIC CRITERIA	RESULTS
Petti, 1978	Children's psychiatric inpatient unit	6-12.5 years no sex breakdown	Parents, children, teachers, and inpatient personnel	BID	43 (59%) of 73 depressed
Carlson and Cantwell, 1979; Carlson and Cantwell, 1980	Children's psychiatric inpatient unit; psychiatric outpatient clinic	12 ± 2.9 years; 62 boys, 40 girls	Parents and children	DSM III, SCDI	28 (27%) of 102 with depressive disorder (DSM III); 50 (49%) of 102 depressed
Kashani et al., 1981	Pediatric inpatient unit	7-12 years; 56 boys, 44 girls	Parents and children	DSM III, BID	7 (7%) of 100 with depressive disorder (DSM III); 9 (9%) of 100 depressive (BID)
Kashani et al., 1982	Children's psychiatric inpatient unit	9-12 years 75 boys, 25 girls	Parents, children and inpatient personnel	DSM III	13 (13%) of 100 with major depressive disorder
Kashani et al., 1982	Surgical hospital	7-12 years; 48 boys, 52 girls	Parents and children	DSM III	23 (23%) of 100 with major depressive disorder

Table 15.4 (cont'd)

AUTHORS	SETTING	AGE AND SEX OF SAMPLE	SOURCES OF DATA	DIAGNOSTIC CRITERIA	RESULTS
Poznanski et al., 1983	Children's psychiatric inpatient unit	8-12 years 24 boys, 6 girls	Children	Global clinical assessment (no criteria given); CDRS	9 (30%) of 30 depressed on clinical assessment; 13 (43%) of 30 depressed (CDRS)

Table 15.5: Prevalence studies of childhood depression in non-clinic samples

AUTHORS	SETTING	AGE AND SEX OF SAMPLE	SOURCES OF DATA	DIAGNOSTIC CRITERIA	RESULTS
Rutter et al., 1970	Isle of Wight	10 and 11 years; exact sex breakdown unavailable	Parents, children and teachers	Not given	3 (0.1%) of 2199 with depression
Albert and Beck, 1975	Parochial suburban school (7th and 8th grades)	11.2–15.1 years; 36 boys, 27 girls	Children	CDI	21 (33%) of 63 with depression
Kashani and Simonds, 1978	Family practice clinic; children born at a university hospital	7–12 years; 51 boys, 52 girls	Parents and children	DSM III	2 (2%) of 103 with major depressive disorder; 18 (17%) of 103 with sadness
Leon et al., 1980	Suburban elementary school (3rd to 6th grade)	Age not given; 73 boys, 65 girls	Parents	Depression Scale of the Personality Inventory for Children	21 (15%) of 138 with depression

Table 15.5 (cont'd)

AUTHORS	SETTING	AGE AND SEX OF SAMPLE	SOURCES OF DATA	DIAGNOSTIC CRITERIA	RESULTS
Kashani et al., 1983	Children born at one hospital, Dunedin, New Zealand	9 years; sex breakdown unavailable	Parents, children and teachers	DSM III for major depressive disorder; RDC for minor depressive disorder	Point prevalence rate: major depressive disorder 1.8%; minor depressive disorder 2.5%

parental checklist data were used to make a diagnosis of depression. In the third (Kashani and Simonds, 1979) data were collected from interviews with parents and children but the nature and structure of the interviews were not specified.
The Isle of Wight Study (Rutter et al., 1970) was a landmark work in child epidemiology but it did not focus on depression. Clear diagnostic criteria for depression were not employed and the diagnostic system used excluded the possibility of making a diagnosis of depression in children with conduct disorder.
The most recent study (Kashani et al., 1983) is the best. The authors used a two-stage sampling procedure on an initial group of 955 nine-year-olds. Data collection in the first stage consisted of parent and child checklist information. The second stage was carried out on those identified by the first stage as possibly depressed and on a random sample of non-identified children. The second stage was composed of a structured interview (K-SADS-E) (Puig-Antich et al., 1980) administered to the children. The diagnosis of major depressive disorder was based on DSM III criteria and of minor depressive disorder on RDC criteria. All information collected from parents, teachers, and the children themselves was available to the psychiatrists making the diagnosis. The point prevalence rates for major depressive disorder and minor depressive disorder were 1.8% and 2.5% respectively. In the case of past depressive disorder, the prevalences of major and minor episodes were 1.1% and 9.7% respectively. Depressed children compared to others were reported by their parents, but not by their teachers, as having more behaviour problems. They also had been referred more often for assessment or treatment of behaviour or emotional problems and had more negative self-perceptions of their academic ability. There was no association between socioeconomic class, cognitive or motor development, and depression.
The epidemiological studies, limited as they are, suggest that in a non-clinic sample, major depressive disorder among prepubertal children is rare. However, children in larger numbers do express part of the full depressive syndrome such as misery and unhappiness. For instance, in the Isle of Wight study (Rutter et al., 1970, p. 192) approximately 25% of the children with neurotic disorder or conduct disorder were described by their parents as exhibiting this symptom. In addition, in the

careful study by Kashani and his associates (1983) almost 10% of the children had in the past fulfilled the RDC criteria for minor depressive disorder. Clearly, investigations are needed not only of children with the full depressive syndrome but of those with some of the symptoms of major depressive disorder.

Etiologic Factors

It is generally acknowledged that integration of biological and psychosocial perspectives are necessary in the research and treatment of psychiatric disorders (Lewis and Lewis, 1981). Affective disorders in adults have served as a model of such a psychobiological approach (Akiskal and McKinney, 1973) which has lead to a richer understanding and more sophisticated treatment of these disorders.

Although psychologic and biologic factors are considered separately, it is likely that they interact in a complex manner in the multifactorial etiology of childhood affective illness.

Biologic Factors

The investigation of biological correlates of childhood depression has been hampered, initially by the longstanding controversy over the existence of the disorder (Rie, 19966) and, more recently, by the poor definition of the limits of the concept of childhood depressive illness (Glaser, 1967; Toolan, 1962). As noted earlier in this chapter, it is now generally accepted that clinical manifestations of childhood depression are analogous to those in adults (Weinberg et al., 1973; Cytryn et al., 1980). Furthermore, standardized operational criteria for childhood affective illness, similar to those for adults, have been provided by DSM III (American Psychiatric Association, 1980). These developments have facilitated research into the biological correlates of major depression in childhood.

There are several reasons why the study and identification of biological correlates of childhood affective disorder are important. First, the presence of these markers provides external validation of the clinical psychiatric syndrome (Puig-Antich, 1980). Second, they may provide some understanding of the pathophysiology of the disorder as their occurrence in association with the illness implies their direct or indirect implication in the pathogenesis of the disorder. Third, provided that the biological marker has adequate sensitivity and specificity (Shapiro et al., 1983), it may be useful as a diagnostic test for prepubertal depressive disorder. Lastly, by studying established biological correlates of adult affective illness in childhood depression, the relationship of mood disorders in these different age groups may be better understood.

Although studies of biological correlates of childhood depression are extremely limited, there are preliminary data on several abnormal biological parameters in childhood depression which have been established in adult affective illness.

Cortisol. Various abnormalities of the hypothalamo-pituitary-adrenal axis have been reported in adult major depressive disorder. These include hypersecretion of cortisol (Carroll et al., 1976a,b), inappropriate cortisol nocturnal secretion (Sachar et al., 1973a), and early escape of plasma cortisol concentrations from suppression with the overnight dexamethasone suppression test (Carroll et al., 1981). These neuroendocrine disturbances are thought to be an indication of abnormal limbic system function, which has a regulatory influence on the hypothalamo-pituitary-adrenal axis (Sachar, 1982), rather than a direct manifestation of stress experienced by the depressed patient. Although recent studies have questioned the specificity of the dexamethasone suppression test (Shapiro et al., 1983), it appears to be of research and, to a lesser extent, of clinical use in a selected group of psychiatric patients with a preponderance of affective illness where the test maintains an adequate sensitivity and specificity (Shapiro et al., 1983).

In a preliminary, uncontrolled study, 2 out of 4 prepubertal children with endogenous major depression, according to Research Diagnostic Criteria (Spitzer et al., 1978), showed evidence of cortisol hypersecretion, which normalized with recovery from depression, when plasma cortisol was measured every 20 minutes over a period of 10 to 24 hours (Puig-Antich et al., 1979b). The same research group confirmed their findings in a larger sample of 15 children with endogenous and 5 children with non-endogenous major depressive disorder (Puig-Antich, 1980). Three of the children with endogenous and none of those with non-endogenous depression showed abnormalities of cortisol secretion. These preliminary data suggest that abnormalities of cortisol secretion similar to those in adult depression occur with reduced frequency in childhood depression.

On the other hand, the data on the dexamethasone suppression test in children are inconclusive. The two studies to date, involving small samples of prepubertal depressed children, have reported contrasting data (Poznanski et al., 1982; Geller et al., 1983a). Dexamethasone nonsuppression was reported in 2 of 14 cases in the one study (Geller et al., 1983a) and in 5 of 9 cases in the other (Poznanski et al., 1982). Reasons for the difference in frequency of nonsuppression are unclear, although the small sample sizes and the larger dose of dexamethasone used in Geller and associates' study (20 µg/kg as compared to 14.9 µg/kg) may account for the reported discrepancy.

Further systematic studies of the dexamethasone suppression test in normal children and those with a variety of psychiatric disorders including depression are necessary. Such works should pay particular attention to the dose of dexamethasone used by taking into account pharmacokinetic variables of dexamethasone which are unique to children (Geller et al., 1983a). The doses used in studies to date have been empirical and largely extrapolated from adult studies. Only with improved studies can the utility of the dexamethasone suppression test in childhood depression be definitively assessed.

Growth Hormone. The response of this hormone to insulin-induced hypoglycaemia has been reported to be blunted in a preliminary study of 20 children with major depressive disorder (Puig-Antich, 1981). Nine of 10 endogenous and 5 of 10 non-endogenous depressed children had a blunted growth hormone response. This finding parallels that in adult depression although the frequency of a blunted growth hormone response is less in a comparably depressed adult sample (Sachar et al., 1973b). However, estrogens potentiate the growth hormone response to a variety of stimuli (Merimee and Fineberg, 1971) so that inclusion of females of different ages and menstrual status in the adult samples may account for the reported difference between children and adults in the frequency of the blunted growth hormone response to insulin-induced hypoglycaemia.

Growth hormone secretion from the pituitary gland is influenced by a number of neurotransmitters, especially the catecholamines and indoleamines (Sachar, 1982). Alteration of the growth hormone response to insulin-induced hypoglycaemia in depression suggests functional abnormalities of one or more neurotransmitters which is consistent with the monoamine hypothesis of affective illness (Schildkraut, 1965). In adults, the growth hormone response to a variety of provocative tests such as clonidine, an alpha-2 noradrenergic receptor agonist (Matussek, 1979), and L-dopa, a dopamine precursor (Sachar et al., 1975), has been measured to identify more specifically the neurotransmitter abnormalities present in depression. Such strategies would be useful in children.

Biogenic Amines. A large number of studies have measured a variety of neurotransmitters and their metabolites in blood, cerebrospinal fluid, and urine of adults with affective disorder (Zis and Goodwin, 1982) to test the biogenic amine hypothesis of affective illness (Schildkraut, 1965). Interpretation of such studies is difficult because factors such as age, sex, diet, and level of motor activity substantially affect these various neurochemicals (Zis and Goodwin, 1982). Furthermore, the extent to which these various measurements represents central nervous system neurotransmitter function is problematic (Post and Goodwin, 1974; Maas et al., 1976). However, certain consistent findings have emerged. These include lower levels of noradrenergic and dopaminergic neurotransmitters and their metabolites in depression as compared to mania (Zis and Goodwin, 1982), and lower levels of urinary 3-methoxy-4-hydroxyphenylglycol (MHPG) in bipolar as compared to unipolar depression which may predict antidepressant response to imipramine (Maas et al., 1972).

Cytryn and McKnew (1979) measured urinary MHPG in 9 chronically depressed prepubertal children and found it to be significantly decreased in comparison to normal age-matched controls. To the extent that urinary MHPG reflects cerebral noradrenergic function, since only 40 percent of MHPG in the urine is thought to be of central nervous system origin (Ebert and Kopin, 1975), these preliminary data suggest that there may be a noradrenergic deficiency in at least a subset of cases of childhood depression, as may be the case in some subtypes of adult depression (Maas et al., 1972).

Studies of neurotransmitters and their metabolites in childhood depression are extremely limited largely because of the difficulty in obtaining specimen samples, particularly cerebrospinal fluid. Nevertheless, further such studies may facilitate understanding of the pathophysiology of affective illness in children.

Sleep Architecture. A variety of sleep electroencephalogram abnormalities have been established as biological correlates of adult major depressive disorder (Kupfer and Foster, 1979; Vogel et al., 1980). These include: (1) decreased REM latency; (2) increased REM density; (3) abnormal temporal distribution of REM sleep; (4) decreased delta sleep; and (5) decreased sleep efficiency. However, the same alterations in these sleep parameters occur with increased age regardless of the presence of depression (Ulrich et al., 1980). In a study of 54 prepubertal children with major depressive disorder, three nights of polysomnography revealed no differences in any sleep parameters between these children and normal as well as non-depressed neurotic controls (Puig-Antich et al., 1982a). These findings confirm those of an earlier study (Kupfer et al., 1977). Puig-Antich and colleagues also reported that REM latency decreased and sleep continuity improved when 28 prepubertal children were studied after recovery from depression in a drug-free state (Puig-Antich et al., 1983). These data suggest that shortened REM latency with recovery may be either a trait marker of prepubertal depressive disorder or else a residual effect of a depressive episode.

The sleep data in childhood depression differ from those in adult depression. In view of the significant age effect on sleep parameters in adults (Ulrich et al., 1980), this difference is likely due to a maturational effect on a biological marker rather than to a true biological difference between childhood and adult depression.

Despite the lack of polysomnographic changes, depressed children are reported to have a higher incidence of sleep continuity complaints than do age-matched, normal controls (Puig-Antich et al., 1982a). Sleep spindle activity, a feature of stage 2 sleep, may be related to the feeling of not sleeping well (Goetz et al., 1983). However, a recent study reported that sleep spindle activity does not differentiate children with major depressive disorder from either age-matched normals or those with non-depressed emotional disorders (Goetz et al., 1983).

Cross-sectional and longitudinal studies of sleep architecture in affectively ill children are required. Particular attention should be paid to differences in specific sleep parameters with age, stage of illness, and response to various antidepressant treatments.

Genetic. Family (Gershon et al., 1975), twin (Bertelsen, 1979), and adoption studies (Mendlewicz and Rainier, 1977) have substantiated the presence of a possible genetic factor in adult affective disorder. Such evidence is not available for childhood depression. Recent studies, however, suggest that children of parents with affective illness have an increased frequency of episodes of depressive symptoms (Cytryn et al., 1982; Welner et al., 1977). In contrast, it has been found that although children of parents with affective disorder had a high rate of psychiatric illnesses, these were not confined to affective disorders (Rutter, 1966; Weissman et al., 1984). This suggests that other factors in addition to genetic transmission account for the high psychiatric morbidity in the offspring of affectively ill adults.

A family history study of 26 children with major depressive disorder indicates that the lifetime morbidity risk for major depression in their first-degree biological relatives over the age of 16 years is 0.42 (Puig-Antich, 1980). In adults with major depressive disorder, this relative risk is only 0.30, suggesting a strong genetic factor in prepubertal major depressive disorder. However, further systematic investigation, using family, twin and adoption study designs, is required to clarify the role of genetic factors in prepubertal depression and its relationship to adult affective illness.

Neuropsychological. The concept that cognitive function is independent of non-brain damaged emotional disturbance in children has, until recently, hampered the investigation of neuropsychological correlates of childhood affective illness (Brumback and Staton, 1980). Recently, preliminary studies have shown that children with prepubertal depression have a wide range of cognitive impairments on an extensive neuropsychological battery. These impairments resolve with treatment of the depression (Brumback and Staton, 1980; Staton et al., 1981). Furthermore, the greatest improvement occurs with reasoning, judgment, visuoperceptual and visuospatial functions, all of which are localized to the right hemisphere and frontal lobes (Staton et al., 1981). In addition, children of manic-depressive parents have been shown to have lower performance I.Q. scores, a manifestation of right cerebral hemi-

sphere function, than controls on the Wechsler Intelligence Scale for children (Kron et al., 1982).
Lateralized specialization of cerebral hemisphere function is well documented (Brumback and Staton, 1982). There is considerable evidence including electroencephalographic, neuropsychological, and head injury data that right hemisphere dysfunction is associated with affective illness in adults (Flor-Henry, 1976, 1979). Therefore, the preliminary data in children (Brumback and Staton, 1980; Kron et al., 1982) are compatible with those in adults and suggest that, regardless of age, depression may be associated with right-sided cerebral dysfunction.
Moreover, certain learning disabilities, attention deficit disorder, and major depressive disorder are all postulated to be manifestations of right cerebral hemisphere dysfunction (Brumback and Staton, 1982). This possible common locus of pathology may account for the frequent concurrence of these disorders. For example, in children referred to an educational diagnostic centre, learning disabilities occurred in up to 55% and attention deficit disorder in approximately 60% of depressed children (Staton and Brumback, 1981). Therefore, cognitive disturbance in depressed children may be a direct result of the depressive illness or may antedate the depression and the associated attention deficit disorder or learning disability.
Further study of cognitive impairment in prepubertal depression is necessary. With increasing recognition of the syndrome, major depressive disorder may become an important consideration in the differential diagnosis of poor school performance and academic failure in childhood.

Psychologic Factors

Psychodynamic. This model stresses the fundamental importance of the early experience of loss and separation in the etiology of depression (Lewis and Lewis, 1981). Various psychoanalytic theorists have elaborated on the response to loss, such as self-reproach against an internalized love object (Freud, 1917), internalized hostility and ambivalence (Abraham, 1924), and the development of the ego state of depression with resultant loss of self-esteem (Bibring, 1953).
Most of the premises of the psychodynamic model are derived from intense clinical observation and do not lend themselves to systematic investigation.

However, studies to date on early loss have failed to show that it is an invariable feature of depressed subjects (Pfohl et al., 1983). Furthermore, not all individuals who experience early loss will later develop depression (Pfohl et al., 1983). Therefore, the role of early loss in the development of depression is unclear but it certainly does not appear to be of primary etiological importance in a large subgroup of adult patients. In the children's area, object loss has been associated with depressive symptoms in children (Kashani et al., 1981), but no systematic data are available on its possible etiologic role in childhood depression.

Behavioural. Seligman observed maladaptive behaviour, particularly passivity, in dogs exposed to inescapable electric shocks (Seligman, 1975). This behaviour was termed 'learned helplessness' and has been postulated as an etiological model of depression where the depressed person views his behaviour as independent of reinforcers which leads in turn to helplessness and giving up. 'Learned helplessness' has been experimentally induced in children without psychiatric illness (Dweck and Reppucci, 1973), and there is preliminary evidence that it may be implicated in the pathogenesis of childhood depression (Petti, 1983).

The behaviour reinforcement model of Lewinsohn and associates postulates that depressed subjects have fewer social skills and, therefore, are unable to elicit positive reinforcement from their environment (Lewinsohn et al., 1976). This model has not been specifically applied to childhood depression.

Cognitive Distortion. This model, described by Kovacs and Beck, states that affective illness is the consequence of negative cognitions originating in early, adverse life experiences (Kovacs and Beck, 1978). Beck described a triad of negative cognitions, i.e. negative self-concept, negative expectations of the future, and negative interpretation of present life circumstances, as being characteristic of the depressed individual (Kovacs and Beck, 1978). These negative ideas are said to become so pervasive that all aspects of daily living are viewed as adverse and hopeless. Hopelessness and pessimism are common features of childhood depression but there is very little evidence that such cognitive factors are of etiopathologic significance in childhood depression.

Other. Other psychologic etiological models of depression have been proposed in adults. These include the sociological model where depression is seen as the result of an adverse social structure (Klerman, 1976), as well as the life stress model where depression is seen as the response to an excess of life stresses (Paykel et al., 1969). There are no experimental data on either of these etiological models in childhood depression. However, stressors and environmental circumstances such as marital discord, parental mental illness, overcrowding and low socioeconomic class are risk factors for childhood psychiatric illness in general and suicide and depression in particular (Rutter, 1981).

Natural History

There is a paucity of studies which examine the natural history of childhood depression or depressive symptoms in childhood. Three reports (Poznanski et al., 1976; Eastgate and Gilmour, 1984; Kovacs et al., 1984) present data on the course of childhood depression. The first (Poznanski et al., 1976, 1981) re-evaluated six and one half years later 10 children who were described originally as 'affectively depressed'. Five of the group were clinically depressed at follow-up. This study has several limitations, including the small number of subjects, the lack of rigorous criteria for the diagnosis of depression initially and at follow-up, and the absence of a blind follow-up evaluation. The second study (Eastgate and Gilmour, 1984) followed up 19 of 36 patients seven to eight years after their initial referral. The 36 patients were 4% of 852 consecutive referrals over a two-year period to a psychiatric department of a children's hospital. All 36 received a diagnosis of depression according to Weinberg criteria (Weinberg et al., 1973; Brumback et al., 1977). At follow-up, 8 of the 19 still had moderate to severe disability including 4 with depression, 1 schizophrenic, and 4 with personality disorders. The loss of almost fifty percent of the original sample at follow-up, the lack of blind evaluation and rigorous diagnostic criteria at follow-up, as well as the lack of a control group, are major weaknesses of the work. The third study (Kovacs et al., 1984), located in a psychiatric outpatient clinic, followed three cohorts of children with different DSM-III diagnoses of depression, namely, adjustment disorder with depressed mood, major depressive disorder, and dysthymic disorder. The first group, adjustment disorder with depressed mood, had the best prognosis with a median recovery time of about five months. After nine months, 90% of the children had recovered from the adjustment disorder. The major depressive disorder cohort had a median recovery time of about seven months and by eighteen months the maximum recovery rate of 92% from the depressive episode was reached. The dysthymic group had by far the worst prognosis. Here the median recovery time was three and one-half years and it took more than six years to reach the maximal recovery rate of 89%. In the entire depressed group of three cohorts, 63% received treatment at some time during the index episode. However, treatment had a beneficial effect on the recovery rate of only one cohort, the major depressive disorder group.

One study (Tesing and Lekowitz, 1982) has examined the stability of depressive symptoms in fourth and fifth grade children by peer, self and teacher ratings over a six-month period. While all correlations were statistically significant, the peer ratings were the most stable ($r = 0.70$) followed by the teacher ($r = 0.60$), and the self-rating ($r = 0.44$).

Much more work needs to be done in learning about the course of childhood disorders in general (Robins, 1979). As can be seen, little is known in this area about childhood depression. It is important to note, however, that there is scanty evidence to suggest that childhood depression or depressive symptoms have any genetic or particular psychopathological link with adult depression (Graham, 1974).

Treatment Approaches

Tricyclic Antidepressants

Tricyclic antidepressants are of undisputed therapeutic benefit in adults with major depression (Morris and Beck, 1974). The evidence for their use in children is equivocal. Early studies reported a response rate to tricyclics of 49 to 95 percent in depressed children (Ling et al., 1970; Weinberg et al., 1973; Ossofsky, 1974). However, these studies suffer from methodological flaws such as absence of diagnostic criteria for depression, poorly controlled or uncontrolled study designs, inadequate measures of response, and the use of both in-patient and out-patient subjects without consideration of the problem of greater non-compliance with treatment in the latter.

A recent, more systematic, open study found a response rate of 6 of 13 prepubertal depressed children (Puig-Antich, 1978). However, although all these studies suggest that tricylcics may be useful in childhood depression, they are not able to determine whether these drugs are more effective than placebo. In the only double-blind, placebo-controlled study reported to date (Puig-Antich, 1982b), the response rate to imipramine did not differ from placebo. The placebo effect is strong in adult depression and may be even more significant in childhood depression where placebo response rates up to 71 percent have been reported (Puig-Antich, 1982b). Furthermore, the majority of studies of tricyclics in children have been carried out together with various forms of psychotherapy. Recent studies in adults have shown that psychotherapy may be equally effective as tricyclics (DiMascio et al., 1979). Therefore, the high response rate attributed to placebo in studies of childhood depression may be the effect of therapies other than drugs and these need to be controlled for in future studies.

Most studies of tricyclic antidepressants in childhood depression have used imipramine. Amitryptiline (Weise et al., 1972), nortryptiline (Geller et al., 1983b) and maprotiline (Kuhn-Gebhardt, 1972) have been reported to be useful, although these data are limited by the methodological inadequacies of the studies.

Two recent reports have emphasized the importance of monitoring drug plasma levels in controlled studies of the effectiveness of tricyclics, particularly imipramine, in childhood depression (Puig-Antich et al., 1979; Preskorn et al., 1982). Preskorn and colleagues found a response rate of 4 of 20 prepubertal depressed children treated with imipramine. These 4 had combined steady-state plasma levels of imipramine and desipramine of 125-225 ng/ml. None with plasma levels below or above this range remitted. Adjustment of dosage in the non-responders resulted in 12 achieving these plasma levels, 11 of whom showed remission by the end of the second 3-week treatment period. These data suggest a curvilinear relationship between drug plasma concentration and clinical response. This is contrary to the linear relationship between drug plasma concentration and response in adults treated with imipramine (Glassman et al., 1977), although the lower limit of the therapeutic range in children of 125 ng/ml (Preskorn et al., 1982) is consistent with that in the adult literature (Gram et al., 1976). The second study (Puig-Antich et al., 1979a) reported a positive correlation between total tricyclic plasma levels and clinical response in a double-blind, placebo-controlled study of imipramine. It was found that responders had significantly higher drug plasma levels than non-responders.

There may be in excess of a seven-fold variation in the steady-state plasma concentration of tricyclics in children on a fixed dose, regardless of age, weight, height and body surface area (Preskorn et al., 1983). Therefore, it is more rational to assess appropriate tricyclic dose for clinical response on the basis of plasma levels rather than on a milligram per kilogram basis. Furthermore, studies comparing imipramine to placebo should employ drug plasma level monitoring as part of the design.

Certain aspects of the pharmacokinetics of tricyclics are different in children as compared to adults. Drug binding to plasma albumin is less in children, leading to relatively larger amounts of circulating free drug (Winsberg et al., 1974). The relatively larger amount of liver tissue in children may account for the enhanced production of demethylated and hydroxylated metabolites in this age group (Zametkin and Rapoport, 1983). Little is known about drug absorption and excretion patterns in children as compared to adults. However, in children imipramine has a shorter half-life of approximately 6-15 hours (Winsberg et al., 1974).

The difference in tricyclic pharmacokinetics in children as compared to adults has implications for clinical use. First, the use of a single daily dose as compared to divided doses of tricyclic may be hazardous because of the production of a high peak of circulating free drug and resultant increased side effects (Winsberg et al., 1974). Second, the increased production of metabolites and the increased amount of circulating free drug may make children particularly vulnerable to tricyclics as there have been increased reports of side effects with increased use of these drugs in the pediatric population (Zametkin and Rapoport, 1983). In addition to side effects such as sedation, dry mouth, tremors, and gastrointestinal disturbance, potentially more serious problems have been reported. These include induction of seizures by therapeutic doses of both imipramine (Brown et al., 1973) and maprotiline (Kuhn-Gebhartdt, 1972), as well as cardiovascular effects such as tachycardia, raised blood pressure, and EKG changes (Preskorn et al., 1983). The EKG changes reported in some (Winsberg et al., 1975; Preskorn et al., 1983), but not all (Rapoport et al., 1974; Martin and Zaug, 1973), studies include conduction defects such as prolongation of the PR, QRS and QT intervals as well as various T wave changes with doses up to 5 mg/kg of imipramine. The majority of these studies did not monitor drug plasma levels. However, Preskorn and colleagues, in their study of imipramine treatment in depressed children, have shown a direct correlation between plasma drug concentrations and cardiac effects (Preskorn et al., 1983). Changes in cardiac rate and conduction were uniformly present when the combined imipramine and desipramine level exceeded 225 ng/ml. The cardiac effects may also be accounted for by the increase in children of 2-hydroxylated imipramine, which has a high affinity for cardiac tissue (Klutch and Hanna, 1976). As in adults, the clinical significance of the cardiovascular effects of tricyclic antidepressants is unclear, and therefore definitive recommendations about EKG monitoring, or continuation of treatment if such EKG changes occur, must await further study.

Serious toxic effects have been reported with tricyclic poisoning in children (Bickel, 1975). These include drowsiness, delirium and coma as well as cardiac arrhythmias and cardiovascular collapse. Fatalities have also been reported.

The mechanism of action of tricyclic antidepressants in childhood depression is presently unknown. There are no data on the effects of these drugs on biogenic amines, neuroendocrine function, or other biological correlates of childhood depression. Such studies would provide valuable information about the pathophysiology of childhood depression and the mechanism(s) of action of antidepressants in this disorder as well as clarifying the possible relationship between depressive illness in children and adults. Two studies have reported that tricyclics cause an immediate and sustained reduction in REM sleep in enuretic children (Millelsen et al., 1980; Rapoport et al., 1980). While this observation may not be pertinent to tricyclic treatment of childhood depression, such an effect on REM sleep is common to all types of antidepressant treatment in adults (Mendelson et al., 1977).

At the present state of knowledge, clinical use of tricyclic antidepressants in children should parallel that in adults. Daily doses of tricyclics to a maximum of 5 mg/kg should be effective in approximately four weeks, although there is a preliminary report that, at least with nortryptiline, a therapeutic effect may take as long as eight weeks in children (Geller et al., 1983). Due to the limited data on the course of affective illness in children, it is unclear how long one should continue a course of antidepressant treatment. However, discontinuation should be gradual so as to avoid withdrawal symptoms of nausea, vomiting, and abdominal pain which have been reported in children (Law et al., 1981).

Lithium. Lithium carbonate has firmly established indications in the acute and prophylactic treatment of manic depressive illness in adults (Schou, 1968). Despite its longstanding use, dating back at least 25 years, no clear consensus has been reached on lithium's effectiveness in childhood psychiatric disorders (Jefferson, 1982). Three main factors account for this lack of established efficacy. First, the existence of a prepubertal form of manic-depressive illness has been controversial (Jefferson, 1982). Second, largely as a result of this controversy, there have been very poor definitions of criteria for the syndrome of manic-depressive illness, making a target population for a trial of lithium treatment extremely difficult to define (Weinberg and Brumback, 1976). Third, despite an extensive literature on the effects of lithium in a variety of childhood psychiatric disorders (Lena, 1979), no randomized, double-blind studies and few adequately controlled studies have been reported (Jefferson, 1982). Most studies have been either single-case reports or open, uncontrolled trials with small, poorly defined samples and inadequate mood and behavioural assessments, making it impossible to draw definite conclusions about the effectiveness of lithium treatment (Youngerman and Canino, 1976). Nevertheless, despite their inadequacies, the studies seem to suggest that lithium is useful in certain childhood psychiatric disorders. Cases of typical childhood manic-depressive illness, although extremely rare, appear to have responded to lithium, suggesting that it is an effective treatment for typical bipolar illness regardless of age (Youngerman and Canino, 1976). The vast majority of cases reported describe a variety of behavioural disorders, episodic or continuous in nature, with varying degrees of affective and psychotic symptoms

(Youngerman and Canino, 1976). Despite their methodological and descriptive flaws, all these studies have a common theme in that, regardless of the range of symptomatology in each case, the presence of an affective component, with or without a family history of affective illness, suggests a treatment response to lithium (Youngerman and Canino, 1976). This has been confirmed in a double-blind controlled trial of lithium in children (McKnew et al., 1981).

Other investigators have noted that hostility and aggression are features common to lithium responders regardless of primary diagnosis (Sheard, 1975; Marini and Sheard, 1977). The anti-aggressive effect of lithium may be non-specific (Shader et al., 1974) and does not imply that aggressive behavioural disorders in childhood are atypical variants of manic-depressive illness. On the other hand, some authors contend that even in such aggressive behavioural disorders, the presence of an affective component predicts better response to lithium (Youngerman and Canino, 1976).

It is apparent that further investigation of lithium's effectiveness in childhood psychiatric disorders is warranted. Evaluation of lithium's efficacy should not be confined to affective illness only, but should involve the whole range of childhood emotional and behavioural disorders as lithium may prove to be a definitive and effective addition to the very limited therapeutic armamentarium available for these disorders.

Very little is known about lithium pharmacokinetics and side effects in children. Lithium has a higher renal clearance in children than in adults (Jefferson, 1982). Therefore, larger lithium doses may be required to maintain equivalent blood levels. In the studies to date, lithium levels were maintained in the range 0.6-1.5 meq/l when reported (Feinstein and Wolpert, 1973; Brumback and Weinberg, 1977). It is unclear whether the same blood levels are required in children as in adults for a therapeutic effect. Systematic investigation of dose range and schedules and therapeutic blood levels for acute and prophylactic treatment are necessary to establish a standardized treatment approach which is safe and effective for children.

Side effects of lithium are reported to be less frequent in children (Lena, 1979). This may be the result of the limited use of lithium in children or a failure to report the occurrence of side effects which do occur. Little is known about the long-term effects of lithium in children. In adults, however, lithium has significant long-term endocrine effects with alterations in thyroid, parathyroid, and pancreatic functions (Mannistro, 1980). Alterations in endocrine function may affect growth and development (Jefferson, 1982). In particular, a single dose of lithium inhibits release of growth hormone in rats (Smythe et al., 1979) but not in human adults (Lal et al., 1978). No data are available for children.

Although a high frequency of proteinuria has been reported, the long-term effects of lithium on renal function in children is unknown (Lena, 1979). Lithium has inhibitory effects on bone size in rats (Birch, 1980) and is known to accumulate in bone in humans (Birch, 1980). It may, therefore, have adverse effects on developing bone and should be used with caution in children.

The long-term renal, endocrine, and bone effects of lithium require further study. This is particularly important in children with affective disorder who face a potentially longer duration of lithium treatment than their adult counterparts.

Other Antidepressants. Other antidepressant treatments have received very little attention in children. There are preliminary data that monoamine oxidase inhibitors may be useful in childhood depression, although the dietary precautions needed for these drugs make their use in children particularly difficult and hazardous (Frommer, 1967; Kelly et al., 1970).

There are several case reports of the effectiveness of ECT in both childhood depression and mania (Carr et al., 1983). Ethical considerations preclude more systematic study of this treatment in children but it may be useful in cases of severe depression or mania refractory to other treatment.

Psychosocial Treatment. A variety of psychologic treatments, including individual psychodynamic or behavioural therapy as well as family therapy, have been reported to be effective in childhood depression (Kahani et al., 1981). However, there are no systematic studies on the effectiveness of psychotherapy in prepubertal depression. The need for well designed studies is obvious in view of the evidence in adults that cognitive behavioural and interpersonal forms of therapy are effective in the treatment of adult depression (DiMascio et al., 1979; Kovacs et al., 1981).

The aim of psychotherapy is to enhance the child's self-esteem, improve his social relationships, and encourage a greater sense of self-mastery and effectiveness. In this regard, educational assistance for these children may be extremely important. Family therapy is often necessary not only to foster parental understanding and decrease rejection of the depressed child but also to ensure greater treatment compliance.

Multimodality treatment programs are most commonly used to treat childhood psychiatric illness in general and childhood depression in particular. Until further study clarifies the relative efficacy of various types of treatments and their differential effects on specific symptoms, multimodality treatment seems indicated.

Concluding Remarks

The increasing acceptance of the existence of a syndrome of childhood depression with a clinical picture similar to adult depressive disorder has resulted in a recent increase in the number of studies in the area. It is evident that a prerequisite for etiologic, natural history, and treatment studies is the development of psychometrically sound instruments for both diagnosis and the measurement of important changes in the clinical picture.

In the biological domain, recent methodological advances have reduced the barriers of obtaining biological measures on children. For example, measurements of plasma metabolites of dopamine are now reliable indicators of cerebral dopamine function, and smaller amounts of blood or easily obtainable specimens of urine and saliva can provide the basis for adequate measurement of biological variables (Jefferson, 1983). This step forward together with the progress in diagnosis augers well for future investigations.

On the clinical side, there is a major need for randomized controlled trials of the effectiveness of combinations of pharmacological and psychosocial treatments of clearly defined groups of children with childhood depression. In the meantime, clinicians in the child psychiatric field have scanty data on which to base a rational, effective treatment plan for patients with childhood depression.

References

Abraham, K. (1927) A short study of the development of the libido, viewed in the light of mental disorders. In: Selected Papers on Psychoanalysis (Jones, E. J., ed.), Hogarth Press, London, pp. 418-515.

Akiskal, H. and McKinney, W. T. Jr. (1973) Depressive disorders: toward a unified hypothesis. Science 182, 20-23.

Albert, N. and Beck, A. T. (1975) Incidence of depression in early adolescence: a preliminary study. J. Youth and Adol. 4, 301-307.

American Psychiatric Association (1980) Diagnostic and Statistical Manual of Mental Disorders (DSM III). American Psychiatric Association, Washington.

Bauersfeld, K. H. (1971) Diagnosis and treatment of depressive conditions at a school psychiatric centre. In: Depressive States in Childhood and Adolescence (Annell, A. L., ed.), Almqvist and Wiksell, Stockholm, pp. 281-285.

Beck, A. T. (1972) Measuring depression: the depression inventory. In: Recent Advances in the Psychobiology of the Depressive Illnesses (Williams, T. A., Katz, M. M., and Shield, J. E., eds), U.S. Government Printing Office, Washington, pp. 299-302.

Bertelsen, A., Harvald, B., and Hauge, M. (1977) A Danish twin study of manic-depressive disorders. Brit. J. Psychiatry 130, 330-351.

Bibring, E. (1953) The mechanism of depression. In: Affective Disorders (Greenacre, P., ed.), International Universities Press, New York, pp. 13-48.

Bickel, M. (1975) Poisoning by tricyclic antidepressant drugs. Int. J. Clin. Pharmacol. 11, 145-176.

Birch, N. J. (1980) Bone side effects of lithium. In: Handbook of Lithium Therapy (Johnson, F. N., ed.), MTP Press, Lancaster, pp. 365-371.

Brown, D., Winsberg, B., Bialer, I., and Press, M. (1973) Imipramine therapy and seizures. Am. J. Psychiatry 130, 210-212.

Brumback, R. A., Dietz-Schmidt, S. G., and Weinberg, W. A. (1977) Depression in children referred to an educational diagnostic center: diagnosis and treatment and analysis of criteria and literature review. Dis. Nerv. Sys. 38, 529-535.

Brumback, R. A. and Staton, R. D. (1980) Neuropsychological study of children during and after remission of endogenous depressive episodes.

Perceptual and Motor Skills **50**, 1163-1167.
Brumback, R. A. and Staton, R. D. (1982) An hypothesis regarding the commonality of right hemisphere involvement in learning disability, attentional disorder and childhood major depressive disorder. *Perceptual and Motor Skills* **55**, 1091-1097.
Brumback, R. A. and Weinberg, W. A. (1977a) Mania in childhood. II-Therapeutic trial of lithium carbonate and further description of manic-depressive illness in children. *Am. J. Diseases of Children* **131**, 1122-1126.
Brumback, R. A. and Weinberg, W. A. (1977b) Relationship of hyperactivity and depression in children. *Perceptual and Motor Skills* **45**, 247-251.
Cantwell, D. P. and Carlson, G. (1979) Problems and prospects in the study of childhood depression. *J. Nerv. Men. Dis.* **167**, 522-529.
Carlson, G. A. and Cantwell, D. P. (1979) A survey of depressive symptoms in a child and adolescent psychiatric population. *J. Am. Acad. Child Psychiatry* **18**, 587-599.
Carlson, G. A. and Cantwell, D. P. (1980a) Masking depression in children and adolescents. *Am. J. Psychiatry* **137**, 445-449.
Carlson, G. A. and Cantwell, D. P. (1980b) A survey of depressive symptoms, syndrome and disorder in a child psychiatric population. *J. Child Psychol. Psychiat.* **21**, 19-25.
Carr, V., Dorrington, C., Shrader, G., and Wale, J. (1983) The use of ECT for mania in childhood bipolar disorder. *Brit. J. Psychiatry* **143**, 411-415.
Carroll, B. J., Curtis, G. C., and Mendels, J. (1976a) Neuroendocrine regulation in depression. I. Limbic system-adrenocortisol dysfunctions. *Arch. Gen. Psychiatry* **33**, 1039-1044.
Carroll, B. J., Curtis, G. C., and Mendels, J. (1976b) Neuroendocrine regulation in depression. II. Discrimination of depressed from non-depressed patients. *Arch. Gen. Psychiatry* **33**, 1051-1058.
Carroll, B. J., Feinberg, M., Greden, J. F., Tarika, J., Albala, A. A., Haskett, R. F., James, N. McI., Kronfol, Z., Lohr, N., Steiner, M., de Vigne, J. P., and Young, E. (1981) A specific laboratory test for the diagnosis of melancholia. *Arch. Gen. Psychiatry* **38**, 15-22.
Ceberoglu, R., Sumer, E., and Polvan, O. (1971) Etiology and pathogenesis of depression in Turkish children. In: *Depressive States in Childhood*

and Adolescence (Annell, A. L., ed.), Almqvist and Wiksell, Stockholm, pp. 133-136.

Chambers, W. J., Puig-Antich, J., and Tabrizi, M. A. (1978) The ongoing development of the Kiddie-SADS (Schedule for Affective Disorders and Schizophrenia for School Age Children). Paper presented at the American Academy of Child Psychiatry Annual Meeting, San Diego, California.

Chambers, W. J., Puig-Antich, J., Tabrizi, M. A., and Davies, M. (1982) Psychotic symptoms in prepubertal major depressive disorder. Arch. Gen. Psychiatry 39, 921-927.

Cohen, J. (1960) A coefficient of agreement for nominal scales. Educational and Psychological Measurement 20, 37-46.

Costello, A. (1984) Personal communciation.

Costello, C. G. (1980) Childhood depression: three basic but questionable assumptions in the Lefkowitz and Burton critique. Psychol. Bull. 87, 185-190.

Cytryn, L. and McKnew, D. H. (1972) Proposed classification of childhood depression. Am. J. Psychiatry 129, 149-155.

Cytryn, L. and McKnew, D. H. Jr. (1974) Factors influencing the changing clinical expression of the depressive process in children. Am. J. Psychiatry 131, 879-881.

Cytryn, L., McKnew, D. H., Bartko, J. J., Lamour, M., and Hamovitt, J. (1982) Offspring of patients with affective disorder. J. Am. Acad. Child Psychiatry 21, 389-391.

Cytryn, L., McKnew, D. H. Jr., and Bunney, W. E. (1980) Diagnosis of depression in children: a reassessment. Am. J. Psychiatry 137, 22-25.

DiMascio, A., Weissman, M. M., Prusoff, B. A., Neu, C., Zwilling, M., and Klerman, G. L. (1979) Differential symptom reduction by drugs and psychotherapy in acute depression. Arch. Gen. Psychiatry 36, 1450-1456.

Dweck, C. S. and Reppucci, N. D. (1973) Learned helplessness and reinforcement responsibility in children. J. Personality and Soc. Psychol. 25, 109-116.

Eastgate, J. and Gilmour, L. (1984) Long-term outcome of depressed children: a follow-up study. Develop. Med. and Child Neurol. 26, 68-72.

Ebert, M. and Kopin, I. J. (1975) Origins of urinary catecholamine metabolites: differential labeling by dopamine-^{14}C. Trans. Assoc. Am. Physicians 28, 256.

Feighner, J. P., Robins, E., Guze, S., Woodruff, R., Winokur, G., and Munoz, R. (1972) Diagnostic criteria for use in psychiatric research. Arch. Gen. Psychiatry 26, 57-63.

Feinstein, S. C. and Wolpert, E. A. (1973) Juvenile manic-depressive illness: clinical and therapeutic considerations. J. Am. Acad. Child Psychiatry 12, 123-136.

Flor-Henry, P. (1976) Lateralized temporal-limbic dysfunction and psychopathology. Ann. N.Y. Acad. Sci. 280, 777-795.

Flor-Henry, P. (1979) On certain aspects of the localization of the cerebral systems regulating and determining emotion. Biol. Psychiatry 14, 677-698.

Freud, S. (1917) Mourning and melancholia. In: The Standard Edition of The Complete Psychological Works of Sigmund Freud, vol. XIV (Strachey, J., ed. and trans.), Hogarth Press, London, 1957, pp. 237-258.

Frommer, E. A. (1967) Treatment of childhood depression with antidepressant drugs. Brit. Med. J. 1, 729-732.

Frommer, E. (1968) Depressive illness in childhood. Brit. J. Psychiatry 2, 117-123.

Geller, B., Perel, J. M., Knitter, E. F., Lycaki, H., and Farooki, Z. Q. (1983a) Nortriptyline in major depressive disorder in children: response, steady-state plasma levels, predictive kinetics and pharmacokinetics. Psychopharmacol. Bull. 19, 62-65.

Geller, B., Rogol, A. D., and Knitter, E. F. (1983b) Preliminary data on the dexamethasone suppression test in children with major depressive disorder. Am. J. Psychiatry 140, 620-622.

Gershon, E. S., Baron, M., and Leakman, J. (1975) Genetic models of the transmission of affective disorders. J. Psychiatric Res. 12, 301-317.

Glaser, K. (1967) Masked depression in children and adolescents. Am. J. Psychotherapy 21, 565-574.

Glassman, A. H., Perel, J. M., Shostak, M., Kantor, S. J., and Fleiss, J. L. (1977) Clinical implications of imipramine plasma levels for depressive illness. Arch. Gen. Psychiatry 34, 197-204.

Goetz, R. R., Goetz, D. M., Hanlon, C., Davies, M., and Weitzman, E. D. (1983) Spindle characteristics in prepubertal major depressives during an episode and after sustained recovery: a controlled study. Sleep 6, 369-375.

Gould, M. S., Wunsch-Hitzig, R., and Dohrenwend, B. (1981) Estimating the prevalence of childhood psychopathology. J. American Acad. Child Psychiatry 20, 462-476.

Graham, P. (1974) Depression in pre-pubertal children. Develop. Med. and Child Neurol. 16, 340-349.

Gram, L., Reisby, N., and Ibsen, I. (1976) Plasma levels and antidepressive effect of imipramine. Clin. Pharmacol. Ther. 19, 318-324.

Herjanic, B. and Campbell, W. (1977) Differentiating psychiatrically disturbed children on the basis of a structured interview. J. Abnor. Child Psychol. 5, 127-134.

Hirsch, M., Paez, P., Chambers, W. J., Tabrizi, M. A., and Puig-Antich, J. (1980) Test-retest of the K-SADS-P. Paper presented at the American Academy of Child Psychiatry Annual Meeting, Chicago.

Hughes, M. C. (1984) Recurrent abdominal pain and childhood depression: clinical observations of 23 children and their families. Am. J. Orthopsychiatry 54, 146-155.

Jefferson, J. W. (1982) The use of lithium in childhood and adolescence: an overview. J. Clin. Psychiatry 43, 174-177.

Kashani, J. H., Barbero, G. J., and Bolander, F. D. (1981a) Depression in hospitalized pediatric patients. J. Am. Acad. Child Psychiatry 20, 123-134.

Kashani, J. H., Cantwell, D. P., Shekim, W. O., and Reid, J. C. (1982) Major depressive disorder in children admitted to an inpatient community mental health center. Am. J. Psychiatry 139, 671-672.

Kashani, J. H., Husain, A., Shekim, W. O., Hodges, K. K., Cytryn, L., and McKnew, D. H. (1981b) Current perspectives on childhood depression: an overview. Am. J. Psychiatry 138, 143-153.

Kashani, J. H., McGee, R. O., Clarkson, S. E., Anderson, J. C., Walton, L. A., Williams, S., Silva, P. A., Robins, R. J., Cytryn, L., and McKnew, D. H. (1983) Depression in a sample of 9-year-old children. Arch. Gen. Psychiatry 40, 1217-1223.

Kashani, J. and Simonds, J. F. (1979) The incidence of depression in children. Am. J. Psychiatry 136, 1203-1205.

Kashani, J. H., Venzke, R., and Millar, E. A. (1981c) Depression in children admitted to hospital for orthopaedic procedures. Brit. J. Psychiatry 138, 21-25.

Kazdin, A. E. (1981) Assessment techniques for childhood depression. J. Am. Acad. Child Psychiatry 20, 358-375.

Kelly, D., Guirguis, W., Frommer, E., Mitchell-Heggs, N., and Sargant, W. (1970) Treatment of phobic states with antidepressants. Brit. J. Psychiatry 116, 387-398.

Klerman, G. L. (1976) Age and clinical depression: today's youth in the twenty-first century. J. Gerentol. 31, 318-323.

Klerman, G. L. and Cole, J. O. (1965) Clinical pharmacology of imipramine and related antidepressant compounds. Pharmacol. Rev. 17, 101-145.

Klutch, A. and Hanna, M. The urinary metabolites of imipramine in behaviour disordered children (submitted).

Kovacs, M. and Beck, A. T. (1977) An empirical-clinical approach toward the definition of childhood depression. In: Depression in Childhood: Diagnosis, Treatment and Conceptual Models (Schulterbrandt, J. G. and Raskin, A., eds), Raven Press, New York, pp. 1-25.

Kovacs, M. and Beck, A. T. (1978) Maladaptive cognitive structures in depression. Am. J. Psychiatry 135, 525-533.

Kovacs, M., Feinberg, T. L., Crouse-Novak, M. A., Paulankas, S. L., and Finkelstein, R. (1984) Depressive disorders in childhood. I. A longitudinal prospective study of characteristics and recovery. Arch. Gen. Psychiatry 41, 229-237.

Kovacs, M., Rush, A. J., Beck, A. T., and Hollon, S. D. (1981) Depressed outpatients treated with cognitive therapy or pharmacotherapy: a one-year follow-up. Arch. Gen. Psychiatry 38, 33-39.

Kron, L., Decina, P., Kestenbaum, C. J., Farber, S., Gargan, M., and Fieve, R. (1982) The offspring of bipolar manic-depressives: clinical features. Adolescent Psychiatry 10, 273-291.

Kuhn-Gebhardt, V. (1972) Results obtained with a new antidepressant in children with a depressive illness. In: Depressive States in Childhood and Adolescence (Annell, A., ed.), Halsted Press, New York, pp. 455-459.

Kupfer, D. J., Coble, P., and Kane, J. (1979a) Imipramine and EEG sleep in children with depressive symptoms. Psychopharmacology 60, 117-123.

Kupfer, D. and Foster, F. G. (1979b) EEG sleep and depression. In: Sleep Disorders: Diagnosis and Treatment (Williams, R. L. and Karacan, I., eds), Wiley, New York, pp. 163-204.

Lal, S., Nair, N. P. V., and Guyda, H. (1978) Effects of lithium on hypothalamic-pituitary dopaminergic functions. Acta psychiatr. scand. **57**, 91-96.

Lang, M. and Tisher, M. (1978) Children's Depression Scale. The Australian Council for Educational Research, Victoria, Australia.

Law, W., Petti, T. A., and Kazdin, A. E. (1981) Withdrawal symptoms after graduated cessation of imipramine in children. Am. J. Psychiatry **138**, 647-650.

Lefkowitz, M. M. (1980) A reply to Costello. Psychol. Bull. **87**, 191-194.

Lefkowitz, M. M. and Burton, N. (1978) Childhood depression: a critique of the concept. Psychol. Bull. **85**, 716-726.

Lefkowitz, M. M. and Tesing, E. P. (1980) Assessment of childhood depression. J. Consulting and Clin. Psychol. **48**, 43-50.

Lena, B. (1979) Lithium in childhood and adolescent psychiatry. Arch. Gen. Psychiatry **36**, 854-855.

Leon, G. R., Kendall, P. C., and Garber, J. (1980) Depression in children: parent, teacher and child perspectives. J. Abnor. Child Psychology **8**, 221-235.

Lewinsohn, P. M., Biglan, A., and Zeiss, A. M. (1976) Behavioral treatment of depression. In: Behavior Management of Anxiety, Depression and Pain (Davidson, O., ed.), Bruner Mazel, New York, pp. 91-146.

Lewis, M. and Lewis, D. O. (1981) Depression in childhood: a biopsychosocial perspective. Am. J. Psychotherapy **35**, 323-329.

Ling, W., Oftedal, G., and Weinberg, W. (1970) Depressive illness in childhood presenting as a severe headache. Am. J. Dis. Children **120**, 122-124.

Lucas, A. R. (1977) Treatment of depressive states. In: Psychopharmacology in Childhood and Adolescence (Weiner, J. M., ed.), Basic Books, New York, pp. 149-168.

Malmquist, C. P. (1971) Depression in childhood and adolescence. New Engl. J. Med. **284**, 887-893.

Mannisto, P. T. (1980) Endocrine side-effects of lithium. In: Handbook of Lithium Therapy (Johnson, F. N., ed.), MTP Press, Lancaster, pp. 310-322.

Marini, J. L. and Sheard, M. H. (1977) Antiaggressive effect of lithium ion in man. Acta psychiatr. scand. **55**, 269-275.

Martin, G. I. and Zang, P. J. (1973) EKG monitoring of enuretic children given imipramine. J. Am. Med. Assoc. 224, 902-903.

Mass, J. W. (1976) Biogenic amines in depression. Arch. Gen. Psychiatry 32, 1357-1361.

Mass, J. W., Fawcett, J. A., and Dekirmenjian, H. (1972) Catecholamine metabolism, depressive illness and drug response. Arch. Gen. Psychiatry 26, 252-262.

Matussek, N. (1979) Neuroendocrinological studies in affective disorders. In: Origin, Prevention and Treatment of Affective Disorders (Schou, M. and Stromgren, E., eds), Academic Press, London, pp. 171-178.

McConville, B. J., Boag, L. C., and Purohit, A. P. (1973) Three types of childhood depression. Can. Psychiatric Assoc. J. 18, 133-138.

McKnew, D. H. Jr. and Cytryn, L. (1979) Urinary metabolites in chronically depressed children. J. Am. Acad. Child Psychiatry 18, 608-615.

McKnew, D. H., Cytryn, L., Buchsbaum, M. S., Hamovit, J., Lamour, M., Rapoport, J. L., and Gershon, E. S. (1981) Lithium in children of lithium-responding parents. Psychiatry Res. 4, 171-180.

McKnew, D. H. Jr., Cytryn, L., Efron, A. M., Gershon, E. S., and Brunner, W. E. (1979) Offspring of patients with affective disorder. Brit. J. Psychiatry 134, 148-152.

Meierhofer, M. (1971) Depression in infancy and childhood. In: Depressive States in Childhood and Adolescence (Annell, A. L., ed.), Almqvist and Wiksell, Stockholm, pp. 159-162.

Mendelsohn, W., Grillen, J. C., and Wyatt, R. (1977) Human Sleep and its Disorders. Plenum Press, New York.

Mendlewicz, J. and Ranier, J. D. (1977) Adoption study supporting genetic transmission in manic-depressive illness. Nature (Lond.) 268, 327-329.

Merimee, T. J. and Fineberg, S. E. (1971) Studies of the sex based variation of human growth hormone secretion. J. Clin. Endocrinol. Metab. 33, 896-902.

Mikkelson, E. J., Rapoport, J. L., Nee, L. E., Gruenau, C., Mendelson, W., and Gillen, C. (1980) Childhood enuresis: sleep pattern and psychopathology. Arch. Gen. Psychiatry 37, 1139-1144.

Morris, J. B. and Beck, A. T. (1974) The efficacy of antidepressant drugs. Arch. Gen. Psychiatry 30, 667-674.

Offord, D. R. and Waters, B. G. (1983) Socialization and its failure. In: *Developmental-Behavioral Pediatrics* (Levine, M. D., Carey, W. B., Crocker, A. C., and Gross, R. T., eds), Saunders, Philadelphia, pp. 650-682.

Orvaschel, H., Puig-Antich, J., Chambers, W., Tabrizi, M. A., and Johnson, R. (1982) Retrospective assessment of prepubertal major depression with the Kiddie-SADS-E. *J. Am. Acad. Child Psychiatry* 21, 392-397.

Orvaschel, H., Sholomskas, D., and Weissman, M. (1980a) Assessing children in psychiatric epidemiological studies. In: *Studies of Children* (Earls, F., ed.), Prodist, New York, pp. 84-95.

Orvaschel, H., Sholomskas, D., and Weissman, M. M. (1980b) *The Assessment of Psychopathology and Behavioral Problems in Children: A Review of Scales Suitable for Epidemiological and Clinical Research (1967-1978)*. NIMH Series AN No. 1, DHHS Publication No. (ADM) 80-1037, U.S. Government Printing Office, Washington.

Ossofsky, H. (1974) Endogenous depression in infancy and childhood. *Comp. Psychiatry* 15, 19-25.

Paykel, E. S., Myers, J. K., Dienelt, M. N., Klerman, G. L., Lindenthal, J. J., and Pepper, M. P. (1969) Life events and depression: a controlled study. *Arch. Gen. Psychiatry* 21, 753-760.

Pearce, J. B. (1978) The recognition of depressive disorder in children. *J. Roy. Soc. Med.* 71, 494-497.

Petti, T. A. (1978) Depression in hospitalized child psychiatric patients. *J. Am. Acad. Child Psychiatry* 17, 49-59.

Petti, T. (1983) Behavioral approaches in the treatment of depressed children. In: *Affective Disorders in Children and Adolescents* (Cantwell, D. and Carlson, G., eds), Spectrum Publications, New York, pp. 417-443.

Pfohl, B., Stangl, D., and Tsuang, M. T. (1983) The association between early parental loss and diagnosis in the Iowa 500. *Arch. Gen. Psychiatry* 40, 965-967.

Polvan, O. and Cebiroglu, R. (1972) Treatment with psychopharmacologic agents in childhood depression. In: *Depressive States in Childhood and Adolescence* (Annel, A., ed.), Almqvist and Wiksell, Stockholm, pp. 467-472.

Post, R. M. and Goodwin, F. K. (1974) Cerebrospinal fluid amine metabolites in affective illness. *Psychotherapy and Psychosomatics* 23, 142-158.

Poznanski, E. O., Carroll, B. J., Banegas, M. C., Cook, S. C., and Grossman, J. A. (1982) The dexamethasone suppression test in prepubertal depressed children. Am. J. Psychiatry 139, 321-324.

Poznanski, E., Cook, S. C., and Carroll, B. J. (1979) A depression rating scale for children. Pediatrics 64, 442-450.

Poznanski, E. O., Cook, S. C., Carroll, B. J., and Corzo, H. (1983) Use of the children's depression rating scale in an inpatient psychiatric population. J. Clin. Psychiatry 44, 200-203.

Poznanski, E. O., Grossman, J. E., Buchbaum, Y., Banegas, M., Freeman, L., and Gibbons, R. (1984) Preliminary studies of the reliability and validity of the children's depression rating scale. J. Am. Acad. Child Psychiatry 23, 191-197.

Poznanski, E. O., Krahenbuhl, V., and Zrull, J. P. (1976) Childhood depression: a longitudinal perspective. J. Am. Acad. Child Psychiatry 15, 491-501.

Preskorn, S. H., Weller, E. B., and Weller, R. A. (1982) Depression in children: relationship between plasma imipramine levels and response. J. Clin. Psychiatry 43, 450-453.

Preskorn, S. H., Weller, E. B., Weller, R. A., and Glotzbach, E. (1983) Plasma levels of imipramine and adverse effects in children. Am. J. Psychiatry 140, 1332-1334.

Puig-Antich, J. (1980) Affective disorders in childhood: a review and perspective. Psychiat. Clin. North America 3, 403-424.

Puig-Antich, J. (1982) Major depression and conduct disorder in prepuberty. J. Am. Acad. Child Psychiatry 21, 118-128.

Puig-Antich, J., Blau, S., Marz, N., Greenhill, L. L., and Chambers, W. (1978) Prepubertal major depressive disorder: a pilot study. J. Am. Acad. Child Psychiatry 17, 695-707.

Puig-Antich, J., Chambers, W., Halpern, F., Hanlon, C., and Sachar, E. J. (1979a) Cortisol hypersecretion in prepubertal depressive illness: a preliminary report. Psychoneuroendocrinology 4, 191-197.

Puig-Antich, J., Goetz, R., Hanlon, C., Davies, M., Thompson, J., Chambers, W. J., Tabrizi, M. A., and Weitzman, E. D. (1982) Sleep architecture and REM sleep measures in prepubertal children with major depression: a controlled study. Arch. Gen. Psychiatry 39, 932-939.

Puig-Antich, J., Goetz, R., Hanlon, C., Tabrizi, M. A., Davies, M., and Weitzman, E. D. (1983) Sleep architecture and REM sleep measures in prepubertal major depressives: studies during recovery from the depressive episode in a drug-free state. Arch. Gen. Psychiatry 40, 187-192.

Puig-Antich, J., Orvaschel, H., Tabrizi, M. A., and Chambers, W. (1980) The Schedule for Affective Disorders and Schizophrenia for School-Age Children - Epidemiologic Version (Kiddie-SADS-E), 3rd ed. New York State Psychiatric Institute and Yale University School of Medicine, New York.

Puig-Antich, J., Perel, J. M., Lupatkin, W., Chambers, W. J., Shea, C., Tabrizi, M. A., and Stiller, R. L. (1979b) Plasma levels of imipramine (IMI) and desmethylimipramine (DMI) and clinical response in prepubertal major depressive disorder. J. Am. Acad. Child Psychiatry 18, 616-627.

Puig-Antich, J., Tabrizi, M. A., Davies, M., Goetz, R., Chambers, W. J., Halpern, F., and Sachar, E. J. (1981) Prepubertal endogenous major depressives hyposecrete growth hormone in response to insulin-induced hypoglycemia. Biol. Psychiatry 16, 801-819.

Rapoport, J. L., Mikkelson, E. J., Zavadil, A., Nee, L., Gruenau, C., Mendelson, W., and Gillen, J. C. (1980) Childhood enuresis, II. Psychopathology, tricyclic concentrations in plasma and antienuretic effects. Arch. Gen. Psychiatry 37, 1146-1152.

Rapoport, J., Quinn, P., Bradbard, G., Riddle, G., and Brookes, E. (1974) Imipramine and methylphenidate treatments of hyperactive boys: a double-blind comparison. Arch. Gen. Psychiatry 30, 789-793.

Reich, W., Herjanic, B., Welner, Z., and Gandhy, P. R. (1982) Development of a structured psychiatric interview for children: agreement and diagnosis comparing child and parent interviews. J. Abnor. Child Psychology 10, 325-336.

Riddle, K. D. and Rapoport, J. L. (1976) A 2-year follow-up of 72 hyperactive boys. J. Nerv. Men. Dis. 162, 126-134.

Rie, H. E. (1966) Depression in childhood: a survey of some pertinent contributions. J. Am. Acad. Child Psychiatry 5, 653-685.

Robins, L. N. (1979) Longitudinal methods in the study of normal and pathological development. In: Grundlagen und Methoden der Psychiatrie, vol. 1 (Kisker, K. P., Meyer, J. E., Muller, C., and Stromgren, E., eds), Springer-Verlag, Heidelberg, pp. 627-684.

Rutter, M. (1966) Children of Sick Parents. Maudsley Monograph No. 16, Oxford University Press, London.

Rutter, M. (1972) Diagnostic validity in child psychiatry. Adv. Biol. Psychiatry 2, 2-22.

Rutter, M., Tizard, J., and Whitmore, K. (1970) Education, Health and Behavior. Longman, London.

Sachar, E. J. (1982) Endocrine abnormalities in depression. In: Handbook of Affective Disorders (Paykel, E. S., ed.), Gilford Press, New York, pp. 191-201.

Sachar, E. J., Altman, N., Gruen, P. H., Glassman, A., Halpern, F. S., and Sassin, J. (1975) Human growth hormone response to levodopa. Arch. Gen. Psychiatry 32, 502-503.

Sachar, E. J., Frantz, A., Altman, N., and Sassin, J. (1973a) Growth hormone and prolactin in unipolar and bipolar depressed patients: responses to hypoglycemia and L-dopa. Am. J. Psychiatry 130, 1362-1367.

Sachar, E. J., Hellman, L., Roffwarg, H. P., Halpern, F. S., Fukushima, D. K., and Gallagher, T. F. (1973b) Disrupted 24 hr pattern of cortisol secretion in psychotic depression. Arch. Gen. Psychiatry 28, 19-25.

Schildkraut, J. J. (1965) The catecholamine hypothesis of affective disorders: a review of supporting evidence. Am. J. Psychiatry 122, 509-522.

Schou, M. (1968) Lithium in psychiatric therapy and prophylaxis. J. Psychiatric Res. 6, 67-95.

Seligman, M. E. P. (1975) Helplessness: On Depression, Development and Death. Freeman, San Francisco.

Shader, R. I., Jackson, A. H., and Dedes, L. M. (1974) The antiaggressive effects of lithium in man. Psychopharmacology 40, 17-21.

Shapiro, M. F. and Lehman, A. F. (1983) The diagnosis of depression in different clinical settings: an analysis of the literature on the dexamethasone suppression test. J. Nerv. Men. Dis. 171, 714-720.

Sheard, M. H. (1975) Lithium in the treatment of aggression. J. Nerv. Men. Dis. 160, 108-115.

Smythe, G. A., Brandstater, J. F., and Lazarus, L. (1979) Acute effects of lithium on central dopamine and serotonin activity reflected by inhibition of prolactin and growth hormone secretion in the rat. Austral. J. Biol. Sci. 32, 329-334.

Spitzer, R. L. and Endicott, J. (1978) Schedule for Affective Disorders and Schizophrenia, 3rd ed. National Institute of Mental Health, Rockville, Maryland.

Spitzer, R. L., Endicott, J., and Robins, E. (1978) Research diagnostic criteria: rationale and reliability. Arch. Gen. Psychiatry 35, 773-782.

Staton, R. D. and Brumback, R. A. (1981) Non-specificity of motor hyperactivity as a diagnostic criterion. Perceptual and Motor Skills 52, 323-332.

Staton, R. D., Wilson, H., and Brumback, R. A. (1962) Cognitive improvements associated with tricyclic antidepressant treatment of childhood major depressive illness. Perceptual and Motor Skills 53, 219-234.

Stewart, M. A. (1970) Hyperactive children. Sci. Amer. 222, 94-98.

Tessing, E. P. and Lefkowitz, M. M. (1982) Childhood depression: a 6-month follow-up study. J. Consulting and Clin. Psychology 50, 778-780.

Toolan, J. M. (1962) Depression in children and adolescents. Am. J. Orthopsychiatry 32, 404-414.

Trotter, R. J. (1981) Psychiatry for the 80's. Science News 119, 348-349.

Ulrich, R., Shaw, D. H., and Kupfer, D. J. (1980) The effects of aging on sleep. Sleep 3, 31-40.

Vogel, G. W., Vogel, F., and McAbee, R. S. (1980) Improvement of depression by REM sleep deprivation: new findings and a theory. Arch. Gen. Psychiatry 37, 247-253.

Weinberg, W. A. and Brumback, R. A. (1976) Mania in childhood, case studies and literature review. Am. J. Dis. Children 130, 380-385.

Weinberg, W. A., Rutman, J., Sullivan, L., Penick, E. C., and Dietz, S. G. (1973) Depression in children referred to an educational diagnostic center: diagnosis and treatment. Behav. Pediatrics 83, 1065-1072.

Weiss, C. C., O'Reilly, P. P., and Hesbacher, P. (1972) Perphenazine-amitriptyline in neurotic underachieving students: a controlled study. Dis. Nerv. Sys. 9, 318-326.

Weissman, M. M., Prusoff, B. A., Gammon, G. D., Merikangas, K. R., Leckman, J. F., and Kidd, K. K. (1984) Psychopathology in the children (ages 6-18) of depressed and normal parents. J. Am. Acad. Child Psychiatry 23, 78-84.

Welner, Z. (1978) Childhood depression: an overview. J. Nerv. Men. Dis. 166, 588-593.

Winsberg, B., Goldstein, S., Yepes, L., and Perel, J. (1975) Imipramine and electrocardiographic abnormalities in hyperactive children. *Am. J. Psychiatry* **132**, 542–545.

Winsberg, B., Perel, J., Hurwic, M., and Klutch, A. (1974) Imipramine protein binding and pharmacokinetics in children. In: *The Phenothiazines and Structurally Related Drugs* (Forrest, I., Carr, J. C., and Usdin, E., eds), Raven Press, New York, pp. 425–432.

Youngerman, J. and Canino, I. A. (1978) Lithium carbonate use in children and adolescents: a survey of the literature. *Arch. Gen. Psychiatry* **35**, 216–224.

Zametkin, A. and Rapoport, J. L. (1983) Tricyclic antidepressants and children. In: *Drugs in Psychiatry*, vol. 1 (Burrows, G. D., Norman, T. R., and Davies, B., eds), Elsevier, New York, pp. 129–148.

Zis, A. P. and Goodwin, F. K. (1982) The amine hypothesis. In: *Handbook of Affective Disorders* (Paykel, E. S., ed.), The Guilford Press, New York, pp. 175–190.

16.

THE CHEMOTHERAPY OF AFFECTIVE DISORDERS IN THE ELDERLY

B. Pitt

Special Considerations

Special considerations in the treatment of affective disorders in the elderly include:
1. Difficulties in diagnosis:
    a) Distinguishing normal from pathological emotional states.
    b) Distinguishing psychological from physical disorder.
    c) Distinguishing functional from organic mental disorder.
    d) Atypical presentations.
2. Concomitant physical disorders and medications.
3. Compliance.
4. The alteration in pharmacokinetics and pharmacodynamics with ageing.
5. Low threshold for adverse drug reactions.

Prevalence

Community surveys (e.g. Kay et al., 1964) of elderly people at home show that depression is relatively common. While 1-2 per cent of those over 65 suffer from a severe form of the disorder, 8-12 per cent show affective disorder of a milder, neurotic or reactive type. In the Duke longitudinal study (Busse, 1978) 20 per cent of subjects reported significant depressive episodes over the course of three years. Weissman and Myers (1978), using the Research Diagnostic Criteria for a community sample of 111 people over the age of 66, found a prevalence of major depression of 5.4 per cent, but a lower prevalence of minor depression (2.7 per cent). Blazer and Williams (1980) found that 14.7 per cent of almost 1,000 people over age 65 in the community

Affective Disorders in the Elderly

exhibited significant dysphoric symptoms. In the United States:United Kingdom Cross National Project's Geriatric Community Study (Gurland et al., 1983) a pervasive state of depression was identified in 12-13 per cent of subjects in New York and London, while the more clinically obvious manic depressive disorder prevailed in 2.5 per cent of the New York elderly population and 1.3 per cent of Londoners.

Diagnosis

Although common, depression is not all that easily diagnosed in old age. For one thing, little is known of the normal lifestyle of the elderly, so that a wide range of behaviour may be interpreted as normal for that age. For another, depressed old people rarely complain of actual depression but instead describe malaise, lassitude, anorexia, insomnia, constipation and various other psychosomatic or hypochondriacal concerns which suggest physical rather than mental disorder. They may complain of a poor or fading memory (which organically demented old people uncommonly do) and indeed exhibit so much cognitive impairment that the phrase 'depressive pseudodementia' (Kiloh, 1961; McAllister, 1983; Wells, 1979) has been used to describe a condition so diagnostically fraught that, as Kiloh has stated, it endangers the patient's safety and the doctor's reputation. Mildly to moderately depressed old people become less active and more introverted and stay indoors, almost housebound, moping, and thus may never consult the doctor at all.

In Barraclough's study (1971) of suicide among the elderly on the South coast of England, the majority of those who took their lives appeared to have been suffering depressive illness of months, rather than years, in duration and to have consulted their doctors a week or two before they died. Although tranquillisers and hypnotics were widely prescribed, few were given antidepressants, either because the doctors were, perhaps, nervous about administering them to the elderly, did not recognise whether or how severely their patients were depressed, or doubted their appropriateness or efficacy. To younger people the elderly may seem so burdened by physical problems, bereavement, impoverishment, isolation, dependency, short expectation of life, inactivity and the loss of the status of being employed and having a role and purpose that any depression is regarded as normal, reactive and

Affective Disorders in the Elderly

remediable only in the unlikely event that their lot can be improved. Yet it is apparently not normal for old people to lament their misfortunes, but rather to 'count their blessings' (DHSS, 1978). After all, many have endured lives of such hardship and insecurity that their present state, with such benefits as electric light, central heating, indoor lavatories, hot running water, radio, television, a pension, a health service and a protected tenancy, seems almost privileged.

In the Edinburgh community study (Williamson et al., 1964) general practitioners were unaware of three quarters of the cases of depression among the elderly living at home. To the possible reasons given already must be added ignorance--it is impossible to diagnose that of which one is unaware, and in the past the education of medical students in psychiatry, let alone psychogeriatrics, was perfunctory in the extreme.

This should improve now that academic departments of psychiatry are so widespread and many teaching hospitals have psychiatrists with a special interest in the elderly on their staffs. But even the better trained doctors may be distracted by the physical disorder which the patient may have as well as depression, and which may indeed be an important factor in the depression, but may be coincidental and not responsible for the most troublesome symptoms. There is a marked tendency among doctors to regard physical disease as more important than and outweighing mental disease.

The fear of missing a physical illness sometimes unbalances judgement. Likewise depression may be underestimated when it accompanies dementia, as it not infrequently does, especially when the dementia is multi-infarct. Dementia is deemed to supercede depression in the hierarchy of mental disorder, but 'organic dementia' may be treatable with considerable relief of distress and disturbed behaviour.

It is typical of illness in the elderly to present atypically, and so it is with depression, which may thus confound diagnosis. Not only may depressed old people mimic dementia, but they may also show such florid behaviour disorder as screaming, soiling, abuse of hypnotics and drugs, taking to bed, histrionic falling, food refusal with alarming weight loss, cantankerous abuse, scratching, biting, importunate emergency calls to family, friends, the doctor, hospital, police and social services and urgent demands for meals-on-wheels, home helps, sheltered housing and a residential or nursing home. There is evidence (Bergmann et al., 1978) that social workers and others tend to respond to such demands by providing the services and thus, perhaps, increasing and continuing dependency (and using a valuable resource inappropriately) while the depression goes unrecognised.

Mania and hypomania are far less common than depression, but do recur or present for the first time in old age and may then be misdiagnosed. An acute manic episode, especially when precipitated by physical illness, or post-operatively or by drugs, e.g. steroids, may resemble delirium, with the pressure of talk, inattention, and distractibility being taken for disjointed incoherence and confusion, especially where the patient is more restless than euphoric. Hypomania may be attributed to eccentricity, a difficult personality or even delinquency (e.g. in a normally reticent old man who becomes sexually disinhibited and starts to steal women's underwear).

The dexamethasone suppression test (DST) may be of some assistance in the diagnosis of major depressive illness in the elderly and in predicting the likelihood of response to chemotherapy or ECT (Carroll et al., 1981), but false positives have been reported in dementia (Spar and Gerner, 1982) and it seems that these are not due to co-existing depression. So the value of the test in distinguishing pseudodementia from organic dementia is limited. Georgotas (1983) suggests that such electro-physiological measures as sleep, EEG and auditory evoked potentials may prove of diagnostic value, but as yet this work is experimental.

The physical disorders which should be distinguished from depressive illness are manifold--anaemia, malignant disease, Parkinson's disease, thyroid dysfunction, diabetes, renal failure and drug-induced lassitude being among the more common--and will usually be detected by the competent, conscientious physician. To diagnose depression when that is the chief cause of distress and disability, the clinician must be aware of its high prevalence in the elderly, and how and under what circumstances it may present. Important pointers are a previous history of affective illness and the relationship of the condition to recent severe life events (Murphy, 1982).

The various dichotomous classifications of depression--endogenous and exogenous or reactive, psychotic and neurotic, typical and atypical, masked and unmasked, primary and secondary, unipolar and

Affective Disorders in the Elderly

bipolar--may be applied to the elderly with varying success. Functional or organic (depression associated with dementia) is another distinction to be made in old age. The suggestion (e.g. Bergmann, 1972) that those whose depression first occurs, or recurs after a long interval, in old age, are less likely to have a family history of affective illness and more likely to be physically ill than those who had their first episodes when younger indicates another possible differentiation, though it was not confirmed by Murphy's (1982) study. However, Jacoby (1981) has shown that people suffering first onset of depression very late in life have brain ventricular enlargement intermediate between that of normal and demented subjects of like age, and a high mortality.

Broadly, it is helpful clinically to perceive depression in old age as more or less <u>severe</u>, and taking an agitated or retarded form (Pitt, 1974). Thus severe agitated depression corresponds to the outmoded involutional melancholia with extreme anguish, importunate pleas for reassurance which cannot be accepted, and delusions of guilt, unworthiness, poverty, doom and bizarre bodily dysfunction. In severe retarded depression the patient has little or nothing to say and refusal of food and fluids threatens life. 'Biological' features--weight loss, diurnal variation of mood (worst in the morning) and late insomnia--are prominent in severe depression, and there is a preoccupation with suicide. These characteristics are to be found in the Diagnostic and Statistical Manual of Mental Disorders, third edition (DSM III) under the diagnostic criteria for a major depressive episode.

Anxiety is prominent in agitated milder depression. It is mainly somatised and is thus the basis of hypochondriasis which, lacking the bizarre quality of the severe form of illness, is more likely to be taken literally by the doctor. Thus Bergmann and Eastham (1974) found 14 per cent of the patients over 65 in a general medical ward to be suffering from this form of depression, to which little attention was being given while their physical symptoms were investigated.

The symptoms are manifold, dizziness, tinnitus, tension headache, burning in the throat and abdomen, dysphagia, fullness, flatulence, diarrhea, constipation, chest pain, shortness of breath, fatigue, backache, tingling, itching, numbness being among them. When investigations prove negative, or fail to detect a physical cause which adequately explains the symptoms, or do not lead to effective treatment, neither the patient nor the doctor is greatly satisfied. When eventually a psychiatric basis is considered (generally 'anxiety state', 'functional overlay' or even 'hysteria'), the usual prescription is a tranquilliser, which may indeed give some symptomatic relief, but it tends to be temporary and there is the risk of dependency and drug-induced lassitude.

Milder retarded depression, characterised by apathy, anhedonia and withdrawal, is easily overlooked and may never be presented to the physician. Former interests dwindle, the effort to converse and be sociable is too much, and there is a tendency to mope indoors, ignoring radio, television, and newspapers. Thus, if questioned the patient is ill-informed and in any case disinclined to try very hard to give correct answers, and this and the slowness of the responses may suggest an early dementia. With this thought in mind the diagnostician, even if a history and evidence of a personality change are obtained, may fall into error.

Aetiological Considerations in Treatment

A logical basis is given for the chemotherapy of depressive illness in old age by certain neurobiochemical effects of ageing. Finch (1977) notes decreases in animal and human brain levels of dopamine and noradrenaline, and increases in dopamine beta-hydroxylase and monoamine oxidase. Thus lower levels of biogenic amines may increase the susceptibility of the aging brain to depression. Also, as Bergmann (1982) points out, elderly people have a different sleep pattern from younger ones, with shorter sleep, and REM latency and high REM density (Kupfer et al., 1978) which may reflect changes in circadian rhythm which may increase vulnerability to depression.

Murphy (1982) found a relationship between physical illness and the onset of depression in 28 per cent of her patients, while only 6 per cent of her normal controls were physically ill--a highly significant difference. Other severe life events were also significantly more common among depressives (separations, deaths, severe illness of or unpleasant disclosure about someone close, enforced change of residence, financial/material loss) as were major social difficulties.

So rare is it to meet depression developing for

the first time in the senium without a family history of the disorder or the recent stress and strain described by Murphy (1982) that if one does so it is wise to look very hard for undisclosed personal problems or occult physical disease, notably malignant (Whitlock et al., 1979).

The logical approach to the treatment of depression in old age, then, encompasses social and psychological supports to try to alleviate and compensate for losses and social problems, and pharmacotherapy which may remedy the postulated biochemical deficits which render the old person liable to react to these stresses with excessive and prolonged depression.

Treating Depression in the Physically Ill
===

Not only is depression difficult to diagnose in the presence of physical illness, which may itself cause anorexia, weight loss, anergy and insomnia, but it is deceptive to treat. That it is worth treating seems probable, given that depression may compound disability, delay rehabilitation and hasten mortality ('turning the face to the fall'). However, in the presence of nausea or malabsorption, or conditions affecting the heart or hepatic and renal function and thus the metabolism and clearance of drugs, the choice, dosage and route of medication pose major problems. Reduction in plasma albumin concentrations and reduced plasma binding occurs commonly in sick old people and may increase the concentration of unbound bioavailable drug. These problems are compounded by possible <u>interactions</u> between drugs given for depression and those given for physical disease. Imipramine, for example, interferes with the absorption of L-dopa (Morgan et al., 1975) and tricyclic antidepressants may block the antihypertensive action of guanethidine, debrisoquine, bethanidine and clonidine and potentiate warfarin.

The elderly, tending to suffer diverse ills at the same time, are at risk of polypharmacy. Williamson and Chopin (1980) found that over 80 per cent of patients admitted to geriatric wards were taking prescribed drugs, and Kelloway and McCrae (1973) that the risk of adverse drug reactions increases linearly with the number of medications used. Lawson and Jick (1976) found a significantly higher adverse drug reaction rate (26 per cent) in American patients admitted to medical wards, who received an average of 9.4 drugs per admission, than

Affective Disorders in the Elderly

in Scottish patients (15 per cent) matched by age, sex, stay in hospital, survival and diagnosis, who received an average of only 4.5 drugs. Stanasek and Franklin (1978) found that the 23 per cent of 3028 veterans attending out-patient clinics who were over 60 received 35 per cent of the potentially interacting drug combinations. Of 12,836 drugs prescribed, 935 (7.2 per cent) were pairs with potential for drug interactions. The elderly are also major self-prescribers of over-the-counter drugs (Williamson and Chopin, 1980). Cooper et al. (1975) described almost a quarter of nursing home admissions as due to drug interactions.

Nevertheless, physically ill or even dying patients may well benefit, in quality of mood and, perhaps, tolerance of pain, improved function and prolongation of life, from the relief of depression by chemotherapy. This is an under, if not virtually unresearched area with few well-founded guidelines. Until these are available a judicious, selective, cautious, gradual approach with careful monitoring is commended rather than no treatment at all.

Compliance

Compliance with medication is a notorious problem in the elderly (Evans and Spelman, 1983). The patient, the prescriber, other people and the prescription itself may all be responsible.

The <u>patient</u> may fail to read or understand the place, purpose and regime of the prescription because of impaired sight or hearing, confusion, distraction by anxiety, or depressive preoccupation. There may be aversion to medication in general or to this particular prescription on the grounds that it is for 'nerves' rather than a bodily ailment or a previous unsatisfactory experience with something similar. Negative placebo responders have great problems in taking drugs, especially antidepressants. There may be a wish for a companion, a service or a change of abode rather than medication. The patient may feel coerced into the consultation, or may dislike the doctor or his/her attitude. Negativism may be part of the mental state (notably in depression) or there may be reluctance to get well and risk relinquishing dependency. Very anxious patients worry inordinately about exactly when to take drugs, e.g. in relationship to meals, and about possible side-effects and interactions. Impatience when (as is usual with antidepressants) there is no benefit after a week or two, or unex-

Affective Disorders in the Elderly

pectedly rapid improvement may both affect compliance. Some patients want to continue to take alcohol, so forego medication. Others may find the cost prohibitive. Abuse of such drugs as tranquillisers, hypnotics and laxatives by the elderly is also non-compliance.

The <u>prescriber</u> who rushes the prescription, fails to explain why the drug is prescribed and how to take it (at all, or in terms which the patient can understand), uses too complicated a regime, fails to take account of other drugs prescribed, gives too little or too much, does not use his or her imagination to consider how the condition and circumstances of this patient might affect the ability to comply, keeps poor records so that (s)he is not always aware of what (s)he and others have/are given/ing and lacks the salesmanship to persuade the patient to put up with the side-effects of antidepressants and keep taking the tablets to reap the benefit is unlikely to secure full compliance with the treatment of depression.

<u>Others</u>, such as spouses, children, siblings and friends, may affect the patient's compliance by discouragement, domination, competition or confusion. Families often abhor medication for a patient's depression and feel that self-control, pulling the self together and even 'a boot in the backside' are more appropriate. Dominant spouses may control the patient's drug-taking according to whims and their own needs for a sicker or healthier partner. Competition and/or confusion may explain the situation where a couple take each other's medications.

Finally, <u>the prescription</u> may be ineffective, be hedged about by alarming precautions (it really does demand salesmanship to persuade a depressed patient to give informed consent to a course of MAOIs), produce such distressing side-effects that the cure is worse than the disease, or be thwarted by 'child-proof' containers which the patient cannot open.

<u>Intelligent non-compliance</u> (Weintraub, 1981) occurs when the patient discerns that, quantitatively or qualitatively, the prescription is wrong.

Among measures which <u>enhance</u> compliance among older patients, in addition to those obvious from what has been set out above, are clear, informative labelling, daily prescriptions, administration by community nurses and at day units, and careful monitoring at home, out-patient clinics and in hospital (including serum assays) of how the drugs prescribed are being taken.

Affective Disorders in the Elderly

Changes in Pharmacokinetics and Pharmacodynamics with Ageing

Ageing affects absorption, distribution, metabolism and excretion of drugs, increasing the plasma half-life by as much as 50 per cent. Much the most important factor increasing drug concentration in the body is the decline in renal clearance from early adulthood onwards (Hansen et al., 1970; Triggs et al., 1975).

<u>Absorption</u> may be reduced by reduced gastric acidity and gastro-intestinal motility and blood flow, but this is of doubtful importance.

<u>Distribution</u> is affected by decreased total body water, serum albumin and lean body mass, and increased body fat (Rossman, 1980). Thus less drug is protein-bound, and more is bio-available in the body water and tissues (Vestal, 1978), increasing the effects of a standard dose. On the other hand, antidepressants are generally lipophilic and therefore accumulated in the increased body fat, which is likely to prolong their action. Central blood flow is diminished but the blood-brain barrier may decrease with ageing, modifying the effects of drugs on the target organ. Most drugs given for depression are <u>metabolised</u> by the liver. With ageing, liver mass and blood flow decrease. Phase I drug metabolism (hydroxylation), catalysed by microsomal oxidase enzyme systems, is slowed by ageing, whereas Phase II, detoxification by conjugation with, for example, glucuronic acid, is much less affected. Environmental factors, notably smoking (Jusho, 1978), may modify these ageing changes.

<u>Excretion</u> by the kidneys is affected by decreased renal plasma flow, glomerular filtration rate and tubular secretory function. Overall, ageing definitely prolongs the actions of most, if not all, psychotropic drugs (Lader, 1982). The formula:

$$\bar{C}_\infty = 1.44 \times \frac{fD \times t_{1/2\beta}}{Vd \times \tau}$$

is used to determine the mean steady state concentration of drug in the blood, $\bar{C}_\infty$, where fD is the absorbed dose, $t_{1/2\beta}$ the elimination half-life, Vd the apparent volume of distribution in the body and τ the dose interval (Friedel, 1980). Nies et al. (1977) found that ageing increased the steady state

Affective Disorders in the Elderly

concentrations of the antidepressants amitriptyline, desipramine, imipramine and mianserin, though not of nortriptyline.

Without a knowledge of the effects of ageing on pharmacodynamics, however, the changes in pharmacokinetics do not suffice to explain drug actions. Thus studies of propranolol showed that age was associated with a two-fold increase in blood propranolol concentrations, but a four-fold decrease in sensitivity to the drug (Wood and Feely, 1984). Generally the response of tissue systems to drugs declines with ageing. In the brain, the number of receptor cells is reduced, as is their binding (Roth, 1975). The increase in adverse drug reactions in the elderly is related to pharmacodynamic changes (Vestal, 1978).

The Place of Chemotherapy in Affective Disorders in Old Age

Once an affective disorder has been diagnosed a decision must be made about how to treat it. Occasionally the process of reaching a diagnosis is sufficiently therapeutic. The patient recognises the nature of the problem, is helped by learning what it is and is not, and feels better able to cope. Sometimes such coping is assisted by psychotherapy and behavioural therapy.

<u>Psychotherapy</u> (Stever, 1982) is appropriate where dynamic problems such as fear of dependency, isolation or death, grief or conflict with the spouse or a member of the family seem to be contributing to the disorder.' Abreaction, insight and mastery may be achieved. Techniques such as Butler's (1968) life review and Goldfarb's (1962) approach to the patient who is frantically searching for aid are useful. Psychotherapy may be given individually, to a couple, a family or in a group. Reasonably articulate, motivated patients able to grasp the concepts involved and no more than moderately depressed are the most suitable.

<u>Cognitive behavioural therapy</u> (Beck, 1967) which aims systematically to change the patient's negative view of life to a more positive outlook may be of value in the elderly (Emery, 1963) and operant conditioning may successfully modify behaviour disorder associated with protracted and atypical depression (Pitt, 1982).

All depressed patients should be treated with empathy and encouraged by informed optimism. <u>Social</u>

measures, befriending, support, rehousing, financial assistance, help at home, introduction to a club or an activities centre may mitigate stress and loneliness.

Electroconvulsive therapy, though unpopular with the public and many patients, is still the most effective treatment for severe depression. It is used when a speedy relief of the suffering of an anguished, psychotic or suicidal patient is needed, where life is threatened by food and fluid refusal, where there has been no response to appropriate medication in proper dosage or where the side-effects of such medication preclude its further use. It is a safe treatment (which may be given to elderly outpatients) with a mortality of about 1/10,000 treatments, though 0.3 per cent of those treated are reported as suffering lasting memory impairment (Fink, 1978). The use of unilateral ECT, over the non-dominant hemisphere, reduces this risk.

For the chronically, severely depressed patient with a refractory depression which used to respond to ECT and/or antidepressants but now does so no longer, psychosurgery, e.g. stereotactic tractotomy (Bridges and Bartlett, 1973) offers the hope of lasting respite. However, the patient's informed consent is required in most countries and often the nature of the mental disorder is such that the patient is not deemed to be sufficiently rational to be informed, or is too gloomy and negative to consent.

Except in the mildest, most reactive cases (e.g. distress after a very recent widowing, or clearly related to current problems and fluctuating as they worsen or improve) there is deemed to be an important place for drugs in the treatment of depression (and always in the treatment of mania and hypomania). It must be admitted, however, that this place has been largely reached by clinical consensus rather than established by systematic clinical trials. Most controlled trials have an upper age limit of 65 or 70, debar even the mildly confused and those with physical illness and on other drugs and thus exclude most of the typical depressives in a psychogeriatric practice.

Jarvik et al. (1983) treated 36 patients over age 65 over nine months in a double blind placebo-controlled study of imipramine and doxepin and found that the benefits of antidepressants clearly outweighed the adverse effects. Whereas only a fifth of those on placebo remitted, a half of those on the drugs got better according to the criteria of clinical evaluation and a reduction by a mean of 7 on the Hamilton Depressive Rating Scale.

Antidepressants have had a rather bad press lately. Their uncomfortable anticholinergic effects, hypotensive and sedative qualities, cardiotoxicity, dangerousness in overdosage and the risk of drug interactions have made many doctors wary of their use in the elderly. Some of these problems have, however, been exaggerated, while the risks to independence and life expectancy, to say nothing of the protracted misery of remaining depressed, have been underestimated, especially by non-psychiatrists. In follow-up studies of two Newcastle community samples (Kay and Bergmann, 1966; Kay et al., 1970) more depressives than normal entered institutions and their mortality (especially that of men) was increased.

Before prescribing it is important to ascertain as far as possible what antidepressants the patient has taken or may now be taking, the dosage and the duration of the course, the desirable and undesirable effects, and any other current medications. If a house call is made it is a good opportunity to track down the medication. If the patient attends a clinic (s)he should be asked to bring the medication along (Blazer and Friedman, 1979). The symptoms it is hoped to relieve should be carefully documented and explained to the patient, e.g. insomnia, agitation, anorexia, anergy are likely to be improved before there is any lifting of the depression. The principle of 'start low, go slow' should be followed, with a gradual increase in dosage until either the patient is better, has clearly not responded, or side-effects are too troublesome. It is important, however, to understand, and to explain to the patient, that what may seem to be side-effects (e.g. a feeling of pressure over the head, muzziness, agitation) may be manifestations of the as yet unrelieved depression. The patient needs to be helped to tolerate the wait for eventual recovery and the early side-effects (provided that they are not quite incapacitating) with the encouragement that they are likely to subside as the benefit of treatment becomes apparent.

While giving the drug once daily, at bedtime, improves compliance, morning hangover may necessitate divided doses. The help of an alert, informed member of the family is most valuable, as may be a dispenser apparatus partitioned two ways, into days and times, if the patient is being treated at home.

The decision to treat in <u>hospital</u> is determined

by the severity of the illness, danger of suicide or self-neglect, physical frailty, a need to ensure compliance, where more intensive therapies such as combined antidepressants or electroplexy are undertaken, and by the lack of adequate help and supervision at home. A day hospital is a useful intermediate facility. Supervision during treatment involves assessing compliance (in which plasma levels are valuable), response, side-effects, the course of the affective illness, and the attitudes of significant people in contact with the patient. Once it is clear that a complying patient who has had long enough on a large enough dose (or, better, at a therapeutic plasma level) to respond is not doing so, it is time to switch to another treatment.

Tricyclic antidepressants (Table 16.1) are the drugs of first choice in the great majority of depressive illnesses in the elderly. Imipramine, the longest established, is in the writer's opinion unsuitable for the elderly because of its liability to cause hypotension and serious falls. Amitriptyline, which has been available for about as long as imipramine, is still widely used. It is an effective antidepressant, so sedative as to be useful for the sleepless depressed as well as in agitated depression, although hangover and drowsiness by day can be troublesome. The most serious drawback, though, is its powerful anticholinergic action, causing dry mouth, constipation, blurred vision, urinary retention, sweating, and, occasionally but most seriously, confusion. (There may be a connection here with the acetylcholine deficiency in Alzheimer's disease, and tricyclics are theoretically inadvisable in depression associated with that disease and in practice usually ineffective.) There is generally a tendency for drowsiness and the anticholinergic side-effects to dwindle after a week or two, after which those who can put up with them may have their reward.

The dose required to achieve a therapeutic level (about 50 ng/ml; Lader, 1982) varies a good deal (Carr and Hobson, 1977). Generally the starting dose should be 25 mg at night in a single or divided dosage according to the patient's condition and circumstances until a satisfactory plasma level has been obtained, side-effects are apparent and becoming troublesome, the depression is lifting, or, after three weeks at a therapeutic level, there is little or no response.

Other tricyclics are more or less sedative or anticholinergic. The dose is similar to that of

Table 16.1: Antidepressant drugs for the elderly: monoamine re-uptake inhibitors

Drug	Dose/Day	Indication	Comments, side-effects
A. Tricyclics			
1. Sedative			
Amitriptyline	25-150 mg	Moderate - severe depression	Anti-cholinergic, cardiotoxic, cause weight gain
Doxepin	25-150 mg	Agitation	
Trimipramine	25-150 mg	Agitation Insomnia	Diurnal somnolence
2. Less sedative			
Nortriptyline	25-150 mg		
Dothiepin	25-150 mg	Most patients	Generally well tolerated
3. Not sedative			
(Imipramine)	25-150 mg	Retarded	Hypotension, results in falling
Clomipramine	25-150 mg	Resistant	Powerful, strongly anticholinergic, may release agitation
4. Stimulant			
Protriptyline	20-60 mg	Retarded	Powerful, strongly anticholinergic, may release agitation
B. Second Generation			
1. Tetracyclics			
Maprotiline	25-130 mg	Most patients	Well tolerated but ? potency
Mianserin	30-120 mg	Agitation, insomnia	Very sedative
2. Nomifensine	50-200 mg	Parkinsonism	Dopamine agonist
3. Trazodone	100-300 mg	Cardiac disease	? potency, sedative

Affective Disorders in the Elderly

amitriptyline except for protriptyline, the most stimulating of the group, which is somewhat lower. In the case of the nortriptyline at least, a 'therapeutic window' effect has been observed (Montgomery et al., 1977) so that too high plasma levels are as ineffective as too low. Jarvik et al. (1983) noted that doxepin was better tolerated by elderly subjects than imipramine, but for both drugs response in the first week of treatment was a good predictor of ultimate remission.

Trimipramine is an exceedingly sedative tricyclic, useful for those who sleep badly in that benefit can be almost immediate. Clomipramine is a powerful antidepressant with anticholinergic effects matching those of amitriptyline, useful when other tricyclics have failed and for atypical depressions in which neurotic (i.e. phobic and obsessional symptoms) are to the fore. This drug can be administered, in a crisis, in an intravenous drip. Probably the most generally useful tricyclics for the elderly, neither too sedative nor too anticholinergic but nevertheless effective, are doxepin, nortriptyline and dothiepin, currently the subject of an extensive multi-centre comparison with amitriptyline in the U.K.

The vexing question of cardiotoxic effects has been ably reviewed by Orme (1984). Studies in Aberdeen (Coull et al., 1970) linked the use of amitriptyline with sudden death, though this was not confirmed by the Boston Collaboration Drug Surveillance Program (1972). Anticholinergic activity causes tachycardia and decreases conduction through the atrio-ventricular node; a quinidine-like action on the myocardium may also delay atrio-ventricular conduction. Thus the P-R and Q-T intervals are prolonged. Hypotension is partly due to these mechanisms and, when tricyclics are given in very high doses, to peripheral adrenoreceptor blockade. The antihypertensive effect of adrenergic blocking drugs like bethanidine and centrally acting drugs like methyldopa may be blocked. Nevertheless Veith et al. (1982) concluded that for most patients with mild cardiac disease the risks of tricyclic therapy have been over-emphasized. Orme states that:

i. Patients with mild heart disease (history of myocardial infarction, mild angina) can probably be treated with any antidepressant.

ii. Great care should be taken in using tricyclics in patients with severe heart disease, suffering from heart failure, bundle branch block, heart block in the electrocardiograms, or who

have recently had a myocardial infarction.
iii. There is as yet no clear evidence that the second generation antidepressants are safer than the older tricyclics.

In overdose, tricyclics may cause collapse, convulsions and cardiac arrest, all very dangerous at any age but especially in the elderly. Giving the depressed patient a large supply of the antidepressant gives the means of recovery and of suicide, which must obviously be taken into consideration in the treatment policy. The time of greatest risk is early in the course, when side-effects may be troublesome and benefits invisible.

The second generation antidepressants (Table 16.1) have been developed in the hope of finding faster-acting, more effective, less toxic and more tolerable substitutes for the tricyclics. Most are at least less toxic, though zimeldine, an interesting specific inhibitor of the membrane uptake pump for 5-hydroxytryptamine, had to be withdrawn in 1983 because of an excess of Guillan Barre syndrome reaction, some cases of which proved fatal. Maprotiline is very like the tricyclics but has an ethylene bridge across and at right angles to the central ring and hence is 'tetracyclic'. It specifically inhibits noradrenaline uptake. It is well tolerated by the elderly (Middleton et al., 1978). Some of the effects of mianserin resulting from the blocking of pre-synaptic α-receptors are most unlike those of the tricyclics (Coppen et al., 1976). Trazodone is a triazolopyridine derivative selectively inhibiting 5-hydroxytryptamine uptake, and nomifensine specifically blocks the uptake of noradrenaline and dopamine, so might be deemed particularly suitable for depression associated with Parkinson's disease. Goldstein et al. (1982) compared nomifensine with amitriptyline in the treatment of 33 depressed geriatric patients and found the former more effective in reactive depression and the latter in endogenous depression. Trazodone has been found as effective as the tricyclics in elderly populations (Gerner et al., 1980) and less likely to affect cognition than amitriptyline (Branconnier and Cole, 1981). Nevertheless, drowsiness can be a troublesome side-effect, as it can be with mianserin. Nomifensine can release agitation and viloxazine was given up by many clinicians because it is so often nauseating. Obviously the advantages of a drug's being weakly anticholinergic are much reduced if there are other effects which the patient can barely tolerate.

Reports are now available of the use of bupropion, a structurally unique (single ring) compound with a specific dopamine re-uptake inhibiting action, in the elderly which suggest that it could be particularly useful. Branconnier et al. (1983) compared the effects of 150 mg/day or 450 mg/day of bupropion with 150 mg/day of imipramine or placebo in 63 elderly patients for 35 days and found the new drug as effective as the old with no more adverse effects than the placebo. Kane et al. (1983) also compared bupropion with imipramine and placebo in a double-blind study of 38 patients over age 55 (not very geriatric!) for four weeks and found that it had antidepressant activity and was well tolerated.

Nevertheless, had the advantages of the second generation antidepressants been overwhelming, they would have rendered the old tricyclics obsolete, and this has clearly not happened. This may be partly because clinicians tend to stick to the drugs they know best, particularly when, despite their side-effects, they know that most tricyclics are well tolerated by the elderly, who often benefit from their use. It is likely also that they are put off by the discovery that 'new improved' drugs can have troublesome side-effects and are costly, and by doubts (especially as they tend to try them out on a small number of patients, several of whom suffer from refractory depression or are physically frail) that they really are as effective as their predecessors.

Monoamine Oxidase Inhibitors (Table 16.2)

These antidepressants have had the worst press of all because of their ability to produce a sometimes fatal hypertensive crisis if the patient ingests food with a high tyramine content (Blackwell, 1963). They also interact with a large number of drugs, potentiating barbiturates, pethidine, morphine, insulin, ganglion blocking agents, and indirectly-acting sympathomimetic amines such as ephedrine and dexamphetamine. Interaction with some tricyclics may cause twitching, convulsions, headache, delirium, hyper-pyrexia and death. Their use in the elderly may be hazardous not only because old people are likely to be taking a number of drugs but also because of a tendency to cause orthostatic hypotension.

Nevertheless they are often better tolerated by the elderly than are the tricyclics. They rarely cause a 'drugged' feeling, and many old people are quite capable of avoiding the prohibited foods:

Table 16.2: Antidepressant drugs for the elderly: monoamine oxidase inhibitors (MAOIs) and others

Drug	Dose/Day	Indication	Comments, side-effects
A. MAO Inhibitors			
1. Stimulant			
Tranylcypromine	10-60 mg	Resistant	Hypertensive crisis if taken with tyramine. Drug interactions Sometimes hypotensive Powerful, early stimulation like dexamphetamine
2. Not stimulant		? Organic	
Phenelzine	15-90 mg	Moderate agitated	Usually well tolerated. May be combined with sedative tricyclics.
Isocarboxiazid	10-60 mg	Resistant	
B. Stimulants		Mainly for mild-moderate retarded	
1. Dexamphetamine	5-30 mg	Organic	Little risk of habituation in this group
2. Pemoline	20-80 mg	Frail, retarded	? More effective than caffeine in tea, coffee, or coca-cola
3. Methylphenidate	10-40 mg	Mildly depressed	
C. Monoamine Precursor			
L-Tryptophan	1-3 mg	Resistant	Adjunct to other drugs, especially MAOIs
D. Neuroleptic			
Fluanxol	0.5-3 mg	Moderate, retarded, frail	Anecdotally effective, well tolerated
E. Mood Regulator			
Lithium carbonate	0.5-3 mg	Recurrent, especially bipolar	Need to monitor serum levels. Toxicity, hypothyroidism, nephrogenic diabetes insipidus, weight gain.

Affective Disorders in the Elderly

Chianti wine, for example, rarely features in their diet, and it is easy not to eat cheese. As levels of monoamine oxidase (MAO) increase with ageing there is a sound theoretical base to their use, and in practice they appear to be useful in the treatment of refractory depression, of moderate agitated (neurotic, atypical) depression, and sometimes of depression associated with dementia. They have, however, been studied far less than the monoamine re-uptake inhibitors. Georgotas et al. (1983) studied the effects of phenelzine for 2-7 weeks on a group of elderly patients with major depressive illness resistant to other treatments and obtained a 65 per cent response, sustained during a follow-up period of at least a year.

Phenelzine (30-90 mg/day, in divided dosage) is the most widely used MAO inhibitor, but some old people better tolerate isocarboxazid, 20-60 mg/day. Tranylcypromine is the most likely to cause dangerous interactions and should generally be saved for refractory depressions (10-60 mg/day). Phenelzine and isocarboxazid generally take two to three weeks to start to lift depression. Tranylcypromine, which often has an early amphetamine-like action, may work within days. The occasional dramatic lifting of a long entrenched depression by tranylcypromine is one of the clinician's delightful surprises, though sometimes the benefit is short-lived.

The second generation MAO inhibitor L-deprenil (an inhibitor of MAO-B, the main substrate of which is phenylethylamine) was compared with placebo in a double-blind controlled study of 14 patients on the drug and 13 on placebo only, and proved more effective (Mendlewicz and Youdim, 1983). The great advantage of such a preparation is that it does not interact with tyramine, but its efficacy in the treatment of depression in the elderly has yet to be demonstrated.

In the treatment of refractory depression tricyclics and MAO inhibitors are sometimes combined (Lader, 1983). Tranylcypromine, imipramine and clomipramine should generally be avoided; specific serotonin re-uptake inhibitors are regarded as dangerous. But the combination of sedative tricyclics (amitriptyline, trimipramine), or even one a little less sedative (dothiepin), with phenelzine seems safe enough. The doses used may be as much as for either drug given alone. Evidence from controlled studies that such combinations are more effective than one or the other drug on its own is as yet lacking, but at the anecdotal level occasional successes are reported. This writer has often used such combinations in a busy geropsychiatric practice (Pitt, 1982), where refractory depression is a frequent problem, and found them useful.

Stimulants (Table 16.2)

The place of these drugs is very small. They are sometimes used for the physically frail and retarded and for the confused, who tolerate tricyclics poorly and for whom MAO inhibitors seem somewhat drastic. The most powerful is dextroamphetamine, which used to be widely employed in the treatment of depression until its habituating effects were appreciated and the tricyclics and MAO inhibitors became available. Side-effects include excitement, insomnia and anorexia. It is of special value in depressed demented patients in whom the risk of habituation is irrelevant. Dosage ranges from 5-10 mg once, twice or thrice daily (Kaufmann et al., 1984). Methylphenidate (Katan and Raskind, 1980) and pemoline are used in apathetic, ancient elderly patients who appear to need 'bucking up', although their effectiveness in such cases has not been clearly shown.

Monoamine Precursors (Table 16.2)

The effect of tricyclics and especially, it seems, of MAO inhibitors may be enhanced by the prescription' of L-tryptophan, a precursor of serotonin (5-hydroxytryptamine). The only side-effect of this amino acid appears to be drowsiness. In moderate agitated depression, L-tryptophan is sometimes used alone. The dosage is usually 1-6 g/day, in divided dosage. Walinder et al. (1975) showed the action of clomipramine to be potentiated by L-tryptophan.

Neuroleptics

The major tranquillisers may ameliorate extreme agitation to the extent that the patient feels much relieved, even though there is no specific antidepressant action. Also they may act more quickly than antidepressants. Chlorpromazine, 50-100 mg three times a day, or thioridazine, up to 200 mg three times a day, may be combined with antidepressants for a while in the treatment of severe agitated depression, though chlorpromazine causes much hypotension in the elderly and both phenothiazines are strongly anticholinergic.
 Paranoia may be prominent and persistent in

severe, psychotic depression and may need treatment in its own right. Trifluoperazine is the most valuable drug for the purpose, in doses ranging from 2-30 mg daily. There is the risk of extra-pyramidal side effects which may require anti-Parkinsonian drugs such as orphenadrine, 50-100 mg twice or thrice a day.

Manic and hypomanic old people generally require medication with haloperidol in doses ranging from 3-9 mg/day in divided doses. Again, there may be the need for anti-Parkinsonian agents. The depot preparation haloperidol decanoate may be useful where there are problems with compliance or as a means of preventing relapse--a dose of 100-200 mg every 1-4 weeks by deep intramuscular injection is used.

Flupenthixol in low dose (Table 16.2) appears to be antidepressant (Trimble and Robertson, 1983) and is useful in mild to moderate agitated or retarded depression. It seems to act a little sooner than the conventional antidepressants, and to have a mildly stimulant action which gives it a place in the frail, confused group for which other stimulants may be prescribed. It is generally well tolerated but of no use in severe depression. The dosage is 0.5-1 mg once or twice a day. It should not be given during the day because the patient may find difficulty in getting to sleep.

Mood Regulators (Table 16.2)

Lithium carbonate with its low therapeutic index and need for good compliance is not an easy drug to administer in old age but has a place in the prophylaxis of frequently recurrent affective disorder (especially bipolar) and, occasionally, in the treatment of mania. Renal clearance and the distribution volume of lithium are substantially reduced in the elderly (Chapron et al., 1982), so the risk of toxicity is increased. Roose et al. (1979) found that in patients older than 60 on maintenance lithium therapy, 13 per cent developed toxicity during a period of 18 months. Side-effects include thirst, polyuria, tremor, gastro-intestinal upsets and weight gain. Longer term effects include nephrogenic diabetes insipidus and hypothyroidism. The toxic picture is one of delirium, fits, coma, circulatory failure and death; this is seen at levels about 2 mmol/litre. The risk of toxicity is increased by any intercurrent illness which reduces fluid intake and renal function, thiazide diuretics, digoxin, antihypertensive agents and nephrotoxic antibiotics.

The writer recalls an elderly person, subject to recurrent bipolar affective disorder (mainly depression) since a puerperal episode more than 40 years ago, who was spending half the year depressed and had ceased to respond to ECT or, to any appreciable extent, to antidepressants. Over the course of two years the prescription of lithium carbonate appeared to abolish her depressions, but during the next few years there were two episodes of dangerous toxicity related to heart failure and her having only one kidney. Nevertheless the lithium treatment was resumed and continued at her request, and she remarked to her daughter on her death-bed (unrelated to the lithium therapy), 'I'm so glad not to be dying depressed'.

There is little convincing evidence in favour of sustained-release preparations. It is usual to start with 250 mg of the salt and to increase, if necessary, in divided doses until a therapeutic blood level of about 0.6 mmol/litre has been obtained. At first, weekly estimations are desirable, but once a steady-state at a satisfactory level has been achieved, monthly and then tri-monthly measurements will suffice. Should an intercurrent illness develop, then lithium levels must be carefully monitored until it is over.

Carbamazepine, an extraordinarily versatile drug with some structural similarities to imipramine, is now being assessed as an alternative mood regulator (Ballenger and Post, 1980) but has yet to be studied in the elderly. The dosage, of the order of 100-200 mg three times a day, should achieve a plasma concentration of 6-10 µg/ml.

Anxiolytics and Hypnotics

Few elderly depressives will not have been prescribed a hypnotic before an antidepressant. Often one can gauge the duration of the depressive illness from the length of that prescription. Benzodiazepines are most commonly used, notably nitrazepam and flurazepam, both of which are unsuitable because of their long half-lives in the elderly (especially flurazepam) and tendency to cause 'hangover'.

It is desirable to persuade the depressed insomniac to use a sedative antidepressant as a hypnotic; amitriptyline, trimipramine and mianserin are particularly appropriate. Otherwise a shorter-acting hypnotic should be used, such as chlormethiazole, 2 capsules (each of which contains 192 mg base), or triazolam, 125-250 µg.

Benzodiazepine tranquillisers may be prescribed alone (though inappropriately) when the prescriber picks up the patient's anxiety but not the underlying depression. Under these circumstances, although the relief is often not well sustained, habituation develops very easily. They may, however, be used as an adjunct to antidepressant therapy when speedy relief of agitation (usually in the moderately depressed) is desired. Diazepam, 2-10 mg up to three times a day, is the most widely used, but has a rather long half-life which may cause some accumulation and sopor, whereas lorazepam, 0.5-2.5 mg up to three times a day, is more rapidly eliminated and seems rather more effective. Once depression has been brought under control by the antidepressant the tranquilliser should be phased out or replaced by one less likely to induce dependency, such as clobazam, 10-20 mg up to three times a day.

Refractory Depression

This pervasive problem in geropsychiatric practice demands an energetic, resourceful approach if the patient is to be spared years of blighted misery. The scheme advocated by Bergmann (1982) commends itself. He asks the question, Has the patient had a full course of at least two tricyclics? If not, unless the drugs are poorly tolerated, a full therapeutic trial of tricyclics should be undertaken. If there is no response, or the side-effects are a major problem, a tetracyclic should be tried. If this is ineffective, L-tryptophan should be added. If there is still no response and the patient has not had a course of ECT in the past three months, this should be given. If there is still no response an MAO inhibitor should be tried. If this is ineffective, combined MAO inhibitor and tricyclic or tetracyclic is the next step. If this fails, all treatment should be stopped, then a trial made of lithium (and/or carbamazepine), and the whole cycle may be repeated. Somewhere along the line a thought should be given to psychosurgery.

How Long to Treat?

Unlike the antibiotics, antidepressants are not deemed usually to cure the condition for which they are given, but rather to relieve it until there is a spontaneous remission. The question of the duration of treatment is under-researched and frequently evaded.

If the patient's illness has been of no more than a few months' duration and recovery is complete, the antidepressant should be continued for at least three months beyond the time of maximum improvement and then gradually stopped over the next two to three months. If the patient relapses, the original dose should be restored and maintained for another three months beyond recovery before reduction. If there is again relapse, the drug had better be continued indefinitely. If there is a history of depression for longer than a year, or if improvement, though useful, is incomplete, it is probably wise not to stop the antidepressant. Although protection is far from complete, the dangers of remaining on an antidepressant long-term are likely to be less than those arising from suffering a relapse into depression.

Prognosis
=========

Post (1962, 1972) showed that while treatment is successful in most patients at first, there is subsequent invalidism, psychological and social, in about half of them. A bad prognosis was associated with older age and an aged appearance, evidence of brain disease, stroke, Parkinsonism, dementia--any serious disabling bodily disease and a history of uninterrupted depression for more than two years. He compared a group treated with ECT plus support only with a later group, most of whom also had tricyclic antidepressants, and found rather fewer who made a lasting recovery (though fewer, too, who were lastingly ill) in the drug-treated group. It is possible, though, that the patients in this group were more severely depressed or refractory, having mostly failed to respond to antidepressants prescribed by their general practitioners.

Murphy (1983) made a one-year prospective study of 124 elderly patients referred to catchment area geropsychiatric services and found that only a third had a good outcome. Poor outcome was associated with severity of initial illness, those with depressive delusions doing particularly badly. Physical health problems and severe life-events in the course of the year worsened prognosis. This study barely addressed the question of how the patients were

Affective Disorders in the Elderly

treated, but all were referred to established, energetic geropsychiatric services which would be unlikely to treat over-tentatively.

Roughly, there seems to be a 'rule of three': a third do well and stay well, a third get better and suffer a relapse, and a third do not do very well at all.

An increased mortality for those who suffer depression in old age, more from illness than suicide (though extreme self-neglect is likely to play a part) has been noted by Jacoby (1981), Kay (1962) and Post (1972), with a tendency to a higher mortality in those where first affective illness is in old age.

Summary

Depression is relatively common in old age but not all that easy to diagnose. Little is known of what is normal behaviour in the elderly--old people tend to somatise their symptoms and suffer from associated physical disorder, may appear confused and commonly present atypical pictures. Doctors have tended to be ill-informed on the topic and most often miss the condition. Mania and hypomania too may be misdiagnosed. The DST is less helpful than in younger patients. Depression in the elderly is moderate or severe, taking an agitated or a retarded form.

Lower levels of brain monoamines and increased monoamine oxidase contribute with physical illness and ill-health and other adverse life events and circumstances to depression in old age.

Possible interactions with other drugs are a special hazard of prescribing antidepressants to the elderly. Nevertheless, the seriously physically ill patient may benefit from chemotherapy for depression. Compliance may be impaired by the patient's misunderstanding, attitude or experience of side-effects. The prescriber needs to explain and 'sell' the treatment. Other people may interfere, or the prescription may be ineffective, daunting or inappropriate.

Pharmacokinetic changes, especially in metabolism and renal clearance and reduction in plasma proteins, tend to make a little drug go a long way, but this may be offset by pharmacodynamic decreases in brain sensitivity.

Psychotherapy, cognitive therapy, social support, ECT and psychosurgery are alternatives but more often complements to chemotherapy for depression. The hazards of drug treatment have been somewhat exaggerated and are a good deal less than the hazards of staying depressed. Previous and current drugs given should be ascertained, target symptoms identified, and a decision made about where to treat and with whose help; close supervision of treatment is essential.

Of the monoamine re-uptake inhibitors, tricyclics are the most widely used despite their anticholinergic side-effects, danger in overdose and occasional cardiotoxicity. The second generation antidepressants are safer but may have different, still troublesome side-effects and may be less effective. There is a place for MAO inhibitors, tryptophan and neuroleptics in the treatment of old age depression, and for lithium in those who suffer frequent recurrences. Stimulants, anxiolytics and hypnotics have a much smaller place.

Refractory depression is a common problem in old age and warrants an energetic, resourceful approach. Only a third of elderly depressives appear to remain well for a year or more after treatment. Older, frailer, afflicted patients with a long history and delusions appear to do least well. There is also an increased mortality.

Affective Disorders in the Elderly

References

Ballenger, J. C. and Post, R. M. (1980) Carbamazepine in manic depressive illness: a new treatment. *Am. J. Psychiatry* **139**, 948-949.

Barraclough, B. M. (1971) Suicide in the elderly. In: *Recent Developments in Psychogeriatrics* (Kay, D. W. K. and Walk, A., eds), Headley Bros., London.

Beck, A. T. (1967) *Depression: Clinical, Experimental and Theoretical Aspects*. Harper and Row, New York.

Bergmann, K. (1972) Psychogeriatrics. *Medicine* (1st series), **9**, 643-652.

Bergmann, K. (1982) Depression in the elderly. In: *Recent Advances in Geriatric Medicine II* (Isaacs, B., ed.), Churchill Livingstone, Edinburgh and London.

Bergmann, K. and Eastham, E. (1974) Psychogeriatric ascertainment and assessment for treatment in the acute medical ward setting. *Age and Ageing* **3**, 174-188.

Bergmann, K., Foster, E. M., Justice, A. W., and Matthews, V. (1978) Management of the demented elderly patient in the community. *Brit. J. Psychiatry* **132**, 441-449.

Blackwell, B. (1963) Hypertensive crisis due to monoamine oxidase inhibitors. *Lancet* **ii**, 849-851.

Blazer, D. and Friedman, S. W. (1979) Depression in late life. *Am. Fam. Physician* **20**, 91-96.

Blazer, D. G. and Williams, C. D. (1980) The epidemiology of dysphoria and depression in an elderly population. *Am. J. Psychiatry* **137**, 439-444.

Boston Collaborative Drug Surveillance Program (1972) Adverse reactions to tricyclic antidepressant drugs. *Lancet* **i**, 529-531.

Branconnier, R. and Cole, J. O. (1981) Effects of acute administration of trazodone and amitriptyline on cognition, cardiovascular function and salivation in the normal geriatric subject. *J. Clin. Psychopharmacol.* **1**, 82-86.

Branconnier, R. J., Cole, J. O., and Ghazuinian, S. (1983) Clinical pharmacology of bupropion in elderly patients. Preliminary observations. *J. Clin. Psychiatry* **44**, 134-136.

Bridges, P. K. and Bartlett, J. R. (1973) The work of a psycho-surgical unit. *Postgrad. Med. J.* **49**, 855-859.

Busse, F. W. (1978) The Duke longitudinal study: 1. Senescence and senility. In: *Alzheimer's Disease, Senile Dementia and Related Disorders* (Katz, R., Terry, R., and Bick, K., eds), Raven Press, New York.

Butler, R. N. (1968) Towards a psychiatry of the life cycle: implication of sociopsychologic studies of the ageing process for the psychotherapeutic situation. *Psychiatry Res. Reports* 23, 233.

Carr, A. C. and Hobson, R. P. (1977) High serum concentrations of antidepressants in elderly patients. *Brit. Med. J.* 2, 1151.

Carroll, B. J., Feinberg, M., Greden, J. F., Tarika, J., Albala, A. A., Haskett, R. F., James, N. M., Kronfol, Z., Lohr, N., Steiner, M., De Vigne, J. P., and Young, E. (1981) A specific laboratory test for the diagnosis of melancholia: standardization, validation and clinical utility. *Arch. Gen. Psychiatry* 38, 15-22.

Chapron, D. J., Cameron, J. R., White, L. B., and Merrall, P. (1982) Observations on lithium disposition in the elderly. *J. Am. Geriatric Soc.* 30, 651-655.

Cooper, J. W., Wellins, I., Fisk, K. H., and Loomis, M. E. (1975) A seven nursing home study. Frequency of potential drug interactions. *J. Am. Pharmaceut. Assoc.* 78, 255-268.

Coppen, A., Cupta, R., Montgomery, S., Ghose, K., Bailey, J., and De Ridder, J. J. (1976) Mianserin hydrochloride: a novel antidepressant. *Brit. J. Psychiatry* 129, 342-345.

Coull, D. C., Crooks, J., Dingwall-Fordyce, I., Scott, A. M., and Weir, R. D. (1970) Amitriptyline and cardiac disease: risk of sudden death identified by monitoring system. *Lancet* ii, 561-564.

Department of Health and Social Security (1978) *A Happier Old Age*. HMSO, London.

Diagnostic and Statistical Manual of Mental Disorders. 3rd edition (DSM III) (1980). American Psychiatric Association.

Emery, G. (1983) Cognitive therapy with the elderly. In: *New Directions in Cognitive Therapy* (Emery, G., Hollon, S., and Bedrosian, R., eds), Guildford Press, New York.

Evans, L. and Spelman, M. (1983) The problems of non-compliance with drug therapy. *Drugs* 25, 63-76.

Finch, C. E. (1977) Neuroendocrine and autonomic aspects of ageing. In: *Handbook of the Biology of Ageing* (Finch, C. E. and Hayflick, L., eds),

Van Nostrand Rheinhold Co., New York.
Fink, M. (1978) Efficacy and safety of induced seizures (EST) in man. Comp. Psychiatry 19, 1-18.
Friedel, R. O. (1984) The pharmacotherapy of depression in the elderly: pharmacokinetic considerations. In: Psychopathology in the Aged (Cole, J. O. and Barrett, J. E., eds), Raven Press, New York.
Georgotas, A. (1983) Affective disorders in the elderly: diagnostic and research considerations. Age and Ageing 12, 1-10.
Georgotas, A., Friedman, E., and McCarthy, M. (1983) Resistant geriatric depressions and therapeutic response to monoamine oxidase inhibitors. Biol. Psychiatry 18, 195-205.
Gerner, R., Eastabrook, W., Stever, J., and Jarvik, L. (1980) Treatment of geriatric depression with trazodone, imipramine and placebo: a double blind study. J. Clin. Psychiatry 41, 216-220.
Goldfarb, A. I. (1962) The psychotherapy of elderly patients. In: Medical and Clinical Aspects of Ageing (Blumenthal, H. T., ed.), Columbia University Press, New York.
Goldstein, S. E., Birnbom, F., and Laliberte, R. (1982) Nomifensine in the treatment of depressed geriatric patients. J. Clin. Psychiatry 43, 287-289.
Gurland, B., Copeland, J., Kuriansky, J., Kelleher, M., Sharpe, L., and Dean, L. L. (1983) The Mind and Mood of Ageing. Croom Helm, London.
Hansen, J. M., Kampmann, J., and Laurssen, H. (1970) Renal excretion of drugs in the elderly. Lancet i, 1170.
Jacoby, R. (1981) Depression in the elderly. Brit. J. Hosp. Medicine, Jan., 40-47.
Jarvik, L. (1983) Affective disorders in late life. Pharmacotherapy. VII World Congress of Psychiatry, Abstract S. 185, p. 59.
Jusko, W. J. (1978) Role of tobacco smoking in pharmacokinetics. J. Pharmacokinet. Biopharmaceut. 6, 7-39.
Kane, J. M., Cole, K., and Sarantakos, S. (1983) Safety and efficacy of bupropion in elderly patients. Preliminary observations. J. Clin. Psychiatry 44, 134-136.
Katon, W. and Raskind, M. (1980) Treatment of depression in the mentally ill elderly with methylphenidate. Am. J. Psychiatry 137, 963-965.
Kaufmann, M. W., Cassem, N. H., Murray, G. B., and Jenike, M. (1984) Use of psychostimulants in medically ill patients with neurological disease and

major depression. Can. J. Psychiatry 29, 46-49.
Kay, D. W. K. (1962) Outcome and cause of death in mental disorders of the aged: a long-term followup of functional and organic psychoses. Acta psychiatr. scand. 38, 249-276.
Kay, D. W. K., Beamish, P., and Roth, M. (1964) Old age mental disorders in Newcastle-upon-Tyne: a study of prevalence. Brit. J. Psychiatry 110, 146-668.
Kay, D. W. K. and Bergmann, K. (1966) Physical disability and mental health in old age. J. Psychosom. Res. 101, 3-12.
Kay, D. W. K., Bergmann, K., Foster, E. M., McKechnie, A. A., and Roth, M. (1970) Mental illness and hospital usage in the elderly: a random sample followed up. Comp. Psychiatry 1, 26-35.
Kellaway, G. S. M. and McCrae, E. (1973) Intensive monitoring for adverse drug effects in patients discharged from acute medical wards. New Zealand Med. J. 78, 525-528.
Kiloh, L. (1961) Pseudo-dementia. Acta psychiatr. scand. 37, 336-351.
Kupfer, D. J., Spiker, D. G., Coble, P. A., and Shaw, D. H. (1978) Electroencephalographic sleep recordings and depression in the elderly. J. Am. Geriatric Soc. 26, 53-55.
Lader, M. (1982) The psychopharmacology of old age. In: The Psychiatry of Late Life (Levy, B. and Post, F., eds), Blackwell, Oxford and London.
Lader, M. (1983) Combined use of tricyclic antidepressants and monoamine oxidase inhibitors. J. Clin. Psychiatry 44, 20-24.
Lawson, D. H. and Jick, H. (1976) Drug prescribing in hospitals: an international comparison. Am. J. Public Health 66, 644-648.
McAllister (1983) Overview: pseudo-dementia. Am. J. Psychiatry 140, 528-533.
Mendlewicz, J. and Youdim, M. B. H. (1983) L-Deprenil, a selective monoamine type B inhibitor, in the treatment of depression: a double blind evaluation. Brit. J. Psychiatry 142, 508-511.
Middleton, R. S. W., Radham, A. D. M. M., and Lloyd, A. H. (1978) Maprotiline vs imipramine in the depression of old age. Brit. J. Clin. Practice 32, 53-56.
Montgomery, S. A., Braithwaite, R. A., and Crammer, J. L. (1977) Routine nortriptyline levels in the treatment of depression. Brit. Med. J. 2, 166-167.

Morgan, J. P., Rivera-Calimlim, L., Messiha, F., Sundaresan, P. R., and Trabert, N. (1975) Imipramine-mediated interference with levodopa absorption from the gastro-intestinal tract in man. Neurology 25, 1029-1034.

Murphy, E. (1982) Social origins of depression in old age. Brit. J. Psychiatry 141, 135-142.

Murphy, E. (1983) The prognosis of depression in old age. Brit. J. Psychiatry 142, 111-119.

Nies, A., Robinson, D. S., Friedman, M. J., Green, R., Cooper, T. B., Ravaris, C. L., and Ives, R. O. (1977) Relationship between age and tricyclic antidepressant plasma levels. Am. J. Psychiatry 134, 790-993.

Orme, M. L. E. (1984) Antidepressants and heart disease. Brit. Med. J. 289, 1-2.

Pitt, B. (1974) Psychogeriatrics. Churchill Livingstone, Edinburgh and London.

Pitt, B. (1982) Psychogeriatrics, 2nd ed. Churchill Livingstone, Edinburgh and London.

Post, F. (1962) The Significance of Affective Symptoms in Old Age. O. U. Press, London.

Post, F. (1972) The management and nature of depressive illness in late life: a followthrough study. Brit. J. Psychiatry 121, 393-404.

Roose, S. P., Bone, S., Haidorfer, C., Dunner, D. L., and Fieve, R. R. (1979) Lithium treatment in older patients. Am. J. Psychiatry 136, 843-844.

Rossman, I. (1980) Bodily changes with ageing. In: Handbook of Geriatric Psychiatry (Busse, F. W. and Blazer, D. G., eds), Van Nostrand and Reinhold, New York.

Roth, G. S. (1975) Altered hormone binding and responsiveness during ageing. Proceedings of the Tenth International Congress of Gerontology 1, 44-45. Excerpta Medica, New York.

Spar, J. and Gerner, R. (1982) Does the dexamethasone suppression test distinguish dementia from depression? Am. J. Psychiatry 139, 238-240.

Stanaszek, W. F. and Franklin, G. E. (1978) Survey of potential drug interactions in an out-patient clinic population. Hospital Pharmacy 13, 255-263.

Stever, J. (1982) Psychotherapy for depressed elders. In: Depression in Late Life (Blazer, D. G., ed.), C.O. Mosby Co., St. Louis.

Triggs, E. J., Nation, R. L., and Long, A. (1975) Pharmacokinetics in the elderly. Eur. J. Clin. Pharmacol. 8, 55-62.

Trimble, M. R. and Robertson, M. M. (1983) Flupenthixol in depression. A study of serum levels and prolactin response. J. Affec. Disorders 5, 81-89.

Veith, R. C., Raskind, M. A., Caldwell, J. H., Barnes, R. E., Gumbrecht, G., and Ritchie, J. L. (1982) Cardiovascular effects of tricyclic antidepressants in depressed patients with chronic heart disease. New Eng. J. Med. 306, 954-959.

Vestal, R. E. (1978) Drug use in the elderly: a review of problems and special considerations. Drugs 16, 358-382.

Walinder, J. (1975) Potentiation of antidepressant action of clomipramine by tryptophan. Lancet i, 984.

Weintraub, M. (1981) Intelligent non-compliance, with special emphasis on the elderly. Contemp. Pharm. Pract. 4, 8-11.

Weissman, M. M. and Myers, J. K. (1978) Affective disorders in a U.S. urban community. Arch. Gen. Psychiatry 35, 1304-1311.

Wells, C. E. (1979) Pseudo-dementia. Am. J. Psychiatry 136, 895-900.

Whitlock, F. and Sisking, M. (1979) Depression and cancer: a follow-up study. Psychol. Med. 9, 747-752.

Williamson, J. and Chopin, J. M. (1980) Adverse reactions to prescribed drugs in the elderly. A multicentre investigation. Age and Ageing 9, 73-80.

Williamson, J., Stokoe, I. H., Gray, S., Fisk, M., Smith, A., McGhee, A., and Stephenson, E. (1964) Old people at home--their unreported needs. Lancet i, 1117-1120.

Wood, A. J. J. and Feely, J. (1984) Effect of age on sensitivity to drugs. In: Clinical Pharmacology and Drug Treatment in the Elderly (O'Malley, K., ed.), Churchill Livingstone, Edinburgh and London.

INDEX

acetylation 396, 406-7, 425
acetylcholine 9-10, 61, 170-4, 269-70, 287-9, 292-99, 312, 315, 317, 327, 488, 490-1, 597-8, 600
S-adenosylmethionine 24
adinazolam 296, 302, 305, 350, 352, 356-7, 366
adrenaline 276-7
adrenocorticotrophic hormone 14
alcohol 62, 73, 85, 87-8, 111, 168, 171, 187, 276-8, 287, 408, 415, 516
alprazolam 296, 399, 403, 405, 411, 421
Alzheimer's disease 64, 85
amiflamine 239
amino acids (see also individual amino acids) 11-12, 15, 115, 170-4, 255, 312-13, 318-20, 327, 348, 358-9, 364, 602, 604, 607, 610
γ-aminobutyric acid (GABA) 12, 115, 170-4, 312, 318-20, 327, 348, 359
amitriptyline 3, 10, 13, 70-1, 119, 126, 128, 153, 243-4, 264-5, 267-72, 278, 280-1, 288-9, 291-4, 298, 342, 350, 352, 358, 387-8, 391-2, 396-7, 399-402, 404-5, 407-9, 413, 415, 418, 422, 450, 454-5, 459, 464-5, 469-473, 475, 477, 479-80, 482-4, 487, 490, 492, 514, 521-2, 563, 594, 597-9, 603, 606
amitriptyline N-oxide 417
amoxepine 267-8, 271-4, 278, 280, 394, 421, 424, 450, 71, 474-5
amphetamine 15, 115, 117, 119, 121, 128-9, 131-2, 161, 174, 232, 276-7, 346, 422, 425, 602, 604
animal models 108-37
Annett's handedness inventory 156
anticholinergics 121, 125, 130, 133, 172
antihistamines 118, 121, 125, 276-7, 411-12
antipsychotics (neuroleptics) (see also individual drugs) 16, 84, 121, 128, 130-1, 133, 168, 172, 174, 276-7, 410, 479

617

Index

antipyrine 408
anxiety 8, 74, 156-7, 187, 241-5, 249, 264, 607
area under the plasma concentration versus time curve (AUC) 384, 388
arecholine 81
aspirin 87, 276
asymmetries 151-175
atomic absorption spectroscopy 495
ATPases 21-2
atropine 117, 275, 295, 491
atypical depressions 8, 241, 243-4, 423, 586-7, 603
AUC (see area under the plasma concentration versus time curve)
axes of DSM 194-5
6-AZAmianserin (ORG 3770) 295, 302, 305

barbiturates 84, 87, 134, 248, 276-7, 409
Bech-Rafaelson Mania Rating Scale (BRMS or BRMAS) 212
Bech-Rafaelson Melancholia Scale (BRMES) 212
Beck Depression Inventory 213, 520
behavioural despair 116-19, 125
Bellevue Index of Depression (BID) 540
benzodiazepines (see also the individual drugs) 84, 115, 118, 121, 128, 130, 133-4, 274, 276-7, 287, 294, 296, 318-19, 396, 399, 403, 405, 409, 411, 413-15, 417, 421, 458, 478-9, 606-7
benztropine 491
bethanechol 269-70

BID (see Bellevue Index of Depression)
binary classification 231
biological markers 2-26, 60-89, 554-6, 558, 587
•bipolar disorders 2, 8-9, 13, 16, 18, 21-2, 65, 73-80, 85, 87-88, 154, 157, 164-8, 174, 187-9, 191, 196, 199, 201, 208, 215-18, 220, 222-3, 231-2, 246, 262-3, 288-9, 296, 320, 535, 538, 556, 588
blood-brain barrier 7, 67, 417
body water 19
bombesin 17
BRMS (see Bech-Rafaelson Mania Rating Scale)
BRMES (see Bech-Rafaelson Melancholia Scale)
bromocriptine 322
bupropion 117, 121, 287-8, 301, 303, 342, 394, 409, 424
butriptyline 458
BW647U 293

caffeine 115, 117
calcitonin 17, 21
calcium 21, 24, 321-3
carbamazepine 12, 17, 84, 130, 318-20, 411-13, 421-2, 492
carpipramine 118
CARS (see Children's Affective Rating Scale)
catechol-O-methyl transferase 13
CATEGO 195
CDI (see Childhood Depression Inventory)

Index

CDRS (see Children's Depression Rating Scale)
Center for Epidemiologic Studies - Depression Scale (CES-D) 186
cerebrospinal fluid (CSF) 2, 4-5, 7, 17-18, 20, 24, 66-9, 111, 153-4, 169, 320, 339, 387, 422
CES-D (see Center for Epidemiologic Studies - Depression Scale)
CGP 11305A 239
chemical ionization 464
childhood depression 283
Childhood Depression Inventory (CDI) 532
Children's Affective Rating Scale (CARS) 541
Children's Depression Rating Scale (CDRS) 540
chloral hydrate 84, 276-7
chloramphenicol 276-7
chlordiazepoxide 115, 118, 478
p-chlorophenylalanine 115, 130, 313, 347, 361, 364-5
chlorpromazine 111, 115, 118, 120, 128, 134, 169, 248, 262, 314-16, 346, 348, 409, 482, 486, 604
chlorprothixene 118, 128
cholecystokinin 17
cholesterol 24-5
choline 10, 317
choline acetyltransferase 170
chronic stress models 119-22
chronic social isolation 121-2
cimetidine 276-7, 411-12
cimoxatone 239
cinanserin 314
citalopram 290-1, 296, 301, 304, 342, 358, 474-478
classification systems for affective disorders 186, 211, 231-7, 262-5, 516-17, 532-46, 585-9
clearance of drugs 387-91, 396-406, 408, 410-13, 415-16, 418-21, 424, 593
clenbuterol 342, 345
clomipramine 4-5, 12, 251, 267-8, 349-52, 387, 393, 396, 398, 402, 406, 412, 450, 459, 464-5, 471-2, 477-8, 482-4, 494, 524, 598-9, 603
clonazepam 318-19
clonidine 15, 127, 250-1, 276, 289, 356, 362
clorgyline 9, 239-44, 247, 250-2, 254-5, 343, 349, 351-2, 360-3
clovoxamine 288-9, 301, 303
cocaine 5
Composite Interview Schedule 196
conjugation 8, 383, 385-6, 415, 418-20, 422
corticotropin-releasing factor (CRF) 85
cortisol 14-15, 23, 82-7, 233, 553
CRF (see corticotropin-releasing factor)
CT scans 162, 168, 174, 608
cyclic nucleotides 5, 250, 323-4, 339, 342-4, 347
Cytryn and McKnew criteria 531-2

danitracene 117
debrisoquine 418, 590

619

Index

dementia 64, 85, 232, 586-7, 608
demethylation 383, 385, 387-8, 402-3, 411-12, 415, 418-19, 421-2, 564
deprenyl 12, 73, 239-41, 245, 247-9, 251-2, 339, 349, 351, 360-2
°depression 2, 8-9, 13-22, 24-5, 61, 64-6, 68-70, 72-82, 86-9, 111-13, 120, 122-3, 126, 128, 130-1, 134-5, 154, 157-60, 162-8, 174, 185-91, 196-7, 199, 201-8, 212-23, 238, 241-4, 246, 262-3, 288-91, 295-6, 298, 316, 318, 320, 322-4, 326, 357, 516, 531, 535-6, 538, 556, 584-9, 591, 595, 603
Depression Scale of the Personality Inventory for Children 550
Depressive Spectrum Disease (DSD) 85, 190
derivatization of antidepressants 453, 456-7, 461-2, 480
desipramine 3, 6, 13, 15, 65, 70, 111, 114-15, 119, 125, 130-1, 264, 267-71, 174, 178-81, 342, 345-7, 349, 351-2, 385, 387, 389-92, 395-7, 399-400, 402-6, 408-11, 415, 417, 419-20, 450, 454-5, 457, 459, 464, 470-1, 475, 480, 483, 487, 490, 492, 494, 524-5, 563, 565, 594
desmethylclomipramine 457, 459, 464, 472, 475, 482, 485, 490, 520
desmethyldoxepin 469

desmethylnortriptyline 473, 492
dexamethasone supression test (DST) 14, 23, 82-6, 88, 233, 553-5, 587, 609
dextrality 152, 156-7, 159-60
DHPG (see 3,4-dihydroxyphenylethylene glycol)
diabetes 23, 587
Diagnostic and Statistical Manual of Mental Disorders (DSM) 187, 194-6, 208-11, 220, 516, 531-2, 534, 541, 545-6, 548, 551, 561, 588
Diagnostic Interview for Children and Adolescents (DICA) 539, 541
Diagnostic Interview Schedule (DIS) 195
diazepam 115, 118, 134, 274, 276, 478
DICA (see Diagnostic Interview for Children and Adolescents)
digitalis 276
digoxin 606
3,4-dihydroxyphenylethylene glycol (DHPG) 70
3,4-dihydroxyphenylalanine (dopa) 7, 11, 18, 276, 287, 313, 590
dimethyltryptamine 153
diphenylhydantoin 321
DISC (NIMH Interview) 541
dopa (see 3,4-dihydroxyphenylalanine)
dopa decarboxylase 15, 556
dopamine 6-7, 9, 16, 66, 115-16, 118, 123-5, 129, 133, 152, 169-73, 241, 251, 287, 289-91, 293, 295-8, 312-14, 316,

Index

318-19, 321, 323,
  327, 360, 365-6, 421,
  556, 589, 598, 601
dopamine β-hydroxylase
  13, 174, 314, 589
dothiepin 293-4, 301,
  304, 393, 398, 401,
  405, 420, 598, 603
double radioisotope
  derivative analysis
  494, 496
doxepin 117, 264, 266,
  268-71, 278, 280,
  291, 342, 384, 393,
  397, 450, 455, 459,
  465, 469, 471, 474,
  483, 487, 595, 598-9
drug interactions 245-8,
  276-8, 407-13, 601
drug models of depression 122-9
DSD (see Depressive
  Spectrum Disease)
DSM (see Diagnostic and
  Statistical Manual of
  Mental Disorders)
DST (see dexamethasone
  suppression test)
duration and frequency
  of affective disorders 214-15, 264-5,
  561-2, 607-8
dysphoria 154, 156, 160,
  585

electroconvulsive shock
  therapy 5-6, 12, 19,
  23, 64, 115, 121, 134,
  164, 338, 343, 345,
  356-7, 365-6, 568,
  587, 595, 606-9
electroencephalography
  25, 79-82, 127, 153,
  165, 168-9, 557, 559,
  587
elderly patients 283,
  298, 401-3, 414,
  584-610
electrochemical detection
  476, 478-9

electron-capture detection 453, 459, 461
electron impact ionization 464
elimination half-life
  ($t_{1/2}$) 278, 282, 296,
  389-96, 401-5, 411,
  415-16, 422-3, 593
endorphins 18-19
enkephalins 18
enzyme immunoassay
  491-3, 496
ephedrine 601
Epidemiologic Studies -
  Depression Scale
  (CEDS-D)
epidemiology of affective disorders 220-3,
  543, 546-553
erythrocyte 10, 12-13,
  21-2, 75-9, 495
euphoria 130-2, 159,
  161, 163-4, 166
extraction of antidepressants 451-3,
  462-3, 466-8, 484-6

Familial Pure Depressive
  Disease (FPDD) 85,
  190
Feighner criteria (see
  St. Louis criteria)
femoxatine 64, 349-50,
  353, 358
fezolamine 289, 301, 303
first-pass metabolism
  384, 408, 412
flame emission photometry 495
flame-ionization detection 453
fluorescence detection
  476, 478, 480
fluorescence polarization immunoassay 496
fluoxetine 64, 126-7,
  291-2, 301, 304
flupenthixol 605
fluphenazine 273, 277,
  411

621

Index

flurazepam 478, 606
fluvoxamine 289-90, 301, 303, 342, 358
folic acid 24
FPDD (see Familial Pure Depressive Disease)
fusaric acid 314

gas chromatography 449, 462, 453-9, 461, 487-8, 491-2, 495-6
genetic factors 1, 26, 68, 75-8, 167, 169, 395-6, 425, 513, 558
glucose 22-3
glutamate decarboxylase 170
glutethemide 84
glycine 12
growth hormone 15, 17, 86, 555, 556
guanethidine 276, 289, 299, 590

haloperidol 115, 118, 121, 134, 273, 276-7, 315-16, 323, 410, 486, 605
Hamilton Depression Rating Scale 74, 212-13, 243, 294, 296-7, 520, 596
Hatotani model 119-20
heroin 80
5-HIAA (see 5-hydroxyindole-3-acetic acid)
high-pressure (performance) liquid chromatography (HPLC) 388, 465, 466-79, 487-8, 490-1, 495-6
histamine 10, 61, 269, 271-2, 287, 289-92, 294-5, 298, 301-2, 315-16, 339, 411
homovanillic acid (HVA) 7, 24, 169, 314
HPA axis (see hypothalamic-pituitary-adrenal axis)

HPLC (see high-pressure liquid chromatography)
hydroxydesmethylclomipramine 419
2-hydroxydesmethylimipramine 279, 385-6, 388, 403-5, 407-8
6-hydroxydopamine 65, 134
2-hydroxyimipramine 279, 385-6, 388, 408, 419-20, 481, 490, 565
5-hydroxyindole-3-acetic acid (5-HIAA) 4-5, 24, 66-9, 153-4, 339, 418
hydroxylation 385-6, 388-9, 391, 395, 399, 403, 410-12, 416-22, 564, 593
p-hydroxymandelic acid 8
hydroxymaprotiline 420
10-hydroxynortriptyline 272, 388, 391, 395, 403-4, 410, 416, 418-19, 473, 477-8, 488
p-hydroxyphenylacetic acid 8
5-hydroxytryptamine (serotonin) 1, 3-5, 7-9, 15-16, 25, 61-2, 64-7, 69, 73, 85, 115-16, 118-19, 123-4, 126-7, 129, 153-4, 156, 169, 172-5, 250-1, 267, 271-2, 287-98, 313, 315, 318-19, 321, 339, 344, 347-54, 356-60, 362-6, 418, 526, 600
5-hydroxytryptophan 115, 118, 126, 134, 364
hyperactivity 544-5
hyperthermia 124
hypothalamic-pituitary-adrenal (HPA) axis 15, 82-6, 89, 553

Index

hypothalamic-pituitary-
 thyroid axis 16
hypothermia 117, 124-5,
 129
hypoxanthine 23-4

ICD (see International
 Classification of
 Diseases)
iminodibenzyl 386, 417
imipramine 5-6, 21,
 61-6, 70-1, 117,
 120-1, 124-6, 128,
 134, 242, 251, 262,
 264, 266-8, 270-2,
 279-81, 290, 293,
 297-8, 338, 342,
 350-2, 357-62, 382-4,
 386-7, 389-92, 396-7,
 399-400, 402-12, 415,
 417, 450, 454-5, 457,
 459, 464-5, 469-70,
 475, 478-9, 483-4,
 487, 490, 492, 523,
 556, 564-5, 590,
 594-5, 597-8, 601
imipramine N-oxide 386,
 389, 417
indalpine 296-7, 302,
 305, 349, 352, 358-60,
 474
indomethacin 84
insulin 15, 17, 22, 555,
 601,
internal standards 461-2,
 464-5, 477, 481
International Classifica-
 tion of Diseases (ICD)
 186, 196
Interview Schedule for
 Children (ISC) 539-40
intravenous administra-
 tion of antidepres-
 sants 265, 599
iprindole 5, 10, 61,
 115, 117, 121, 126,
 342, 344-5, 349-53
iproniazid 238-9, 338,
 382, 243, 262
ISC (see Interview Sche-
 dule for Children)

isocarboxazid 238-9,
 241-2, 244, 249,
 602-3
isoleucine 11
isoniazid 412
isoproterenol 346

Katz model 120-1
17-ketosteroids 14
kiddie-SADS 539,
 541-2, 545, 551
kindling 129, 133, 320

learned helplessness
 12, 109, 113-16, 119,
 125, 560
lecithin 317
leucine 11
Lilly 51641 240
lithium 10, 12, 17,
 20-2, 74-9, 84, 87,
 130-4, 218, 254-5,
 312, 314-15, 320-6,
 358, 403, 413, 416,
 422, 494-5, 566-8,
 602, 605-7, 610
lofepramine 465, 525
loxapine 273
lorazepam 115, 134, 294,
 415
LSD (see lysergic acid
 diethylamide)
lysergic acid diethyl-
 amide (LSD) 130,
 360-1
luteinizing hormone 18

magnesium 21, 231, 323
mania 1, 2, 7, 9, 14,
 16, 19-21, 61, 66,
 74, 80, 83, 86-8,
 129-33, 156, 158,
 161, 165-8, 172, 174,
 186, 188, 190, 192,
 198-201, 210-15,
 217-19, 222, 246,
 263, 312-27, 556,
 587, 595, 605
Mania Rating Scale (MRS)
 212

623

Index

Manic State Rating Scale (MS) 212
maprotiline 3-4, 265, 271, 295, 351, 394, 396, 420-1, 423-4, 450, 454, 459, 464-5, 482, 493, 524, 563, 565, 600
mass spectrometry 388, 458, 462-6, 475, 487-8, 490, 495
melatonin 346
5-MeODMT (see 5-methoxy-N,N-dimethyltryptamine)
meprobamate 84
metanephrine 69
methadone 459
methaqualone 84
5-methoxy-N,N-dimethyltryptamine (5-MeODMT) 354, 356, 364
3-methoxy-4-hydroxyphenylethylene glycol (MHPG, MOPEG) 4, 69, 70-3, 119, 247, 264, 339, 355, 418-19, 423, 556
3-methoxytyramine 8
methylation 602
α-methyldopa 278-9, 417, 599
methylhistamine 10
methylphenidate 276-7, 317, 411, 604
α-methyl-para-tyrosine 115, 125, 130, 313, 357, 362
methysergide 126, 314
metoprolol 416
MHPG, MOPEG (see 3-methoxy-4-hydroxyphenylethylene glycol)
mianserin 5, 10, 61, 115, 117, 121, 125-8, 294-5, 302, 305, 340, 342, 345, 347, 349, 351-2, 356-7, 365, 394, 405, 412-13, 424, 458, 465, 478, 525, 594, 598, 600, 606
minerals (see also the individual minerals) 19-21, 24, 76, 321-3
Minnesota Multiphasic Personality Inventory (MMPI) 68
MMPI (see Minnesota Multiphasic Personality Inventory)
moclobemide 239
monoamine oxidase 1-3, 8-9, 11-13, 73-5, 84, 115, 117, 121, 125-8, 130-1, 134, 153-6, 238-55, 266, 276, 287-9, 294, 297, 338, 343, 345, 362, 382, 403, 423, 425, 455, 462, 589, 603
monoamine oxidase inhibitors (see also the individual drugs) 1-3, 8-9, 11-12, 23, 73, 84, 115, 117, 121, 125-8, 130-1, 134, 238-55, 266, 276, 338-9, 343, 347, 349, 352, 360-4, 366, 382, 396, 403, 407, 412, 415, 422-3, 425, 455, 461-2, 568, 601-3
Montgomery and Asberg Depression Rating Scale 213, 519-20
morphine 130, 132, 297, 601
MRS (see Manic Rating Scale)
MS (see Manic State Rating Scale)

nafasadone 297, 302, 305
nalorphine 132
naloxone 322
natural history of childhood depression 561
negative contrast 134
neostigmine 9

Index

neuroleptics (see antipsychotics)
new antidepressants (see also the individual drugs) 5, 9-10, 61, 64, 115, 117, 121, 125-8, 286-306, 342, 345, 347-53, 358-60, 394, 409, 415, 420, 423-4, 478, 482, 525-6, 600
Newcastle criteria 521, 525
nialamide 11, 239, 343, 250, 343
nisoxetine 342
nitrazepam 606
nitrogen-phosphorous detection 453, 459
nomifensine 7, 121, 297-8, 302, 306, 391, 394, 412, 421, 423-4, 482-3, 485, 487, 526, 600
noradrenaline (norepinephrine) 1-2, 5, 7, 9, 15-16, 61, 65-6, 69-73, 85, 111, 115, 118-20, 123-5, 127, 129, 152, 169, 171-4, 241, 247-8, 250-2, 267, 271, 276-8, 287-93, 295-99, 312-14, 317, 319, 321, 338-41, 344-53, 355-7, 359-63, 365-6, 418, 420, 425, 556, 589, 600
norepinephrine (see noradrenaline)
normetanephrine 8, 6, 9, 313
northiaden 405
nortriptyline 5, 13, 264, 267-8, 270, 272, 278, 280-1, 342, 383-4, 387, 389, 390-2, 395-7, 399-400, 402-5, 407-10, 416-18, 420, 454, 461, 470, 475, 478, 480-4, 486, 492, 514, 520-3, 562, 566, 594, 598-9
norzimelidine 420, 423, 472-3, 526

obsessive-compulsive disorder 83, 85, 187
opioids 18-19, 87, 322
oral contraceptives 15, 276-7, 412
orphenadrine 605
outcome in affective disorders 213-19, 242-4, 264-5, 288-99, 315-16, 323-4, 512, 517-18, 561-9, 594-604, 608-9
oxaprotiline 295-6, 302, 305
oxazepam 121, 415, 458
oxyphenylbutazone 399

P450 280, 383, 388, 408, 411, 414
panic disorder 83, 85, 242, 274
pargyline 128, 134, 239-40, 247, 249, 251-2, 343
parkinsonism 232, 262, 361, 425, 587, 598, 600, 608
paroxetine 298-9, 302, 306
Peer Nomination Inventory for Depression (PNID) 539, 542-3
pemoline 602, 604
perphenazine 410, 486
personality disorders 83, 87, 187, 198, 204
PET (see positron emission tomography)
PGO spikes 124-5
pharmacokinetics 280-2, 291-2, 295-7, 299, 325, 384-426, 514-15, 520-6, 563, 564, 567, 584, 593-4, 609

625

Index

phenelzine 240-4,
 248-50, 253, 255,
 403, 425, 462
phenylacetic acid 8
phenylalanine 11-12
phenylbutazone 276
phenytoin 84, 276
phloretin 77
phobias 75, 83, 187, 298,
 204, 208, 242-3, 423,
 534, 537, 545
phosphorous 21
physostigmine 9, 81,
 130, 172, 270, 275-6,
 317
pilocarpine 269
pimozide 115, 118, 314,
 316
piribidel 314
pizotifen 117
placebo 515, 517-18,
 563-4, 601
plasma levels 2, 4, 11,
 18, 20-1, 70, 76, 82,
 248, 251, 277-8,
 281-3, 355, 364, 387,
 389-91, 395-402,
 405-7, 409, 411,
 415-16, 419-21, 424,
 482, 490-1, 412-27,
 523, 563-4, 590, 597
platelets 62, 64, 66,
 68, 73-5, 153-4, 240,
 249, 423, 490
PNID (see Peer Nomination Inventory for Depression)
polypharmacy 590-1
positive contrast 134
positron emission tomography (PET) 161
postmortem brain tissue
 4, 6, 62, 64, 67-8,
 170-1
post-partum depression
 8, 11
potassium 19, 321, 323
Present State Examination (PSE) 195, 516
probenecid 5, 7, 67
prochlorperazine 128

progabide 12
projective technqiues
 539, 542
prolactin 18, 86, 318,
 322, 358
propranolol 321, 325,
 347, 411, 594
prostaglandins 24
protein binding 276,
 383, 390, 401, 405,
 413-14, 590, 593
Protirelin Test 86-89
protriptyline 268-71,
 278, 280, 282, 388,
 390, 393, 396, 398,
 401, 409, 423, 455,
 478, 487, 492, 599
PSE (see Present State Examination)
psychological factors
 553, 558-61, 568-9
psychosurgery 595, 607,
 609
psychotherapy 263,
 568-9, 594, 609
ptosis 124-5
purines 23-4

quinidine 276
quinuclidinyl benzilate
 (QNB) 488-91

radioimmunoassays 481-8,
 492, 496
radioreceptor binding
 assays 488-91, 496
rapid eye movement (REM)
 sleep 10, 17, 25,
 79-82, 253, 343, 346,
 557, 565, 589
RDC (see Research Diagnostic Criteria)
reactive depression 65,
 75, 188, 196, 517,
 538, 587, 595
receptors 5-7, 9-10, 16,
 61-6, 69, 118, 125,
 127, 133-4, 250-1,
 267, 269-72, 275-6,
 287-99, 301-2, 313,
 315-16, 323-4,

Index

339-47, 349-53, 355-7, 359-63, 365-6, 411, 488-90, 556, 600
refractory affective disorders 265, 317, 512, 515, 517, 568, 595, 598, 602-3, 607-8, 610
REM sleep (see rapid eye movement sleep)
Research Diagnostic Criteria (RDC) 186, 194-6, 199, 291, 551, 553-4, 584
reserpine 1, 3, 9, 117, 123-5, 128, 130-1, 233, 263, 313, 338
RO 4-1284 123-4, 130-1

SADS (see Schedule for Affective Disorders and Schizophrenia)
salbutamol 121, 342
SCDI (see Short Children's Depression Inventory)
Schedule for Affective Disorders and Schizophrenia (SADS) 186, 194
schizoaffective disorders 4, 82-3, 85, 157, 159, 167-8, 196, 209, 215, 321
schizophrenia 16, 20, 73-4, 80-3, 85, 87-8, 131, 156, 167-70, 174, 187, 196, 209, 215-16, 218, 323, 262, 338, 561
scopolamine 117, 121, 276
SDD (see Sporadic Depressive Disease)
secondary affective disorders 190-1, 205
sedation 124-5
separation-induced despair 110, 112
separation-induced vocalisations 111-12
serotonin (see 5-hydroxytryptamine)

Short Children's Depression Inventory (SCDI) 539, 548
side effects of drugs 12, 244-8, 252-4, 264-5, 267, 269-75, 280, 282, 287-306, 320, 325-6, 514, 523, 564-5, 567-8, 596-602, 604-5
silation of glassware 451
sinistrality 152-3, 156-7, 160, 167
sleep disorders 18, 25, 64, 79-82, 130, 264, 557, 589, 590
smoking 276-7, 407-8, 593
sodium 19-21, 76, 321, 323
somatostatin 16
spiroperidol 134, 340, 357
Sporadic Depressive Disease (SDD) 190
Stewart's criteria 544
St. Louis Criteria (Feighner Criteria) 187, 194-5, 197, 516
suicide 4, 6, 14, 19, 66-7, 69, 84-5, 153-4, 346, 533, 537, 595
sulpiride 118

$t_{1/2}$ (see elimination half-life)
tardive dyskinesia 16, 172, 280
Taylor Manifest Anxiety Scale 156
tetrabenazine 123-4
tetrahydrobiopterin 25
therapeutic window 11, 282, 395, 521, 599
thin-layer chromatography 479-81, 494, 496
thioridazine 411, 491
thiothixene 410

Index

thyroid-releasing hormone 15-16, 18, 86-9
thyrotropin-stimulating hormone 15-17, 86-9
thyroxine 86
tomoxetine 292, 301, 304
trace amines (see also the individual amines) 7-9, 74, 247-8, 251-3, 382, 407, 601-3
tranylcypromine 241-2, 245-6, 249-50, 254-5
trazodone 117, 121, 125, 271, 297, 342, 364-5, 394, 421, 424, 450, 474, 526, 600
tricyclic antidepressants (see also the individual drugs) 1, 3-6, 9-10, 12-13, 15, 21, 61, 62-6, 70-1, 84, 88, 111-12, 114-15, 117-21, 124-8, 130-1, 134, 153, 242-4, 251, 262-83, 288, 290-2, 294, 297-9, 313, 338, 342, 345-52, 354-9, 362, 364-6, 382-426, 450, 454-5, 457, 459, 461, 464-5, 469-75, 477-94, 514, 520-5, 556, 562-6, 590, 594-5, 597-9, 601, 603, 606-8
trifluoperazine 273, 486, 605
trihexyphenidyl 276-7, 491
triiodothyronine 86, 277
trimipramine 268, 271, 280, 424, 470, 598-9, 603, 606
tryptophan 11, 15, 115, 255, 313, 358, 364, 602, 604, 607, 610
tryptophan hydroxylase 313
tryptophan oxygenase 15
tyrosine 11-12
tyrosine hydroxylase 313

ultraviolet detection 476, 478-80, 493
unipolar disorders 8, 13, 18, 24, 74-5, 77, 80, 85, 87-8, 164-6, 187-90, 192-3, 199, 205, 213, 215-17, 222, 231-2, 262-3, 290, 535-6, 538, 556, 587
urine 70-3, 385, 399, 423

valine 11
valproate 12, 318
vanadium 22
vanillylmandelic acid (VMA) 3, 70
vasopressin 18
verapamil 322
viloxazine 61, 117, 121, 293, 301, 304, 474, 478, 600
Vitamin B_6 15
VMA (see vanillylmandelic acid)

warfarin 413, 590
WB-4101 488-9
Weinberg criteria 531-2, 544

xanthine 23-4

yohimbine 129

zimelidine 290, 342, 345, 347, 349-50, 352, 358-60, 394, 420, 423-4, 471-3, 482, 526, 600

Date Due

~~DEC 0 8 1989~~			
DEC 7 1990			
~~DEC 0 9 1994~~			
~~DEC 1 9 1995~~			
MAY 0 3 1996			
DEC 1 2 1997			
APR 2 1998			
MAY 0 9 1998			
MAY 0 8 1999			
MAR 2 9 2001			
APR 2 7 2001			

BRODART, INC.   Cat. No. 23 233   Printed in U.S.A.